Basic Science IN Obstetrics AND Gynaecology

FOURTH EDITION

Commissioning Editor: *Pauline Graham*
Development Editor: *Lulu Stader*
Project Manager: *Joannah Duncan*
Designer: *Stewart Larking*
Illustration Manager: *Merlyn Harvey*
Illustrator: *Amanda Williams*

Basic Science IN Obstetrics AND Gynaecology

A TEXTBOOK FOR MRCOG PART I
FOURTH EDITION

Edited by

Phillip Bennett BSc PhD MD FRCOG
Professor of Obstetrics and Gynaecology

Catherine Williamson BSc MD FRCP
Professor of Obstetric Medicine

Queen Charlotte's and Chelsea Hospital,
Institute of Reproductive and Developmental Biology,
Imperial College London, London, UK

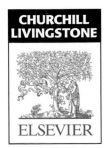

Edinburgh London New York Oxford Philadelphia St Louis Sydney Toronto 2010

CHURCHILL
LIVINGSTONE
ELSEVIER

First edition 1986
Second edition 1992
Third edition 2002
Fourth edition 2010

ISBN: 9780443102813

British Library Cataloguing in Publication Data
A catalogue record for this book is available from the British Library

Library of Congress Cataloging in Publication Data
A catalog record for this book is available from the Library of Congress

Notice
Knowledge and best practice in this field are constantly changing. As new research and experience broaden our knowledge, changes in practice, treatment and drug therapy may become necessary or appropriate. Readers are advised to check the most current information provided (i) on procedures featured or (ii) by the manufacturer of each product to be administered, to verify the recommended dose or formula, the method and duration of administration, and contraindications. It is the responsibility of the practitioner, relying on their own experience and knowledge of the patient, to make diagnoses, to determine dosages and the best treatment for each individual patient, and to take all appropriate safety precautions. To the fullest extent of the law, neither the Publisher nor the Editors assume any liability for any injury and/or damage to persons or property arising out or related to any use of the material contained in this book.

The Publisher

Printed in China

Contents

Contributors

Dawn Adamson
BSc(Hons) MBBS MRCP PhD
Consultant Cardiologist
Department of Cardiology
University Hospital of Coventry and Warwickshire
Coventry, UK

Physiology

Annette Briley SRN RM MSc
Consultant Midwife/Clinical Trial Manager
Biomedical Research Centre, Guy's and St Thomas' NHS
Foundation Trust
Maternal and Fetal Research Unit, Kings College London
London, UK

Clinical research methodology

Louise C Brown PhD MSc BEng
Division of Surgery, Oncology, Reproductive Biology and
Anaesthetics
Imperial College London
London, UK

Statistics and evidence-based healthcare

Peter H Dixon PhD BSc
Maternal and Fetal Disease Group
Institute of Reproductive and Developmental Biology
Faculty of Medicine, Imperial College London,
Hammersmith Hospital
London, UK

Structure and function of the genome

Kate Hardy BA PhD
Professor of Reproductive Biology
Institute of Reproductive and Developmental Biology
Faculty of Medicine, Imperial College London,
Hammersmith Hospital
London, UK

Embryology

Andrew JT George MA PhD FRCPath FRSA
Professor of Molecular Immunology
Department of Immunology, Division of Medicine,
Faculty of Medicine, Imperial College London,
Hammersmith Hospital
London, UK

Immunology

Mark R Johnson PhD MRCP MRCOG
Professor of Obstetrics
Department of Maternal and Fetal Medicine
Imperial College School of Medicine
Chelsea and Westminster Hospital
London, UK

Endocrinology

Anna P Kenyon MBChB MD MRCOG
Clinical Lecturer
Institute for Women's Health
University College London
London, UK

Physiology

Sailesh Kumar
DPhil FRCS FRCOG FRANZCOG CMFM
Consultant/Senior Lecturer
Centre for Fetal Care
Queen Charlotte's and Chelsea Hospital
Imperial College London
London, UK

Fetal and placental physiology

Fiona Lyall BSc PhD FRCPath MBA
Professor of Maternal and Fetal Health
Maternal and Fetal Medicine Section
Institute of Medical Genetics
University of Glasgow
Glasgow, UK

Biochemistry

Vivek Nama MD MRCOG

Clinical Research Fellow
Maternal Medicine Department
Epsom & St Helier University Hospitals NHS Trust
Carshalton, Surrey, UK

Drugs and drug therapy

Sara Paterson-Brown FRCS FRCOG

Consultant in Obstetrics and Gynaecology
Queen Charlotte's and Chelsea Hospital
London, UK

Applied anatomy

Geoffrey L Ridgway
MD BSc FRCP FRCPath

Consultant Clinical Microbiologist and Honorary Senior
Lecturer
University College London Hospitals NHS Trust
London, UK

Microbiology and virology

Neil J Sebire
MB BS BClinSci MD DRCOG FRCPath

Consultant in Paediatric Pathology
Department of Histopathology
Camelia Botnar Laboratories
Great Ormond Street Hospital
London, UK

Pathology

Hassan Shehata MRCPI MRCOG

Consultant Obstetrician & Obstetric Physician
Epsom & St Helier University Hospitals NHS Trust
Carshalton, Surrey, UK

Drugs and drug therapy

Andrew Shennan MBBS MD FRCOG

Professor of Obstetrics
Maternal and Fetal Research Unit
King's College London
St Thomas' Hospital
London, UK

Clinical research methodology

David Talbert PhD MInstP

Senior Lecturer in Biomedical Engineering
Division of Maternal and Fetal Medicine
Imperial College School of Medicine
Hammersmith Hospital
London, UK

Physics

Paul Taylor

Department of Microbiology & Virology
Royal Brompton and Harefield NHS Trust
Royal Brompton Hospital
London, UK

Microbiology and virology

Dorothy Trump MA MB BChir FRCP MD

Professor of Human Molecular Genetics
Academic Unit of Medical Genetics
University of Manchester
St Mary's Hospital
Manchester, UK

Clinical genetics

David Williams MBBS, PhD, FRCP

Consultant Obstetric Physician
Institute for Women's Health
University College London Hospital
London, UK

Physiology

Preface

The way in which junior obstetricians and gynaecologists are being trained has undergone an unprecedented evolution in the eight years since the last edition of this book. Likewise, the MRCOG Part 1 examination has evolved to reflect the exciting advances in reproductive biology, the increased emphasis upon translating basic science discoveries to the bedside, and more modern ways of assessing knowledge. A new edition of this book is therefore timely. This book has been hugely popular since it was first published under the editorship of Geoffrey Chamberlain, Michael de Swiet and the late Sir John Dewhurst, and we are pleased to continue their excellent work. We have brought in several new authors to completely revise topics that were covered in the previous editions and have introduced new chapters on molecular genetics, clinical genetics and clinical trials to reflect the growing importance of these topics in clinical practice. New multiple choice questions and extended matching questions have been devised to match the format of the examination.

We are grateful to the previous editors and authors whose work formed the foundation of the current edition. We hope that this text will continue to help future obstetricians and gynaecologists to leap one of the first hurdles in their career paths and will also be a useful source of information to facilitate their ongoing understanding of basic science as it applies to clinical practice.

Phillip Bennett and Catherine Williamson
London 2010

Acknowledgements

The editors thank the previous editors, Geoffrey Chamberlain, Michael de Swiet and the late Sir John Dewhurst, the past and present contributors and the production and editorial team at Elsevier. We are also very grateful to Mrs Ros Watts for being an efficient interface between us, the contributors and the editorial team.

Chapter One

1

Structure and function of the genome

Peter Dixon

CHAPTER CONTENTS

This chapter will provide a basic introduction to the human genome and some of the tools used to analyse it. Genomics and molecular biology have developed rapidly during the last few decades, and this chapter will highlight some of these advances, in particular with respect to the impact on our knowledge of the structure and function of the genome. The basic science described in this chapter is fundamental to the understanding of the field of clinical genetics, which is described in the following chapter.

Chromosomes

Inheritance is determined by genes, carried on chromosomes in the nuclei of all cells. Each adult cell contains 46 chromosomes, which exist as 23 pairs, one member of each pair having been inherited from each parent. Twenty-two pairs are homologous and are called *autosomes*. The 23rd pair is the sex chromosomes, X and Y in the male, X and X in the female.

Each cell in the body contains two pairs of autosomes plus the sex chromosomes for a total of 46, known as the diploid number (symbol N). Chromosomes are numbered sequentially with the largest first, with the X being almost as large as chromosome 1 and the Y chromosome being the smallest. This means that each cell (except gametes) has two copies of each piece of genetic information. In females, where there are two X chromosomes, one copy is silent (inactive), i.e. genes on that chromosome are not being transcribed (see below).

Each individual inherits one chromosome of each pair from their mother and one from their father following fertilization of the haploid egg (containing one of each autosome and one X chromosome) by the haploid sperm (containing one of each autosome and either an X or a Y chromosome). The sex of the individual is therefore dependent on the sex chromosome in the sperm: an X will lead to a female (with the X chromosome from the egg) and a Y chromosome will lead to a male (with an X from the egg).

Chromosomes are classified by their shape. During metaphase in cell division chromosomes are constricted and have a distinct recognizable 'H' shape with two chromatids joined by an area of constriction called the centromere. For 'metacentric' chromosomes the centromere is close to the middle of the chromosome and for 'acrocentric' chromosomes it is near to the end of the chromosome. The area or 'arm' of the chromosome above the centromere is known as the 'p arm' and the area below is the 'q arm'. For acrocentric chromosomes, the p arm is very small consisting of tiny structures called 'satellites'. Within the two arms regions are numbered from the centromere outwards to give a specific 'address' for each chromosome region (Fig. 1.1). The ends of the chromosomes are called telomeres. Chromosomes only take on the characteristic 'H' shape during a metaphase when they are undergoing division (hence giving the two chromatids).

Chromosomes are recognized by their banding patterns following staining with various compounds in the cytogenetic laboratory. The most commonly used stain is the Giemsa stain (G-banding) which gives a characteristic black and white banding pattern for each chromosome.

In the cell, the chromosomes are folded many hundreds of times around histone proteins and are usually only visible under a microscope during mitosis and meiosis. DNA is composed of a deoxyribose backbone, the 3-position (3′) of each deoxyribose being linked to the 5-position (5′) of the next by a phosphodiester bond. At the 2-position each deoxyribose is linked to one of four nucleic acids, the purines (adenine or guanine) or the pyrimidines (thymine or cytosine). Each DNA molecule is made up of two such strands in a double helix with the nucleic acid bases on the inside. This is the famous double helix structure that was first proposed by Watson and Crick in 1953. The bases pair by hydrogen bonding, adenine (A) with thymine (T) and cytosine (C) with guanine (G). DNA is replicated by separation of the two strands and synthesis by DNA polymerases of new complementary strands. With one notable exception, the reverse transcriptase produced by viruses, DNA polymerases always add new bases at the 3′ end of the molecule. RNA has a structure similar to that of DNA but is single stranded. The backbone consists of ribose, and uracil (U) is used in place of thymine (Fig. 1.2).

Gene structure and function

DNA is organized into discrete functional units known as genes. Genes contain the information for the assembly of every protein in an organism via the translation of the DNA code into a chain of amino acids to form proteins. DNA that encodes a single amino acid consists of three bases, or letters. With four letters and three positions in each 'word', there are 64 possible

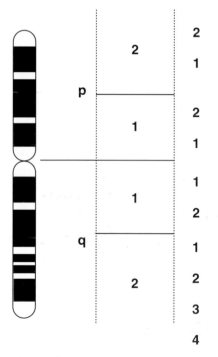

Figure 1.1 • Diagrammatic representation of the X chromosome. Note that the short arm (referred to as p) and the long arm (referred to as q) are each divided into two main segments labelled 1 and 2, within which the individual bands are also labelled 1, 2, 3, etc. (Courtesy of Dorothy Trump.)

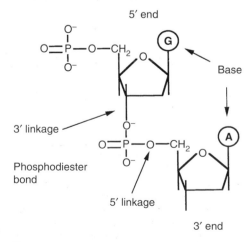

Figure 1.2 • The sugar phosphate backbone of DNA.

combinations of DNA, but in fact only 20 amino acids are coded for (Table 1.1). Therefore, the third base of a codon is often not crucial to determining the amino acid – a phenomenon known as wobble.

A diagram of a typical gene structure is shown (Fig. 1.3). Each gene gives rise to a message (messenger RNA), which can be interpreted by the cellular machinery to make the protein that the gene encodes.

Genes are split into exons, which contain the coding information, and introns, which are between the coding regions and may contain regulatory sequences that control when and where a gene is expressed. Promoters (which control basal and inducible activity) are usually upstream of the gene, whereas enhancers (which usually regulate inducible activity only) can be found throughout the genomic sequence of a gene. The two base pair sequences at the boundary of introns and exons (the splice acceptor and donor sites), identical in over 99% of genes, are known as the splice junction (Fig. 1.3); they signal cellular splicing machinery to cut and paste exonic sequences together at this point. The first residue of each gene is almost always methionine, encoded by the codon ATG.

Recent estimates based on the genome sequence put the number of genes at <30 000, a huge reduction from earlier estimates. This means that the vast majority of

Table 1.1 The genetic code

1st position	2nd position				3rd position
	T	C	A	G	
T	Phe	Ser	Tyr	Cys	T
	Phe	Ser	Tyr	Cys	C
	Leu	Ser	STOP	STOP	A
	Leu	Ser	STOP	Tyr	G
C	Leu	Pro	His	Arg	T
	Leu	Pro	His	Arg	C
	Leu	Pro	Gln	Arg	A
	Leu	Pro	Gln	Arg	G
A	Ile	Thr	Asn	Ser	T
	Ile	Thr	Asn	Ser	C
	Ile	Thr	Lys	Arg	A
	Met	Thr	Lys	Arg	G
G	Val	Ala	Asp	Gly	T
	Val	Ala	Asp	Gly	C
	Val	Ala	Glu	Gly	A
	Val	Ala	Glu	Gly	G

Note that in RNA thymidine (T) is replaced by uracil (U).

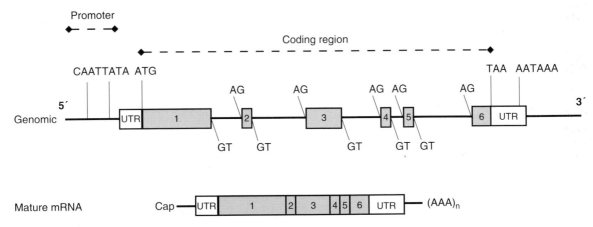

Figure 1.3 • Schematic representation of generalized gene structure. The upper panel shows the genomic organization of a typical gene (with a variety of key features indicated) and the lower panel the mRNA resulting from the transcription of this gene. Key features indicated include the consensus splice sites GT (donor) and AG (acceptor), the initiation codon (ATG), the stop codon (TAA) and polyadenylation signal (AATAAA). Typical promoter motifs are indicated (CAAT and TATA) together with 5′ and 3′ untranslated regions (UTR). Mature mRNAs have a protective 5′ cap (a guanosine nucleotide connected to the mRNA by means of a 5′ to 5′ triphosphate linkage).

human DNA does not contain a coding sequence (i.e. exons), but is rather an intronic sequence: structural motifs and regulatory regions. This is distinct from lower organisms, e.g. bacteria, where >95% of the DNA is a coding sequence. Just exactly why this 'unused' DNA is present remains somewhat enigmatic. The other implication of this finding is that the huge complexity of humans compared to other organisms with similar numbers of genes must arise from more subtle regulation of gene expression, rather than greater numbers of different genes.

The central dogma of molecular biology

The central dogma of molecular biology concerns the information flow pathway in cells and can be simply summarized as: 'DNA makes RNA makes protein, which in turn can facilitate the two prior steps'. These steps are now explained in more detail.

Transcription

'Transcription' is the process of the information encoded in DNA being transferred into a strand of messenger RNA (mRNA). During transcription the RNA polymerase, which constructs the complementary mRNA, reads from the DNA strand complementary to the RNA molecule. This is known as the anti-sense strand while the opposite strand, which has the same base pair composition as the RNA molecule (with thymidine (T) in place of uracil (U) as men-

tioned previously), is the sense strand. Gene sequences are expressed as the sequence of the sense strand of DNA, although it is in fact the anti-sense strand which is read (Fig. 1.4). The vast majority of genes consist of a 5′ untranslated region (UTR) containing response elements to which proteins may bind that influence transcription. The 5′ regions of genes are frequently characterized by elements such as the TATA and CAAT boxes (Fig. 1.3) and are often richer in GC pairs than elsewhere in the genome. This is frequently the case around the 5′ ends of 'housekeeping' genes that are constitutively expressed in the majority of tissues. There then follows the transcribed sequence. The expressed coding parts of the gene are known as the exons, while the intervening sequences are known as introns. The coding portion of the gene is often interrupted by one or more non-coding intervening sequences, although numerous examples of single exon genes exist. Initially, the RNA molecule transcribes both introns and exons and is known as heavy nuclear RNA (hnRNA). The exons are perfectly spliced out (as marked by the splice boundary sequences) and a protective cap added before the now mature mRNA exits the nucleus. Hence, cytoplasmic mRNA consists only of coding regions flanked by untranslated regions at the two ends. A polyadenine (poly A) tail is added to most mRNA molecules at their 3′ end, facilitated by the polyadenylation signal found past the stop codon in the coding sequence. This tail, found on the great majority of expressed mRNAs, serves to protect the RNA from degradation prior to translation by the ribosome (see below).

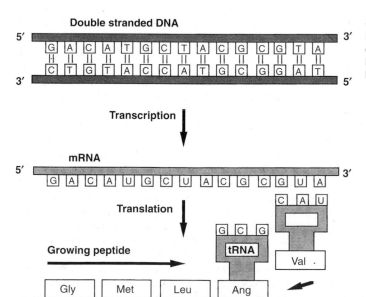

Figure 1.4 • Transcription and translation. Double-stranded DNA is transcribed forming a complementary single-stranded molecule of RNA. The mRNA is translated by tRNA (transfer RNA) to form the peptide chain.

Translation

The term 'translation' describes the process whereby the cellular machinery reads the mRNA code and creates a chain of polypeptides (i.e. a protein). Once in the cytoplasm, the mRNA message is translated into protein by a ribosome. Ribosomes, consisting of a complex bundle of proteins and ribosomal RNA, attach to mRNA at the 5' end. Protein synthesis begins at the amino terminal and amino acids are sequentially added at the freshly made carboxyl end. Amino acids are brought into the reaction by specific transfer RNA (tRNA) molecules. Each tRNA is a single-stranded molecule which folds in a way that allows complementary base pairing between parts of the same strand. The specific configuration allows the tRNA molecule to bind to its specific amino acid. There remains, unpaired, at one end of the molecule, three bases which are complementary to the codon coding for the amino acid. This anticodon binds to the codon of the mRNA and places the amino acid in the correct sequence of the protein (Fig. 1.4). Usually, several ribosomes translate a single mRNA molecule at any one time.

Replication

'Replication' is the process whereby DNA is copied or replicated to permit transmission of genetic information to offspring. DNA replication is performed prior to cell division, when an identical copy must be made for each daughter cell resulting from division. Replication occurs before mitosis, the normal form of cellular division where resulting cells have identical DNA to the original. Meiosis, the second form of cellular division, occurs during gametogenesis, and results in haploid cells, i.e. cells with half the usual complement of DNA. In meiosis the resulting cells (gametes) are haploid, i.e. carry only a single copy of the genomic sequence.

It is important to note that since this dogma was first established in 1958 by Crick, a number of exceptions have been identified. For example retroviruses (e.g. HIV-1) can cause information to flow from RNA to DNA by integrating their genome (carried as RNA) into that of the host. A second example is ribozymes, which are functional enzymes composed solely of RNA and hence have no need to be translated into protein.

Regulation of gene expression

When a gene is actively being transcribed into mRNA and then translated into a protein, it is said to be 'expressed'. Gene expression can be controlled at several levels. Transcription of DNA into mRNA is generally regulated by the binding of specific proteins, known as transcription factors, to the region of DNA just upstream, or 5', of the coding sequence itself. Other proteins can bind enhancer sequences that may be within the gene or a long way upstream or downstream.

The promoter contains specific DNA sequence motifs which bind transcription factors. In general, transcription factors become active when the cells receive some form of signal and then translocate to the nucleus, where they bind to specific sequences in the promoters of specific genes and activate transcription. Other genes, often known as housekeeping genes, have a constant level of expression and are not induced in this way.

Many different types of transcription factor exist with different modes of action. Typical examples of two types will be considered here, namely intracellular nuclear hormone receptors (which are transcription factors) and cell surface receptors, which are capable of activating transcription factors.

Members of the nuclear hormone receptor super-family, such as the progesterone receptor and the thyroid hormone receptor, are present mainly in the cytoplasm of the cell. When a steroid hormone crosses the lipid bilayer of the cell membrane, it binds to the receptor which is usually dimerized to form pairs of receptor molecules. The receptor/hormone dimer complex then translocates to the nucleus and binds to response elements in the promoters of target genes, where it activates (or indeed represses) transcription. This process also involves the recruitment of many other co-factors to the dimer complex which are also involved in regulation of the expression of the target gene.

Cell surface receptors, subsequent to binding of ligands, can activate pathways leading to the formation of active transcription factors. For example activation of tyrosine kinase-linked receptors on the cell surface may lead to a series of phosphorylation events within the cell, culminating in the phosphorylation of the protein Jun. Jun will then combine with the protein Fos to form a dimer transcription factor called AP-1, which can bind to specific AP-1 binding sites in the promoters of responsive genes.

In another example of cell surface receptor action, the 'inflammatory' transcription factor NFκB exists in the cytoplasm of cells as dimers bound to an inhibitory protein IκB. Mediators of inflammation, such as the inflammatory cytokine interleukin 1β, bind to cell surface receptors and activate a chain of biochemical events that result in the phosphorylation and subsequent breakdown of IκB. Uninhibited NFκB dimers then translocate to the nucleus to activate genes whose promoters contain NFκB DNA binding motifs.

Gene expression can also be controlled by regulation of the stability of the transcript. Most mRNA molecules are protected from degradation by the presence of their poly-A tail. Degradation of mRNA is controlled by specific destabilizing elements within the sequence of the molecule. One type of destabilizing element has been well characterized. The Shaw–Kayman or AU-rich sequence (ARE) is a region of RNA, usually within the 3′ untranslated region, in which the motif AUUUA is repeated several times. Rapid response genes, whose expression is rapidly switched on and then off again in response to some signal, often contain an ARE within their 3′ untranslated region. Binding of specific proteins to the ARE leads to removal of the mRNA's poly-A tails and then to degradation of the molecule.

Epigenetics

The field of epigenetics is concerned with modifications of DNA and chromatin that do not affect the underlying DNA sequence. In recent years, the importance of these modifications has come to light and this is now a very active area of research.

Epigenetic modification of DNA

The principal epigenetic modification of DNA is methylation, whereby a methyl group ($-CH_3$) is added to a cytosine, converting it to 5-methylcytosine. This can only occur where a cytosine is next to a guanine, i.e. joined by a phosphate linkage, and is usually described as CpG to distinguish it from a cytosine base-paired to a guanine via hydrogen bonds across the double helix.

Methylation, particularly in the 5′ promoter regions of genes that are often GC-rich, is associated with silencing. Humans have at least three DNA methyl transferases, and the process is critical to imprinting (parent of origin-dependent gene expression) and X inactivation. Abnormal DNA methylation is being increasingly recognized as playing a role in cancer cell development.

Epigenetic modification of histones

Histone proteins are associated with DNA to form nucleosomes, which make up chromatin. Two of each histone protein (2A, 2B, 3 and 4) form the octameric core of the nucleosome, with H1 histone attached and linking nucleosomes to form the 'beads on a string' structure. Chromatin structure plays an important role in regulation of gene expression, and this structure is heavily influenced by modifications of the histone proteins. These modifications usually occur on the tail region of the protein, and include methylation, acetylation, phosphorylation and ubiquitination. Combinations of modifications are considered to constitute a code (the so-called histone code), which it is hypothesized, control DNA–chromatin interaction. A comprehensive understanding of these mechanisms has not

yet been elucidated; however some functions have been worked out in detail. For example, deacetylation allows for tight bunching of chromatin, preventing gene expression.

Mitochondrial DNA

In addition to the genomic DNA present within cells, another type of DNA is present – mitochondrial DNA. The mitochondria are small organelles within cells that have a unique double-layered membrane and are the energy source for cellular activity and metabolism via production of adenosine triphosphate (ATP). They have their own genome (mtDNA), consisting of a single circular piece of DNA of 16 568 base pairs and encoding 37 genes. Mitochondria are only ever inherited maternally because all the mitochondria in a zygote come from the ovum and none from the sperm. Mitochondrial DNA can be used for confirming family relatedness through analysis of the maternal lineage. In addition, mitochondrial DNA has been successfully and reproducibly extracted from ancient DNA samples, largely due to the high copy number compared with nuclear DNA. Mutations in mitochondrial DNA are responsible for a number of human diseases (see Ch. 2).

Studying DNA

The vast majority of DNA samples used for genetic analysis originate from a peripheral blood sample, usually collected in a 10 mL tube containing an anticoagulant, e.g. EDTA. From this sample, large quantities of DNA are easily extracted from the leucocytes using one of the many commercial kits available. This has replaced the older method of phenol/chloroform extraction. Alternatively, if only a small amount of DNA is required, buccal swabs can be used to collect DNA. As this is non-invasive, it has considerable advantage, for example where patients are needle-phobic, or where DNA is required from small children. It is also possible to extract usable quantities of DNA from very small amounts of tissue or blood from archive samples such as formalin-fixed paraffin-embedded sections.

Mendelian genetics and linkage studies

The majority of advances in recent years in disease gene identification have come from the field of Mendelian disease. This refers to diseases (e.g. cystic fibrosis or muscular dystrophy) where the inheritance pattern follows classical Mendelian principles, i.e. those established by Gregor Mendel at the end of the nineteenth century. His work, long before the existence of DNA was known, established simple rules for inheritance of characteristics (phenotypes). That is, a disease can be dominant (requiring only one mutant allele to have the disease), recessive (requires two) or X-linked (one mutant allele on the X chromosome and hence much more common in males). Since the first gene was identified by linkage/positional cloning in 1986, well over 1000 Mendelian disease genes have been identified, initially by the use of linkage studies.

Linkage studies rely on the use of large, phenotypically well-characterized families. Typically, 12 or more affected family members are required for tracing autosomal dominant diseases, but far smaller families with as few as three affected individuals can be used for recessive diseases. Family members are typed for polymorphic markers throughout the genome in order to detect which regions the affected individuals share, and hence are more likely to contain the disease gene. The marker of choice for these studies is usually short tandem repeats (STRs) which are more commonly known as microsatellites. These markers are repeat sequences that most commonly consist of dinucleotide base repeats, e.g. $(CA)_n$, but they may also comprise tri- or tetranucleotide repeats. These markers exhibit length polymorphism, such that they are different lengths in different individuals, and can be heterozygous. For example an individual may carry at one marker position one repeat of five units and one of seven. These different repeat lengths are easily detectable by common molecular biology techniques. If a disease gene is close to a particular marker, i.e. linked, it will almost always be inherited with it. Thus, if affected individuals all show the same length repeat at a particular marker, the disease gene may be close by. Statistical analysis is used to formalize the results and give likelihood ratios, the LOD score, or the location of a disease locus.

In the recent past, linkage studies were followed by positional cloning to identify a disease gene. This method of gene identification is so called because genes are identified primarily on the basis of their position in the genome, with no underlying assumptions about the protein they encode. After the linkage of a disease had been achieved, a physical map of the linked region was constructed. This was done using large-scale cloning vectors such as YACs (yeast artificial chromosomes) or BACs (bacterial artificial chromosomes), which contain inserts of up to a megabase (1 000 000 base pairs) of the human genome. Libraries of the whole genome were screened with the microsatellite markers used that had been linked to the disease and a series of overlapping clones, or contig, of the linked region constructed. Once this had been established, these clones would be searched for genes which when identified would be screened for mutations in affected patients. This search would have utilized a variety of methods such as direct library hybridization or exon trapping to identify genes within the contig. Much of this work however is now unnecessary due to the greatest advance in the field of human genetics in the last few years – the completion of the sequence of the human genome.

The sequencing of the genome

The completion of the human genome sequencing project has transformed the field of genetics. In brief, BAC (see above) libraries were constructed from the DNA of a handful of anonymous donors, and arranged in order around the genome using genetic markers with established positions. Each BAC was then sequenced and, by the use of high-powered computers, the sequence was assembled, first into the original BAC and then, by matching overlaps, to build up a sequence for the entire genome. The genome centres involved in this project utilized vast numbers of sequencing machines and a production-line environment to achieve the throughput required. In addition to the publicly funded consortium, a private company also produced a complete human genome sequence using a slightly different methodology.

Individual labs and researchers now have access to the entire genome dataset from the publicly funded project freely available on the internet. This information is an invaluable resource and has greatly accelerated research into the molecular aetiology of genetic disease. Once the position of a disease gene has been confirmed (linkage), scientists can now employ an in-silico (i.e. computer-based) approach to identifying the disease gene. Practically, this involves searching databases for all the identified genes in a region and then sequencing them in affected individuals to look for mutations. These 'positional candidates' are often prioritized using other sources of information such as tissue expression pattern or predicted function. Once mutations have been identified, functional studies of mutant forms of the protein to determine the exact nature of the molecular aetiology of the disease in question are often pursued.

Completion of this project has enabled genome centres to focus on two other areas: that of whole-genome sequencing of other organisms for comparative purposes, and so-called 'deep resequencing' to identify the spectrum of genetic variation in human populations.

Analysis of complex traits

The vast majority of so-called 'genetic' disease does not fall into the category of Mendelian disease. Rather, it is caused by so-called complex genetic disease or traits, where a number of genetic factors interacting with the environment result in a disease phenotype. It is this area of genetics that current research is most focused upon.

An example of such a disease in obstetrics is pre-eclampsia (see later chapters). It is important to note that in this type of genetic disease the mutant gene may only be having a small effect on disease susceptibility, and for each disease a large number of genes together with environmental influences may be playing a role.

Methods of analysis of complex traits can be broadly divided into two areas: family-based studies and case–control studies. Family-based studies are usually based upon microsatellite typing approaches (see above), whereas association studies (otherwise known as case–control studies) generally employ another kind of genetic marker, single nucleotide polymorphisms (SNPs). SNPs are much more frequent throughout the genome (every 1000 bases or so) and although they have a lower information content than microsatellites can be used for much finer mapping studies, thanks to their more frequent occurrence.

Family-based studies rely on large collections of nuclear families, parent–offspring trios and/or affected or discordant sibling (sib) pairs. The term discordant refers to disease status, i.e. a discordant sib pair comprises one affected and one unaffected individual. Unaffected family members act as controls.

The dissection of complex traits using these approaches has been problematic for many years for a variety of reasons. These include insufficient sample size (i.e. underpowered studies), inappropriate controls (in association studies) and a lack of knowledge about the underlying structure of the genome (i.e. the patterns of linkage disequilibrium, or the underlying non-random association of markers). In addition, very little was known on a genome-wide scale about the pattern of naturally occurring human variation. However, with a more complete understanding of the structure of the genome, and ever-larger sample resources, significant and reproducible associations of genetic variation with common human disease are emerging. Technology has played a role too, with it now being possible to type many thousands of SNPs in a single experiment using DNA array technologies.

Molecular biology techniques

The manipulation of DNA, RNA and proteins at a molecular level is collectively referred to as molecular biology. This term encompasses a huge range of techniques some of which are outlined here. All of these techniques are in routine use in clinical and research labs around the world.

Restriction endonucleases

One of the key tools used to manipulate DNA is restriction endonucleases. These enzymes, which have been isolated from a wide range of bacteria, cut or restrict DNA at a certain site determined by the base sequence. The reaction occurs under certain conditions, i.e. at the correct temperature and in the correct buffer (usually supplied by the manufacturer). These known recognition sites can be used to manipulate DNA for cloning, blotting, etc. The enzymes have usually been isolated from microorganisms, and their name reflects the organism from which they have been isolated. For example, the common restriction enzyme EcoRI, which cuts or restricts DNA at the sequence GAATTC, was isolated from *Escherichia coli* RY13. *Note*: the recognition of the restriction site depends upon double-stranded DNA, and the cleavage can result in an overhang of a few bases ('sticky ends') or a straight cut across both strands ('blunt ends').

The polymerase chain reaction

The polymerase chain reaction (PCR) is the bedrock of molecular biology and refers to a procedure whereby a known sequence of DNA (the target sequence) can be amplified many millions of times to generate enough copies to visualize, clone, sequence or manipulate in many other ways. A known DNA sequence is amplified first by using a uniquely designed pair of primers at the start (5′) and end (3′; on the reverse strand) of the sequence to be amplified. The primers are thus small pieces of DNA, known as oligonucleotides (oligos), and are usually synthesized by commercial companies for relatively minimal cost. The primers are used in combination with a buffer, a source of deoxyribose nucleotide triphosphate (dNTP) building blocks, the target DNA and Taq polymerase. This polymerase, first isolated from *Thermophilus aquaticus*, is able to replicate DNA at high temperatures. Once prepared, the reaction is placed into a thermal cycler. The reaction proceeds through a number of repeated cycles where the DNA template is denatured, the primers anneal and the polymerase extends the products. Cycling of these three temperatures (one for each of the above steps) results in an exponential amplification of the target sequence. Following amplification, products can be visualized by agarose gel electrophoresis (see below).

Many other commonly used applications are based around the principles of PCR. For example, reverse transcription PCR (RT-PCR), which can be applied to RNA analysis. This technique uses reverse transcriptase enzymes isolated from retroviruses to generate DNA copies of template RNA to detect expression of a particular gene. This approach is further enhanced by quantitative RT-PCR, where relative or absolute expression levels of a particular message can be measured.

Another development of PCR is whole genome amplification, which relies on the use of specialist polymerases to amplify the entire genome in a single reaction, a very useful tool when the amount of sample available is limited.

Electrophoresis

DNA molecules are slightly negatively charged and hence, under the right conditions, will migrate towards a positive charge. This phenomenon can be exploited to visualize DNA. For example the results of a PCR reaction (see above) can be assessed in this way, or a sample of genomic DNA digested with a restriction enzyme can be separated. DNA samples are loaded onto an agarose gel (a sieving mixture of seaweed extract) in the range of 0.5–4% (depending on the size range of DNA to be separated) in a tank containing running buffer (commonly Tris/borate/EDTA). Under an electric current the DNA will migrate at a rate proportional to its size. The samples can then be visualized under a UV light box after the addition of ethidium bromide, or one of the newer less toxic alternatives (e.g. Sybersafe). Larger DNA molecules and RNA samples can also be visualized by electrophoresis. Slightly different conditions are used to protect the RNA, which is inherently more unstable than DNA, and specialized running equipment is need to separate DNA molecules >10 kb in size.

Blotting

DNA (in the case of Southern blotting), RNA (northern) and protein (western) can be fixed to nylon membranes for further analysis, e.g. for screening with a radioactively labelled probe (DNA/RNA) or with an antibody raised to an epitope of interest (proteins). This is a fairly straightforward and routine procedure, which enables a range of downstream experiments to be carried out. For example, a genomic DNA digest can be screened with a radiolabelled or biotinylated probe for a gene sequence of interest, or an antibody raised against a particular protein can be used to screen for that protein in cellular extracts.

Sequencing

DNA sequencing is now a rapid and straightforward process. The sequence of an amplified fragment of DNA is determined using a variation of the PCR method incorporating fluorescently labelled bases which can be read by a laser detection system. In this application, a PCR cycle is performed using only one primer, either forward or reverse, and the labelled nucleotides. This results in linear amplification of product with consecutive lengths of sequence with a fluorescent tag corresponding to the final base of the fragment. When run on a slab gel or capillary and read by a laser, the sequence is determined by the sequential reading of each base. Recent advances in the use of capillary-based machines with multiple channels have resulted in a huge increase in throughput and capacity, and facilitated the rapid acceleration in efforts to sequence the entire human genome.

Cloning vectors and cDNA analysis

As outlined above, the human genome sequence now makes it unnecessary to clone genes from a candidate region before mutation analysis. However, cloning is still a critical part of the analysis of gene function subsequent to mutation detection. For example, using some of the techniques outlined above in the molecular biology section, the expression pattern of a gene can be studied, factors that induce transcription can be identified, and so on. Many of these techniques rely on the use of cDNA clones. These are vectors of much smaller size than YACs and are carried and propagated in bacteria as plasmids or phage. They may also be introduced into cell lines by transfection. The vectors contain an insert of DNA, which corresponds to the full-length mRNA of the gene in question; this is known as copy DNA (cDNA) and contains only the exonic material of the gene. Clones may be screened from libraries or in many cases purchased from commercial sources. Isolation and propagation of these clones in a suitable host strain of bacteria allows detailed analysis of gene function.

Expression studies

A detailed explanation of protein analysis is beyond the scope of this chapter. Key concepts to understand are that proteins can be expressed in mammalian and bacterial systems, their interactions studied and function analysed. A recent approach gaining popularity is to use short interfering RNA (siRNA) to 'knock-down' genes of interest in both *in-vitro* and *in-vivo* systems. In this approach, a vector is introduced which expresses short pieces of carefully designed RNA. These RNA molecules interact with cellular machinery and interfere with endogenously expressed mRNA by targeting it for degradation. This results in the reduction, or knocking down, of the expression of the target gene by up to 80% of the original expression level.

In-silico analysis

The free availability of the human genome sequence via the internet has greatly enhanced the use of computer analysis for molecular biology. This has led to an enormous rise in the discipline of 'bioinformatics', which can be simply defined as deriving knowledge from computer analysis of biological data.

A variety of molecular biology databases, also freely available over the web, provide a large amount of useful information. In addition to the human genome sequence already discussed, a huge range of structural and functional databases, together with organism- and disease-specific databases, polymorphism databases and enzyme databases, can be used to aid research (for example, see Table 1.2).

The 'post-genomic' era

Following the completion of the sequencing of the human genome, and the ongoing projects to completely sequence the genome of a range of other organisms, focus has shifted into a broad range of fields that consider and analyse cells or whole organisms in their entirety, the so-called 'post-genomics' era. This approach is sometimes referred to as systems biology; broadly it encompasses a range of methodologies to analyse whole systems (be it cells, tissues or whole organisms). The range of techniques used in this field is collectively known as the 'omics' topics. Some of these are as follows:

Proteomics (the large-scale study of proteins). The total protein make-up of a biological sample can be determined using, for example, automated gas chromatography/mass spectrophotometry systems (GC/MS). These systems, which combine separation methods (GC) and identification methods (MS), are enhanced through automation and pattern-matching techniques to facilitate rapid and accurate identification of protein content.

Transcriptomics (high-throughput analysis of total mRNA populations). The total mRNA population (or transcriptome) of two groups can be compared by isolating RNA and hybridizing it to a chip which has oligos for every identified gene arrayed on its surface. The output of these experiments can, for example,

determine changes in gene expression under different conditions, or can be used to analyse changes in gene expression during carcinogenesis.

Metabonomics (the analysis of all metabolites in a cellular system). This discipline is concerned with quantitative changes in metabolites, i.e. molecules changing during the process of normal or abnormal metabolism. This may be analysed using proteomic methodology and nuclear magnetic resonance spectroscopy (NMR) methods.

The molecular basis of inherited disease – DNA mutations

DNA mutations occur during cellular replication and division and can result in a range of alterations from large-scale chromosomal abnormalities (which are considered in more detail in Ch. 2) down to single base changes, also called 'point mutations' (which will be considered in general terms here and in more detail in Ch. 2). An important distinction to make is between somatic and germ-line mutations. Somatic mutations occur in sub-populations of cells and are not inherited. Examples of such somatic mutations are those seen in a variety of cancer cell populations, where cancerous cells accumulate a number of somatic mutations as they develop into tumours. Germ-line mutations, as the name implies, are present in the germ-line (i.e. sperm and oocytes) and are inherited down generations. In the rest of this section, only germ-line mutations will be considered.

Variation in genomic DNA sequence arises from errors in DNA replication. This variation is often repaired by cellular machinery, or occurs in non-coding regions of the genome. However, when variations, or polymorphisms, occur within genes and affect protein function, they are considered mutations. A variety of

Table 1.2 Examples of online databases used by molecular biologists

	URL	Description
DNA	http://genome.ucsc.edu/ http://genewindow.nci.nih.gov:8080/home.jsp http://www.ncbi.nlm.nih.gov/BLAST/	Gateway to whole genome sequences including human Graphical database of human genome with known polymorphisms annotated Web tool for sequence alignment
RNA	http://bioinfo.mbi.ucla.edu/ASAP/ http://microrna.sanger.ac.uk/sequences/ http://itb1.biologie.hu-berlin.de/~nebulus/sirna/	Alternative splicing database Micro RNA database Human short interfering RNA database
Protein	http://www.ebi.ac.uk/swissprot/ http://srs6.bionet.nsc.ru/srs6/ http://www.gpcr.org/7tm/	Annotated protein sequence database Database of 3D structure of protein functional sites Database of G-protein-coupled receptors

Wild-type

```
... ... TGT CAT CAT GCC ATG ... ...
... ... Cys His His Ala Met ... ...
```

Missense

```
... ... TGT CAT GAT GCC ATG ... ...
... ... Cys His Asp Ala Met ... ...
```

Nonsense

```
... ... TGA CAT CAT GCC ATG ... ...
... ... STOP
```

Deletion

```
                  ▽
... ... TGT CAT CAG CCA TG. ... ...
... ... Cys His Gln Pro FS FS FS
```

Insertion

```
                  ▽
... ... TGT CAT CAA TGC CAT ... ...
... ... Cys His Gln Cys His FS FS
```

Polymorphism

```
... ... TGT CAT CAC GCC ATG ... ...
... ... Cys His His Ala Met ... ...
```

Figure 1.5 • Examples of mutations in DNA sequence and their effect upon the protein. In each case, the result of a base change in the DNA sequence (upper strand) is shown on the protein sequence (lower strand). FS, frameshift.

small-scale mutation types are illustrated (Fig. 1.5). This figure illustrates a variety of effects that are possible on encoded proteins by small changes in the DNA sequence. It is important to remember that common variation occurs throughout the human population; for example single nucleotide polymorphisms (SNPs) occur about once every 1000 bases. This causes individuals to be polymorphic (i.e. carry different alleles at the same loci).

The severity of a mutation, i.e. the degree of effect on protein function, often, but not always, correlates with the extent of changes to the protein caused by the change in DNA sequence. For example, a missense mutation will alter only one amino acid, whereas a nonsense mutation will cause a premature truncation of the protein. In some cases, the missense amino acid will not have a great effect.

Due to the degenerative nature of the DNA code (Table 1.1), some changes occur within coding regions that do not result in an amino acid change. These changes are deemed polymorphisms (Fig. 1.5).

The application of this knowledge leads to the related clinical speciality, that of the clinical genetics field, which is considered in more detail in Chapter 2.

Chapter Two

2

Clinical genetics

Dorothy Trump

CHAPTER CONTENTS

The specialty of Clinical Genetics is concerned with the investigation and diagnosis of patients of all ages with disorders that may be inherited. In some cases, this will also involve longer-term surveillance and treatment. Genetic risk assessment and non-directive counselling are an important part of the clinical workload and may involve both the proband and also other family members. Unlike other medical specialties clinical genetics deals with families rather than individuals and even medical case notes are kept for a whole family rather than for each individual. Appointments are often for 30 or 45 min slots and may include several family members together for coordination of genetic testing, risk assessment or screening in genetic multisystem conditions. The clinical genetics team consists of consultants and specialist registrars working closely with genetic counsellors and in close collaboration with laboratory diagnostic genetic scientists and cytogeneticists. For many families their care will involve individuals from all of these groups.

Genetic disorders may be broadly classified into three areas:

1. Chromosomal disorders
2. Single gene disorders
3. Multifactorial disorders.

This chapter will deal with each of these and will also cover more unusual mechanisms of disease including genetic imprinting and mitochondrial disorders. Diagnostic techniques and interpretation of results will be summarized.

Chromosome abnormalities

The normal diploid human genome consists of 46 human chromosomes which are arranged in 23 pairs (Fig. 2.1).

Patient A.C.

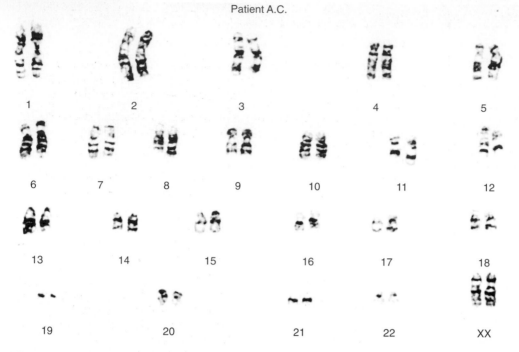

Figure 2.1 • A normal female 46,XX G-banded karyotype illustrating the banding patterns which permit identification of each individual chromosome.

Chromosomes are recognized by their banding patterns following staining with various compounds in the cytogenetic laboratory. The most commonly used stain is the Giemsa stain (G-banding) which gives a characteristic black and white banding pattern for each chromosome, often likened to a supermarket bar code. This allows the cytogeneticist to identify each chromosome in a karyotype, to count the number of chromosomes present and to identify major structural abnormalities such as deletions, duplications or translocations (see later). Testing of patients is usually performed from a blood sample taken into a heparinized bottle. Lymphocytes are cultured for 48–72 h and colchicine is used to arrest cell division in metaphase. The chromosomes are then stained and examined by eye. Additional tests, such as fluorescent *in situ* hybridization (see later), may also be performed. Occasionally additional testing may be performed on other tissues such as skin.

Chromosome abnormalities may be grouped into abnormalities of chromosome number (aneuploidy) and abnormalities of chromosome structure. It is estimated that between 50% and 70% of miscarriages occur due to a chromosome abnormality.

Aneuploidy

Aneuploidy is the term for an abnormal number of chromosomes and includes polyploidy, trisomy and monosomy and additional structurally abnormal (marker) chromosomes (Table 2.1). Abnormal numbers of sex chromosomes are often thought of as a separate group (Table 2.2 and below).

Polyploidy

Polyploid cells contain whole extra copies of the haploid genome (i.e. one set of all the chromosomes). Triploidy, in which 69 chromosomes are present, occurs in 1–3% of conceptions and usually results in spontaneous abortion. There are reports of live births of affected infants, usually with growth restriction and congenital malformations, who die within the first few hours of life. The additional set of chromosomes can come from either the father (type 1 or diandry) or from the mother (type 2 or digyny). Type 1 polyploidy is usually the result of simultaneous fertilization by two sperm, whereas type 2 occurs when a diploid egg is fertilized. Diploid eggs may be the result of non-disjunction of all chromosomes during meiosis or the fertilization of a nucleated primary oocyte. Partial hydatidiform mole is a consequence of type 1 (diandry) triploidy. Diploid/triploid mosaicism is a well recognized dysmorphic syndrome with body or facial asymmetry and skin – or pigmentation defects, obesity and syndactyly of the fingers and toes. Tetraploidy (92 chromosomes) is rare, and survival to term very rare.

Table 2.1 Numerical abnormalities of autosomes

Condition	Karyotype	Clinical picture
Polyploidy	69,XXX or 69,XXY	Usually spontaneous abortion. Occasional live born, die soon after birth. Growth retardation, congenital malformation, mental retardation.
Diandry polyploidy	69,XXX or 69,XXY extra chromosomes from father	Usually spontaneous abortion. Can lead to partial hydatidiform mole.
Trisomy		
Trisomy 21 (Down syndrome)	47,XX + 21 or 47,XY + 21	Characteristic facial dysmorphology, mental retardation, congenital cardiac anomalies, duodenal atresia.
Trisomy 13 (Patau syndrome)	47,XX + 13 or 47,XY + 13	Cleft lip and palate, microcephaly, holoprosencephaly, closely spaced eyes, post-axial polydactyly. Death usually within few weeks of birth.
Trisomy 18 (Edward syndrome)	47,XX + 18 or 47,XY + 18	Low birth weight, small chin, narrow palpebral fissures, overlapping fingers, rocker bottom feet, congenital heart defects, death usually within few weeks of birth.
Monosomy		Monosomy of autosomes not viable.

Trisomy

Trisomy is the presence of an extra chromosome. This can arise as a result of non-disjunction, when homologous chromosomes fail to separate at meiosis resulting in a germ cell containing 24 chromosomes rather than 23. Trisomy of any chromosome can occur, but all except trisomies 21, 18, 13, X and Y are lethal *in utero*. The risk of non-disjunction increases with maternal age, particularly for chromosome 21.

Trisomy 21 is the commonest of the viable trisomies affecting around 1 in every 650 live births in the absence of prenatal screening. The majority of Down syndrome occurs due to non-disjunction trisomy 21 and is associated with maternal age. Around 5% of Down syndrome is associated with a chromosome translocation. The risk of non-disjunction Down syndrome increases with maternal age with a live-born risk in a 25-year-old woman of under 1 in 1000; in a 30-year-old woman, the risk (1 in 900) is similar to the population risk and rises to 1% at a maternal age of 40. Tables of risk are available and screening is offered to pregnant women in the UK. The clinical features of Down syndrome are summarized in Table 2.1.

Trisomies 13 (Patau syndrome) and 18 (Edward syndrome) are much rarer. The risk does increase with maternal age but is much lower than for Down syndrome at all ages. These trisomies cause severe congenital malformations (Table 2.1) and mental retardation, usually resulting in death within the first few months of life.

Monosomy

The absence of one of a pair of chromosomes is usually lethal to the embryo and therefore rare in live-born infants. The only exception is monosomy X or Turner syndrome (see below).

Sex chromosome anomalies

Aneuploidy of sex chromosomes generally has less severe consequences than aneuploidy of autosomes. The features of these syndromes are summarized in Table 2.2. Trisomy of the sex chromosomes is often undetected, particularly in Klinefelter syndrome (47,XXY) until a karyotype is performed. Monosomy, resulting in Turner syndrome (45,X), is the only viable monosomy and has an incidence in newborn females of approximately 1 in 2500. The features are summarized in Table 2.2. A much larger number of affected pregnancies miscarry and monosomy X accounts for about 18% of chromosomal abnormalities seen in spontaneous abortion. Absence of the X chromosome leaving only the Y is incompatible with embryonic development and will always result in early abortion.

Table 2.2 Sex chromosome anomalies

Condition	Karyotype	Clinical picture
Triple X syndrome	47,XXX	Slender body habitus, mild learning difficulties, as a group reduction in IQ, individually may not be noticeable.
Tetrasomy X	48,XXXX	Mental retardation more severe than 47,XXX (mean IQ around 60).
Klinefelter syndrome	47,XXY	1 in 1000 newborns but often not diagnosed until much later. Tall, small testes, gynaecomastia, sparse facial hair, infertility, mild reduction in IQ.
XYY syndrome	47,XYY	Often undiagnosed, can cause mild learning difficulty, behavioural problems.
Turner syndrome	45,X	Often causes spontaneous miscarriage, short stature, webbing of neck, congenital heart defect, wide-spaced nipples, gonadal dysgenesis leading to delayed or absent puberty.

Tetrasomy (48,XXXX) and pentasomy (49,XXXXX) of sex chromosomes are compatible with normal physical development but affected individuals usually have some degree of mental retardation. It appears that the greater the number of X chromosomes, the greater the degree of mental impairment. Whatever the number of X chromosomes, the presence of a normal Y chromosome always produces the male phenotype.

Mosaicism

Mosaicism occurs when an individual has two cell populations each with a different genotype such as diploid/triploid mosaicism (see above). This may occur if there is non-disjunction during early cleavage of the zygote or in anaphase lagging in which one chromosome fails to travel along the nuclear spindle to enter the nucleus and becomes lost, resulting in a normal/monosomy mosaicism. Turner syndrome is often mosaic and may explain the occasional report of fertility in Turner syndrome.

Structural chromosome abnormalities

Structural chromosome abnormalities are very variable and occur when there are breaks in chromosomes. The nature of the chromosomal abnormality will depend upon the fate of the broken pieces.

Chromosome deletions

The absence of part of a chromosome leads to monosomy for that stretch of chromosome and the consequences depend on the region involved and the size of the deletion. Any part of either the long or the short arm of a chromosome may be lost. Terminal deletions involve the end of the chromosome; interstitial deletions occur within one of the arms. Identification of the missing portion can be made by examination of the G-banding pattern. The deletion is described in the karyotype report as 'del' followed by the missing region

(see nomenclature below). Recognizable syndromes are associated with certain chromosome deletions such as 5p- which causes *cri du chat*, a condition associated with severe mental retardation and a characteristic cry from birth which is said to sound like a cat.

There is an increasing number of microdeletion syndromes recognized. In these conditions, such as 22q- or Di George syndrome, the chromosome deletion is too small to be detected by eye using G-banding. Instead specific tests are required to test for the presence of two copies of that portion of the chromosome using fluorescent *in situ* hybridization or FISH (see later).

A chromosome with a deletion at both ends may circularize to form a ring chromosome. Ring formation always indicates that some chromosomal material has been lost, although identification of which portion is missing may be difficult. FISH studies can be helpful in the investigation of this.

Chromosome duplications

Duplicated material may occur within a chromosome, may be attached to the chromosome elsewhere or may be attached to another chromosome. Because there is little or no loss of genetic material, duplications are more often compatible with life than other chromosomal abnormalities and are therefore found more frequently. The duplicated region may be in tandem with the original or inverted (i.e. upside down with respect to the original). The phenotype will depend on the region involved and the size of the duplication. Some duplications are known to occur without phenotypic effect and can be classified as polymorphisms.

Chromosome inversions

When a segment of chromosome is reversed in its orientation, this is described as an inversion ('inv' on the karyotype report). This may be confined to one single arm of the chromosome (paracentric inversion) or include both arms on either side of the centromere (pericentric inversion). Inversions may not be associated with a phenotype since there is neither loss nor gain of chromosomal material, but if the break occurs within a gene or within the controlling region associated with a gene then a phenotype may occur.

Isochromosome

These chromosomes consist of either two long arms or two short arms and occur if the centromere divides transversely rather than longitudinally during meiosis (Fig. 2.2). This abnormality has been often described in the X chromosome and may result in the Turner phenotype.

Translocations

Translocations occur when chromosomes become broken during meiosis and the resulting fragment becomes joined to another chromosome.

Reciprocal translocations: In a balanced reciprocal translocation (Fig. 2.3), genetic material is exchanged between two chromosomes with no apparent loss. The portions exchanged are known as 'translocated segments' and the rearranged chromosome is called a 'derivative', reported as 'der', and is named according to its centromere. Provided that there is no loss of genetic material, the translocation is balanced (i.e. no loss or gain of genetic material) and usually results in normal development. Rarely, the breaks occur within a gene or separate a gene from its controlling element which may then lead to a phenotype. Often, there is loss of DNA at the break point that is too small to be detected by G-banding; this usually occurs in non-coding DNA and is inconsequential, but rarely may interrupt a gene and cause a phenotype. Reciprocal translocations are usually specific to a family but there are several which are

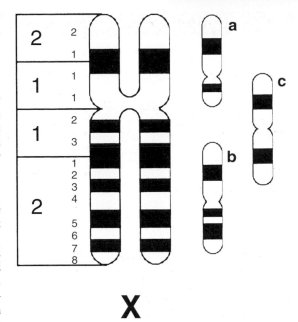

X

Figure 2.2 • Chromosome deletion and isochromosome formation. The large X chromosome at metaphase is seen on the left; (a,b) deletion of the long arm at different points; (c) isochromosome formation; only the two short arms of the X chromosome are represented here since division has been transverse instead of longitudinal and the isochromosome for the short arm of the X has been formed.

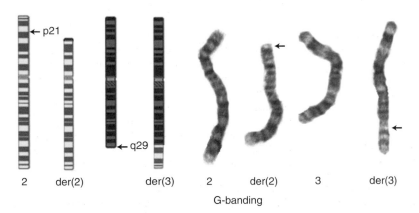

2   der(2)   der(3)   2   der(2)   3   der(3)

G-banding

Figure 2.3 • Reciprocal translocation between chromosomes 2 and 3. A portion of the short arm of chromosome 2 has been exchanged with a small portion of the long arm of chromosome 3. The panel on the left shows this in diagrammatic form. The middle panel is the result of G-banding. The right panel shows chromosome painting with chromosome 2 in pink and chromosome 3 in turquoise. This is a balanced translocation. (Figure provided by Dr L Willett, East Anglian Genetics Service, Cytogenetics Laboratory.)

known to occur more commonly. Around 1 in 500 individuals carry a reciprocal translocation and are usually unaware of this. Individuals who carry a balanced translocation are at risk of having recurrent miscarriages or indeed a child with congenital abnormalities and/or learning difficulties as the offspring might inherit an unbalanced form of the translocation. Reciprocal translocations are found in approximately 3% of couples with recurrent miscarriage.

During meiosis, homologous chromosomes pair. When a reciprocal translocation is present, the four chromosomes (i.e. the two derivative and two normal) come together as a four chromosome structure known as a 'quadrivalent'. Two of these chromosomes then pass into the gamete. There are thus four possibilities: the gamete contains the two normal chromosomes and will result in a normal karyotype in the offspring; the gamete contains the two derivative chromosomes and will result in offspring with the reciprocal balanced translocation like the parent or one of the two derivates, and the other normal chromosomes pass into the gamete (or vice versa) resulting in offspring with monosomy for one region of the genome and trisomy for another. This can result in either miscarriage or, if the chromosome segments are not large, a viable offspring with congenital abnormalities. The phenotype depends on the segments of chromosome involved. The risk of a live-born infant with an unbalanced translocation is specific to each reciprocal translocation and is difficult to calculate depending on which segments of chromosomes are involved, how large they are and whether there are reports of other live-born infants with the same karyotype. It is important to note this is not a 1 in 4 risk.

Robertsonian translocations: Acrocentric chromosomes have very short p arms consisting of satellites (see above). Breakage of the short arm of two acrocentric chromosomes near to the centromere may result in loss of the short arms and junction of the long arms resulting in a large chromosome consisting of both centromeres and long arms (Fig. 2.4). When an individual carries a Robertsonian translocation, they therefore

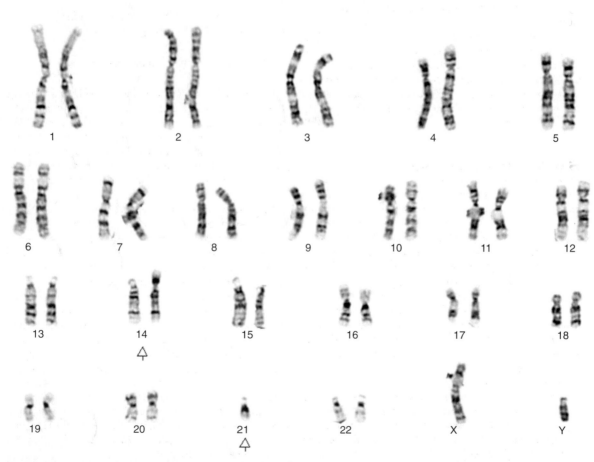

Figure 2.4 • Robertsonian translocation between chromosomes 14 and 21. (Figure provided by Dr L Gaunt, Manchester Regional Genetics Service, Cytogenetics Laboratory.)

have 45 chromosomes. Since only satellite material has been lost, there is no phenotype associated with a Robertsonian translocation. However, when these individuals have children, there is a risk of both the Robertsonian and one of the normal homologous chromosomes being inherited from that parent, resulting in trisomy for this chromosome. One common Robertsonian translocation involves chromosomes 11 and 21. There is a risk of the child inheriting the homologous chromosome 21 in addition to the Robertsonian chromosome, resulting in trisomy 21 (Down syndrome). This is 'translocation Down syndrome'.

Chromosome nomenclature

There is an agreed format for describing chromosome abnormalities and this forms the basis of reports from cytogenetics laboratories. Take the reciprocal translocation in Figure 2.3 as an example: 46,XY,t(2;3)(p21;q29). The total number of chromosomes is given first (i.e. 46), the sex chromosomes are indicated next (i.e. XY indicating male). A translocation is indicated by the letter 't' and is followed in parentheses by the number of chromosomes concerned, with 'p' or 'q' relating to the involvement of long or short arms (i.e. chromosome 2p and chromosome 3q). The regions of the chromosome are indicated by their numerical address (i.e. chromosome 2p21 has swapped position with chromosome 3q29). Deletions are indicated by the term 'der' and duplications by 'dup' followed by the region involved.

Single gene disorders

Genetic disorders occurring due to faults or mutations in single genes can be inherited in a number of ways. The vast majority follow Mendelian patterns of inheritance and are either dominant or recessive, autosomal or sex-linked. A small number of disorders are caused by mutations in mitochondrial genes and these follow a maternal inheritance pattern (see later). There are two copies of autosomal genes in the genome, one inherited from each parent. For an autosomal dominant disease, a mutation in one of the gene copies (or alleles) is enough to cause the phenotype or disease, whereas a recessive disease is caused when mutations occur in both gene copies.

Genes encode proteins and a change in the sequence of a gene can have serious consequences for the encoded protein. A single base-pair change can lead to: (1) a change in the protein sequence, i.e. an incorrect amino acid being inserted into the protein, which can lead to misfolding and either degradation within the cell or interference with its function; (2) a premature stop codon which causes production of a truncated protein which might lack its functional domain or can lead to nonsense-mediated decay resulting in no protein being produced or (3) problems with splicing the exons together leading to incorrect sequence in the messenger RNA and thus in the protein (see Ch. 1). Deletions and insertions can also occur which may involve a single base, several or many bases. These will all interfere with the sequence of the protein.

Autosomal dominant diseases

In autosomal dominant diseases a mutation in only one of the two gene copies is required to cause the disease. An affected individual will therefore usually carry only one mutated copy of the relevant gene and has another normal copy of the gene. There is therefore a 50% risk of transmission of the mutation to his or her offspring. Individuals who are affected with an autosomal dominant disease will often therefore have a number of other affected family members in several generations. Typical features of autosomal dominant inheritance are:

* An equal ratio of affected males and females
* Transmission of the disease from either sex to either sex
* Possibility of affected individuals in every generation.

Despite the presence of a normal allele the mutant allele causes the disease phenotype (i.e. it is dominant). This may simply be due to a lack of the normal level of functioning protein, i.e. a dosage effect or 'haplo-insufficiency'. Alternatively, this can occur because the mutant protein interferes with the function of the normal protein, described as a 'dominant negative' effect.

If autosomal dominant diseases were fatal in early life or had a significant effect upon reproductive efficiency, it would be expected that natural selection would cause them to die out. In general, autosomal dominant diseases are less severe than recessive diseases. They can also display variable expression, whereby the phenotype may be more or less severe in different individuals (e.g. neurofibromatosis type 1). On occasion, the phenotype may become so mild that the disease appears to skip a generation (e.g. autosomal dominant deafness). In some conditions, there may be rare individuals who have the mutation but exhibit none of the features of the disease. This is called non-penetrance. Some autosomal dominant diseases have a late age of onset and occur in adult life, after reproductive maturity has been reached. For example Huntington disease, a neurodegenerative disorder, usually occurs after the age of 30.

If a child is diagnosed with an autosomal dominant condition and there is no family history of the condition then the mutation may have occurred in the child for the first time. However, because some conditions are known to exhibit variable expression, it is extremely important to examine both parents for any features of the disease in order to give accurate figures for the risk of recurrence in another child. If either parent is affected, the risk will be 50%, but if neither has the condition, the risk is very low. This is not zero since occasionally a parent can have germinal mosaicism, i.e. one parent has a small proportion of germ cells with the mutation.

It is now possible to offer prenatal genetic diagnosis for some autosomal dominant diseases (see later).

Examples of more common autosomal dominant conditions include:

- Achondroplasia
- Myotonic dystrophy
- Huntington disease
- Marfan syndrome
- Neurofibromatosis type 1
- Multiple polyposis of the colon
- Osteogenesis imperfecta
- Autosomal dominant polycystic kidney disease
- Tuberose sclerosis.

Autosomal recessive diseases

An autosomal recessive disorder occurs only when an individual has mutations of both copies of the relevant gene. The individual may have the same mutation affecting both the maternal and paternal copy of the gene, e.g. when there is a common mutation causing the disease, such as sickle cell disease. This individual is said to be 'homozygous' for the mutation. If the individual has a different mutation on each copy of a gene then they are described as a 'compound heterozygote'. This occurs more often in diseases such as cystic fibrosis where many different mutations can cause the disease. Individuals who have only one mutated copy of the gene and another normal copy of the gene will be unaffected and unaware that they carry the disease. Very occasionally in some conditions, these 'carriers' may exhibit some symptoms; for example, individuals who are heterozygous for the sickle cell mutation may become symptomatic under extreme conditions, especially if they also carry thalassaemia mutations or the haemoglobin C mutation. Carriers of autosomal recessive diseases are unlikely to have any family history and their carrier status is often detected following the birth of an affected child.

For an individual to be affected, both parents must be carriers. For such a couple there will be a 1 in 4 risk of having an affected child each time they have a child. There will also be a 1 in 2 chance of a child being a carrier (and therefore unaffected) and a 1 in 4 chance

of a child being unaffected and not a carrier. It follows therefore that the *unaffected* sibling of an affected child has a 2 in 3 risk of being a carrier. Consanguinity increases the likelihood of autosomal recessive disease since there is a greater chance that both parents carry the same mutation.

Examples of recessive conditions include:

- Cystic fibrosis
- Congenital adrenal hyperplasia
- Usher syndrome
- Galactosaemia
- Spinal muscular atrophy
- Phenylketonuria.

Because they are frequently encountered in obstetric practice, three autosomal recessive diseases are worth considering in greater detail: (1) cystic fibrosis, (2) sickle cell disease and (3) the thalassaemias.

Cystic fibrosis

Cystic fibrosis is the most common autosomal recessive disorder in the UK Caucasian population. The gene encodes a chloride channel protein called cystic fibrosis conductance transmembrane regulator (CFTR). Mutations in this gene lead to thick sticky secretions resulting in lung disease (recurrent bacterial infections), pancreatic insufficiency and male infertility. Patients often present in infancy, with respiratory and gastrointestinal problems, and failure to thrive. In some regions of the UK, population screening is now under way, testing the levels of trypsinogen in blood from the newborn with Guthrie test cards (raised in cystic fibrosis). Life expectancy is reduced, but with great improvements in management and the possibility of lung transplants, this is increasing and many children born today with cystic fibrosis will live to their mid-20s or 30s. This is important as families may have a much more pessimistic understanding of life expectancy based on past experience. Women with cystic fibrosis are now attending for genetic counselling prior to having their own children. Diagnosis is often still made by sweat testing, a measurement of chloride concentration in sweat, which is abnormally high in cases of cystic fibrosis. This is now coupled with DNA analysis of the *CFTR* gene. Approximately 1 in 25 individuals in the UK Caucasian population is a cystic fibrosis carrier and therefore 1 in 625 couples are at risk of having an affected child. The risk that carrier parents will produce a child with cystic fibrosis is 1 in 4; therefore the birth prevalence is approximately 1 in 2500. It is now possible to test for mutations in the gene. The gene is large and >700 different mutations have been reported as causing cystic fibrosis. Some of these are more common than others with, for example the ΔF508 mutation (a deletion of 3 base pairs removing one amino acid from the protein) accounts for approximately 70% of mutations in Caucasians. Genetic testing is comprehensive but is still unable to detect all disease alleles. This means that only one mutation may be detected in some affected individuals – not because the diagnosis is incorrect but due to the limitations of the technique. Sweat testing is therefore critical to making the diagnosis in these cases.

Prenatal diagnosis following chorionic villous sampling (CVS) is now possible for couples who both carry a cystic fibrosis mutation providing these mutations are known.

Thalassaemias

Haemoglobins have a tetrameric structure, made up of four globin chains. In adult and fetal haemoglobins, two of these chains are always α. The type of haemoglobin is determined by the type of chain linked to these α chains: adult HbA has β chains and adult HbA2 has δ chains, fetal HbF has γ chains. There are two types of γ chain, differing by only a single amino acid, glycine or alanine at position 136. HbF is a mixture of the two types. Embryonic haemoglobin may have either α or ζ chains combined with either γ or ε.

The α and ζ genes are close together on chromosome 16. There are two α genes, α1 and α2. Just upstream from these are two pseudogenes Ψα and Ψζ. Pseudogenes are DNA sequences which have homology to their functioning counterparts but are not functional, having been disabled at some time during evolution. The ζ gene is just a little further upstream. Similarly the β genes are close together on chromosome 11 in the order: 5′ ε Γγ Aγ Ψβ δβ 3′. The gene Ψβ is also a pseudogene. The α gene family all have an identical intron arrangement as do the β family, since each family was formed by a series of duplication events.

Alpha thalassaemia is caused by reduced synthesis of the alpha chain of haemoglobin. Disease severity is determined by the number of functioning α genes and alpha thalassaemia has two clinically distinct phenotypes: Hb Bart hydrops fetalis (Hb Bart) syndrome and haemoglobin H (HbH) disease. Hb Bart syndrome is the most severe form, caused by mutations or deletions affecting all four α globin alleles (copies of the α globin genes) causing a lack of production of α haemoglobin. This leads to oedema and intrauterine hypoxia resulting in stillbirth or death in the neonatal period. The γ chains combine to produce Hb Barts (γ4) and with the ζ chains to produce Hb Portland (ζ2γ2). HbH disease occurs when only one of the four α globin genes is functioning and causes a microcytic hypochromic haemolytic anaemia, hepatosplenomegaly and mild jaundice.

The α0 thalassaemias are caused by large deletions which may span both of the α genes. The deletion usually begins in the α1 gene and may include part or all of the α2 gene and sometimes the adjacent pseudogenes. Molecular genetic diagnosis of α-thalassaemias is generally performed by a combination of PCR and Southern blotting with hybridization to α-globin gene-specific DNA probes.

Alpha thalassaemia is thus inherited in an autosomal recessive manner. For parents who are carriers there will be a 25% risk of a child having Hb Bart hydrops fetalis, a 50% chance of having alpha thalassaemia trait and a 25% chance of being unaffected and not a carrier. Prenatal testing is available.

Beta thalassaemia is caused by reduced synthesis of the haemoglobin beta chain which results in microcytic hypochromic anaemia, nucleated red blood cells, and reduced haemoglobin A (HbA). Affected individuals (thalassaemia major) have anaemia and hepatosplenomegaly, and without treatment affected children fail to thrive and have a shortened life expectancy. Carriers (thalassaemia minor) are symptom free but have a mild microcytic hypochromic picture in peripheral blood. There are many different molecular pathologies that cause β-thalassaemia and disease severity can be affected by modifying factors.

Sickle cell disease

Sickle cell disease is a haemoglobinopathy in which there is anaemia coupled with a tendency for red cells to deform into a characteristic sickle shape under conditions of low oxygen tension. Sickled erythrocytes tend to block small capillaries leading to recurrent episodes of lung, spleen and bone infarction. This causes extreme pain. The haemolysis can lead to chronic anaemia and jaundice. The sickle mutation is a single base-pair substitution that leads to a single amino acid change from valine to glutamine in the β-globin molecule. Diagnostic testing is often by haemoglobin analysis. The disease is inherited as an autosomal recessive condition and prenatal diagnosis can be offered.

Sex-linked inheritance

A female has two X chromosomes and a male has one. X inactivation results in only one allele being active in female cells. X inactivation begins in early embryogenesis and is random, although once an individual cell has set its inactivated X chromosome, all daughter cells have the same X chromosome switched off. Because, in general, X inactivation is random, in an adult the maternal and paternal X chromosomes will each appear to show approximately 50% expression in any particular tissue.

X-linked recessive diseases

Where disease is due to mutation of a gene on the X chromosome, females who inherit the mutation will be protected from its effects by the presence of the normal homologue on their other X chromosome. They will therefore be unaffected although, since expression of the 'normal' chromosome will be limited to 50%, it is often possible to detect female carriers of an X-linked disease by measurement of the gene product. For example, female carriers of classic haemophilia may be found to have reduced circulating factor VIII concentrations. The main characteristics of an X-linked family pedigree include:

- Usually only males are affected (see later)
- Females may be carriers
- Male-to-male transmission of the disease is not possible
- The disease is invariable in phenotype
- There is a 50% risk that the sons of a carrier female will be affected
- There is a 50% risk that the daughters of a carrier female will be carriers
- All the daughters of an affected male will be carriers.

New mutations are more common in X-linked than in autosomal diseases. New mutations may occur either in an affected male or in a carrier female. Females may, rarely, be affected by X-linked recessive diseases. This may occur if a female is homozygous for a mutation, i.e. affected father and carrier mother, in Turner syndrome (female with only one X chromosome), in skewed X inactivation (by chance there is much more inactivation of the normal allele resulting in expression of the mutant allele) and in X–autosome translocations (part of the X chromosome is translocated to an autosome), which can interfere with random inactivation. Examples of recessive X-linked conditions include:

- Factor IX deficiency
- Duchenne muscular dystrophy
- Glucose-6-phosphate dehydrogenase deficiency
- Haemophilia (factor VIII deficiency).

X-linked dominant diseases

X-linked dominant diseases are rare. The only significant conditions are vitamin D resistant rickets, incontinentia pigmenti, and the Xg blood group. Family pedigrees are similar to those of autosomal dominant diseases with the exception that a father cannot pass on the disease to his son. Because there is some protection against the disease in females, from the homologous 'normal' chromosome, X-linked dominant diseases tend to be more severe in males. So, for example, incontinentia pigmenti is lethal in the hemizygous male.

Y-linked diseases

There are currently no known examples of Y-linked disease. Sexual development depends upon the effect of the sex chromosomes on gonadal differentiation, the correct functioning of the differentiated testis and the response of the end organs to substances produced by the testis. In the normal situation, the presence of a Y chromosome causes differentiation of the undifferentiated gonads to testes. The Y chromosome carries a gene which functions as a testicular differentiating factor (TDF). Studies of individuals who were XX, but carried a small translocation from their father's Y chromosome onto X, showed that TDF must be on the long arm of the Y chromosome just below the X–Y homology region. A gene in this region has been found and called the 'sex determining region of Y' (SRY). Mutations in the SRY cause failure of testicular development and result in XY females. Although the mutation in the SRY in an XY female may have arisen in the father, XY females are not fertile and the mutation cannot be further propagated.

Mitochondrial inheritance

The genes in the mitochondrial genome can mutate and the consequences are difficult to predict, as these will depend on how many of the mitochondria within the cell have the mutation and how many do not. This is called heteroplasmy and is analogous to mosaicism in an organism. When cells divide, the mitochondria replicate and are distributed randomly in the daughter cells. This means daughter cells can have a different proportion of mutant mitochondria than the parent cells. Within an individual, there can be great variation in this proportion between tissues and cells – leading to a variable phenotype.

Mitochondrial diseases are rare and have a characteristic inheritance pattern as they are always maternally inherited. The embryo derives all its mitochondria from the egg, i.e. the mother. When the mother has a mitochondrial mutation then all maternal offspring are usually affected and the males never transmit mitochondrial mutations. Mitochondrial diseases characteristically affect muscle and nervous systems and the phenotype is very variable. Examples of mitochondrial diseases include:

- Leber's hereditary optic neuropathy (LHON)
- Chronic progressive external ophthalmoplegia (CPEO)
- Myoclonic epilepsy with ragged red fibres (MERRF)
- Mitochondrial myopathy, encephalopathy, lactic acidosis with stroke-like episodes (MELAS).

Genomic imprinting

The male and female parental contributions to the genome are not fully equivalent. There is increasing evidence that the function of some genes or chromosomal regions may differ depending upon whether it is maternally or paternally derived. For example, it appears that in early development it is mostly paternally derived genes that control the development of the placental tissues, while maternally derived genes play a more important role in development of the embryo. Genomic imprinting has been especially found to be associated with genes that are concerned with growth, such as the insulin-like growth factor receptor. The differences between the maternally and paternally derived chromosomes appear to remain fixed through successive mitotic divisions. This has been termed genomic imprinting. Genomic imprinting must affect a chromosome in a way that survives mitosis but not meiosis. At meiosis, the chromosome must be newly imprinted depending upon the sex of its 'host'.

A current theory for the mechanism of imprinting is selective methylation of the genome. In females, X inactivation depends, at least in part, on the methylation of CG-rich regions adjacent to the gene on the inactive chromosome. Treatment of cells with a demethylating agent can reactivate these genes. Methylation of the inactive X chromosome is analogous to imprinting, although it affects the entire chromosome rather than parts of it and is not dependent on the sex of parental origin.

The concept of genomic imprinting suggests that in certain cases a genetic defect will only produce a phenotype if inherited from a particular parent. For example, a chromosomal deletion in a region concerned with placental development may have no effect if inherited maternally, but may cause failure of placental development if inherited paternally. Examples of chromosome deletion syndrome where this seems to apply are the Prader–Willi and Angelman syndromes. The Prader–Willi syndrome is characterized by hypotonia in infancy, developmental delay, obesity and hypogonadism. It is associated with deletions of chromosome 15q11–13. In some cases, the deletion is detectable by cytogenetic studies; in other cases it is submicroscopic and can only be detected by using DNA probes. In individuals who have Prader–Willi syndrome, the deleted chromosome is always paternally derived. Angelman syndrome is characterized by a happy disposition, mental retardation, ataxic movements, a large mouth and protruding tongue, and seizures. Angelman syndrome is also associated with deletions of 15q11–13 but in this case the deleted chromosome is always maternally inherited. It is possible that similar differences in phenotype may be seen with other deletions depending upon the parental origin. When siblings have the same disorder but have phenotypically normal parents, it is often assumed that this represents an autosomal recessive inheritance. But it is possible that these may represent chromosome deletions in imprintable regions which have no effect in the parent but, since the imprinting status changes with meiosis, it does have an effect in the offspring.

In certain autosomal dominant conditions, there is a difference in the expression, severity or age of onset of the disease depending upon the sex of the affected parent. The clearest example of the effects of genomic imprinting on a single gene disease is the hereditary glomus tumour. This rare, benign tumour has an autosomal dominant inheritance but is only seen in individuals who have inherited the disease from their father. The gene is presumably imprinted in the female germ cell line so that it is not expressed in the offspring of affected mothers. The disease might appear to jump a generation when inherited by a female, whose sons would not exhibit the disease but whose grandchildren could do so.

Uniparental disomy

Uniparental disomy is when both of a pair of homologous chromosomes are inherited from the same parent. If the two chromosomes are identical, with the aneuploid event occurring at the first meiotic division, this is termed heterodisomy. If the two are non-identical homologues, with the aneuploid event occurring at the second meiotic division, it is termed isodisomy. The mechanisms of haploid uniparental disomy are not fully understood at present. If it arose only when a gamete with an extra chromosome met with a gamete with that chromosome missing it would be a very rare event. It is more likely that it arises by combination of a disomic gamete with a normal gamete. The cell-selective pressure to eject one of the three homologues may cause the extra chromosome to be lost in early development and, in some cases, this may leave two homologues from the same gamete.

There are numerous recognized cases of disomy of the sex chromosomes, 47,XXX and 47,XXY, as these are easily identified by cytogenetic studies. Diploid isodisomy is very infrequently recognized, since this requires analysis of DNA polymorphisms. There is a reported case of the father-to-son transmission of haemophilia A. This is usually impossible, since the male offspring of an affected male inherit only his Y chromosomes and the haemophilia defect is on the X chromosome. In this particular case, it was found that the male child had inherited both X and Y chromosomes from his father. There are also cases of cystic fibrosis in which only one parent was a carrier and the child had uniparental disomy for chromosome 7. These cases were identified by the study of DNA polymorphisms around the cystic fibrosis locus.

Multifactorial inheritance

A number of common disorders appear to have a pattern of inheritance which involves a combination of genetic factors or of both genetic and environmental factors. This is termed 'multifactorial inheritance' or 'complex trait' and includes:

- Major neural tube defects (spina bifida and anencephaly)
- Congenital heart disease
- Cleft lip and palate
- Hypertension
- Pre-eclampsia
- Diabetes mellitus
- Atopy.

The reasons for suspecting a combination of genetic and environmental factors in their causation comes from observations of monochorial twins discordant for disease and on the tendency for certain diseases to recur in the same family but with a pattern not consistent with simple monogenic inheritance. For more information on the analysis of complex traits, see Chapter 1.

Genetic testing and interpretation of a genetic result

Genetic investigations include karyotyping (i.e. chromosome analysis) and fluorescent *in situ* hybridization (FISH) which detects small deletions or gene testing for mutations. In order to understand and interpret results from these tests, it is important to understand how the investigations are performed and their limitations.

Chromosome analysis

Karyotyping is usually performed on a sample of peripheral blood which has to be collected into heparin. Lymphocytes are cultured and induced to divide so the chromosomes can be visualized. Cells from other tissues can also be used, with fibroblasts from skin biopsy samples being a common source. For prenatal diagnosis, chorionic villi or fetal cells (skin, etc.) that are shed into the amniotic fluid can also be used. 'Banding' techniques allow chromosomes to be visualized and identified (Fig. 2.1). This involves staining the chromosomes with a DNA-specific dye, most commonly Giemsa, which gives G-banded (black and white striped) chromosomes. Regions with the highest concentration of genes are pale staining and the dark bands contain more condensed chromatin. Cytogeneticists in the laboratory can identify individual chromosomes and whether these look normal or have unusual features, e.g. areas missing or additional material. The limitation of what can be detected in this way is approximately 4 Mb (4 million base pairs). Any abnormality smaller than this is likely to be missed.

Molecular cytogenetics: FISH

Fluorescent *in situ* hybridization (FISH) can be used to test for the presence or absence of specific chromosome regions and is often used to detect small chromosome deletions such as Williams syndrome. This involves using a specific DNA probe which recognizes the region to be tested. The probe is labelled with a fluorescent dye and is hybridized to the chromosomes on a microscope slide. It will only stick to its matched region. In a normal cell this will give two signals (one from each chromosome) and in a cell with a deletion will give only one signal. This can also be used for a quick diagnosis of a trisomy such as Edward syndrome (as three signals will be seen).

Chromosome painting is a similar technique but uses a large collection of probes specific to a whole chromosome. This can be used to identify abnormal additional chromosome material attached to a chromosome (e.g. an unbalanced translocation).

Mutation testing

Mutation testing is now often used to confirm a genetic diagnosis. This is restricted, however, to genes that can be tested: genes that have been shown to cause a particular disease and those genes for which genetic testing is available. Genetic laboratories have been known to receive blood samples with the request 'genes please'! This cannot be done. The lab needs to know which gene and for which disease.

Genetic testing for mutations can be performed in a number of ways: either the gene can be fully sequenced or one of a number of screening techniques is used to detect likely mutations and then that region of the gene is sequenced. When interpreting a genetic result, it is important to know which of these has been used. If a mutation is detected, then a diagnosis has been confirmed. However if no mutation has been detected then the diagnosis may still be correct even if no mutation has been found. This is because of the limitations of the testing. Sequencing the full gene will pick up most mutations but some of the screening techniques may only pick up a proportion of mutations, e.g. 70% of mutations, i.e. leaving 30% undetected. The interpretation of a negative result depends therefore on the technique used to give that result. Laboratory reports will describe this and the detection rate of the technique. Many will also interpret the result in full. A negative result may not mean the patient has no mutation in that gene. If there is any doubt, discuss the result with the laboratory or your local clinical genetics team.

Chapter Three

3

Embryology

Kate Hardy

Oogenesis, spermatogenesis and organogenesis

Oogenesis

During fetal life the developing ovaries become populated with primordial germ cells (oogonia), which continue to divide by mitosis until a few weeks before birth. After this time, no new oocytes are produced, and the female is born with all the oocytes she will ever have (approximately 1 000 000), which are not replaced. From early in gestation, fetal oogonia enter meiosis, reaching the first prophase stage, whereupon they become arrested and remain so for up to 50 years until just before ovulation. During this arrest, the oocyte with the surrounding layer of flattened granulosa cells is known as a *primordial follicle*. These primordial follicles are scattered throughout the cortex of the ovaries, surrounded by interstitial connective tissue. The majority of ovarian oocytes become atretic by puberty, leaving only about 250 000 available in the reproductive phase of life. Of these, only about 400 will be ovulated.

In the ovary there is continual recruitment of small numbers of primordial follicles to start folliculogenesis, which is a lengthy process taking 6 months or longer. This recruitment continues until the supply of primordial follicles is exhausted, around the time of the menopause. Folliculogenesis encompasses recruitment of a cohort of primordial follicles from the resting pool, initiation of follicle and oocyte growth; this is followed by final selection and maturation of a single preovulatory follicle, with the remaining follicles being eliminated by atresia. During this time, the oocyte grows from 35 μm to 120 μm in diameter, undergoes meiosis to produce a haploid gamete, produces large amounts of stable RNA to support early embryonic development and acquires the nuclear and cytoplasmic maturity to undergo fertilization and embryogenesis.

Following recruitment, the granulosa cells of the primordial follicle become cuboidal in shape and undergo cell division. When the follicle reaches the secondary stage, with two layers of granulosa cells, a layer of theca cells develops around the follicle. The theca and granulosa cells of the follicle, which are epithelial in nature, create a specialized microenvironment for the developing oocyte. At the same time, the granulosa cells secrete a glycoprotein coat around the oocyte, known as the *zona pellucida*. Later on, this will provide species-specific sperm receptors at fertilization, and protect the embryo before implantation. Microvilli extend from the granulosa cells through the zona pellucida to the plasma membrane of the oocyte and are intimately involved in the transfer of nutrients and signalling molecules between the two.

When there are several layers of granulosa cells and the oocyte is fully grown, a fluid-filled cavity (the antrum) appears, and starts expanding. The oocyte itself is pushed to one side and is surrounded by two or three layers of tightly knit granulosa cells, the corona radiata. From now until ovulation, follicular development is subject to endocrine control, predominantly by follicle stimulating hormone (FSH). At the beginning of each menstrual cycle, there is a group of about 20 small antral follicles, only one of which will ovulate 2 weeks later. The rest of the group undergo atresia, and die by apoptosis.

After antrum formation, the rate of cell division in the granulosa cell population slows down, and these cells differentiate and become steroidogenic, utilizing theca-derived androgen to produce increasing amounts of oestradiol. In the mid-follicular phase, a dominant follicle emerges and its secretion is responsible for about 95% of circulating oestradiol levels in the late follicular phase. During the final maturation of the follicle, the corona cells become columnar and less tightly packed. The primary oocyte resumes meiotic maturation in response to the onset of the mid-cycle surge of luteinizing hormone (LH). The germinal vesicle breaks down and the first polar body, containing one of each pair of homologous chromosomes (23 in total) and a minute amount of cytoplasm, is extruded. The oocyte (now termed a secondary oocyte) is ovulated while proceeding through the second meiotic division, where it arrests again at metaphase II, and is only stimulated to complete meiosis at fertilization. Each of the 23 chromosomes consists of two chromatids. At fertilization the pairs of chromatids separate, with 23 being retained in the oocyte and 23 being expelled in the second polar body. With the entry of the sperm containing its complement of 23 chromosomes, diploidy is restored.

Spermatogenesis

By comparison with the mature ovum, the mature spermatozoon is very small, the head piece measuring only 4–5 μm in length. Maturation of an ovum is a prolonged process starting in fetal life and involving two substantial resting phases before producing the definitive cell in the adult female. By contrast, the spermatozoon is produced in 70–80 days in a continuous process of development and maturation, which only occurs after puberty in the male. Spermatozoa develop from the basic germ cells of the male, the spermatogonia, which line the basal lamina of the seminiferous tubules interspersed with Sertoli cells. As the spermatozoa develop through the phases of primary spermatocyte, secondary spermatocyte and spermatid, they progress towards the lumen of the tubule into which the mature form is shed.

Spermatogenesis depends on the hormonal drive of the two principal gonadotrophins from the pituitary gland. FSH provides the impetus for the early development stages and the interstitial cell-stimulating hormone (ICSH) aids the later stages and also provokes the Leydig cells to produce testosterone. Spermatogonia constantly divide by mitosis, providing an endless supply of stem cells, only some of which increase in size and develop into primary spermatocytes, each containing 46 chromosomes. Like the primary oocytes these primary spermatocytes undergo a reduction division, known as the first meiotic division, in which the two daughter cells receive 23 chromosomes and are known as secondary spermatocytes. Whereas the first meiotic division of the oocyte produces one secondary oocyte and one polar body, the same division in the male produces two equal secondary spermatocytes of the same size and cytoplasmic content. Each of the secondary spermatocytes undergoes a further meiotic division to form two equal spermatids, each with 23 chromosomes.

The various generations of spermatogonia, spermatocytes and spermatids are linked in small groups by cytoplasmic bridges, possibly as an aid to nutrition and also to ensure synchronous development. The occasional occurrence of twinned mature sperm may represent failure of separation of these bridges. The individual spermatids undergo substantial metamorphosis known as spermiogenesis in order to produce mature spermatozoa. The nuclear material migrates to form the dense sperm head covered by the acrosomal cap (Fig. 3.1). The acrosomal cap is itself developed from vacuoles in the Golgi apparatus that fuse to form the acrosomal vesicle, which spreads out over the nucleus. The very important function of the acrosomal contents in penetrating the ovum is considered under Fertilization. The cytoplasm is gradually reduced, leaving the head piece almost totally full of nuclear

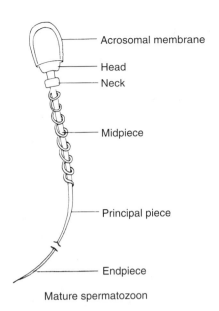

— Acrosomal membrane

— Head

— Neck

— Midpiece

— Principal piece

— Endpiece

Mature spermatozoon

Figure 3.1 • Diagram of a mature spermatozoon showing its principal features.

material. Meanwhile the centriole divides into two, from which the axial filament or flagellum develops. Most of the mitochondria form a sheath for the proximal part of the middle piece of the spermatozoon, whereas the tail piece develops a thin fibrous sheath.

The ripe spermatozoa are released into the lumen of the tubule together with the residual fragments of cytoplasm, mitochondria and Golgi apparatus, which separate from the sperm and eventually degenerate. The mature spermatozoon thus consists of a head piece covered by an acrosomal membrane, and a tail divided into four sections, the neck, midpiece, principal piece and endpiece. The DNA is confined to the nucleus in the head piece, and this alone penetrates the ovum at fertilization. The remainder of the spermatozoon is responsible for its movement. The fully formed spermatozoa are passed through the tubules of the testis to the epididymis. Taken from this source they are known to have the capacity for fertilization *in vivo* and *in vitro*. During ejaculation the spermatozoa are ejected through the vas deferens and prostatic urethra, where they combine with local secretions to form the seminal fluid.

Early embryogenesis: fertilization, transportation and implantation

The complicated process of fertilization implies the union of the mature germ cells, the ovum and spermatozoon. In humans there is a ready supply of spermatozoa constantly available from the normal healthy male after the age of puberty. An average ejaculate will consist of 2–5 mL of seminal fluid with an average

sperm density of 60×10^6/mL. It is true that the sperm density may decline if ejaculation is repeated more frequently than every 48 h but this is seldom a factor in infertility.

By contrast, the normal healthy female will only bring one ovum to maturity and ovulation in each 28-day cycle. Other follicles do develop partially in the same cycle but rarely will more than one reach full maturity. When this does occur, it provokes the potential for binovular twinning. The timing of ovulation is regulated by the cyclical release of gonadotrophins from the pituitary. The ovum is released at the site of a slightly raised nipple on the follicle known as the stigma. As previously described, it oozes out in a sticky envelope of cumulus cells loosely packed around it. The fimbrial end of the ipsilateral fallopian tube gently folds over the ovary and comes to rest over the stigma so that the ovum is taken up into the tube directly. Although this is the normal pattern, it is also possible for the ovum to move over the peritoneal surface of the pelvis behind the uterus to reach the fimbrial end of the contralateral tube.

Once inside the tube, the ovum is wafted medially by the rhythmical action of the cilia, which line the lumen. This movement is augmented by the finely tuned muscular activity of the fallopian tube, which by a combination of peristalsis and shunting squeezes the contents towards the uterus. The whole process is temporarily halted for up to 38 h when the ovum reaches the ampulla of the tube. There appears to be a physiological valve mechanism which prevents further passage of the ovum, and is possibly only released by the rising concentration of the progesterone from the newly formed corpus luteum. When the valve is released, the ovum is moved on once again by the combination of cilial and muscular activity.

This temporary hold-up of the ovum in the ampulla allows additional time for fertilization, and means that sexual intercourse need not coincide precisely with ovulation. Furthermore, spermatozoa have the capacity to retain their potency in the tube for at least 48 h after ejaculation with the implication that, providing coitus occurs within 2 days before or after ovulation, fertilization of the ovum is possible.

Sexual intercourse occurs at random in humans although the female may be more responsive at ovulation time, when the cervical glands produce a copious watery secretion which not only serves to lubricate the vagina but also assists the ascent of the spermatozoa. Normal ejaculation will occur into the upper vagina where the semen forms a coagulum for about 20 min before liquefying. The coagulum prevents immediate loss of fluid from the vagina after sexual intercourse. The surface cells of the vagina are rich in glycogen, especially when under the influence of oestrogen in the follicular phase of the menstrual cycle. Döderlein's bacilli convert glycogen to lactic acid with the result that the vagina becomes weakly acidic and, as such, is hostile to spermatozoa. However, the seminal fluid is alkaline and acts as a buffer for the sperm until they can reach the cervical fluid, which is also alkaline. At mid-cycle the flow of cervical mucus will raise the pH of the upper vagina and facilitate the activity of the sperm. The early progress of the spermatozoa is dependent on the propulsive effect of the tail piece which acts as a flagellum, thus poor motility of the sperm in the seminal sample is an important cause of male infertility. In addition, the passage of the spermatozoa is aided by low-grade contractions of the uterus, which produce a slight negative pressure in the cavity serving to draw the sperm upwards. Spermatozoa have the ability to pass through the uterus and fallopian tubes with amazing rapidity. It is possible to aspirate viable sperm from the pouch of Douglas within 30 min of artificial insemination in the upper vagina. Because the ovum is temporarily held up at the ampulla, the majority of fertilizations occur at that site. Experimental work in which the fallopian tubes have been cut into sections after insemination have defined the section of the tubes in which most newly fertilized ova are found.

Capacitation is an imprecise term coined to explain the concept of some indeterminate change, which is said to occur to the sperm during the first 6 h in the female genital tract, and without which fertilization was thought to be impossible. With recent advances in extracorporeal fertilization, it is clear that spermatozoa have the ability to fertilize an ovum almost immediately, and without any contact with the genital tract. When a spermatozoon reaches the cumulus around the ovum, a quite definite change occurs in the acrosomal cap. The outer acrosomal membrane fuses with the plasma membrane surrounding the spermatozoon and, as they coalesce, fine pores open up with the release of various lytic enzymes which have the ability to break up the cumulus cells and penetrate the zona pellucida, through a narrow channel. The first spermatozoon to reach the cell membrane of the ovum fuses with it, and the head piece containing the nucleus passes into the cytoplasm of the oocyte, where it appears as the male pronucleus. It is easily discernible by light microscopy next to the nucleus of the oocyte, which forms the female pronucleus. The tail piece of the spermatozoon is left behind outside the cell membrane of the oocyte.

As soon as the head piece has penetrated the oocyte, cortical granules release their contents into the space between the egg and the zona pellucida, changing the cell membrane and preventing further penetration by any other spermatozoa. Thus only one spermatozoon out of many million produced in a single ejaculation is needed for fertilization, but, despite this fact, low-density semen of <20 million/mL is associated with relative infertility. *In vitro*, however, a much lower sperm density, even as low as 500 000 million/mL, is compatible with fertilization providing the motility and morphology are normal.

Following fertilization, the ovum continues to move towards the uterus aided as before by the muscle activity of the tube and to a lesser extent by the cilia, which are sparser at the medial end of the tubes where the glandular secretory cells are more numerous. The early development of the fertilized ovum depends on the nutrients derived from the secretions from these cells. It takes about 4 days to traverse the fallopian tube and reach the uterine cavity, which is also lined by a spongy secretory endometrium receptive to implantation of the blastocyst. The first 4 or 5 days after fertilization produce the most remarkable series of changes in the oocyte, all of which have now been followed clearly during *in-vitro* experiments. The second meiotic division of the oocyte is only completed after fertilization, with the extrusion of the second polar body (see Oogenesis above). Following fertilization, nuclear membranes re-form around the two sets of haploid chromosomes, one from the oocyte and one from the sperm, resulting in the formation of female and male pronuclei, which each contain 23 chromosomes. The pronuclei migrate towards each other, but it is not until the time of the first cleavage division that the maternally derived and paternally derived chromosomes finally come together on the first mitotic spindle. The embryo now has 23 pairs of chromosomes, with each pair consisting of one chromosome from the mother and one from the father. The genetic features of the offspring are thus ordained.

Within 30 h of fertilization, the first cell division occurs, in which the fertilized ovum splits equally into two separate cells (Fig. 3.2). This process is known as 'cleavage'; each of the daughter cells, or blastomeres, contains a nucleus with a full complement of 46 chromosomes. Within 12 h, a second cleavage occurs when each of the daughter cells divides into two again by mitotic division. Subsequent cleavage of successive generations of cells follows in quick succession and not always synchronously, so that at any particular time there may be an uneven number of cells. During the

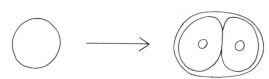

Figure 3.2 • Diagrammatic representation of the first cleavage division.

preimplantation period there is no growth; blastomeres cleave to form successively smaller daughter cells until, just before implantation, they attain the size of adult somatic cells. During early cleavage the cells are spherical, loosely attached to each other, and totipotent (i.e. able to contribute to any embryonic or extraembryonic lineage). During the first few cleavage divisions the embryo is dependent on maternal stores of RNA laid down during oogenesis, and the genetic material brought in by the sperm is not active. Between the 4- and 8-cell stages the 'embryonic' genome is activated.

When the embryo has between 16 and 32 cells, after the fourth cleavage division, it undergoes a process known as compaction. The cells maximize their intercellular contacts with each other, and flatten onto each other. It becomes impossible to discern the cell outlines and the embryo becomes known as a morula (Fig. 3.3), Latin for a mulberry, which it resembles. At the morula stage, the embryo moves from the fallopian tube to the uterine cavity, at which stage a fluid-filled cavity (the blastocoele) develops between the cells and a blastocyst is formed.

After morula formation, the cells differentiate for the first time, when the embryo has around 32 cells. The outer cells become polarized and epithelial, forming zonular tight junctions with each other to make a watertight seal. Sodium is actively pumped into the interstitial spaces inside the embryo, which in turn draws in water through the cells by osmosis, with the formation of a blastocoele cavity. This outer epithelial layer is known as the trophectoderm, which gives rise mainly to the extraembryonic membranes and the placenta. The inner cells remain totipotent, and form an acentrically positioned clump of cells (the inner cell mass) on the inner surface of the trophectoderm. These cells give rise to the fetus.

In-vitro studies of human preimplantation embryo development have shown that human embryos have variable morphology and developmental potential. About 75% of embryos have varying numbers of cytoplasmic membrane-bound fragments, and blastomeres are frequently uneven in size. Only about 50% of embryos cultured *in vitro* will reach the blastocyst stage, with the remaining embryos arresting development mainly between the 4-cell and morula stages. The reasons for this embryonic arrest are unclear, but may reflect a combination of suboptimal culture conditions, chromosomal abnormalities or inadequate oocyte maturation. It is becoming apparent that a large proportion (about 20%) of human embryos have gross chromosomal abnormalities, and nearly 70% of embryos have one or more blastomeres with two or more nuclei. These factors, combined with a sensitivity to the environment, may contribute to the low rates of implantation (approximately 25%) following *in-vitro* fertilization and transfer of embryos at the 2- to 4-cell stage. High levels of embryonic arrest, coupled with low implantation rates, suggest that in the human there are very high levels of embryonic loss during the first 2 weeks following fertilization.

The blastocyst implants into the secretory endometrium of the uterus about 6 days after fertilization. The trophoblast cells produce a proteolytic enzyme which allows invasion into the endometrium. As this occurs, the basal cytotrophoblast divides rapidly, producing a more superficial syncytium of cells, the syncytiotrophoblast, which interlocks into the spongy network of the endometrium. By the end of 10 days, the early embryo has burrowed into the endometrium to such an extent that it is completely covered. It extracts nutrients from the endometrial secretions and is already producing human chorionic gonadotrophin (hCG), which may be measured in maternal serum or urine. The trophoblast cells go on to form the placenta which is described later in this chapter.

Early development of the embryo

The few cells known as the inner cell mass which are heaped up on one wall of the trophoblast start a rapid development from the 10th day following conception. The mass is partially divided by a waist and takes on the shape of a cottage loaf. In the centre of each half of this inner cell mass a fluid cavity forms; that in the upper half is called the amniotic vesicle, later becoming the amniotic sac, and that in the lower half is called the endocervical vesicle, later becoming the yolk sac. Only two layers of cells lie between the two fluid cavities of the amniotic sac and yolk sac. The layer of

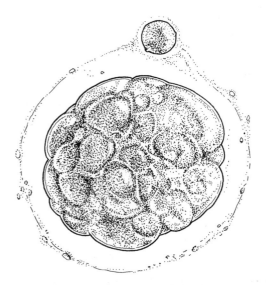

Figure 3.3 • The morula stage of development.

cells adjacent to the amniotic sac consists of tall columnar cells that form the embryonic ectoderm. From these few cells, all the ectodermal tissues of the fetus develop, that is the skin and all its appendages, and also the neural tube and its derivatives (the brain, spinal cord, nerves, autonomic ganglia and adrenal medulla).

The layer of cells adjacent to the yolk sac forms the embryonic endoderm, and from these few cells all the endodermal tissues of the fetus develop, that is the lining of the gut and the epithelial cells of the gut derivatives (the thyroid, parathyroid, trachea, lungs, liver and pancreas).

Between the ectoderm and endoderm a third layer of cells grows principally from ectodermal proliferation. This middle layer forms the embryonic mesoderm and, from it, all the mesodermal tissues of the fetus develop, that is the bones, muscles, cartilage and subcutaneous tissues of the skin.

Organogenesis

Development of the germ layers

The three layers of ectoderm, mesoderm and endoderm initially take the form of a flat circular sandwich, but later there is a disproportionate growth of the ectoderm at opposite poles so that the embryonic plate elongates into an oval, each end of which curves towards the yolk sac thus forming the head fold and tail fold. The amniotic sac enlarges until it completely surrounds the developing embryo and yolk sac.

On the dorsal or amniotic surface of the ectoderm a groove develops in the middle from the head to the tail of the embryo. Its edges grow over and eventually unite and close to change the groove into a tube – the neural tube – from which the nervous system will develop (Fig. 3.4). Meanwhile, the mesodermal layer is growing laterally, the part nearest the midline becom-

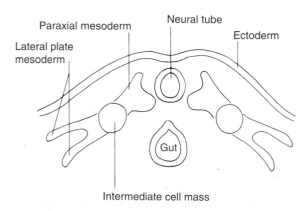

Figure 3.4 • Diagram to indicate the formation of the neural tube, the paraxial mesoderm, intermediate cell mass and lateral plate mesoderm.

ing the paraxial mesoderm, the part further out becoming the intermediate mesoderm, and the part that is most lateral becoming the lateral plate mesoderm (Fig. 3.4).

Growth of the endoderm is at first lateral and then ventral, eventually folding round to form the gut tube. A portion of the yolk sac is incorporated in the foregut and also in the hindgut. At first, the midgut is in direct continuity with the diminishing yolk sac but as the lateral folds of the embryo grow round they constrict the opening to the yolk sac, which eventually becomes separated from the gut altogether and forms a tubular stalk, the vitellointestinal duct. Occasionally, the connection with the gut may persist as Meckel's diverticulum.

The lateral plate of the mesoderm divides into the somatopleure, which remains adjacent to the ectoderm, and the splanchnopleure, which grows round the developing gut. The space between the somatopleure and splanchnopleure forms the coelomic cavity (Fig. 3.5), later the pleural and peritoneal cavities.

The paraxial and intermediate mesoderm become segmented into discrete masses of cells, or somites, progressively along the length of the embryo. The paraxial mesoderm somites develop into the vertebrae, dura mater, muscles of the body wall and part of the dermis of the neck and trunk. The intermediate mesoderm develops in a ventral direction towards the coelomic cavity and forms the origins of the urogenital system. The limb buds develop from the lateral plate mesoderm, pushing out a covering of ectoderm. The nerve supply to the limb buds comes off the neural tube at the level at which they originate.

Much of the early development of the embryo is at the head end, where the coverings of the neural tube develop with the brain. Also a condensation of mesoderm occurs at the cranial end of the coelomic cavity, and this forms the pericardial cavity and the primitive heart tubes. A further accumulation of mesoderm caudal to the developing heart is called the septum transversum and is destined to become the centre of the diaphragm.

As the head fold grows more quickly on the dorsal surface than on the ventral surface, it begins to curl round the developing heart and diaphragm (Fig. 3.6). The foregut also curves round behind the pericardium and reaches the surface at the pit between the forebrain and pericardium known as the stomatodeum (Fig. 3.6). The thin buccopharyngeal membrane at this point breaks down at the 3rd week of embryonic life leaving a continuous channel between mouth, lined with ectoderm, and foregut or pharynx, lined with endoderm. A small outpouch in the roof of the mouth grows up into the developing brain. This is Rathke's pouch, which develops into the anterior lobe of the pituitary gland.

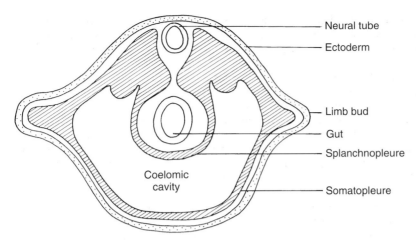

Figure 3.5 • Diagram showing division of the mesoderm into splanchnopleure and somatopleure to form the coelomic cavity.

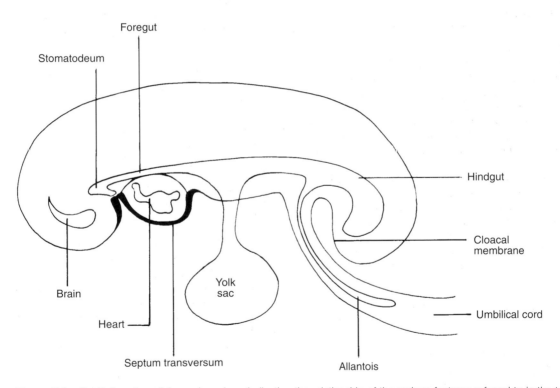

Figure 3.6 • Sagittal section of the early embryo indicating the relationship of the various features referred to in the text.

Pharyngeal region

The lower part of the face (mandibles) and the whole of the neck region is developed from condensations of mesoderm into a series of symmetrical arches which grow round the sides of the pharynx and eventually meet ventrally in the midline thus becoming horseshoe shaped. In fish, these are the gill arches and the spaces between them are the gills, but in humans the condensations of ectoderm and endoderm between the pharyngeal arches remain intact, and a very thick layer of mesoderm interleaves between them (Fig. 3.7). In each pharyngeal arch there develops a cartilage bar and surrounding muscle supplied by segmental blood vessels and nerves. Between the arches, a series of pharyngeal pouches develops.

Various structures develop from each of the pharyngeal arches and their adjacent pouches. Around the first arch, the upper and lower jaws, the palate, incus, malleus, anterior two-thirds of the tongue and muscles of mastication develop. The first pouch is extended laterally as the Eustachian tube and the middle ear.

The second pharyngeal arch structures include part of the hyoid bone, the stylohyoid ligament, the styloid process and stapes, as well as the muscles of facial expression served by the seventh cranial nerve. The second pouch contributes to the tympanic cavity and

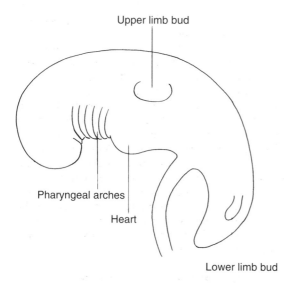

Figure 3.7 • Diagram showing embryonic development at the stage of preliminary pharyngeal arches.

forms the tonsil and supratonsillar fossa. The third pharyngeal arch gives rise to the lower part of the hyoid bone and stylopharyngeus muscle served by the ninth cranial nerve. The posterior third of the tongue and anterior part of the epiglottis are covered with mucous membranes derived from this arch. In the third pharyngeal pouch, the inferior parathyroids and the thymus gland develop. The fourth and sixth pharyngeal arches give rise to the laryngeal cartilages, while the fifth arch regresses. From the fourth pouch, the superior parathyroid glands are formed.

Each of the pharyngeal arches has its own blood vessels and nerve supplying the structure derived from it. Each nerve divides into an anterior and posterior division, which in certain situations may supply the adjacent arch structures. Not all the pharyngeal arch arteries survive; the first and second regress apart from the small maxillary and stapedial arteries, and the fifth disappears altogether. The third arch arteries form part of the internal carotid artery, while the right fourth arch artery forms the right subclavian artery and the left fourth arch artery forms the arch of the aorta. The sixth arch arteries form the pulmonary arteries, and also the ductus arteriosus on the left side (Fig. 3.8). From the floor of the pharynx, three important midline structures develop: the tongue, the thyroid and the respiratory system.

The muscles of the tongue develop from three occipital myotomes, but the connective tissue, lymph glands and mucosa are derived from the first and third pharyngeal arches, supplying the anterior two-thirds and posterior one-third, respectively. Between the two components the thyroglossal duct exists in the fetus but is usually obliterated before birth. From the distal end of the duct grows the thyroid gland.

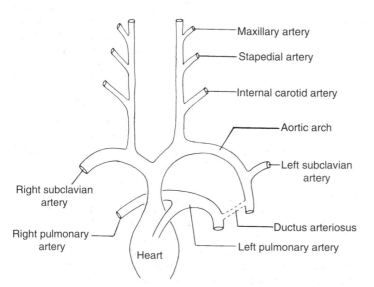

Figure 3.8 • The arterial development from the pharyngeal arch arteries as described in the text.

At the caudal end of the ventral aspect of the pharynx a fossa develops and this gradually grows away from the pharynx as the trachea. From this, the bronchi and primitive lungs are derived. The cartilage of the fourth and sixth arches contributes to the bones of the larynx which border the opening to the trachea.

The development of the pharyngeal region, face and mouth is a complex one, sometimes occurring imperfectly. Among the more common developmental abnormalities that may arise are failure of fusion of the palate or maxillary processes giving rise to cleft palate or hare lip. Failure of occlusion of the second pharyngeal pouch may give rise to a branchial cyst, and failure of regression of the thyroglossal duct may produce thyroglossal cysts. At birth, the ductus arteriosus normally closes, but occasionally fails to do so.

Cardiovascular system

Angiogenic tissue is recognizable in the very early presomite embryo, and will soon develop into the heart and blood vessels of the fetus. A beating fetal heart tube can be recognized with ultrasound techniques by the 32nd day of intrauterine life. The heart is formed as a pair of heart tubes developing from an accumulation of angiogenic cells in the area of the pericardial mesoderm. These left and right endocardial heart tubes fuse to form a single chamber within the pericardial mesoderm. The caudal end of the tube receives blood from the confluence of the vitelline, umbilical and cardinal veins, which run into the left and right sinus venosus. The cranial end of the heart tube leads into the bulbus cordis and on to the newly formed aorta. The two ends of the heart tube are soon fixed to the pericardium, so that further growth of the bulbus cordis and ventricle causes the tube to bend up on itself and form an S shape.

The atrium expands laterally and also moves up in front of, or ventral to, the bulbus cordis. The two lateral expansions become the left and right auricles. The atrium now receives blood through an opening on its dorsocaudal part from the sinus venosus. Blood leaves the atrium through an opening on the ventral surface, the atrial canal, which leads to the ventricle. Next, endocardial cushions appear on the dorsal and ventral surfaces of this atrial canal and eventually fuse, dividing the canal but leaving two small orifices, the atrioventricular canals. The division of the atrium into two cavities is brought about by the growth of two septa which eventually overlap and close the foramen ovale at birth. Throughout fetal life, the foramen is patent conducting blood from right to left.

A more complex development of septa occurs in the ventricle and the truncus arteriosus, to form a left and right ventricle, and an aortic and pulmonary artery. Dorsal and ventral ridges arise on the walls of the ventricular cavity, eventually fusing to divide the right and

left ventricle. Failure of fusion leaves a patent interventricular foramen. The proximal bulbar septum is formed from right and left bulbar ridges and it divides the aorta from the pulmonary artery. Finally, the heart valves are formed from endothelial projections at the atrioventricular orifices, and also at the distal end of the bulbus cordis at the pulmonary and aortic orifices. The total development from heart tube to completion occurs between the 4th and 7th weeks of intrauterine life.

Fetal circulation

Oxygenation of fetal blood occurs in the placenta before it returns in the umbilical vein which joins the left branch of the portal vein. It bypasses the capillaries of the liver by going through the ductus venosus, which is obliterated after birth and becomes the ligamentum venosum. The oxygenated blood enters the inferior vena cava and is transported to the right atrium and thence through the patent foramen ovale to the left atrium and on to the left ventricle. From the left ventricle, the blood flows into the aorta and through the fetal vascular network. Blood returning from the head of the fetus passes through the superior vena cava to the right atrium and straight on to the right ventricle and pulmonary artery. However, it does not enter the pulmonary circulation, being short-circuited by the ductus arteriosus to the aorta. Aortic blood is carried via the umbilical arteries back to the placenta for reoxygenation. At birth, the three short circuits, the ductus venosus, foramen ovale and ductus arteriosus, close.

Alimentary system, pulmonary and peritoneal cavities

The gut, which develops in continuity with the pharynx, may be subdivided into three sections, each with its own blood supply. The foregut extends as a tube, the oesophagus, to the stomach which forms as a sac at the 5th week of intrauterine life. Below the stomach the liver grows out from the ventral aspect of the foregut. At first it is a hollow diverticulum growing up into the septum transversum, but later it produces two solid buds of cells which form the left and right lobes of the liver. The foregut structures are supplied by blood from the coeliac artery (Fig. 3.9). The midgut starts in the duodenum at the level of the entry of the bile duct. From it, the pancreas develops initially as a ventral and dorsal part, the former arising from the bile duct and the latter from the duodenum itself. The two parts subsequently fuse and the two ducts form a common opening to the duodenum. The midgut extends down to the splenic flexure of the colon, and is supplied with blood from the superior mesenteric artery. This part of the gut grows far more rapidly than the vertebral column and therefore produces a large ventral loop held in place by an extensive dorsal mesentery, through

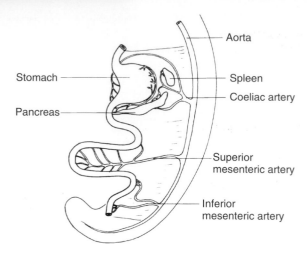

Figure 3.9 • The vascular supply to the developing alimentary system.

which the blood vessels run. Fixation of folds in the lower part of the loop produces the characteristic position of ascending and transverse colon in the adult, while the ileum retains its mesentery, and mobility.

The hindgut forms the descending colon and rectum, and is supplied by the inferior mesenteric artery, although the anal canal is also supplied by middle and inferior rectal arteries. The hindgut opens into the dorsal part of the cloaca. The spleen, which takes its blood supply from the splenic branch of the coeliac artery, arises from cellular islands in the coelomic epithelium, and is not a derivative of the foregut.

Respiratory organs

In the midline of the ventral surface of the primitive pharynx a groove appears at the 4th week of intrauterine life. The groove lengthens and becomes tubular as it grows away from the pharynx. From the growing end of the tube, two lung buds develop, filling the pleural coeloms; these form the connective tissues of the bronchi and lungs. The lining of the respiratory passages is endodermal in origin. The lung buds start to appear before the laryngotracheal groove is converted into a tube. They then subdivide into lobules, three on the right and two on the left, which in turn will form the lobes of the mature lungs. The air sacs do not appear until the 6th month of intrauterine life. Growth of the trachea and lung buds proceeds in a caudal direction so that by full term the bifurcation of the trachea is at the level of the fourth thoracic vertebra.

The pleural coeloms form the pleural cavities, which are separated from the pericardial cavity by the pleuropericardial membrane, and from the peritoneal cavity by the developing diaphragm.

The diaphragm itself develops from the septum transversum, the pleuroperitoneal membrane, the

costal margin and the gastrohepatic ligament. There is a very small contribution from the dorsal mesentery behind the oesophagus, and from the mesoderm around the aorta.

Central nervous system

The cells of the central nervous system develop from the dorsal surface of the embryonic plate. A shallow neural groove develops in the primitive ectoderm and later becomes covered, thus forming the neural tube. The anterior end forms the forebrain limited by the lamina terminalis. The side walls of the foremost part of the neural tube develop into the hypothalamus, while the two cerebral hemispheres originate as two hollow diverticula, the cerebral vesicles. They grow forward and laterally from the hypothalamus. The cavities of the cerebral hemispheres form the lateral ventricles of the mature brain and interconnect through the interventricular foramen.

The midbrain, brain stem and cerebellum develop by further cell proliferation at the cranial end of the neural tube, while the caudal section develops into a spinal cord. When the neural tube closes over, a rapid proliferation of neural cells occurs throughout the length of the brain stem and spinal cord. These cells then undergo functional differentiation arranging themselves into distinct bundles to become the visceral and somatic, and efferent and afferent pathways.

As the tube closes, some neural cells are excluded on the dorsal aspect and form the neural crest between the spinal cord and the ectodermal surface. Some of these cells migrate laterally either side of the midline to become the cell bodies in the autonomic ganglia including the suprarenal medulla, and the posterior root ganglia (Fig. 3.10).

At the level of the brain stem, the central canal is wider and flatter as it opens up into the fourth ventricle. The distribution of afferent and efferent pathways is similar to that in the cord but the afferent groups lie more laterally. In addition, special branchial afferent and efferent nerve cell groups appear supplying the pharyngeal arch derivatives as the cranial nerves (Fig. 3.11).

Failure of closure of the neural tube on its dorsal aspect gives rise to the variety of neural tube defect abnormalities, most commonly seen at the caudal end as an open spina bifida.

Skeletal system

All the bones in the body are derived from embryonic mesenchyme. Some of the bones are preformed in cartilage before undergoing ossification, while others are ossified directly from membranous precursors. The vertebrae are formed from the segmental sclerotomes around the notochord and neural tube. These sclerotomes are derived from the mesodermal

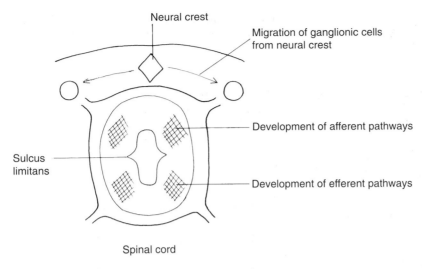

Figure 3.10 • Early development of the spinal cord.

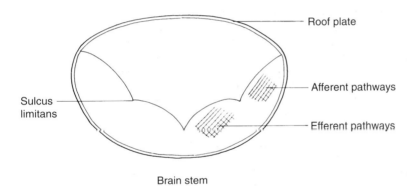

Figure 3.11 • Diagram showing spinal cord development at the level of the brain stem.

somites. Each vertebra is preformed as a cartilaginous ring in which three centres of ossification appear, one for the body and one for each half of the neural arch. The process is complete by the 8th week of intrauterine life. The notochordal remnant eventually disappears in the centre of each vertebral body, but persists as the nucleus pulposus of the intervertebral discs.

The ribs are also preformed in cartilage and develop from the costal processes of the primitive vertebral arches. The sternum forms from two sternal plates which develop to link the central ends of the upper nine ribs on each side. The two plates pass through a cartilaginous phase before undergoing ossification and fusion to form the definitive single sternum.

The skull develops from the mesenchyme that envelops the cerebral vesicles. The vault of the skull and part of the base are ossified directly from membranous bone, while the major part of the base, excluding the orbital part of the frontal bone and the lateral part of the greater wing, is preformed in cartilage.

The limbs appear as small limb buds at the end of the 4th week of intrauterine life (see Fig. 3.7). The upper limb buds develop a little in advance of the lower ones. Each bud is derived from several primitive somites and carries with it the corresponding ventral ramus of the spinal nerve. The central mesenchyme forms the cartilaginous skeleton, which eventually ossifies to form the limb bones. The muscles pertaining to the skeleton are derived from the surrounding mesoderm. The feet and hands appear very similar to start with, as flat extensions of the limb buds. Later, the mesenchyme condenses into distinct digits, and failure of this phase gives rise to webbing of the fingers or toes.

The joints between bones evolve from the residual core of mesenchyme which does not differentiate into membranous bone. This mesenchyme may develop into fibrous tissue as the fibrous joints between the skull bones, or it may become cartilaginous as in the cartilage joints. Synovial joints occur when the mesenchyme loosens out and a cavity forms in the centre, while some of the cells liquefy to fill the space.

Muscles, skin and appendages

It has already been observed that the muscles of the limbs develop from the mesenchyme of the limb buds, and the muscles of the head and neck develop from the mesenchyme of the pharyngeal arches. The muscles of the trunk all develop from the dorsolateral part of the somites known as the dermomyotome. Spindle cells proliferate from it to form the muscle plate while the remainder forms the skin plate. The muscle plate or myotome divides into a dorsal part supplied by the dorsal ramus of the corresponding spinal nerve, and a ventral part supplied by the ventral ramus. The dorsal part develops into the muscle groups of the back, and the ventral part forms the muscles of the body wall.

Some of the myotome derivatives degenerate and disappear while others may fuse and form fibrous aponeuroses, as seen in the anterior abdominal wall. Involuntary muscles of the gut, ureters, bladder and uterus are developed from the splanchnopleuric mesoderm *in situ*. The skin plate or dermatome develops into the true dermis, while the overlying ectoderm forms the epidermis, hairs, nails, sweat glands and sebaceous glands.

The dermis and subcutaneous areolar tissue develop towards the end of the 3rd month, and the dermal papillae appear in the 4th month. The primary nailfolds are also seen in the 3rd month, and the sweat glands appear about 1 month later. The mammary glands develop as a collection of modified sweat glands at the cranial end of the milk ridge or nipple line. Occasionally, supernumerary nipples and even gland tissue may develop caudally in the same line. The epithelial lining of the ducts and glands is derived from the ectoderm, while the connective tissue and fat are developed from the underlying mesenchyme.

Development of the genital organs

The genital organs develop in close association with those of the urinary tract. Both arise in the intermediate mesoderm on each side of the root of the mesentery beneath the epithelium of the coelom.

The pronephroi, a few transient tubules in the cervical region, appear first and quickly degenerate. As these regress, they are succeeded by a pair of parallel elongated structures, the mesonephroi, located on either side of the vertebral column in the thoracic and upper lumbar regions and which are drained by the mesonephric (Wolffian) ducts. These ducts pass down the body to reach the cloaca.

The mesonephros develops as a long bulge into the dorsal wall of the coelom in the thoracic and upper lumbar regions. It will later degenerate to a different extent in the two sexes (Fig. 3.12). Two important structures appear on the coelomic surface of the mesonephros: (1) the genital ridge from which the gonad will form; (2) the paramesonephric (Müllerian) duct alongside the Wolffian duct.

The genital ridge appears as a swelling on the medial aspect of the mesonephros; at first it covers the whole extent of the latter, but later contracts to the central part only. The paramesonephric duct forms laterally as an invagination of the coelomic epithelium overlying the mesonephros, which closes to form a tube, or duct. This occurs in embryos of some 10 mm crown–rump length (5–6 weeks).

Uterus and tubes

The paramesonephric ducts on each side extend caudally to reach the dorsal wall of the urogenital sinus by about 9 weeks (Fig. 3.13). At that time, the mesonephric and paramesonephric ducts are both present and capable of development (indifferent stage). From this point on in the female the paramesonephric (Müllerian) duct continues to develop and the mesonephric (Wolffian) one to degenerate; in the male the opposite occurs (Fig. 3.12). As the paramesonephric ducts progress caudally their lower portions come together in the midline and fuse; from this fused part the uterus and cervix develop, and from the separate, unfused, upper part the fallopian tubes develop.

During the 4th month (12–16 weeks) proliferation of mesoderm around the fused lower parts of the ducts forms the muscular walls of the uterus and cervix.

Vagina

Vaginal development is more complex (Figs 2.14, 2.15). At the Müllerian tubercle, where the paramesonephric ducts reach the urogenital sinus, a considerable growth of tissue occurs and the sinusal tubercle becomes thickened. This tissue growth forms the vaginal plate (Fig. 3.14), which is thus composed of sinus epithelium and paramesonephric ducts. The vaginal plate grows rapidly, pushing the remnants of the mesonephric duct, which had also reached the urogenital sinus, cranially. From this vaginal plate, the vagina forms. At first it is a solid organ, but at about 16–18 weeks the central core begins to break down to form the vaginal lumen (Fig. 3.15). Because of the great growth of the plate, it is not possible to be sure how much vagina is developed from the paramesonephric ducts and how much from the urogenital sinus.

External genitalia

The early development of the external genitalia is similar in males and females. At about the 5 mm stage (4 weeks) the primitive cloaca becomes divided by a transverse septum (the urorectal septum) into an anterior primitive urogenital sinus and a posterior rectal portion. From the upper part of the cloaca to approximately the level of the Müllerian tubercle, this septum

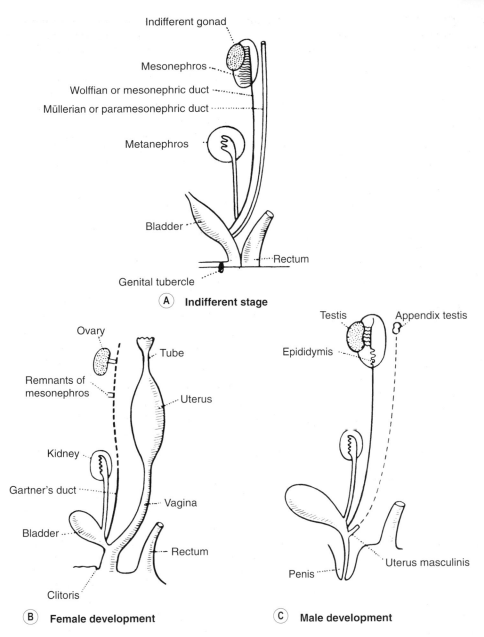

Indifferent gonad

Mesonephros

Wolffian or mesonephric duct

Müllerian or paramesonephric duct

Metanephros

Bladder

Rectum

Genital tubercle

(A) **Indifferent stage**

Ovary

Tube

Remnants of mesonephros

Uterus

Kidney

Gartner's duct

Vagina

Bladder

Rectum

Clitoris

(B) **Female development**

Testis   Appendix testis

Epididymis

Uterus masculinis

Penis

(C) **Male development**

Figure 3.12 • Diagrammatic representation of genital tract development. (A) Indifferent stage. (B) Female development. (C) Male development.

grows downwards; below that, the septum grows inwards from each side. Shortly after division is complete the urogenital portion of the cloacal membrane breaks down.

Soon afterwards the urogenital sinus is seen to be made up of three parts (Fig. 3.16). In its lower portion there is an expanded urogenital sinus above which is a narrow pelvic part (the pelvic urethra) which reaches as far cranially as a point where the Müllerian ducts reach the sinus wall. The superior portion of the urogenital sinus, above the pelvic urethra, forms the presumptive bladder, which extends superiorly and is continuous with the allantois. On the external surface of the embryo, the genital tubercle can be seen, which is a conical projection encircling the anterior part of the cloacal (or urogenital) membrane; the tubercle can be seen before cloacal division is complete (6 weeks). As division of the primitive cloaca (described above)

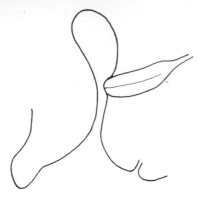

Figure 3.13 • The paramesonephric ducts which have reached the dorsal wall of the urogenital sinus by about 9 weeks.

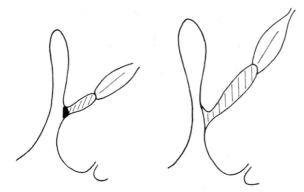

Figure 3.14 • Formation of the vaginal plate. This vaginal plate displaces the lower end of the fused Müllerian ducts cranially as indicated by the hatched areas.

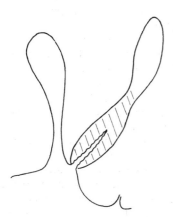

Figure 3.15 • The solid vaginal plate is beginning to break down to form the vaginal lumen at around 16–18 weeks.

reaches completion, the urorectal septum fuses with the cloacal membrane, creating the perineum, which separates the anus from the urogenital region. The urogenital, or cloacal, membrane breaks down, opening the urogenital sinus to the amniotic fluid. Externally, on either side of the urogenital sinus may be seen two pairs of eminences – a medial pair called the genital folds and a lateral pair called the labioscrotal swellings. These are formed by the proliferation of mesoderm around the lower portion of the sinus.

Until approximately 10 weeks, the external appearances of the male and female are similar and it is not possible to determine the sex of a fetus. Then, differentiation occurs. The bladder and urethra are formed from that part of the vesicourethral division of the urogenital sinus while, in the female, the pelvic and inferior portions become shallow and, ultimately, form the vestibule of the vagina (Fig. 3.16B). The genital tubercle remains small and becomes the clitoris; the genital folds form the labia minora and the labioscrotal swellings enlarge to become the labia majora. The primitive perineum does not lengthen. In males, the genital tubercle enlarges to become the penis; the genital folds fuse to form the phallic portion of the male urethra and the labioscrotal swellings enlarge and fuse to form the scrotum.

Finally, proliferating mesoderm spreads ventrally around the lower part of the body wall uniting with its fellow part from the opposite side to complete the development of the clitoris or penis and the anterior surface of the bladder and anterior abdominal wall below the umbilicus.

Gonads

The first sign of a primitive gonad may be seen at about 5 weeks.

The gonad has a triple origin from:

1. The coelomic epithelium of the genital ridge
2. The underlying mesoderm
3. The germ cells which enter it from an extragonadal source.

We have seen that the gonad begins as a bulge on the medial aspect of the mesonephric ridge. First, there is proliferation of the coelomic epithelium at that point and further proliferation of the mesenchyme beneath that epithelium. By 5–6 weeks, cords of coelomic epithelium can be seen projecting into the substance of the developing gonad and breaking up the mesenchyme into loose strands. Rapid development of these cords follows and in the deeper layers they become branched and complex. During these early stages, primordial germ cells can be seen lying between the cords. These germ cells have originated from beneath the epithelium of the yolk sac, from which site they migrate via the hindgut and the dorsal mesentery to enter the genital

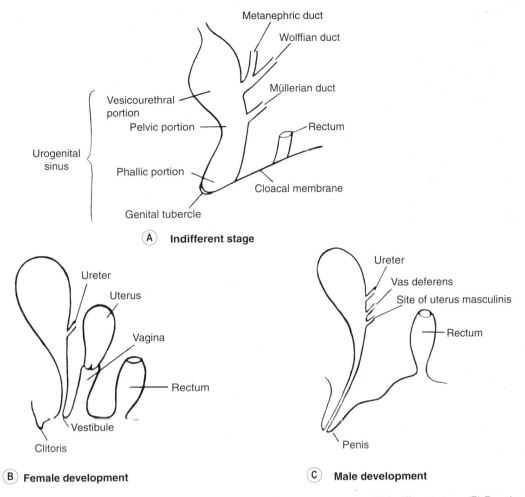

Figure 3.16 • Diagrammatic representation of lower genital tract development. (A) Indifferent stage. (B) Female development. (C) Male development.

ridge. They can be seen in the region of the genital ridge at approximately 4 weeks. At this stage, therefore, the sex cords which have developed from the coelomic epithelium, the primitive mesenchymal tissue and the primordial germ cells all lie together in the developing gonad, which is at its indifferent stage.

Gonadal differentiation can be seen first in the testis at about 7 weeks. There is then great development of the sex cords and a decrease in number and size of the cells of the outer cellular layer from which primordial germ cells disappear. The cells of this outer zone later become differentiated into spindle-shaped fibroblasts and ultimately form the tunica albuginea. The rete testis and the straight and seminiferous tubules arise from the sex cords, while the interstitial cells develop from the mesenchyme.

The ovary cannot be identified until some time later. The outer zone remains more cellular and it is possible to distinguish three groups of cells: the larger primor-

dial germ cells, the supporting cells, which may now be called pregranulosa cells, and more spindle-shaped cells which have formed from the mesenchyme of the genital ridge. This is a phase of tremendous growth and, in particular, the germ cells differentiate into oogonia and increase markedly in number. By 20 weeks, they have almost reached 7 million in number, after which many die by a process known as atresia.

Histological examination of the developing ovary shows that there is a gradient, from the surface of the ovary inwards, of differentiation of oocytes from oogonia, entry of oocytes into meiosis and formation of follicles. Germ cells at the inner cortex–medulla boundary are the first to undergo these processes, so that it is possible simultaneously to see dividing oogonia in the outer cortex and fully formed follicles deeper in the ovary. By 20–24 weeks, follicle formation is taking place, whereby oocytes become surrounded by flattened pregranulosa cells. An interesting feature is that those germ cells which do not succeed in surrounding themselves with a protective layer of pregranulosa cells die. This destruction along with atresia of some follicles, which have passed into the early stage of development, results in many germ cells being eliminated, so that perhaps only 1–2 million remain at birth.

Development of the placenta

The ovum is fertilized in the fallopian tube and enters the uterine cavity as a morula which rapidly sheds its surrounding zona pellucida and converts into a blastocyst. The outer cell layer of the blastocyst then proliferates to form the primary trophoblastic cell mass (Fig. 3.17A), from which cells infiltrate between those of the endometrial epithelium; the latter degenerate and the trophoblast thus comes into direct contact with the endometrial stroma, this process of implantation being complete by the 10th or 11th postovulatory day. In the 7-day blastocyst, the trophoblast forms a peripheral plaque which rapidly differentiates into two layers, an inner layer of larger clear mononuclear cytotrophoblastic cells with well-defined limiting membranes and an outer layer of multinucleated syncytiotrophoblast (Fig. 3.17B), this latter being a true syncytium. That the syncytiotrophoblast is derived from the cytotrophoblast, not only at this early stage but also throughout gestation, is now well established for, even when the trophoblast is growing rapidly, DNA synthesis and mitotic activity occur only in the nuclei of the cytotrophoblastic cells. It would appear that the syncytiotrophoblast is formed by fusion of cytotrophoblastic cells for, although no intercellular membranes can normally be seen in the syncytial layer, remnants of such membranes can occasionally be found on electron microscopy. Cells with a cytoplasmic complexity intermediate between that of the cytotrophoblast and syncytiotrophoblast can also be identified by electron microscopy; these intermediate-type cytotrophoblastic cells appear to be ones which are beginning to differentiate into syncytiotrophoblasts but have not yet lost their limiting plasma membranes.

Between the 10th and 13th postovulatory days, a series of intercommunicating clefts, or lacunae, appears in the rapidly enlarging trophoblastic cell mass (Fig. 3.18); these are probably formed as a result of engulfment within the trophoblast of endometrial capillaries. The lacunae soon become partially confluent to form the precursor of the intervillous space and, as maternal vessels are progressively eroded, this becomes filled with maternal blood; at this stage, the lacunae are incompletely separated off from each other by trabecular columns of syncytiotrophoblast which, between the 14th and 21st postovulatory days, tend to become radially orientated and come to possess a central cellular core that is produced by proliferation of cytotrophoblastic cells at the chorionic base. These trabecular columns are not true villi but serve as the framework from which the villous tree will later develop, the placenta at this stage being a labyrinthine rather than a villous organ and the trabeculae being therefore best known as primary villous stems. Continued growth of the cytotrophoblast leads to its distal extension into the region of decidual attachment and, at the same time, a mesenchymal core appears within the villous stems, this being formed by a distal extension of the extra-embryonic mesenchyme. Later, the villous stems become vascularized, the vessels arising from the mesenchyme within the core and not, as previously thought,

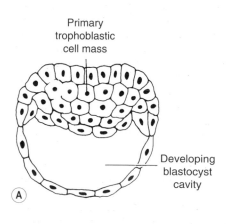
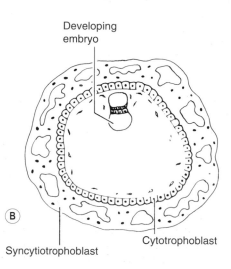

Figure 3.17 • Diagrammatic representation of (A) formation of primary trophoblastic cell mass and (B) the differentiation of this into the cytotrophoblast and syncytiotrophoblast.

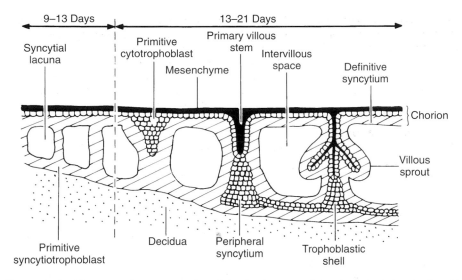

Figure 3.18 • Diagrammatic representation of the development of the placenta during the first 21 days of gestation.

being formed as a downward extension of the chorio-allantoic arteries. In due course, the vessels within the stems establish functional continuity with others differentiating from the body stalk and inner chorionic mesenchyme.

The distal part of the villous stems is formed almost entirely by cytotrophoblast, which is not invaded by mesenchyme and not vascularized but which is anchored to the decidua of the basal plate. These cells, which form the cytotrophoblast cell columns, proliferate and spread laterally to form a continuous cytotrophoblastic shell which splits the syncytiotrophoblast into two layers: the definitive syncytium on the fetal aspect of the shell and the peripheral syncytium between the shell and the decidua. The definitive syncytium persists as the limiting layer of the intervillous space but the peripheral syncytium eventually degenerates and is replaced by a layer of fibrinoid material (Nitabuch's layer). The establishment of the trophoblastic shell is a mechanism to allow for rapid circumferential growth of the developing placenta and this leads to an expansion of the intervillous space into which sprouts extend from the primary villous stems. These offshoots consist initially only of syncytiotrophoblast but as they enlarge they pass through the stages previously seen during the development of the primary villous stems, i.e. intrusion of cytotrophoblast, formation of a mesenchymal core and eventual vascularization. These sprouts form the primary stem villi and, as these are true villous structures, the placenta is, by the 21st day of gestation, a vascularized villous organ. The primary stem villi grow and divide to form secondary and tertiary stem villi and these latter eventually break up into the terminal villous tree.

During the early weeks of gestation, cytotrophoblastic cells from the trophoblastic shell break through the peripheral layer of syncytiotrophoblast and spread into the underlying decidua. Many of these cells go on to colonize the adjacent myometrium where they often fuse to give the typical multinucleated giant cells of the placental bed; the function of, and the role played by, this interstitial extravillous trophoblast is currently unknown. Groups of cytotrophoblastic cells also grow, however, into the lumen of the spiral arteries and extend as far as the deciduo-myometrial junction; these cells, which form the endovascular trophoblast, replace the endothelium and invade the walls of the intradecidual portion of the spiral vessels and appear to destroy the muscular and elastic tissue of the media, the vessel wall eventually being replaced by fibrinoid material which appears to be derived partly from fibrin in the maternal blood and partly from proteins secreted by the trophoblastic cells. Because the walls of the intradecidual portions of the spiral vessels are markedly weakened as a result of this process of trophoblastic invasion, these vessels dilate considerably under the pressure of the maternal blood (Fig. 3.19), this being an important factor in allowing for a greatly augmented blood flow.

Between the 21st postovulatory day and the end of the 4th month of gestation, those villi orientated towards the uterine cavity degenerate and form the chorion laeve, while the thin rim of decidua covering this area gradually disappears to allow the chorion laeve to come into contact with the parietal decidua of the opposite wall of the uterus. The villi on the side of the chorion towards the decidua basalis proliferate and progressively arborize to form the chorion frondosum,

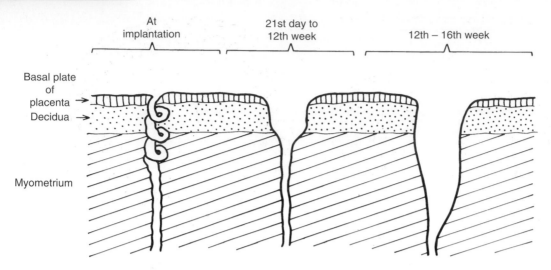

Figure 3.19 • Diagrammatic representation of the conversion of the spiral arteries into uteroplacental arteries.

which develops into the definitive placenta. During this period, there is some regression of the cytotrophoblastic elements in the chorionic plate and in the trophoblastic shell where the cytotrophoblastic cell columns degenerate and are largely replaced by fibrinoid material (Rohr's layer); clumps of cells remain, however, as the cytotrophoblastic cell islands. Although there is cytotrophoblastic regression in the basal plate, during the 4th month of gestation a further proliferation of endovascular cytotrophoblast occurs, a wave of these cells moving in retrograde direction to involve the intramyometrial segments of the spiral vessels. Again, this is where they replace the endothelium, invade and destroy the medial muscular and elastic tissue and lead to deposition of fibrinoid material in the wall; these changes extend almost to the origin of the spiral vessels from the radial arteries and, when complete, result in the transformation of the coiled spiral arteries of the placental bed into dilated, funnel-shaped, flaccid uteroplacental arteries. These arteries can accommodate the progressively increasing blood flow to the placenta (Fig. 3.19).

The placental septa appear during the 3rd month of gestation; they protrude into the intervillous space from the basal plate and divide the maternal surface of the placenta into between 15 and 20 lobes. These septa are simply folds of the basal plate, being formed partly as a result of regional variability in placental growth and partly by the pulling up of basal plate into the intervillous space by anchoring columns which have a poor growth rate. As the basal plate is formed principally by the remnants of the cytotrophoblastic shell embedded in fibrinoid material, it follows that the septa will have a similar composition, although some decidual cells may also be carried up into the folds. The septa are therefore simply an incidental by-product of the architectural refashioning of the placenta and have no physiological or morphological importance.

The lobes between the septa are not functional or structural subunits of the fetal placenta, this role being played by the lobules; each placental lobule is derived from a single secondary stem villus which breaks up just below the chorial plate into tertiary stem villi which sweep down towards the basal plate to form a hollow globular structure. The terminal villous tree, derived from the tertiary stem, is mainly in the outer shell of the hollow globule and the centre of the lobule is relatively empty and villus free. The term cotyledon, if used at all, is best defined as that part of the villous tree which has arisen from a single primary stem villus; such a primary stem villus may give rise to a varying number of secondary stem villi and hence the number of lobules in a cotyledon varies from two to five.

Each fetal lobule is supplied by a single uteroplacental artery, this being not coincidental but due to the preferential formation of the lobules in relationship to the opening of a maternal vessel. The blood from the uteroplacental artery, driven by the maternal head of pressure, flows up, rather like a fountain, in the central hollow core of the lobule towards the chorial plate (Fig. 3.20). Towards the apex of the lobule the driving pressure force becomes dissipated and the blood disperses laterally to flow back towards the basal plate in the outer shell of the lobule. Hence, it is only in the outer shell of the lobule that the maternal blood comes into contact with the terminal villi and only here is there a true physiological intervillous space, this being probably of capillary dimensions throughout.

By the end of the 4th month of gestation the placenta has achieved its definitive form and undergoes no further anatomical modification. Growth continues, however, until term and this is due principally to con-

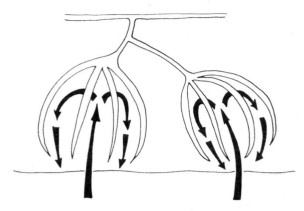

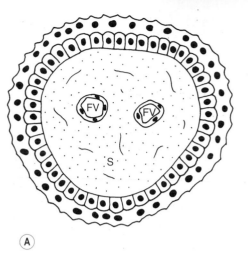

(A)

Figure 3.20 • Diagrammatic representation of the flow of maternal blood (black arrows) through the fetal lobule.

tinuous arborization of the villous tree and formation of fresh villi. This continuing growth is accompanied by a progressive alteration in the morphological appearances of the most distal villi of the tree, these being the only villi that are concerned with maternofetal transfer. In the first trimester, the villi are large and have a regular circumferential mantle of trophoblast which consists of an inner layer of cytotrophoblastic cells and an outer layer of syncytiotrophoblast; the villous stroma is formed of loose mesenchymal tissue in which, towards the end of the first trimester, small centrally placed fetal vessels are present (Fig. 3.21). During the second trimester the villi are smaller, the trophoblastic covering is less regular and the cytotrophoblastic cells less numerous; more collagen is present in the stroma and the fetal vessels are becoming larger in diameter and are beginning to move towards the periphery of the villus. In the third trimester the villi are much smaller in diameter, the trophoblastic layer is irregularly thinned and the cytotrophoblastic cells are few and inconspicuous. Much of the trophoblastic irregularity is due to the formation of thinned anuclear areas of syncytiotrophoblast, these, the vasculosyncytial membranes, being areas of trophoblast specially differentiated for gaseous transfer. The fetal villous stromal vessels are sinusoidally dilated and occupy most of the cross-sectional area of the villus; they have moved peripherally and lie in an immediately sub-trophoblastic position. These villous changes represent a form of functional maturation and are not an indication of ageing; the net result of these intermediate changes is to:

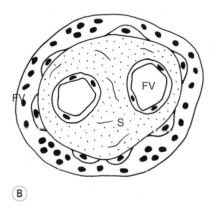

(B)

* increase the surface area of trophoblast in contact with the maternal blood in the intervillous space
* approximate the fetal and maternal circulation
* increase the maternofetal concentration gradient
* provide optimal conditions for maternofetal transfer.

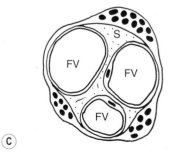

(C)

Figure 3.21 • Diagrammatic representation of the histological appearances of the placental villi in (A) the first trimester, (B) the second trimester and (C) at term. FV, fetal vessels; S, villous stroma.

Placental bed

The term placental bed is applied to the decidua and myometrium, which directly underlie the placenta. As previously described, the placental bed is extensively colonized by extravillous cytotrophoblastic cells during the early stages of gestation. The intravascular component of this extravillous trophoblastic cell population plays a crucial role in converting the spiral arteries of the placental bed into uteroplacental vessels while the interstitial component intermingles with the basal decidual cells and infiltrates between the myometrial fibres.

In the past, the magnitude of this trophoblastic invasion of the placental bed was markedly underestimated, largely because on simple light microscopy it is difficult to distinguish decidual from cytotrophoblastic cells; these two cell populations can, however, be differentiated by staining for cytokeratins, the decidual cells reacting negatively and the trophoblastic cells positively. The use of cytokeratin stains has shown that a high proportion of the apparent decidual cells in the placental bed are, during early pregnancy, extravillous trophoblast; the number of these cells does, however, diminish as pregnancy progresses and at term relatively few trophoblastic cells survive in the placental bed, these commonly being fused into multinucleated cells.

The function of the interstitial trophoblastic cells in the placental bed is unknown but their principal secretory product is, unlike villous trophoblast, human placental lactogen rather than human chorionic gonadotrophin. The extravillous trophoblastic cells also differ from their villous counterparts in their ability to express a class 1 major histocompatibility antigen, which is, however, of an unusual nature and not necessarily functioning as a transplantation antigen.

The maternal component of the placental bed includes decidualized endometrial stromal cells and two leucocytic populations, macrophages and granular lymphocytes. The macrophages are prominent throughout pregnancy and may well play an immunological role while the granular lymphocytes are most conspicuous in the early months of gestation and may be of importance in the processes of implantation and placentation.

Residual endometrial glands are present in the placental bed but are usually attenuated or compressed into slits and only identifiable with epithelial markers.

Development of membranes and formation of amniotic fluid

Membranes

The conversion of the early morula to a blastocyst is accomplished by the formation of a central fluid-filled cavity. This largely separates the primary trophoblastic cell mass, from which the placenta and extraplacental chorion develop, from those cells which give rise to the embryo and contribute to the formation of the yolk sac and amnion; these latter cells form the eccentrically situated inner cell mass which remains in contact with the cytotrophoblast on the inner aspect of the blastocyst wall (Fig. 3.22). During the 8th and 9th postovulatory days the inner cell mass arranges itself into a bilaminar disc, the inner layer (i.e. that facing the blastocyst cavity) forming the primitive embryonic endoderm and the outer, which is in contact with the cytotrophoblast, forming the primitive embryonic ectoderm. The amniotic cavity first appears as a slit-like space between the embryonic ectoderm and the adjacent cytotrophoblast; this enlarges to form, by the 12th postovulatory day, a small cavity, the base of which is formed by embryonic ectoderm and the walls and roof of which are formed of cytotrophoblast (Fig. 3.23). At

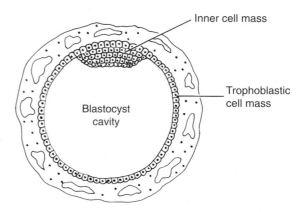

Figure 3.22 • Diagrammatic representation of the blastocyst and inner cell mass.

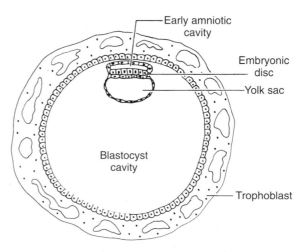

Figure 3.23 • Diagrammatic representation of early stage in the formation of the amniotic cavity.

the same time, endodermal cells migrate out from the deeper layer of the embryonic disc to line the blastocyst cavity and thus form the primary yolk sac. The extraembryonic mesenchyme subsequently appears (Fig. 3.24), possibly derived from the trophoblast, and separates off the primary yolk sac from the blastocyst wall; the extraembryonic mesenchyme also intrudes between, and largely separates off, the roof of the amniotic sac and the trophoblast of the chorion. A connection between the two is, however, maintained for a time by the persistence of a column of cells, the amniotic duct, which provides a pathway for the continuing migration of cells of trophoblastic origin into the amniotic epithelium. Mitotic activity at the margin of the embryonic ectodermal disc suggests that the ectoderm is also a continuing source of supply of amniotic epithelial cells.

The extraembryonic mesenchyme forms a loose reticulum in which small cystic spaces appear; these gradually enlarge and fuse to form the extraembryonic coelom which splits the extraembryonic mesenchyme into two layers, one opposed to the trophoblast and also covering the amnion (the parietal extraembryonic mesenchyme) and the other covering the yolk sac (the visceral extraembryonic mesenchyme) (Fig. 3.25). The progressively enlarging extraembryonic coelom also separates the amnion away from the inner aspect of the chorion, except at the caudal end of the embryo where an attachment of extraembryonic mesenchyme persists to form the body stalk from which the umbilical cord will eventually be derived.

Subsequently, the amniotic space enlarges at the expense of the extraembryonic coelom and the developing embryo bulges into the expanding amniotic cavity (Fig. 3.26). Meanwhile, the yolk sac becomes partially incorporated into the embryo where it gives rise to the gut; that part of the yolk sac remaining outside the embryo communicates with the primitive gut. This communicating channel, however, gradually becomes elongated and attenuated to form the vitelline duct, the extraembryonic yolk sac becoming progressively removed further away from the embryo to be eventually incorporated into the lower end of the body stalk.

Further expansion of the amniotic sac leads to more or less complete obliteration of the extraembryonic coelom with eventual fusion of the extraembryonic mesenchyme covering the amnion with that lining the chorion. At the same time, the extraplacental chorion (the chorion laeve) ceases to produce syncytiotrophoblast and the cytotrophoblastic component undergoes a partial regression. Hence, the single fused amniochorionic membrane is now fully formed and will consist of, from fetal to maternal side, amniotic epithelium, condensed extraembryonic mesenchyme, a loose reticular layer which possibly represents the vestige of the extraembryonic coelom, extraembryonic mesenchyme and trophoblast.

Amniotic fluid

Amniotic fluid volume can now be measured by ultrasound techniques, although measurements were achieved previously by dilution studies. At 12 weeks, it is approximately 50 mL and at 16 weeks, when amniocentesis is often carried out, it is about 150 mL. The volume increases to 900 or 1000 mL in late pregnancy, falling again just before term to 800–900 mL.

Initially the fluid is formed from the primitive cells around the amniotic vesicle. Later there is a transudate

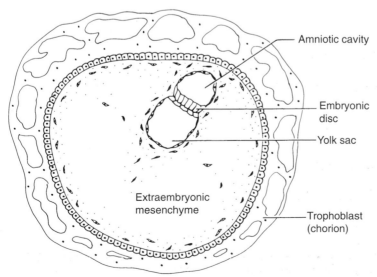

Figure 3.24 • Diagrammatic representation of relationship between developing amniotic cavity and extraembryonic mesenchyme.

Amniotic cavity

Embryonic disc

Yolk sac

Extraembryonic mesenchyme

Trophoblast (chorion)

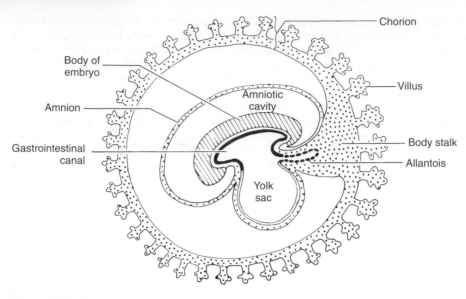

Figure 3.25 • Diagrammatic representation of the relationship between the expanding amniotic cavity and the developing embryo.

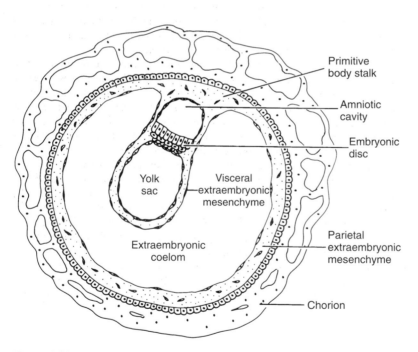

Figure 3.26 • Diagrammatic representation of relationship between developing amniotic cavity, extraembryonic mesenchyme, extraembryonic coelom and primitive body stalk.

of fetal extracellular fluid, which is passed through the fetal skin and umbilical cord. There is also some diffusion of fluid across that part of the amniotic membrane which covers the placenta. In the second trimester, as the skin becomes keratinized and waterproof, there is an increasing contribution from fetal urine and fetal lung secretions. As the fetus develops an ability to swallow, a circulation of fluid occurs whereby urine excreted from the kidneys is passed through the bladder into the amniotic pool. This fluid is then swallowed, digested and re-excreted. Additional contributions to the amniotic pool continue to come from amniotic membrane secretions. At term there is an exchange of 500 mL/24 h, most of which is swallowed and re-excreted by the fetus, and up to 250 mL is transferred to the mother through the membranes.

A reduced liquor volume is found in conjunction with fetal renal agenesis and also with lower urinary tract obstruction. It also occurs to a lesser extent with growth restriction associated with insufficient placental function. Excessive liquor volumes are found where there is any dysfunction of fetal swallowing, and also in cases of open spina bifida lesions, where the spinal fluid may leak out. Polyhydramnios is also found in some cases of twinning, in some diabetic pregnancies, and in the rare presence of a haemangioma of the placenta.

Composition of amniotic fluid

As a result of its mixed origins, amniotic fluid is heterogeneous in composition. Some cells and cellular debris, as well as other insoluble material, are suspended in a clear solution with an osmolarity of approximately 275 mmol/L at term. The osmolarity decreases as pregnancy progresses.

The cells found in amniotic fluid at term are of three main types: fetal epithelial cells, amniotic cells and dermal fibroblasts. The epithelial cells and amniotic cells grow poorly in culture, but the fibroblasts grow well and are used for karyotyping and other analyses. In the presence of renal tube defects, glial cells are also found.

Nitrogenous waste, in the form of urea, creatine and uric acid, increases in concentration from the end of the first trimester until term, and reflects the increasing function of the fetal kidneys. Amino acids are found in about the same concentration as in maternal plasma.

Proteins increase in concentration as pregnancy progresses, but the concentrations level off after 30 weeks of gestation. They are mainly albumen and globulins in a ratio of 6:4. There is virtually no fibrinogen or protein-bound lipids. α-Fetoprotein is found in early pregnancy but in a concentration 10 times lower than in fetal blood. Higher levels of α-fetoprotein may indicate an open neural tube defect, whereas abnormally low levels may be associated with Down syndrome.

Lipids in the amniotic fluid increase to a concentration of about 400 mg/L at term, half of which is in the form of free fatty acids. There are small amounts of phospholipids, cholesterol and lecithin, the latter, being secreted from the lungs, is used as an indicator of surfactant maturation.

Carbohydrates are present in amniotic fluid in concentrations approximately half those found in maternal serum. Glucose predominates, with only smaller quantities of fructose and sucrose. Concentrations of lactate, citrate, pyruvate and α-ketoglutarate are similar to those in maternal blood.

Inorganic salts are found in concentrations almost identical with those in maternal extracellular fluid. Thus sodium and chloride concentrations are high while potassium, calcium, magnesium and phosphate are low. At term, the sodium concentration is 127 mmol/L and potassium 40 mmol/L.

Various enzymes and hormone assays have been recorded, although in some cases considerable variations have been noted. Oestrogens, mainly oestradiol, are found in their conjugated forms. Progesterone and its metabolite pregnanediol are also present. Cortisone and 17-hydroxycortisone are found in trace amounts only. Insulin levels rise towards term, and are much higher in diabetic pregnancies.

Pigment from bilirubin and meconium may stain the amniotic fluid. Bilirubin normally decreases towards term, except in cases of fetal haemolysis. Meconium may be present in late pregnancy, and in labour it is often taken to be an indication of fetal distress but its presence only correlates with biochemical evidence of fetal hypoxia in about 20% of cases.

The partial pressure of oxygen (PO_2) at 2–15 mmHg is lower than that of the maternal arterial blood, whereas the partial pressure of carbon dioxide (PCO_2) at 55–60 mmHg is higher. Compared with blood, the amniotic fluid pH is slightly acidic at 7.0. This fact may be used as a diagnostic test on vaginal fluid when there is doubt about rupture of the membranes and amniotic fluid leakage. The amniotic fluid is thought to have some antibacterial activity, possibly generated by the pH, and also by the presence of lysozyme, peroxidase and α-interferon.

Chapter **Four**

4

Fetal and placental physiology

Sailesh Kumar

Introduction

The concept of the fetus as a patient owes much of its development to, first, our improved understanding of embryonic and fetal physiology and biochemistry, and second, the identification and appreciation of the function of various genes that influence normal fetal growth and development. Many of the advances in fetal physiology come from animal studies; however, simple extrapolation of findings can sometimes be misleading and non-representative in humans. Nevertheless, animal work in the 1950s and 1960s was crucial in helping understand normal fetal physiology. It is very likely that further advances in molecular biology as well greater understanding of gene structure and function will enable various aspects of fetal and placental function to be clarified in the future. This chapter summarizes current knowledge about various fetal and placental systems as well as perturbations that can result in disease.

Fetal growth

Fetal growth and development are complex processes that rely on a series of multiple interacting maternal and uteroplacental factors that ultimately determine the size of the fetus. Both genetic (particularly maternal genes) and environmental factors influence this process. In particular, maternal height, which appears to be a reflection of uterine capacity and therefore for fetal growth, is of particular importance. In embryonic and early gestation, there is an increase in cell number followed by an increase in cell size which becomes more pronounced after 32 weeks of pregnancy.

Adequate maternal nutrition is essential to ensure appropriate fetal growth. Increased caloric intake in the second and third trimesters is important for both fetal and placental growth. Protein intake appears to be particularly important. A Cochrane systematic review found that balanced protein–energy supplementation was able to reduce the risk of small for gestational age neonates by approximately 30%. Glucose is also an important nutrient in the control of fetal growth. Studies in diabetic women have shown that very tight glycaemic control results in smaller babies, whereas hyperglycaemia increases the risk of macrosomic infants. The fetus can exert its own influence on maternal nutrient intake just as fetal sex is known to affect fetal growth, with male babies, being larger, on average than female babies. Fetal sex-specific signals may have influence over growth but, as yet, the nature of these signals is not understood. Other maternal factors that can modulate fetal growth include the following.

Maternal smoking and drug use

This is clearly associated with low birth weight and adverse perinatal outcome. Smoking reduces birth weight by approximately 150–200 g and produces largely symmetrical growth restriction. Smoking results in high maternal levels of carbon monoxide which in turn leads to high fetal levels and subsequent tissue hypoxia as well as the vasoconstrictive effects of nicotine which influences uteroplacental perfusion. Other components of cigarette smoke have been shown to impair activity of placental transporters suggesting an independent effect with fetal growth restriction.

Maternal hypoxia

Altitude is a strong predictor of maternal hypoxia and therefore of fetal size. Its effect is greater on the fetal abdominal circumference rather than head measurements, and mean birth weight can be reduced by as much as 400 g (Krampl et al 2000). The combination of pregnancy and maternal hypoxia can modulate the immune response resulting in higher levels of pro-inflammatory cytokines (TNF, IL-6) and lower levels of anti-inflammatory cytokines (IL-10). In addition maternal hypoxia can also reduce uterine and placental blood flow resulting in not only fetal hypoxia but also a reduction in nutrient transport to the feto-placental unit.

Maternal inflammatory conditions

Many autoimmune conditions or other chronic inflammatory diseases can have an adverse effect on fetal growth. Many mechanisms are responsible, not least a combination of reduced feto-placental blood flow, relative hypoxia and the presence of pro-inflammatory substances. Such conditions include pre-eclampsia, infections, SLE and chronic renal disease.

The placenta and fetal growth

At term, the total placental surface area for gas and nutrient exchange is almost 11 m^2. In fetal growth restriction, both placental volume and villous surface area are reduced. Several aspects of placental function and development are important in achieving optimal fetal growth. These include adequate trophoblast invasion, increase in uteroplacental blood flow, maternal–fetal transfer of glucose, lipids, amino acids and other macro/micro nutrients and the production, transfer and proper function of various growth regulating hormones.

The IGF (insulin-like growth factors) axis

IGF-I and IGF-II are polypeptides similar to that of insulin. They have mitogenic properties, inducing somatic cell growth and proliferation as well as the ability to influence the transport of amino acids and glucose across the placenta. In animal studies, both IGF-I and IGF-II are required for fetal and placental growth. The IGFs bind to two different receptors – type 1 and type 2 IGF receptors, which have differing affinities for the two hormones.

Serum concentrations of IGF-I and IGF-II are higher in pregnant compared with non-pregnant women with concentrations increasing even further by the third trimester. Fetal concentrations of IGF-I and IGF-II increase substantially with advancing gestation, with the greatest rise in IGF-I. The actions of both IGFs are modulated by IGF binding proteins (IGFBP) of which there are six. IGFBP-1 is the major regulator of IGF-I during pregnancy and is produced mainly in the decidua. Phosphorylation and proteolysis of IGFBPs are mechanisms responsible for altering the bioavailability of IGFs during pregnancy. Pregnancy-associated plasma protein-A (PAPP-A) is secreted by the decidua into the maternal circulation during pregnancy and cleaves IGFBP-4, a potent inhibitor of IGF-I, thereby increasing its concentrations. Low circulating levels of PAPP-A (usually detected on first trimester aneuploidy screening) have been associated with an increased risk of fetal growth restriction. Most IGFs in the fetal circulation originate from fetal tissues that express IGFs and their binding proteins which allow the fetus to modulate their levels in both an autocrine and paracrine manner.

Fetal circulation

Development

The fetal heart develops from the splanchnic mesoderm and in its earliest and most rudimentary form is represented by two tubes which subsequently fuse and then canalize. Repeated rotations and septations then occur, which ultimately result in a four-chamber organ.

The myocardium increases by cell division until birth and subsequent growth is due to cell hypertrophy. A fetal heart beat can be detected by 22 days, and by 8 weeks of gestation some degree of neurogenic regulation occurs as a result of innervation by the sympathetic and parasympathetic nervous systems. However, the fetal myocardium, in general, shows immaturity of structure, function and sympathetic innervation relative to the adult heart.

The fetal heart has a limited capacity to increase its output as it normally operates at the top of its cardiac function curve. An increase in fetal heart rate can increase the cardiac output, albeit modestly, but bradycardia can significantly compromise its function.

Distribution and pattern of the fetal circulation

Many of the data on distribution and volume of fetal blood flow come from animal studies, particularly studies of the chronically catheterized sheep fetus. However, with advances in prenatal ultrasound, Doppler studies of the human fetal circulation have enabled us to evaluate fetal blood flow in normal and compromised fetuses with some degree of accuracy. In the fetus, the right and left ventricles pump blood into the arterial circulation in parallel. The characteristic anatomical feature of the fetal circulation, in contrast to the adult, is the presence of several vascular shunts (foramen ovale, ductus venosus and ductus arteriosus), which ensure that most of the blood bypasses the fetal lungs and is shunted towards the organ of gas exchange, the placenta.

The blood volume in the human fetus is estimated to be approximately 10–12% of body weight compared with 7–8% in the adult. The main reason for this is the large reservoir of blood within the placenta. It is estimated that the feto-placental blood volume in human fetuses is in the region of 110–115 mL/kg and the estimated volume in the fetal body is approximately 80 mL/kg. The systemic systolic pressure in human fetuses increases from 15–20 mmHg at 16 weeks to 30–40 mmHg at 28 weeks. A similar increase is also seen for diastolic pressure which is ≤5 mmHg at 16–18 weeks and 5–15 mmHg at 19–26 weeks. Umbilical venous pressure, in contrast, changes only slightly (4.5 mmHg at 18 weeks to 6 mmHg at term).

Approximately 40% (200 mL/kg per min) of fetal cardiac output is distributed to the placental circulation and a similar volume will return to the heart via the umbilical venous system. After entering the intra-abdominal portion of the umbilical vein, a portion of umbilical venous flow supplies the liver but the rest passes through the ductus venosus and into the heart. The ductus venosus is a slender trumpet-like shunt that connects the intra-hepatic portion of the umbilical vein

to the inferior vena cava at its inlet into the heart. The inlet of the ductus venosus has a restrictive diameter of 0.5 mm at mid-gestation and about 2 mm beyond that. Changes in the umbilical venous pressure cause the blood to accelerate from a mean of 10–22 cm/s in the umbilical vein to 60–65 cm/s as it enters the ductus venosus and flows towards the inferior vena cava and heart. Blood flow through the thoracic inferior vena cava represents approximately 65–70% of venous return to the heart and the ductus venosus accounts for about a third of this. There is preferential streaming of blood from the ductus venosus in a dorsal and leftward direction in the inferior vena cava so that this blood flows through the foramen ovale and left atrium and hence through the left ventricle and aorta. This more highly oxygenated blood (SaO_2 60%) therefore perfuses the coronary arteries and the head and neck vessels. Despite the preferential streaming of blood in the inferior vena cava and through the foramen ovale there is still some mixing of blood in the right atrium which passes into the right ventricle. However, the blood in the left atrium (SaO_2 70%) is still of significantly higher saturation compared with that in the right atrium (SaO_2 20%).

Blood returning to the heart from the inferior and superior vena cava and coronary sinus flow preferentially through the right atrium and into the right ventricle. This blood then enters the pulmonary artery but rather than flowing into the pulmonary bed is diverted through the ductus arteriosus into the descending aorta. Almost 40% of the cardiac output is directed through this shunt. The lungs receive approximately 13% of cardiac output at mid-gestation and 20–25% after 30 weeks. Patency of the ductus arteriosus is regulated by both dilatory and constrictive factors and by the impedance of the pulmonary vascular bed which is under the control of prostaglandin I_2. There is a degree of basal tonic constriction that is augmented by endothelin. Circulating prostaglandins, particularly prostaglandin E_2, are crucial in maintaining patency and nitric oxide also has a dilatory effect prior to the third trimester. Sensitivity to prostaglandin antagonists is highest in the third trimester and is enhanced by glucocorticoids and fetal stress. It is therefore particularly vulnerable to prostaglandin synthase inhibitors such as indometacin, which may cause severe and prolonged constriction. The ductus arteriosus closes within 2 days of birth. The main trigger for its closure is the increase in arterial oxygen concentrations which rise when the fetus makes the transition to extrauterine life and regular respiration is established.

Changes at birth

In the human newborn, the ductus venosus is functionally closed within a few hours, although it takes almost 3 weeks to obliterate permanently. This may take longer in pre-term infants or in cases of persistent pulmonary hypertension or cardiac malformations. The foramen ovale is also functionally closed shortly after birth but permanent closure is a slow process and normally does not occur for up to 12 months. As discussed earlier, the ductus arteriosus closes rapidly after birth in response to rising blood oxygen tension and appears to be permanent after approximately 15 h. Within minutes after the onset of respiration, pulmonary vascular resistance decreases and pulmonary blood flow increases approximately 10-fold. Right ventricular output is therefore directed more to the lungs and the right and left sides of the heart begin to pump in series converting to a more adult pattern of circulation. High cardiac output after birth is required principally to sustain global body perfusion and to support the increase in metabolism required to maintain thermoregulation.

Response to stress

Blood flow to the fetal brain, heart and adrenal glands is maintained or increased when oxygen delivery to the fetus decreases. These vital organs depend largely on aerobic metabolism to meet energy requirements and therefore preservation of blood flow during periods of hypoxic stress is an important adaptive mechanism. Similarly, during fetal haemorrhage, blood flow to these organs does not fluctuate, despite a decrease in the arterial oxygen tension. Blood flow to the lower half of the fetus (kidneys, skin, muscle, bone, gastrointestinal tract) and pulmonary bed all reduce during periods of either acute or chronic stress. In late gestation, neurohormonal mechanisms are activated in response to hypoxia and acidaemia and are important regulators of perfusion to these various organ systems.

A hypoxic insult late in pregnancy (cord compression, placental abruption) activates the chemoreceptors in the carotid and aortic bodies causing an immediate vagal response with bradycardia, and simultaneous vasoconstriction mediated by the sympathetic nervous system. An endocrine response follows to maintain vasoconstriction and tachycardia (adrenaline and noradrenaline) and the renin–angiotensin system is activated and renin and angiotensin II levels rise further maintaining vasoconstriction and blood pressure. Other hormones that are released include adrenocorticotrophic hormone (ACTH) and vasopressin from the pituitary gland, atrial natriuretic peptide, cortisol, neuropeptide Y and adrenomedullin. Chronic hypoxia causes fetal adaptation towards decreased cellular oxygen demand, reduced fetal growth and a gradual return of neurohumoral factors and fetal acid–base status towards normal baseline levels. However, this adaptation in fetal homeostasis may have long-term consequences with increased risks for metabolic (diabetes, hyperlipidaemia) and cardiovascular (hypertension, heart disease) diseases in adulthood.

Renal function and amniotic fluid dynamics

The human kidney (metanephros) develops from the Wolffian duct and the metanephric mesenchyme, which are both derived from the intermediate mesoderm. The metanephros begins to develop after the Wolffian duct has extended caudally along the body axis and has produced an outgrowth called the ureteric bud. The ureteric bud is an epithelial tissue that invades the metanephric mesenchyme and induces the mesenchymal cells that surround it to condense to form a cap of closely associated cells. The condensed mesenchymal cells then induce the ureteric bud to branch and form two new ureteric tips and themselves begin to form pre-tubular aggregates that undergo a mesenchyme-to-epithelial transition to form an epithelial tubule. These tubules develop into nephrons, the excretory units of the kidney, by means of several stages of development. The branches of the ureteric bud eventually form the collecting duct system, which collects urine into the renal pelvis and urinary bladder. During ureteric bud branching, tubule induction is repeated to generate approximately 500 000–1 000 000 nephrons in the human kidney. In humans, fetal glomeruli develop by 8–9 weeks, tubular function commences after the 14th week and nephrogenesis is largely complete by birth.

In normal pregnancies there is an inverse relationship between fetal urinary creatinine and sodium levels as gestation progresses. This is a reflection of the increasing maturition of the renal tubular system (Fig. 4.1). After 20 weeks, the kidneys provide over 90% of the amniotic fluid.

Amniotic fluid

There is a wide variation in amniotic fluid volume throughout gestation (Brace & Wolf 1989) with a gradual increase as pregnancy progresses before decreasing after 36 weeks of gestation. The late decrease in amniotic fluid is a normal phenomenon rather than an aberration. Amniotic fluid volume is the net result between inflow and outflow of fluid into the amniotic cavity. In early gestation, the most likely source of amniotic fluid is active transport of solute by the amnion into the amniotic space with water moving passively along. Later in pregnancy, fetal urine, secretions from the respiratory tract, transfer of fluid across the chorionic plate and umbilical cord (intramembranous flow), and movement of fluid directly between the amniotic cavity and maternal blood across the wall of the uterus (transmembranous flow) all contribute to

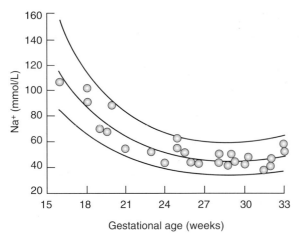

Figure 4.1 • Urinary sodium levels in a cohort of 26 normal fetuses (*Source*: Nicolini U, Fisk N M, Rodeck C H et al 1992 Fetal urine biochemistry: an index of renal maturation and dysfunction. British Journal of Obstetrics and Gynaecology 99:46–50).

Table 4.1	Daily amniotic fluid dynamics in the human fetus
Inflow	**Outflow**
Urine flow (1000–1200 mL)	Swallowing (500–1000 mL)
Lung fluid (340 mL) (50% swallowed)	Intramembranous (200–500 mL)
Pharyngeal fluid (10 mL)	Transmembranous (10 mL)

amniotic fluid volume. Large amounts of fluid enter and leave the amniotic cavity each day.

Although fetal urine is present in the amniotic space as early as 8–11 weeks of gestation, it is the major contributor of amniotic fluid only later in pregnancy. At term, fetal urine flow may be as much as 1000–1200 mL/day. Any condition that prevents either the formation of urine (renal agenesis, renal dysplasia) or its egress into the amniotic sac (bladder outlet obstruction, fetal growth restriction) will cause oligohydramnios. Conversely, any condition that causes increased fetal urine production (maternal diabetes) may cause polyhydramnios. Fetal swallowing plays an important role in maintaining amniotic fluid volume during the latter half of the pregnancy. Obstruction to the upper gastrointestinal tract (oesophageal atresia, duodenal atresia) or any condition that impairs fetal swallowing will result in polyhydramnios. Table 4.1 shows the various contributions to the inflow and outflow of amniotic fluid in the human fetus.

During the first trimester, amniotic fluid has an electrolyte composition and osmolality similar to that of fetal and maternal blood. As fetal urine begins to enter the amniotic cavity, amniotic fluid osmolality decreases compared with fetal blood. This reaches a nadir of 250–260 mmol/kg water near term compared with fetal blood osmolality of 280 mmol/kg water. This low osmolality is a result of extremely hypotonic fetal urine (60–140 mmol/kg water) in combination with a lesser volume of isotonic lung fluid.

Fetal lung development

Lung development is divided into three periods: embryonic, fetal and postnatal. It first appears as a ventral bud off the embryonic foregut which undergoes progressive branching into the surrounding mesenchyme. Fetal lung development is divided into four stages: pseudoglandular, canalicular, saccular and alveolar. In human fetuses, the saccular stage merges with the alveolar stage from 32 weeks of gestation.

Pseudoglandular stage occurs between the 5th and 17th week of gestation and is characterized by progressive division and branching of the airways. In addition, pulmonary microangiogenesis also develops in conjunction with the airways. By the end of this stage, airways, arteries and veins have developed in a pattern corresponding to that found in the adult.

Canalicular stage occurs between 16 and 26 weeks of gestation. During this stage, prospective gas exchange regions are formed with development of the air–blood barrier and differentiation of pulmonary epithelia into type 1 and type 2 pneumocytes and the initiation of synthesis/secretion of alveolar surfactant. There is also in-growth of capillaries into the gas exchange zones resulting in an increased potential for gaseous transfer. At the end of the canalicular stage, airways down to the last prospective respiratory bronchioles are present, to which are attached several irregularly shaped saccules.

Saccular stage occurs from 25 weeks of gestation to term. During the saccular stage, there is a progressive increase in lung volume and epithelial surface area. Elastic tissue starts to appear in the interductal and intersaccular wall, which is an important precursor for alveolar formation.

Alveolar stage occurs between 36 weeks and 2 years of age. More than 80% of alveoli are formed postnatally. There are many factors that can interfere with normal alveolar development. These include mechanical ventilation of the pre-term infant, glucocorticoids, pro-inflammatory cytokines (TNFα, IL-6), chorioamnionitis and hyperoxia or hypoxia. Vitamin A and thyroxine stimulate alveolarization.

Surfactants

Surfactants are a complex mixture of lipids (90%) and proteins (5–10%) which are synthesized by type 2 pneumocytes and secreted into the alveolar spaces. They have the ability to lower alveolar surface tension and therefore prevent collapse of air spaces once respiration is established. Surfactant deficiency causes the classical condition of hyaline membrane disease. Surfactant lipids also play an important role in lung fluid absorption and maintenance of lung liquid balance.

There are several factors that stimulate production of surfactant in the fetus. Glucocorticoids in particular have long been known to accelerate synthesis and secretion of all major components of surfactant. This is the basis for antenatal administration of maternal glucocorticoids to enhance fetal lung maturity. Other factors that stimulate surfactant production include thyroid hormones, which appear to act both independently and in concert with glucocorticoids. Maternal diabetes, in contrast, is associated with delayed fetal lung maturation and this appears to be mediated by fetal hyperglycaemia and hyperinsulinaemia.

Changes at birth

Prior to labour, lung fluid secretion falls and the onset of labour stimulates the production of adrenaline by the fetus and thyrotrophin-releasing hormone by the mother, causing fetal pulmonary epithelial cells to begin reabsorption of lung fluid. After birth, there is an acceleration of active pulmonary fluid absorption, and most is cleared from the full-term newborn lung within 2 h of commencing spontaneous breathing. This is achieved by the active transport of sodium ions out of the alveolar lumen and into the interstitium. With the introduction of air into the lungs, an air/liquid interface, facilitated by surfactant, forms the alveolar lining. After birth, there is a dramatic fall in pulmonary arteriolar resistance and an increase in pulmonary blood flow when the lungs are inflated at birth. Once the alveoli are aerated, breathing needs less effort, requiring minimal negative intrathoracic pressure to maintain a normal tidal volume (Laplace's law). Tactile stimulation and the change in temperature that occurs after birth are also potent stimulants for the transition to extrauterine respiration.

Fetal brain development

Development of the human central nervous system involves several complex steps including neuroectodermal induction, neurulation, cell proliferation and migration, apoptosis, neurogenesis and elimination of excess neurones, synaptogenesis, stabilization and selective elimination of synapses, gliogenesis and myelination (Table 4.2). This is an extremely complex process controlled by a myriad of substances and influenced by both genetic and environmental factors.

Brain injury in the pre-term infant includes many lesions, such as germinal matrix and intraventricular haemorrhage, post-haemorrhagic hydrocephalus and

Table 4.2 Milestones during human brain development

Induction of neuroectoderm	3rd week
Neurulation	3rd–4th week
Formation of the prosencephalon and hemispheres	5th–10th week
Neuronal proliferation	10th–20th week
Neuronal migration	12th–24th week
Neuronal apoptosis	28th–40th week
Neurogenesis	15th–20th week onwards
Synaptogenesis and synaptic stabilization	20th week onwards for many years
Glial formation	20th–24th weeks onwards
Myelination	36th–38th week onwards for 2–3 years
Angiogenesis	5th–10th weeks onwards for several years

periventricular leukomalacia (PVL). PVL now represents the most important brain lesion determining long-term neurodevelopmental outcome in a premature baby. It is characterized by multifocal areas of cystic necrosis forming cysts in the deep periventricular white matter. These cysts are frequently bilateral and correlate well with the development of spastic cerebral palsy. In addition, other more diffuse white matter injury in these babies results in a very high incidence of a broad spectrum of cognitive and learning disabilities.

The placenta

The human placenta has essentially two components: a large fetal portion that develops from the chorionic sac and a smaller maternal portion that is derived from the endometrium. Development of the placenta depends critically on the differentiation of the specialized epithelial cells (cytotrophoblasts) to ensure that the maternal–fetal interface allows adequate nutritional supply to the fetus and, at the same time, elimination of waste products into the maternal circulation. After approximately 6 days post-fertilization, the blastocyst implants into the primed endometrium. As soon as implantation takes place, rapid trophoblast proliferation occurs, resulting in the formation of two distinct layers: an inner mononuclear (cytotrophoblast) and an outer multinucleated syncytiotrophoblast layer.

The syncytiotrophoblast produces various lytic enzymes, which enable digit-like processes to invade the endometrial stroma to complete implantation. Initially, the developing embryo obtains its nutrition from glycogen and lipid-laden stromal cells which degenerate adjacent to the invading syncytiotrophoblast. However, the development of an adequate utero-placental circulation is critical for the maintenance of the embryo, and by the end of the 3rd post-conception week all the necessary anatomical arrangements are in place for feto–maternal exchange. Lacunar networks, which are filled with maternal blood, form through the fusion of individual syncytiotrophoblast lacunae, providing a rich source of nutrition for the embryo.

The intervillous space is derived from these networks and is fed by maternal blood which enters via 80–100 spiral arteries. The terminal villi of the placenta are constantly bathed in maternal blood within the intervillous spaces and this arrangement provides an extremely large area for the exchange of metabolic and gaseous products between the maternal and fetal blood streams. There is normally no intermingling of blood between these two compartments.

Normal physiological placental vascular adaptation in pregnancy involves conversion of the muscular walls of the maternal spiral arteries into large low-pressure capacitance vessels which can then accommodate the massive increase in blood flow that the developing fetus and placenta require. This is achieved by cytotrophoblast invasion into the spiral arteries (endovascular invasion), which leads to the loss of the endothelial lining and most, if not all, of the musculoelastic tissue. By the end of the second trimester, the maternal spiral arteries are lined exclusively by cytotrophoblasts and endothelial cells are no longer apparent, in either the endometrial or myometrial segments.

Nutrient transport across the placenta

The placenta is a metabolically active organ and manages to extract 40–60% of the total glucose and oxygen supplied by the uterine circulation. Various nutrients and metabolites are transferred across the placenta to the fetus by passive diffusion (oxygen, carbon dioxide, urea, fatty acids), facilitated diffusion (glucose, lactate), active transport (amino acids, fatty acids), as well as endocytosis or exocytosis. Facilitated diffusion involves transfer down a concentration gradi-

ent by a carrier molecule without the requirement of additional energy. Active transport, in contrast, requires both carrier proteins and additional energy. In general, placental transfer increases throughout gestation as the fetal growth rate increases.

Endocrine function of the placenta

The placenta is an important endocrine organ responsible for the secretion of a large number of hormones including oestrogen, progesterone, human chorionic gonadotrophin, placental variant of human growth hormone, human placental lactogen, insulin-like growth factors and glucocorticoids.

The placenta in perinatal disease

Abnormal villous development is a prominent feature in early-onset fetal growth restriction with absent/reversed end diastolic flow in the umbilical arteries. Defects in all trophoblast differentiation pathways (endovascular, interstitial and chorionic villous) seem to play a role in the pathogenesis of severe early-onset disease. Similar changes are seen in pre-eclampsia and maternal thrombophilia, which also have additional thrombotic lesions characteristic of the disease.

Fetal origins of adult disease

Events *in utero* may influence long-term adult health. This concept is known as fetal programming or the developmental (fetal) origins of adult disease. Adaptation of the fetus to a hostile intrauterine environment is believed to lead to changes in body structure, physiology and metabolism that persist into extrauterine life. While these adaptations may be suitable for *in-utero* conditions, they are inappropriate after birth. Poor nutrition in early life (either fetal or infant) leads to alterations in the development of key organ systems such as the pancreas, resulting in insulin resistance and adult diabetes. The presence of additional factors, such as obesity, can further increase the risk of disease. Small size at birth has been linked to the development of Syndrome X (the combination of non-insulin-dependent diabetes mellitus, hypertension and hyperlipidaemia). Alterations in beta-cell development and function during fetal undernutrition may result in decreased production of insulin, which becomes pathological in adult life.

References

Brace R A, Wolf E J 1989 Normal amniotic fluid volume changes throughout pregnancy. American Journal of Obstetrics and Gynecology 161:382–388

Krampl E, Lees C, Bland J M et al 2000 Fetal biometry at 4300 m compared to sea level in Peru. Ultrasound in Obstetrics and Gynecology 16:9–18

Chapter Five

Applied anatomy

Sara Paterson-Brown

CHAPTER CONTENTS

Introduction

This chapter will address general anatomical principles as well as covering detailed anatomy relevant to the obstetrician and gynaecologist and the MRCOG exams. Particular attention is given to how this knowledge should be applied clinically, and readers are advised to refer to more detailed comprehensive anatomy books to supplement this applied anatomy approach.

Body tissues and cells

These are composed of four elements:

* Epithelium
* Connective tissue
* Muscle
* Nerve.

Epithelium can be simple or stratified:

1. Simple means it is one layer thick and this is seen with absorptive or secretory surfaces:
   Simple squamous – flat cells, e.g. endothelium
   Simple cuboidal – collecting ducts
   Simple columnar – gut lining/fallopian tubes.
2. Stratified means it has multiple layers and this affords protection:
   Stratified squamous – and if this is also keratinized it comprises skin – vagina
   Stratified cuboidal – (2–3 cells thick), e.g. excretory duct
   Stratified transitional – cuboidal cells right up to surface, i.e. surface cells remain large, e.g. urinary epithelium.

Other histology details are addressed in the relevant sections of the text.

The nervous system

The central nervous system comprises the brain and the spinal cord, while the peripheral nervous system includes the cranial and spinal nerves. Both central and peripheral systems have somatic (aware/voluntary) and autonomic (unaware/involuntary) components.

The somatic nervous system

This both transmits sensory information (afferent pathways) and innervates skeletal muscle (efferent pathways). The sensory cells are derived from the neural crest and are bipolar with their cell bodies lying in the dorsal root ganglia (*Note* there is no synapse in dorsal root ganglia), while the motor cells grow out in the ventral root from the neural tube (i.e. single myelinated cells with no synapses before their end organs). Somatic nerves do not cross the midline (Fig. 5.1).

Spinal nerves consist of:

- Posterior primary rami sequentially supplying erector spinae and overlying skin
- Anterior primary rami supply the rest of the body's muscles and skin and are often involved in forming nerve plexuses before branching and joining together for more distal distribution (cervical, brachial, lumbar and sacral plexuses).

Autonomic nerves often 'hitch a ride' on these nerves (as they do on blood vessels).

The autonomic nervous system

Unlike the somatic nervous system, this is involuntary and regulates the body's internal environment. It has the distinctive feature of comprising two neurones in its motor pathway which synapse outside the central nervous system: one neurone grows out from the CNS and is myelinated (preganglionic) while the postganglionic neurone (derived from neural crest cells) is unmyelinated. Two components (sympathetic and parasympathetic) form the autonomic system and tend to oppose each other to maintain internal homeostasis.

The sympathetic nervous system originates from the thoracolumbar regions and the ganglia form a chain bilaterally down each side of the vertebral column, while the parasympathetic nerves have craniosacral outlets and their ganglia are situated distally near their target organs. These differences together with pharmacological features are illustrated in Figure 5.2.

In addition to these efferent autonomic motor neurones, there are afferent fibres which are conveyed via the sympathetic and parasympathetic nerves, but they are independent of them and do not relay in the ganglia. Like other sensory fibres, their cell bodies lie in the dorsal root ganglia from where they ascend centrally to the hypothalamus and thence to the orbital and frontal gyri of the cerebral cortex (Fig. 5.1).

Clinical application

In normal circumstances, we are unaware of autonomic afferent impulses but if sufficiently strong they can cause the sensation of visceral pain (intestinal colic, uterine pain, etc.) which can also produce referred pain in the dermatome of the relevant segmental supply (e.g. cervix S2 and S3, ovary T10 and T11, body of the uterus lower thoracic and upper lumbar roots). Dermatomes are shown in Figure 5.3.

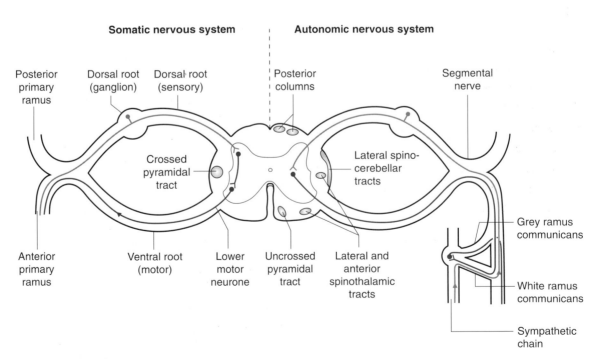

Figure 5.1 • Diagrammatic representation of a transected spinal cord showing the somatic and autonomic neurone pathways and the main tracts running within the cord.

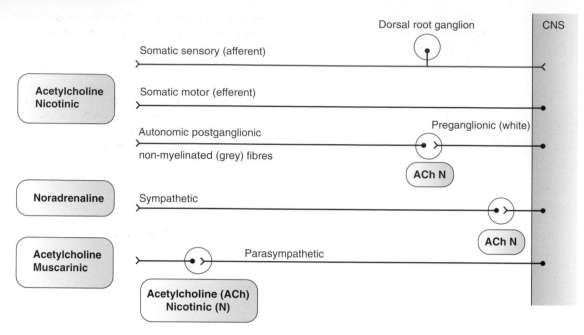

Figure 5.2 • Diagrammatic representation of the neurone arrangements and neurotransmitters of the somatic and autonomic nervous systems.

Sympathetic (thoracolumbar) nervous system

These cells are derived from the lateral horn of T1–L2 but the preganglionic fibres travel up and down to form a chain of ganglia extending from the cervical to the coccygeal region (i.e. the root value of the autonomic component may be different from the spinal component with which it emerges). Postganglionic neurones then form sympathetic nerve plexuses, the main ones being:

- Cardiac plexus (below the aortic arch)
- Pulmonary plexus (at the root of the lungs)
- Coeliac plexus (on the coeliac axis and around the origin of the superior mesenteric artery)
- Superior hypogastric plexus (anterior to the aortic bifurcation)
- Inferior hypogastric plexus (lateral to the rectum, cervix and vaginal fornix).

The peripheral distribution of the sympathetic fibres includes branches for somatic distribution which travel with each spinal nerve to supply the corresponding segmental skin, and the visceral distribution which tends to reach its end organ by means of the arterial pathways.

Approximate segmental supplies:

T1–2 head and neck
T1–4 thoracic viscera

T2–5 upper limb
T4–L2 abdominal viscera
T10–L2 pelvic viscera
T11–L2 lower limb

Note: Thoracic, lumbar and sacral splanchnic nerves emerge from the sympathetic plexuses while the *p*elvic splanchnics, in contrast, are *p*arasympathetic (S23 – nervi erigentes). These parasympathetic preganglionic fibres join the sympathetic fibres (from the inferior hypogastric plexus) for distribution within the pelvis and are described in more detail later.

Sympathetic effects

These are essentially of fight and flight:

- Vasoconstrictor (except to coronary arteries which it dilates)
- Increases the heart rate
- Dilates the bronchial tree
- Relaxes the detrusor muscle
- Contracts smooth muscle sphincters
- Dilates the eye (by relaxing the ciliary muscle)
- Relaxes the small intestine.

The adrenal medulla

This is derived from neural crest cells and comprises approximately 10% of the adrenal gland (the remainder

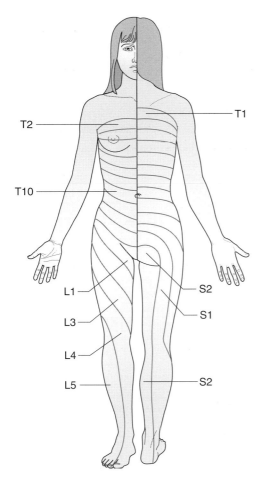

T2
T1
T10
L1
S2
L3
S1
L4
L5
S2

Figure 5.3 • An approximate pattern of anterior and posterior dermatomes.

being the cortex). The myelinated preganglionic sympathetic fibres from the splanchnic nerves travel via the coeliac plexus and synapse directly with the medullary (chromaffin) cells which secrete catecholamines.

Parasympathetic (craniosacral) nervous system

Unlike the sympathetic, the parasympathetic system has no somatic distribution and is purely visceral. Four cranial nerves and two sacral roots are involved.

Cranial: III, VII, IX, X

The vagus is particularly important, travelling widely. It forms a plexus round the oesophagus and the fibres from each side mix and thence continue as anterior and posterior nerves. The vagus contributes to the:

- Cardiac, pulmonary and oesophageal plexuses
- Stomach and liver (via the anterior vagus)

- Small and large intestine as far as the splenic flexure (travelling via the superior mesenteric artery).

Sacral: S2 and S3

Preganglionic cell bodies lie in the lateral horn of the grey matter in the spinal cord from where they pass out as nervi erigentes to intermingle with the inferior hypogastric plexus to supply the:

- Gut beyond the splenic flexure (travel via the inferior mesenteric artery)
- Bladder
- Genital organs
- Pelvic blood vessels.

Parasympathetic effects

- Decreases the heart rate
- Bronchoconstrictor
- Increases glandular secretions
- Increases peristalsis
- Stimulates detrusor contractions
- Relaxes sphincters.

The spinal cord and meninges

This extension of the central nervous system begins in the medulla oblongata at the foramen magnum and ends at L1/L2. The nerve roots that continue after the spinal cord has terminated at the conus medullaris comprise the cauda equina, while the filum terminale (the extension of pia mater) inserts into the coccyx. As the length of the spinal cord is shorter than the vertebral column, nerve roots arise at increasingly higher levels than their corresponding vertebrae and travel increasingly longer distances within the vertebral column before exiting from their respective vertebral foramina.

The membranes of the cord are termed the meninges and they comprise neuroepithelium of which there are three layers. From outside inwards these are:

1. Dura mater (under which lies the subdural space)
2. Arachnoid mater (under this is the subarachnoid space containing cerebrospinal fluid)
3. Pia mater.

Both pia and arachnoid are continued out along the spinal nerve roots, while the dura forms a tough sheath for the cord ending at S2, and it extends out over each nerve root blending with its sheath.

The epidural (extradural) space lies between the dura mater and the spinal canal, and is filled with fat and vessels (lymphatic and blood).

The spinal cord has neuronal cell bodies in its grey matter, and its external white matter comprises axonal tracts (Fig. 5.1).

Afferent neurones include those for:

- Touch and vibration – cell bodies in dorsal root ganglia, tracts in posterior columns
- Pain and temperature – cell bodies in contralateral posterior horn, axons in lateral and anterior spinothalamic tracts
- Proprioception – axons in lateral spinocerebellar tracts

Efferent neurones are motor and pass along the:

- Lateral cerebrospinal (or corticospinal) tract. These neurones originate in the motor cortex but the fibres cross before descending in what is also referred to as the crossed pyramidal tract
- Anterior cerebrospinal (or direct pyramidal) tract. These neurones are uncrossed.

Spinal nerve roots and their plexuses

Each pair of spinal nerves emerges from the vertebral column as illustrated in Figure 5.1, and branches proceed to supply the skin in a pattern which can be mapped out diagrammatically (Fig. 5.3).

Clinical application

Pain can be referred to the dermatome which is supplied by the same nerve root as the area in question. Some spinal nerves merge and re-divide with other nerve roots before proceeding. This produces nerve plexuses and these occur in the cervical, brachial, lumbar and sacral regions. Although the cervical/brachial plexus can be relevant in situations of obstetric trauma to the neonate (in the clinical situations of shoulder dystocia), detailed knowledge of it is beyond the remit of this chapter. The relevant clinical message is to respect the fetal neck and avoid undue traction on it (which can stretch and damage the nerve roots).

The lumbar and sacral plexuses are described in the relevant regional anatomy sections (pp. 81 and 84).

Anatomy of the brain

The brain develops from the neural tube and its cavity persists in the three resulting components:

- The forebrain
  - the cerebral hemispheres, each with their lateral ventricle
  - the deeper diencephalon surrounding the third ventricle
- The midbrain
  - connects the forebrain to the hind brain
  - the aqueduct (of Sylvius) runs through it

- The hindbrain
  - pons, medulla oblongata and cerebellum
  - the fourth ventricle
- The midbrain, pons and medulla comprise the brain stem.

The thalami

The two thalami lie laterally in the diencephalon forming the lateral walls of the third ventricle. The internal capsule lies laterally, separating them from the basal ganglia. The thalamus is sensory in function and relays impulses on to the cerebral cortex via the internal capsule. It also connects to the hypothalamus.

The hypothalamus

The hypothalamus is also in the diencephalon forming the floor of the third ventricle and is concerned with the autonomic nervous system. It contains many cell types, in particular the supraoptic and paraventricular nuclei whose axons connect it to the posterior lobe of the pituitary via the pituitary stalk. It also connects with the basal nuclei caudally and via long axons to the sympathetic and parasympathetic cells in the lateral horns of the spinal cord.

The pineal gland

The pineal gland lies posterior to the thalamus at the posterior end of the third ventricle and is innervated by the sympathetic nervous system. It is most active at night, produces melatonin and tends to have an inhibitory effect on other endocrine glands and gonads. It calcifies with age and may be visible on a skull X-ray after the age of 40 years.

The pituitary gland

The pituitary gland is composed of two parts; both are derived from ectodermal tissue but of different origins:

- The small posterior pituitary is derived from a downgrowth of ectodermal neural plate and these neurones have their cell stations in the hypothalamus. These neurosecretory cells produce oxytocin and antidiuretic hormone (ADH)
- The larger anterior pituitary (pars tuberalis) forms from Rathke's pouch growing up from the roof of the mouth and consists of glandular cells:
  - chromophobes – account for 50% of the anterior pituitary
  - eosinophilic/acidophilic cells produce growth hormone (GH) and prolactin

○ basophilic cells produce adrenocorticotrophic, follicle stimulating, luteinizing and thyroid stimulating hormones (ACTH, FSH, LH, TSH).

This gland occupies the pituitary fossa with:

- The diaphragma sellae and optic chiasma above
- The cavernous sinuses laterally
- The body of the sphenoid below.

Clinical application

Pituitary tumours (including prolactinomas) can grow upwards to press on the medial sides of the optic nerves in the lower anterior part of the optic chiasma causing temporal hemianopia (tunnel vision).

The lymphatic system

Lymphatic vessels

The extracellular tissues of the body are constantly gaining fluid and debris (from capillary leakage, cell death, etc.) and the function of the lymphatics is to remove this and return it to the venous circulation. The lymphatic capillaries have the same basic structure as vascular capillaries but their distribution is not uniform throughout the body. The lymphatics in the limbs tend to be superficial, while those of the viscera tend to drain via channels on the posterior abdominal and thoracic walls.

The lymphatic vessels return the lymph to the venous system via two main channels:

- *The right lymphatic duct* drains the right thorax, upper limb, head and neck
- *The thoracic duct* drains all lymph from the lower half of the body.

The pre- and para-aortic lymphatics drain into the cisterna chyli which is an elongated sac-like vessel that lies over the body of L1 and L2 behind the inferior vena cava and between the aorta and the azygous vein. It becomes the thoracic duct as it ascends through the diaphragm at the level of T12. It starts on the right side of the oesophagus, but as it ascends through the thorax the thoracic duct passes behind the oesophagus (at T5) to reach its left side, then superiorly it passes over the left subclavian artery and the dome of the left pleura to drain into the confluence of the left subclavian with the left internal jugular veins.

Lymphatics, like blood vessels (and unlike somatic nerves), can cross the midline, but in contrast they pass to and from lymph nodes (afferent and efferent lymphatics) and they comprise an anastomosing low-pressure system.

Lymphatic tissue

These comprise concentrations of lymphocytes and occur in mucosal and submucosal collections in the gut (e.g. Peyer's patches in the ileum) as well as in the thymus, the spleen and lymph nodes themselves.

The anatomical clinical importance of this system relates to the drainage patterns of each group of nodes, which is summarized in Table 5.1, but also described for the individual organs in their relevant regional anatomy sections.

The vascular system

Fetal circulation and changes after birth

Oxygenated blood

- *The ductus venosus* bypasses the liver taking oxygenated blood from the left branch of the portal vein (from the umbilical vein) to the inferior vena cava (IVC)
- This flows into the right atrium and is directed towards the *foramen ovale* passing through into the left atrium and thence out to supply the head and neck.

Deoxygenated blood

- Flows back from the superior vena cava and is directed through the tricuspid valve to the right ventricle
- *The ductus arteriosus* bypasses the lungs taking blood from the left branch of the pulmonary trunk to the aorta distal to its three main primary branches
- The blood in the descending aorta then passes out to the placenta via the umbilical arteries which branch off from the internal iliac arteries.

Changes at and after birth

- The pressure changes due to inflation of the lungs and the increased flow through the pulmonary arteries close the foramen ovale
- The ductus arteriosus muscular wall contracts and closes, and is effectively obliterated within 2 months, becoming the ligamentum arteriosum
- The ductus venosus becomes the ligamentum venosum (passing round the caudate lobe of the liver)
- The intra-abdominal umbilical vein becomes the ligamentum teres
- The umbilical arteries become obliterated and form the medial umbilical ligaments (not to be confused with the median umbilical ligament which is the obliterated remains of the urachus).

Table 5.1 Lymphatic drainage patterns

Lymph node group	Location	Tissues/structures drained
Superficial inguinal nodes	Longitudinally along the great saphenous vein and horizontally distal to the inguinal ligament	Anterior abdominal wall (below umbilicus) Upper part of uterus and round ligament Lower third of vagina, vulva, perineum and anus Superficial part of leg and buttock
Deep inguinal lymph nodes	Lie medial to the femoral vein	The superficial inguinal nodes Deep part of leg Clitoris
Deep femoral lymph node of Cloquet	Lies in the femoral canal	Vulva
External iliac nodes	Along the external iliac arteries	Deep inguinal lymph nodes Bladder Lower uterus and cervix
Internal iliac nodes	Along the internal iliac arteries	Urethra and deep perineum Cervix and upper two-thirds of vagina Lower rectum
Common iliac nodes	Along the common iliac arteries	Internal and external iliac nodes Abdominal part of the ureter Fallopian tubes and upper uterus
Obturator nodes	Along the obturator artery	Cervix
Para-aortic nodes	Lie alongside the aorta near the origins of the paired arterial branches	Common iliac nodes Posterior abdominal wall Lumbar region Kidneys and ovaries
Pre-aortic nodes	Anterior to the aorta around the origin of coeliac, superior and inferior mesenteric arteries	Pelvis and abdomen corresponding to ventral aortic arterial branches

The arterial system

The aorta

The aorta (Fig. 5.4) enters the abdomen behind the diaphragm between its crura at T12 and descends to divide into the common iliac arteries at L4. It has three ventral branches which give rise to the portal circulation, while the other branches are systemic.

Three ventral branches

- The coeliac artery (axis/trunk) is very short (1 cm long) arising at level L1
- The superior mesenteric artery arises at level L2
- The inferior mesenteric artery arises at level L3.

Three terminal branches

- The right and left common iliac arteries arise at level L4
- The median sacral artery continues over L5.

Four pairs of branches

- Phrenic arteries
- Suprarenal arteries
- Renal arteries
- Gonadal arteries.

Four lateral pairs

- The four lumbar segmental arteries.

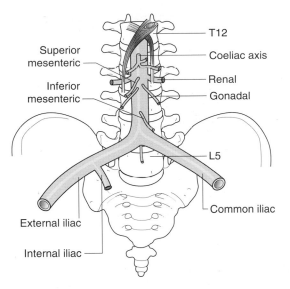

Figure 5.4 • The abdominal aorta and its branches.

The common iliac arteries

The common iliac arteries diverge from in front of the fourth lumbar vertebra and then divide into internal and external iliac arteries in front of the sacroiliac joint.

The external iliac artery is essentially involved in the blood supply to the leg (becoming the femoral artery when it passes behind the inguinal ligament), but it gives two important branches off just above the inguinal ligament: the inferior epigastric and the deep circumflex iliac arteries

The internal iliac artery divides into anterior and posterior branches to supply the pelvis and buttock, respectively. Details of these vessels are given in the section on the pelvis.

Details of individual vessels and their relations are given in the relevant regional anatomy sections.

The venous system

This is a relatively low-pressure valved system for draining blood back to the heart. Flow fluctuates with the arterial pulse while muscle pumps further encourage flow in the limbs and inspiration increases flow in the inferior and superior vena cavae (IVC and SVC) centrally. Excepting the portal circulation, veins generally follow the pattern and path of arteries and have sympathetic innervation.

The inferior vena cava

The common iliac veins join to form the IVC (Fig. 5.5) behind the right external iliac artery at L5. The IVC ascends through the abdomen on the right of the aorta piercing the central tendon of the diaphragm at T8. It receives:

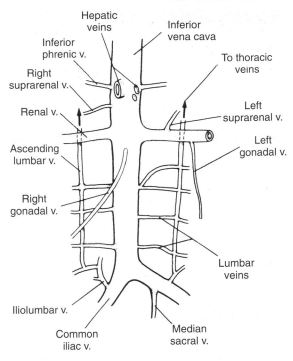

Figure 5.5 • The inferior vena cava and its tributaries.

- Segmental lumbar veins
- The right gonadal vein (the left gonadal vein drains into left renal vein)
- The renal and suprarenal veins
- The hepatic veins
- The inferior phrenic veins.

Collateral venous drainage pathways

There is an extensive network of potential collateral circulations which open when thrombosis of the IVC occurs.

Superficial venous channels which can eventually drain to the superior vena cava are:
- Epigastric
- Circumflex iliac
- Superficial epigastric and lateral thoracic (via thoracoepigastric vein)
- Internal thoracic
- Posterior intercostals
- External pudendal
- Lumbovertebral.

Deep channels which provide deep anastomoses are:
- Azygous
- Hemiazygous
- Lumbar.

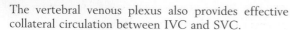

The vertebral venous plexus also provides effective collateral circulation between IVC and SVC.

Clinical application

This collateral circulation is so efficient that, even when there is substantial obstruction to venous flow by a large deep vein thrombosis in the iliac vessels, there can be an absence of clinical symptoms or signs.

The portal venous drainage and portosystemic venous anastomoses

The portal venous system drains blood to the liver from the abdominal part of the alimentary canal (except the anus), the spleen, pancreas and gall bladder. The superior and inferior mesenteric veins join the splenic vein behind the pancreas to form the portal vein which carries blood to the liver, which in turn is drained by the hepatic veins which pass into the IVC. This pathway may be obstructed causing portal hypertension and then collaterals open up between the portal and the systemic venous systems:

- Lower oesophagus – tributaries of: left gastric with hemiazygous/azygous
- Anal wall – superior rectal with middle and inferior rectal
- Caput medusa – tributary from left branch of portal vein (paraumbilical) with epigastrics
- Retroperitoneal veins of abdominal wall with veins of the ascending colon and the bare area of the liver
- Very rarely a patent ductus venosus.

Vertebral column

Venous drainage from both the internal and the external vertebral plexus drain to regional segmental veins providing potential communication with systems which also drain segmentally. This is a largely valveless system and therefore the spread of malignancy is possible (especially likely from breast, uterus, prostate and thyroid):

- Pelvic viscera via the lateral sacral vessels
- Abdomen via the lumbar veins
- Breast via the posterior intercostals
- Neck via the vertebral vein.

The musculoskeletal system

Types of joint

- Fibrous (bone/fibrous tissue/bone), e.g. skull sutures although these ossify in later life
- Cartilaginous:
  - primary (bone/hyaline cartilage/bone), e.g. epiphyses or costochondral junctions
  - secondary (bone/hyaline cartilage/fibrocartilage/ hyaline cartilage/bone) – these only occur in the midline, e.g. pubic symphysis, intervertebral joints
- Synovial joints that allow movement, e.g. hip joint. The sacroiliac joint is also a synovial joint but atypical in that the movement allowed is extremely limited.

The vertebral column

The vertebral column has 33 vertebrae (7 cervical, 12 thoracic, 5 lumbar, 5 sacral and 4 coccygeal). The five sacral vertebrae are fused to form the sacrum, and the coccygeal components can be variably fused.

There are 31 pairs of spinal nerves whose nerve roots travel variable distances within the vertebral column to exit the spine by passing across the disc of the vertebra above (therefore problems with, for example, L4 disc will affect L5 nerve root).

The pelvis

The bony pelvis comprises the sacrum and the os innominatum.

- The sacrum is composed of five fused vertebrae (with four sacral foramina). It articulates with the fifth lumbar vertebra above, the coccyx below and the ilium laterally
- The os innominatum is made up of three bones: ilium, pubis and ischium, which are joined by cartilage in the young, but by bone in adulthood. They meet in a Y-shaped junction in the acetabulum to which they all contribute.

Clinical application

Movement at the pelvic joints is minimal in the non-pregnant state, but there is considerable joint relaxation during pregnancy. In some women, instability can occur with sacroiliitis or pubic symphysis dysfunction which can be extremely debilitating. Limiting abduction of the legs in these conditions is crucial in preventing further deterioration or even permanent instability, and pain-free abduction distances should be measured (knee to knee) and recorded prior to labour so that nursing of the woman (when pain-free with an epidural) does not silently cause more damage.

Obstetric pelvic definitions and dimensions

The pelvic inlet is oval being widest transversely, the pelvic mid-cavity is circular, while the outlet is oval being widest anteroposteriorly. Normally, the fetal head enters the pelvis transversely due to the shape of the inlet and subsequent rotation of the fetal head during the descent through the pelvis in labour takes advantage of the bony dimensions, but the rotation itself is caused by the muscular pelvic gutter (Table 5.2).

The pelvic inlet

The pelvic inlet is oval shaped and is widest from side to side. It divides the bony pelvis into the false pelvis above (made up mainly of the ala of the ilium on each side which forms the lower lateral portion of the abdomen), and the true pelvis below (the pelvic cavity). The boundaries of the pelvic inlet include:

- The promontory of the sacrum
- The arcuate line of the ilium
- The iliopubic eminence
- The pectineal line
- The pubic crest
- The symphysis pubis.

The pelvic outlet

The pelvic outlet is widest from front to back and lies between:

- The lower border of the symphysis pubis anteriorly
- The ischial tuberosities laterally
- The tip of the last sacral vertebra posteriorly.

The true obstetric conjugate extends from the sacral promontory to the upper border of the pubic symphysis. The diagonal conjugate extends from the sacral promontory to the lower border of the pubic symphysis. The important landmarks of the pelvis are indicated in Figures 5.6 and 5.7.

The male and female pelvis

General differences in structure between the male and female pelvis relate to the heavier thick-set skeleton of the male, with more obvious and well marked muscle attachments and larger joint surfaces compared with the female, but there are also notable sex differences (Table 5.3).

Variations in pelvic shape (Fig. 5.8)

- Gynaecoid – normal female
- Android – normal male
- Anthropoid – the pelvic brim is longer anteroposteriorly than transversely
- Platypelloid – the pelvic brim is much wider transversely and foreshortened anteroposteriorly
- Rachitic pelvis – typical of rickets and the result of vitamin D deficiency. The sacral promontory projects forwards reducing the anteroposterior diameter
- The contracted pelvis – can be symmetrical associated with a small stature, or asymmetrical due to a variety of disease processes
- A narrow (gothic) subpubic arch foreshortens the effective pelvic outlet because the narrow anterior triangle (the waste space of Morrison) cannot accommodate the fetal head. In such circumstances, more space is required posteriorly to enable vaginal delivery (Fig. 5.9).

Ligaments of the pelvis

The vertebropelvic ligaments (Figs 5.6, 5.7):
- Iliolumbar – this V-shaped ligament extends from the transverse process of L5 to the iliac crest

Table 5.2	Approximate pelvic obstetric dimensions (cm)		
	Transverse	**Oblique**	**Anteroposterior**
Inlet	13	11	11
Mid-pelvis	12	12	12
Outlet	10.5	11.5	12.5

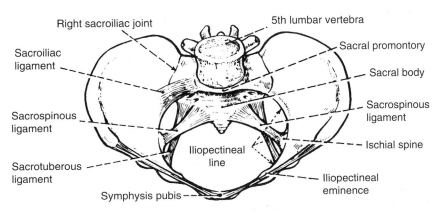

Figure 5.6 • Important landmarks of the pelvis.

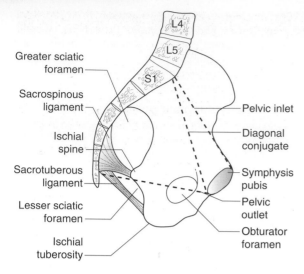

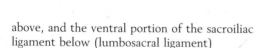

Figure 5.7 • Lateral view of the pelvis showing the obstetric conjugates.

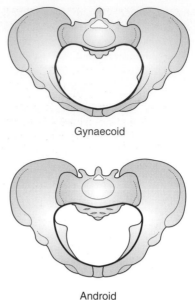

Gynaecoid

Android

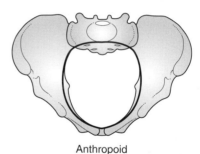

Anthropoid

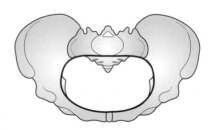

Platypelloid

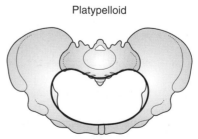

Rachitic

Figure 5.8 • Diagrammatic representation of different pelvic shapes.

above, and the ventral portion of the sacroiliac ligament below (lumbosacral ligament)

- Sacrospinous ligament runs from the lower lateral aspect of the sacrum and the upper lateral aspect of the coccyx to insert into the ischial spine
- Sacrotuberous ligament is extremely strong opposing the forward tilting of the sacral promontory. It also originates from the lower lateral aspect of the sacrum and the upper lateral aspect of the coccyx inserting into the inner aspect of the ischial tuberosity.

The sacrospinous and sacrotuberous ligaments convert the greater and lesser sciatic notches into foramina (Fig. 5.7).

The fetal skull

The skull base develops in cartilage, the vault in membrane. The fetal cranium consists of two frontal bones, two parietal bones and one occipital bone. These are separated by sutures and fontanelles and provide landmarks for defining the presentation of the fetal head in labour:

- Occiput describes the area behind the posterior fontanelle
- The vertex describes the parietal eminences between anterior and posterior fontanelles
- The bregma is the area around the anterior fontanelle
- The sinciput is the area in front of the anterior fontanelle which is further divided into

Table 5.3 Differences between the male and female pelvis

Sex differences	Female	Male
Sacral curve	Short, wide and flat Curved in the lower part	Long and narrow General curve

Articular surfaces of the sacrum	Laterally with two sacral bodies
	Superiorly with L5: oval and occupies
	   one-third of alar surface
		Laterally with three sacral bodies
		Superiorly with L5 and occupies half of
		   the alar surface

Pelvic inlet	Oval	Heart shaped
Pelvic canal	Short and almost cylindrical	Long and tapered
Pelvic outlet	Comparatively large	Comparatively small
Subpubic angle	Approx 80–90°	50–60°
Obturator foramen	Triangular	Oval

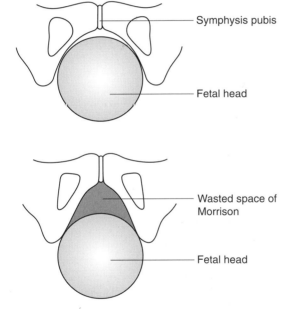

Figure 5.9 • Illustration of the effect of a narrow subpubic arch and the waste space of Morrison.

brow and face (above and below the root of the nose).

The presenting diameter of the fetal skull varies according to its presentation:

- Occipital and face presentations have the smallest diameters (suboccipitobregmatic and submentobregmatic, respectively) both being of the order of 9.5 cm
- Vertex is most common with the occipitofrontal diameter of 11.5 cm

- Brow is the largest with the mentovertical diameter of 13 cm.

Moulding during labour slides the parietal bones under each other and the occipital and frontal bones under the parietal bones, and can reduce dimensions by 1–1.5 cm (Fig. 5.10).

Relevant regional anatomy of the thorax

Surface anatomy

Knowledge of the surface anatomy of the chest can be extremely valuable clinically:

- *The angle of Louis*, which is the ridge produced by the manubriosternal joint, lies at the level of thoracic vertebra T4, but more useful is the site of the second costochondral junction marking the second rib from which subsequent intercostal spaces can be defined. These features also mark the upper limit of the surface markings of the heart
- *The 4th intercostal space* marks the dome of the diaphragm and the uppermost edge of the liver.

Ribs

Ribs generate a negative pressure for respiration (−5 to −15 mmHg)

- True ribs (ribs 1–7) articulate with the sternum
- False ribs (8–10) – their costal cartilages articulate with the rib above
- Floating ribs (11 and 12) have muscle attachments only.

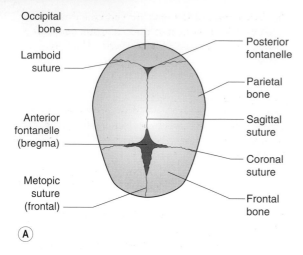

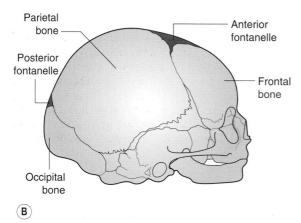

Figure 5.10 • Essential landmarks of the fetal skull: (A) from above and (B) lateral view.

The intercostal muscles which comprise three layers – external, internal and innermost – run between neighbouring ribs. The neurovascular bundles run along the lower inside border of each rib (i.e. superiorly in each intercostal space) between the internal and innermost intercostal muscles.

Clinical application

- When aspirating or inserting a chest drain, the position of the neurovascular bundle should be remembered and access should be achieved by running the needle or drain over the rib rather than under it. The fifth intercostal space in the mid-axillary line is usually used, but in pregnancy it is best to go up one space to allow for the raised diaphragm

- The higher level of the diaphragm in pregnancy is also relevant in situations of trauma to the chest which is more likely to involve intra-abdominal organs
- The parietal pleura is innervated segmentally from the intercostal nerves and therefore when inflamed produces pain which is referred to the cutaneous distribution of that nerve. Thus anterior abdominal wall pain can arise from pleural irritation mimicking an abdominal event.

The diaphragm

This is a musculotendinous structure which separates the thorax from the abdomen. It arises from:

- The xiphisternum
- The lower six ribs and their costal cartilages
- The medial and lateral arcuate ligaments
- The first three lumbar vertebrae on the right/ first two on the left (right and left crus) and fuses into a trifoliate central tendon below the pericardium.

The motor nerve supply is from the phrenic nerve (C3<u>4</u>5), and sensory supply is from the lower six intercostal nerves. The blood supply comes from the lower intercostal arteries superiorly, and the phrenic arteries (branches of aorta) inferiorly.

The three main openings in the diaphragm and their vertebral levels are as follows:

1. The aortic opening at the level of T12 transmits the aorta with the thoracic duct and the azygous vein (from left to right).
2. The oesophageal opening which passes through the right crus of the diaphragm at the level of T10, and also transmits the left gastric artery and both vagi.
3. The inferior vena cava runs through the central tendon at the level of T8 together with the right phrenic nerve.

Other structures which penetrate the diaphragm include the greater and lesser splanchnic nerves and the sympathetic chain.

The abdomen

Surface anatomy

The transpyloric plane is an important landmark because of its anatomical relationships. It lies a patient hand-breadth below their xiphoid and is at the level of the first lumbar vertebra and the ninth costal cartilage and marks the termination of the spinal cord. Structures in this plane include the:

- ○ Pylorus of stomach
- ○ Duodenojejunal flexure
- ○ Fundus of the gall bladder
- ○ Renal hila
- ○ Neck of pancreas.

The subcostal plane joins the lowest costal margins on both sides and marks the tenth rib and the level of the third lumbar vertebra.

The plane of the iliac crests marks the bifurcation of the abdominal aorta at the level of the fourth lumbar vertebra.

The umbilicus is an inconsistent landmark, but in the slim adult lies at the lower part of the third lumbar vertebra, the third part of the duodenum and the origin of the inferior mesenteric artery.

McBurney's point lies two-thirds laterally along a line drawn from the umbilicus to the anterior superior iliac spine. It guides the positioning for an appendicectomy incision (non-pregnant) and needle entry for a paracentesis must pass lateral to this point to avoid the inferior epigastric vessels.

Langer's (cleavage or tension) lines of the skin result from the collagen fibre arrangements, and incisions placed along these heal with minimum scarring. On the anterior abdominal wall, they lie transversely.

The dermatomes of the anterior abdominal wall are relevant in situations of referred pain, and in the assessment of regional anaesthesia. They are illustrated in Figure 5.3.

The abdominal wall

This is essentially muscular, maintaining tone and imposing a positive intra-abdominal pressure (+5 mmHg), despite respiration.

- A muscular cylinder joins two bony rings (costal margin and pelvis) which are joined/splinted apart by the vertebral column
- The superior bony ring is closed off by the muscular diaphragm
- The inferior ring is closed off by the muscular pelvic 'diaphragm'/pelvic floor.

Clinical application

At laparoscopy the intra-abdominal pressure should always be noted together with its fluctuation with respirations. The Veress needle and trocar should be angled inferiorly at 45° from the umbilicus in the midline, thus avoiding the aorta (which has already terminated) and the iliac vessels (which have diverged).

The muscles of the abdominal wall can be thought of as straight (anterior and posterior) and flat (lateral) muscles (Fig. 5.11).

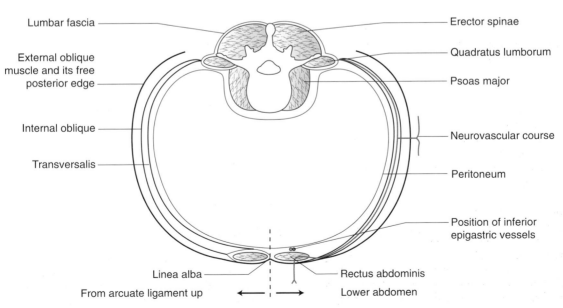

Figure 5.11 • Transverse section through the abdomen showing the muscular arrangements and fascial coverings of the rectus abdominis muscle at different levels (see text) and illustrating the neurovascular plane and course.

Straight muscles
Posteriorly: Quadratus lumborum
Attachments
- Medial half of the lower border of the 12th rib
- Transverse processes of L1–5
- Iliolumbar ligament and posterior aspect of iliac crest.

Nerve supply
- Segmental from T12 to L4 ventral rami.

Anteriorly: Rectus abdominis
Attachments
- 5th–7th costal cartilages plus xiphisternum in horizontal plane
- Pubic crest (and interdigitates across the midline).

Nerve supply
- Segmental T7–T12.

Pyramidalis is a vestigial muscle absent in 20% of the population, which lies anterior to the lower fibres of the rectus abdominis muscle within the rectus sheath. It is supplied by the subcostal nerve.

Flat (lateral) muscles (all innervated segmentally from T7 to L1)
External oblique
Runs downwards, forwards and medially (like the direction your hands take when in your pockets).
Attachments
- Angles of lower eight ribs
- Anterior half of iliac crest and anterior superior iliac spine
- Pubic tubercle and pectineal line on ipsilateral side (lacunar ligament)
- Contralateral pubic tubercle (reflected part of the inguinal ligament – this forms the floor of the inguinal canal).

The external oblique muscle has two free edges
- Posteriorly
- Inferiorly (the inguinal ligament).

Internal oblique
Runs upwards, forwards and medially, i.e. at 90° to external oblique.
Attachments
- Anterior two-thirds of iliac crest
- Internal border of lateral two-thirds of inguinal ligament (conjoint tendon)
- Lower 3–4 ribs and their costal cartilages.

Transversus (transverse abdominis/transversalis)
Runs across laterally.
Attachments
- Inner aspects of costal cartilages of lower six ribs
- Anterior two-thirds of iliac crest
- Internal border of lateral third of inguinal ligament (conjoint tendon).

The conjoint tendon forms from the fibres of internal oblique and transversus abdominis which extend from their inguinal ligament attachment to arch medially and insert into the pubic crest lying behind the superficial inguinal ring.

The neurovascular plane lies between transversalis and internal oblique muscles, and the segmental lateral cutaneous nerves pierce the internal and external oblique muscles laterally to supply the external oblique muscle and skin. The nerve/vessel then continues anteriorly to enter the rectus sheath, supplying it and the anterior skin.

The rectus sheath
The rectus sheath is formed from the aponeuroses of external oblique, internal oblique and transversalis and ends in the linea alba in the midline which extends from the xiphisternum to pubic symphysis.

Superiorly, the internal oblique aponeurosis splits lateral to the rectus muscle (posteriorly it fuses with the aponeurosis of transversus abdominis passing behind rectus abdominis, anteriorly it fuses with the aponeurosis of external oblique and passes in front of rectus abdominis), rejoining in the midline at the linea alba. Midway between the umbilicus and symphysis this arrangement changes and all the aponeuroses pass in front of the rectus, the free edge of the lower posterior aponeurosis at this level is called the *arcuate ligament*. Inferiorly, the posterior aspect of the rectus muscle is separated in the lower third from the peritoneum only by the extraperitoneal connective tissue in which the inferior epigastric vascular bundle travels (Fig. 5.11).

Contents of the rectus sheath (Fig. 5.11)
- Rectus abdominis muscle
- Pyramidalis muscle
- Superior epigastric artery and vein (from internal thoracic)
- Inferior epigastric artery and vein (from external iliac)
- Lower six thoracic nerves and posterior intercostal vessels.

Inferior epigastric artery
The inferior epigastric artery is important for four reasons:
1. It is vulnerable to trauma if a finger is hooked under the rectus muscle when exposing

peritoneum on entering the abdomen or when inserting the lateral laparoscopic port.

2. It is an important landmark for inguinal hernia (direct herniae are medial to this vessel, and the deep inguinal ring lies lateral to it (see Fig. 5.13).
3. In 20% of people an abnormal obturator artery arises from it.
4. Can become arteriosclerotic and fracture causing iliac fossa pain (diagnostic problem).

The inguinal region

The free inferior edge of the external oblique aponeurosis (between its attachments to the iliac spine and the pubic tubercle) comprises the inguinal ligament. The inguinal canal extends from the deep inguinal ring (which is a defect in the transversalis fascia) to the superficial inguinal ring (which is formed by the diverging fibres of external oblique) overlying the pubic tubercle.

Surface markings of inguinal area (Fig. 5.12):

* *The mid-inguinal point* is halfway between the anterior superior iliac spine and the symphysis pubis, and is the point at which the external iliac artery becomes the femoral artery
* *The midpoint of the inguinal ligament* is halfway between the anterior superior iliac spine and the pubic tubercle, and marks the deep inguinal ring. *Note* that this is lateral to the femoral artery, but medial to the inferior epigastric artery.

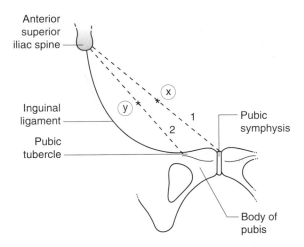

Figure 5.12 • Surface markings of the inguinal area. 1, Straight line from anterior superior iliac spine to pubic symphysis. 2, Straight line from anterior superior iliac spine to pubic tubercle. x, mid-inguinal point. y, midpoint of the inguinal ligament.

The inguinal canal

Contents of the inguinal canal:

* Round ligament or spermatic cord
* Ilioinguinal nerve (supplies the labia)
* Genital branch of the genitofemoral nerve (supplies the labia).

The spermatic cord

The spermatic cord is formed when the testis passes through the inguinal canal descending into the scrotum. It has three coverings: the internal spermatic fascia derives from transversalis fascia, the cremasteric fascia derives from internal oblique and the external spermatic fascia derives from external oblique. The cord consists of:

* Vas deferens (ductus deferens)
* Three nerves
  ○ genital branch of genitofemoral (supplies cremaster muscle)
  ○ ilioinguinal (supplies scrotum and groin)
  ○ sympathetic
* Three arteries
  ○ testicular (from aorta)
  ○ artery to the vas (from inferior vesical)
  ○ cremasteric (from inferior epigastric)
* Lymphatics (which drain to para-aortic nodes)
* Pampiniform venous plexus
* Processus vaginalis (this is the obliterated peritoneal connection with the tunica vaginalis of the testis).

Figure 5.13 illustrates the left inguinal region from behind and demonstrates the inguinal triangle (of Hesselbach) which is the position of direct inguinal herniae which are always acquired (compared with congenital indirect herniae which pass through deep inguinal ring).

The femoral region

In the femoral region (Fig. 5.13), the femoral vessels pick up fascia from transversalis (anteriorly) and psoas (posteriorly) as they pass beneath the inguinal ligament to enter the leg producing the femoral sheath. The femoral nerve lies lateral to (and outside) the sheath, while medial to the femoral vein within the sheath is a space called the femoral canal, which contains the lymph node of Cloquet draining the clitoris or glans penis. The femoral ring is the superior opening to the femoral canal and the site through which herniation can occur.

The borders of the femoral ring are:

* Inguinal ligament anteriorly
* Lacunar ligament medially
* Pectineus muscle posteriorly
* Femoral vein laterally.

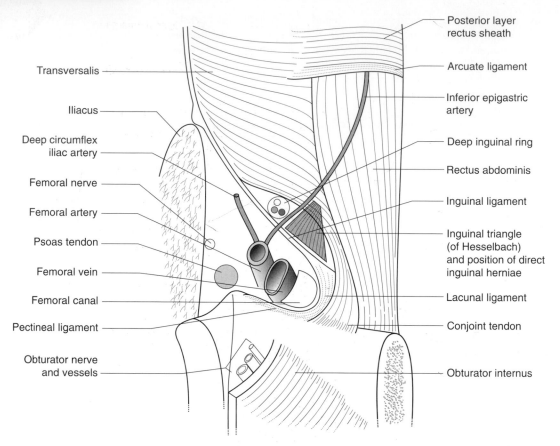

Transversalis

Iliacus

Deep circumflex iliac artery

Femoral nerve

Femoral artery

Psoas tendon

Femoral vein

Femoral canal

Pectineal ligament

Obturator nerve and vessels

Posterior layer rectus sheath

Arcuate ligament

Inferior epigastric artery

Deep inguinal ring

Rectus abdominis

Inguinal ligament

Inguinal triangle (of Hesselbach) and position of direct inguinal herniae

Lacunal ligament

Conjoint tendon

Obturator internus

Figure 5.13 • The posterior aspect of the left anterior abdominal wall showing the relationship of the structures described in the text, and illustrating the course of the inferior epigastric artery and the relative positions of the deep inguinal ring and the femoral sheath and canal.

The femoral triangle

The femoral triangle is bordered by the inguinal ligament, the medial edge of sartorius and the medial border of adductor longus. The adductor longus, pectineus, iliacus and psoas major form the floor of the triangle which contains the femoral vein and artery, the femoral nerve and its branches, and fat and lymph nodes. The apex of the triangle leads on under sartorius to the adductor (subsartorial or Hunter's) canal.

Deeper posterior abdominal muscles

Psoas

This triangular muscle arises from the transverse processes of the lumbar vertebrae, lies on quadratus lumborum and passes across the posterior abdominal wall diagonally inferolaterally to exit under the inguinal ligament and insert into the lesser trochanter of femur. Its nerve supply is from the ventral rami of the first three lumbar nerves.

The relations of psoas (Fig. 5.14)

Posteriorly
• Lumbar arteries and external vertebral venous plexus.

Anteriorly
• Ureter
• Sympathetic trunk
• Genitofemoral nerve
• Gonadal vessels.

Within

Lumbar plexus: the nerves having three main routes of exit:
• Medially: obturator and lumbosacral trunk
• Through the centre: genitofemoral nerve
• Laterally: iliohypogastric, ilioinguinal, femoral, lateral cutaneous nerve of thigh.

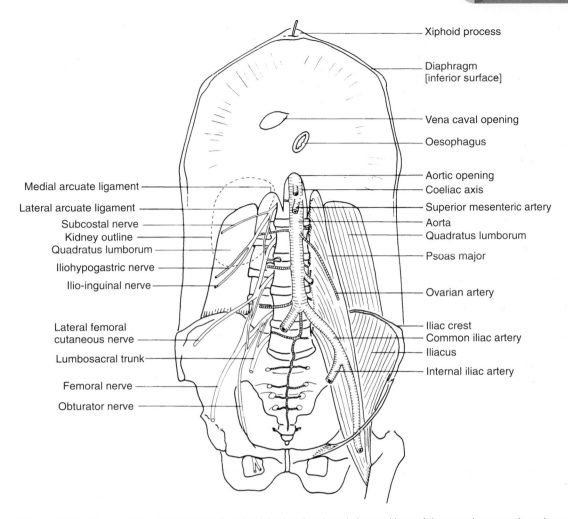

Figure 5.14 • The posterior abdominal wall and pelvis showing the relative positions of the muscles, vessels and nerves.

Peritoneal reflections

The peritoneum lines the abdomen and its contents and tends to fuse with underlying viscera (serosa) while remaining loosely attached to the internal abdominal wall (parietal peritoneum). With the development of intra-abdominal structures the peritoneum is reflected or folded producing:

- Folds – on the posterior surface of the anterior abdominal wall (where obliterated umbilical vessels and urachus run)
- Mesentery – which are double layers of peritoneum which have been reflected off the dorsal surface of the abdomen by developments of the gut. They include the mesenteries to the small intestine, transverse and sigmoid colons,

and the appendix, and they all contain vessels and nerves to supply the gut suspended from them

- The lesser omentum – which connects the stomach to the liver, while the greater omentum hangs down from the stomach lying over the transverse colon, and fusing with its mesentery (Fig. 5.15)
- Ligaments – these double layers of peritoneum are associated with the liver, stomach and spleen, and the uterus (broad ligament).

The final arrangement of the intra-abdominal structures distinguishes those things which are plastered down by their peritoneal covering (retroperitoneal) from those which are suspended from a mesentery (Figs 5.15, 5.16).

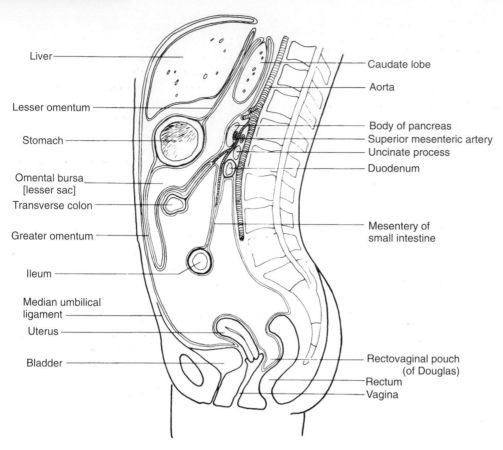

Figure 5.15 • Longitudinal section through the abdominal cavity illustrating the peritoneal reflections.

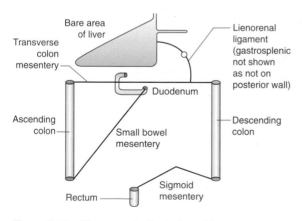

Figure 5.16 • Diagrammatic illustration of the retroperitoneal structures and the position of the roots of the mesenteries produced by the peritoneal reflections off the posterior abdominal wall.

Retroperitoneal structures (Fig. 5.16)

- The bare area of the liver
- Duodenum
- Ascending colon
- Descending colon
- Rectum (almost entirely)
- Kidneys and ureter
- Adrenals
- Major vessels (IVC, aorta, iliac).

Clinical application

- Structures suspended from a mesentery can twist but the sigmoid volvulus with its narrow base is most prone to this in the abdomen. In the pelvis, testicular torsion is a well recognized surgical emergency, but ovaries can similarly twist (although this is most commonly associated with ovarian cysts, it can also occur with normal ovaries)

- Aortic compression is rarely needed but is a potentially life-saving manoeuvre in the management of massive postpartum haemorrhage. If the abdomen is already open, the small bowel needs to be pushed up towards the right hypochondrium together with its mesentery and pressure placed on the abdominal aorta just below the mesentery (if the abdomen has not been opened then pressure applied above the forwardly tilted fundus of the uterus at the approximate level of the umbilicus can also be effective)
- If bleeding from vessels within the broad ligament occurs, rather than producing any sort of tamponade the peritoneal layers just peel away and massive haemorrhage can occur relatively silently (concealed bleeding with minimal if any intra-abdominal pain).

The greater and lesser sacs

The abdominal cavity comprises the general peritoneal cavity (or greater sac) and the omental bursa (or lesser sac) which lies behind the stomach and its peritoneal attachments (Fig. 5.15).

Lesser sac
Relations of the lesser sac:

Anteriorly
- The stomach centrally
- Lesser omentum superiorly
- Greater omentum inferiorly
- Gastrosplenic part of greater omentum on left side
- Caudate lobe of liver on right side.

Posteriorly
- The fused posterior greater omental layer with the transverse mesocolon
- Peritoneum over the neck and body of pancreas
- Left adrenal gland.

Laterally
- Limited to the left by the lienorenal ligament
- Opens into the greater sac by the epiploic foramen (of Winslow) on right.

The epiploic foramen (Fig. 5.17)
This 2.5 cm vertical slit affords communication between the greater and lesser sac. Its borders are:

Superiorly
- The caudate process of the liver.

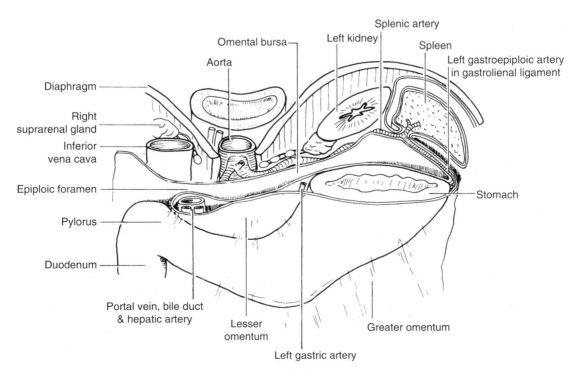

Figure 5.17 • The relations of the lesser sac and the epiploic foramen.

Inferiorly
- The first part of the duodenum.

Posteriorly
- The IVC.

Anteriorly
- The right free edge of the lesser omentum which contains:
  - the portal vein
  - the hepatic artery
  - the common bile duct
  - autonomic nerves
  - lymphatics and nodes.

The liver

This is the largest gland in the body weighing approximately 1500 g which forms from an outgrowth of foregut. It develops in the septum transversum and protrudes into the abdomen dividing the ventral mesentery into two: anteriorly the falciform ligament is produced, posteriorly the lesser omentum.

The liver is divided into the larger right lobe and the small left lobe, and between these two on the visceral (inferior) surface lie the quadrate lobe anteriorly and the caudate lobe behind. The porta hepatis lies across this visceral junction between the lobes and comprises from – in front backwards – the common hepatic duct, the hepatic artery and the portal vein.

The alimentary tract

The foregut extends from the mouth to the point where the bile duct enters the duodenum. The midgut continues on from this point to two-thirds of the way along the transverse colon. The hindgut continues from here to the rectum.

Blood supply to the gut

Blood supply to the gut is directly from the ventral branches of the aorta:
1. *The coeliac axis* supplies the abdominal portion of the foregut. It is surrounded by the sympathetic coeliac plexus and branches almost immediately into the:
   - Left gastric artery which passes left then curves round lesser curve of stomach
   - Common hepatic artery which passes right and gives off the right gastric artery (which anastomoses with the left gastric) and the gastroduodenal artery which divides into the right gastroepiploic artery (which passes

round the greater curve of the stomach) and the superior pancreaticoduodenal artery
   - Splenic artery which passes over the pancreas giving off short gastric arteries and then the left gastroepiploic artery which anastomoses with its right namesake.
2. *The superior mesenteric artery* supplies the midgut. It arises behind the body of the ancreas and the splenic vein anterior to the left renal vein and passes inferiorly over the third part of the duodenum towards the root of the small bowel mesentery. Its branches in order are:
   - Inferior pancreaticoduodenal artery
   - Middle colic, right colic and ileocolic
   - Jejunal and ileal branches from within the mesentery.
3. *The inferior mesenteric artery* supplies the hindgut. It arises below the duodenum and passes on the left psoas muscle inferiorly diagonally across the left infracolic compartment giving off the left colic and sigmoid arteries. It then enters the pelvis crossing the bifurcation of the left common iliac vessels where it lies medial to but is separated from the ureter by the inferior mesenteric vein. It terminates as the superior rectal artery (which anastomoses with the middle rectal from the internal iliac and the inferior rectal from the internal pudendal artery).

Figure 5.18 shows the relations of these vessels near their origins.

Specific features of note in the alimentary tract

Meckel's diverticulum
A Meckel's diverticulum exists in 2% of the population. This antimesenteric ileal diverticulum occurs about 30 cm proximal to the ileocaecal valve and is usually about 5 cm long. The remains of the vitellointestinal duct may persist as a fibrous band which runs from the tip of the diverticulum to the umbilicus.

The appendix
The peritoneal attachments have already been described, but although the ascending colon is retroperitoneal the caecum is often freely mobile being covered with peritoneum which has been reflected off the posterior abdominal wall. The vermiform appendix, which arises from the posteromedial aspect of the caecum just distal to the ileocaecal junction, can lie in this retrocaecal recess. The appendix has its own small triangular mesentery (mesoappendix) containing the appendicular vessels, nerves, lymph vessels and often a lymph node (Fig. 5.19).

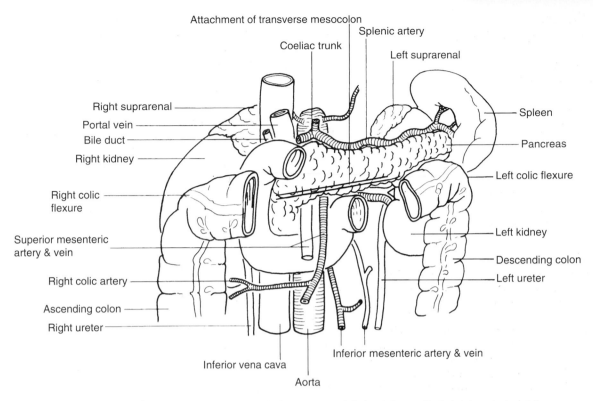

Right suprarenal
Portal vein
Bile duct
Right kidney

Right colic flexure

Superior mesenteric artery & vein

Right colic artery

Ascending colon

Right ureter

Attachment of transverse mesocolon
Coeliac trunk
Splenic artery
Left suprarenal

Spleen
Pancreas
Left colic flexure

Left kidney
Descending colon
Left ureter

Inferior vena cava
Aorta
Inferior mesenteric artery & vein

Figure 5.18 • Diagrammatic view of the upper abdominal contents and their relations with the major arteries of the alimentary canal.

Clinical applications

Due to the different positions of the appendix, the clinical presentation of acute appendicitis can vary (e.g. retrocaecal is relatively sealed versus the freely mobile appendix which can produce frank intra-abdominal peritonitis). In pregnancy, this is further complicated because:

• Signs can be relatively subtle
• Progression of pathology can be rapid due to the failure of the omentum to 'access' the problem and seal it off.

The upward displacement of the caecum by the gravid uterus can mean that the problem is localized in mid or even upper abdomen. The surgical incision for appendicectomy in pregnancy should therefore be over the point of maximum tenderness (Fig. 5.20).

Retroperitoneal organs

Adrenal glands

The medulla originates from neural crest cells (ectoderm) which develop into chromaffin cells that secrete catecholamines, while the larger cortex origi-

nates from mesoderm and secretes adrenocortical hormones.

The blood supply comes from branches of the phrenic and renal arteries and a small branch direct from the aorta. Venous drainage is by a single vein which passes into the IVC on the right, and the renal vein on the left. Lymphatic drainage is to the para-aortic nodes.

The urinary tract

Kidneys

The kidneys lie on the posterior abdominal wall within fat of the retroperitoneum. They lie between T12 and L3 with the right kidney being slightly lower than the left. The suprarenal glands sit on their superomedial poles. The hilum is a deep vertical slit on the medial aspect transmitting from anterior to posterior the renal vein, renal artery and the renal pelvis, as well as lymphatics and sympathetic nerve fibres.

Papillae of renal tissue indent each of a dozen or so minor calyces where urine drains from the collecting tubules, and these in turn drain into two or three major calyces which drain into the renal pelvis and thence via the ureter to the bladder.

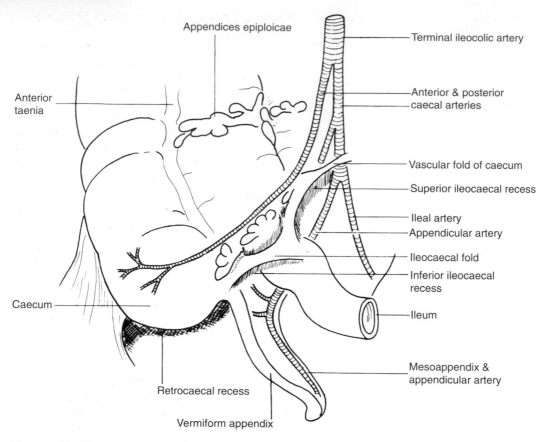

Figure 5.19 • The arrangements of the peritoneal folds and blood supply of the caecum and appendix.

Each kidney receives its blood supply directly from the aorta by means of the paired right and left renal arteries. The right renal artery passes behind the IVC to reach the right kidney. Venous drainage by the accompanying renal veins passes straight into the IVC. The left renal vein is longer than the right passing in front of the aorta below the origin of the superior mesenteric artery to reach the IVC.

Lymphatic drainage passes directly to para-aortic nodes.

Ureter: its course and relations in the abdomen

The ureter is retroperitoneal throughout its course extending from hilum of kidney to the bladder with abdominal, pelvic and intravesical portions. In the abdomen, it passes inferiorly from the renal pelvis on the medial border of psoas (in line with the tips of the transverse processes of L2–5) to enter the pelvis anterior to the common iliac bifurcation in front of the sacroiliac joint.

Blood supply
As it descends, the ureter takes its supply from small branches, in turn from the renal, gonadal, internal iliac and inferior vesical vessels.

Nerve supply
* Sympathetic via T10–12 (renal, aortic, superior hypogastric plexuses)
* Parasympathetic via S2–4
* Lymphatic drainage includes internal, external and common iliac and para-aortic nodes.
  The bladder is described in the pelvic section.

Ovarian arteries

These arise anterolaterally just below the renal branches and the right one passes posterior to the third part of the duodenum. They run retroperitoneally inferiorly towards the bifurcation of the common iliac artery where they cross the ureter and enter the pelvis in the infundibulopelvic fold. They have no branches in the abdomen, but supply twigs to the corresponding ureter,

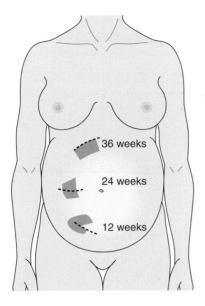

Area of tenderness and maybe rebound tenderness

----- Site of incision

Figure 5.20 • Diagrammatic illustration of the changing position of the appendix (and the approximate site of an incision for an appendicectomy) as pregnancy advances.

Table 5.4 The relations of the ovarian arteries	
The right artery crosses the inferior vena cava and is crossed by: • the middle colic vessels • the caecal vein • terminal ileal vein • ileocolic vein	The left artery is crossed by: • the left colic and sigmoid branches of the inferior mesenteric vessels • the descending colon
The right veins drain into the IVC	The left vein ends in the left renal vein

and they are accompanied by veins and lymphatics. There relations are summarized in Table 5.4.

The common iliac arteries

The common iliac arteries lie retroperitoneally anterior to the common iliac veins and the sympathetic trunk on the psoas muscles. The left artery is crossed by the superior rectal vessels and both are crossed by the ureter as they divide into internal and external iliac arteries (see Fig. 5.22). The latter are crossed near their origin by the ovarian vessels and then by the genital branch of the genitofemoral nerve, the deep circumflex iliac vein and the round ligament before passing under the inguinal ligament to become the femoral artery.

The inferior epigastric and deep circumflex iliac arteries

The inferior epigastric and deep circumflex iliac arteries arise immediately above the inguinal ligament before the external iliac becomes the femoral artery. The inferior epigastric artery passes up and medially behind the conjoint tendon to run deep to the rectus abdominis muscle to enter the rectus sheath and anastomose with the superior epigastric artery (a terminal branch of the internal thoracic). The deep circumflex iliac artery runs laterally up to the anterior superior iliac spine and thence along the crest.

The femoral vessels

The femoral vessels have four cutaneous branches arising just below the inguinal ligament:

* *Superficial circumflex iliac* (runs upwards deep to the inguinal ligament to anastomose at the anterior superior iliac spine)
* *Superficial epigastric* (passes superficial to the inguinal ligament to run towards the umbilicus)
* *Superficial external pudendal* (passes medially anterior to the round ligament to supply the labium majus)
* *Deep external pudendal* (passes medially behind the round ligament to supply the labium majus).

There are accompanying veins of the same names which drain into the great (long) saphenous vein, which in turn drains into the femoral vein approximately 3 cm inferolateral to the pubic tubercle.

Lumbar plexus

Figure 5.21 illustrates the lumbar plexus which involves the anterior primary rami from L1 to L5, and Figure 5.14 illustrates its anatomical relations on the posterior abdominal wall.

This plexus forms in the substance of the psoas major muscle and all except the subcostal nerve emerge to lie on quadratus lumborum underneath the anterior lumbar fascia. All nerves emerge from the lateral border of psoas except:

* The genitofemoral nerve which emerges anteriorly
* The obturator nerve and the lumbosacral trunk which emerge medially.

The lumbar plexus supplies:

* The thigh muscles
* Sensory to the parietal peritoneum
* Anterior abdominal wall (via iliohypogastric and ilioinguinal).

Iliohypogastric and ilioinguinal nerves

The iliohypogastric and ilioinguinal nerves pass from the lateral border of psoas anterior to quadratus lumborum behind the kidney. Both perforate the transver-

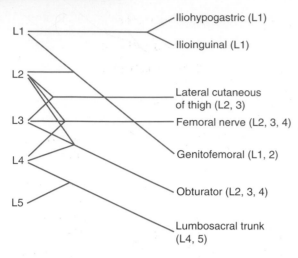

Figure 5.21 • The lumbar plexus represented diagrammatically as it forms from the anterior primary rami of the lumbar nerve roots.

Table 5.5   Structures which cross the genitofemoral nerve

Right	Left
Ureter	Ureter
Gonadal vessels	Gonadal vessels
Iliocolic artery	Left inferior colic artery
Mesentery of the small intestine	Inferior mesenteric vein
Right infracolic compartment	Left infracolic compartment

sus aponeurosis to run between that and the internal oblique, giving off lateral cutaneous branches and ending as cutaneous branches: the iliohypogastric terminating above the pubis, the ilioinguinal, running at a lower level, passing via the inguinal canal to the mons and labium majus.

Genitofemoral nerve

The genitofemoral nerve pierces the psoas anteriorly to run retroperitoneally on its anterior surface behind the ureter. Its genital branch passes through the deep ring to enter the inguinal canal, while the femoral branch runs on the external iliac artery to pass beneath the inguinal ligament to enter the femoral sheath, which it pierces to supply the skin over the femoral triangle. Its relations are summarized in Table 5.5.

Lateral cutaneous nerve of the thigh

The lateral cutaneous nerve of the thigh pierces the inguinal ligament just medial to the anterior superior spine.

Femoral nerve

The femoral nerve (L2–L4) emerges from the psoas to run in the gutter between it and iliacus deep to the iliac fascia and supplying both muscles. It passes behind the inguinal ligament lateral to the femoral artery into the thigh to supply the quadriceps muscles and overlying skin.

Obturator nerve

The obturator nerve emerges medial to psoas at the pelvic brim and passes under the internal iliac vessels on obturator internus to continue along the side wall of the pelvis to the obturator foramen which it passes through above the obturator vessels to supply the adductor compartment of the thigh and both the hip and the knee.

Lumbosacral trunk

The lumbosacral trunk (L4, 5) emerges from the medial border of psoas, crosses the ala of the sacrum, the sacroiliac joint and the upper border of piriformis where it joins S1.

Clinical applications

- The lateral cutaneous nerve of the thigh can be vulnerable to a nerve entrapment syndrome (like carpal tunnel) as it pierces the inguinal ligament due to oedema in pregnancy
- The obturator nerve, separated from the normally situated ovary only by peritoneum, can be irritated by ovarian pathology causing referred pain down the inside of the thigh (Fig. 5.22).

The pelvis

Surface anatomy

Bilateral dimples above the buttocks
- Centre of the sacroiliac joint
- Posterior superior iliac spine
- Level of S2
- Level of the end of the dural canal and of the spinal meninges.

Relations of the sacroiliac joint
- Psoas muscle/tendon
- Genitofemoral nerve
- Common iliac bifurcation
- Ureter
- Inferior mesenteric artery and apex of sigmoid mesocolon on the left
- Iliac branches of iliolumbar artery.

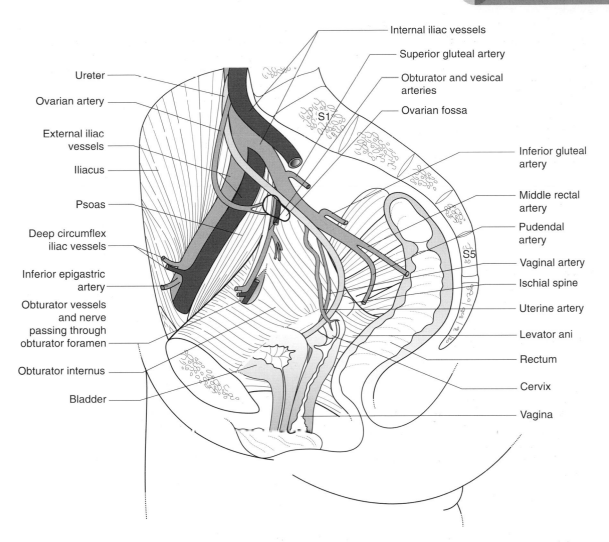

Internal iliac vessels
Superior gluteal artery
Obturator and vesical arteries
Ovarian fossa
Inferior gluteal artery
Middle rectal artery
Pudendal artery
Vaginal artery
Ischial spine
Uterine artery
Levator ani
Rectum
Cervix
Vagina

Ureter
Ovarian artery
External iliac vessels
Iliacus
Psoas
Deep circumflex iliac vessels
Inferior epigastric artery
Obturator vessels and nerve passing through obturator foramen
Obturator internus
Bladder

S1
S5

Figure 5.22 • The side wall of the female pelvis showing the course and relations of the ureter, vessels, nerves and the ovarian fossa.

Blood supply to the pelvis (Fig. 5.22)

For descriptive purposes the arterial tree is described, but the venous drainage mirrors this pattern.

Internal iliac artery

The internal iliac artery passes into the pelvis between the internal iliac vein and the ureter, to divide into posterior and anterior divisions at the upper margin of the greater sciatic foramen. The posterior trunk has three branches which are all parietal: the ascending iliolumbar and the lateral sacral branch off before the largest superior gluteal artery passes with the superior gluteal nerve through the greater sciatic foramen above piriformis to supply the buttock.

Anterior trunk

The anterior trunk continues towards the ischial spine and has nine branches:
1. Three vesical:
   ○ The superior vesical (supplies the lower ureter and upper bladder)
   ○ This continues as the obliterated umbilical artery (medial umbilical ligament) to the umbilicus
   ○ The inferior vesical artery (supplies the ureter and base of the bladder).
2. Three other visceral:
   ○ The middle rectal (supplies muscle of the lower rectum)
   ○ Vaginal arteries

○ The uterine artery – passes medially in the base of the broad ligament where it crosses the ureter to reach the cervix from where it passes upwards in the broad ligament to supply the uterus and tube ending by anastomosing with the tubal branch of the ovarian artery.

3. Three parietal branches:

○ The obturator artery runs with its nerve (above) and vein (below) to the obturator foramen

○ The internal pudendal artery passes out of the pelvis through the greater sciatic foramen below piriformis to curve round the ischial spine to enter the perineum through the lesser sciatic foramen and pudendal canal

○ The inferior gluteal artery passes out of the pelvis to the buttock below piriformis through the greater sciatic foramen.

Sacral plexus

Forms on piriformis and converges and divides on route to the greater sciatic foramen.

Posterior divisions

- Superior gluteal (L4–5, S1)
- Inferior gluteal (L5, S1–2)
- Common peroneal part of sciatic (L4–5, S1–2)

These supply the extensor compartment of the lower limb

- Posterior cutaneous nerve of thigh (S1–3)
- Perforating cutaneous nerve (S2–3)

(goes through the sacrotuberous ligament)

- Piriformis (S2).

Anterior divisions

- Tibial component of sciatic (L4–5, S1–3)
- Nerve to quadratus femoris (L4–5, S1)

These supply the flexor compartment of the lower limb

- Nerve to obturator internus (L5, S12)
- Pudendal nerve (S2–4)
- Perineal branch of S4
- Parasympathetic visceral S2–4 pelvic splanchnics (nervi ergentes).

Muscles of the pelvis

These comprise two groups:

1. Those of the lower limb (piriformis and obturator internus).

2. The pelvic floor (pelvic diaphragm and the superficial muscles).

Pelvic muscles of the lower limb

Piriformis

Piriformis arises from the lateral mass of the middle three sections of sacrum. The sacral plexus lies on it as it passes transversely leaving the pelvis through the greater sciatic foramen to enter the buttock and then insert into the greater trochanter. It serves to help stabilize the hip and is innervated by its named nerve from the posterior division of the sacral plexus.

Obturator internus

Obturator internus arises from the inner surface of most of the anterolateral wall of the pelvis including the thick membrane which covers most of the obturator foramen. This fan-like muscle then converges into a tendon which passes out of the pelvis into the buttock through the lesser sciatic foramen to insert into the greater trochanter. It is innervated by its named nerve from the anterior division of the sacral plexus.

Pelvic diaphragm

The floor of the pelvis (Fig. 5.23), the pelvic diaphragm, is a muscular sling supporting the pelvic contents and exerting sphincteric actions on the rectum and vagina which pass through it. Its deep aspect relates to the pelvic viscera, while superficially its perineal aspect forms the inner wall of the ischiorectal fossa (see Fig. 5.25). It arises from the:

- Body of the pubis
- Ischial spines
- Fascia over obturator internus.

Levator ani

The levator ani is comprised of two parts:

Pubococcygeus

This arises from the pubis and anterior half of the 'white line' obturator internus fascia in front of the obturator canal. It has three parts:

1. The more posterior fibres insert into the coccyx and anococcygeal raphe.
2. More anterior fibres sling around the rectum producing puborectalis (no raphe).
3. Anterior fibres insert into the perineal body producing pubovaginalis/levator prostate.

Iliococcygeus

Arises from the posterior half of the 'white line' fascia over obturator internus and some ischium and inserts into the anococcygeal body and raphe and the coccyx.

Coccygeus has the same attachments as the sacrospinatous ligament – this degenerating muscle used to wag the tail.

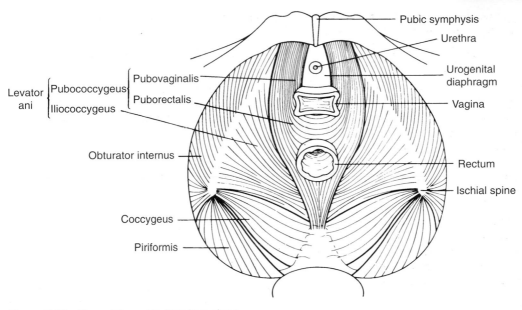

Figure 5.23 • View of the pelvic floor from above.

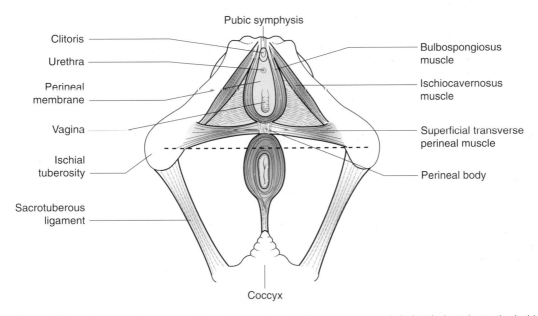

Figure 5.24 • Diagrammatic representation of the perineum showing the urogenital triangle (anterior to the ischial tuberosities) and the anal triangle (posteriorly) and the arrangements of the superficial muscles.

The perineum (Fig. 5.24)

Urogenital triangle

The anterior perineum (urogenital triangle) lies superficial to the anterior pelvic diaphragm and is bordered by a line joining the ischial tuberosities (this passes just anterior to the anus) and ischiopubic rami.

The perineal membrane is a tough fascia sheet which attaches to the sides of this triangle and is penetrated by the urethra and by the vagina in the female. The space between this membrane and the levator ani comprises the deep perineal pouch, which contains the:

- External urethral sphincter
- Deep transverse perineal muscles

- The glands of Cowper (in the male)
- Areolar tissue.

The superficial perineal pouch exists superficial to the perineal membrane and contains:

- Bulbospongiosus muscle (pierced by the vagina with the Bartholin's glands in the female, and surrounding the corpus spongiosum in the male)
- Ischiocavernosus muscles
- Superficial transverse perineal muscle.

Perineal body

The perineal body is a fibromuscular pyramid-shaped mass (base inferiorly) which lies in the midline at the junction of anterior and posterior perineum separating the lower vagina from the anal canal and is the point of attachment for:

- The external anal sphincter
- Bulbospongiosus
- Transverse perineal muscles (superficial and deep)
- Pubococcygeal fibres of the levator ani.

Anal triangle

The posterior perineum (anal triangle) lies between the ischial tuberosities and the coccyx and comprises:

- The anus and its sphincters
- The levator ani
- The ischiorectal fossae.

The ischiorectal fossae (Fig. 5.25)

The ischiorectal fossae occur bilaterally but communicate posteriorly behind the rectum with each other. Their borders are as follows:

- Superficially, skin
- Anteriorly, the anterior perineum
- Posteriorly, the sacrotuberous ligament and gluteus maximus
- Medially, the fascia over levator ani and the external anal sphincter
- Laterally, the ischial tuberosity with obturator internus and its fascia which contains the pudendal canal (of Alcock) with the pudendal vessels and nerve.

Contents:

- Ischiorectal pad of fat
- Pudendal canal (laterally)
- Transversely, the inferior rectal vessels/nerves (pudendal branches)
- Posteriorly, perineal branch S4 and perforating cutaneous nerve.

Clinical application

- Vaginal delivery can cause trauma in this area with haemorrhage which can be concealed – beware of pain out of proportion to the apparent level of injury sustained and examine carefully for fullness and tension which can be felt through the skin between anus and ischial tuberosity, or through

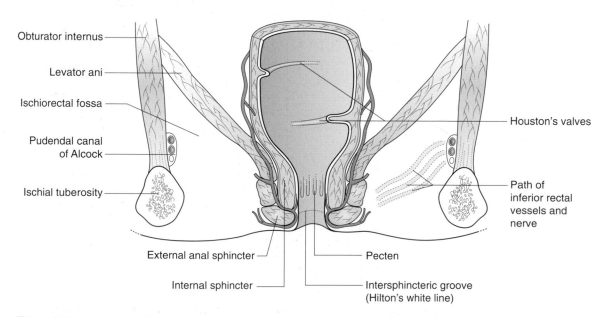

Obturator internus

Levator ani

Ischiorectal fossa

Pudendal canal
of Alcock

Ischial tuberosity

Houston's valves

Path of
inferior rectal
vessels and
nerve

External anal sphincter

Pecten

Internal sphincter

Intersphincteric groove
(Hilton's white line)

Figure 5.25 • Illustration of the relations of the ischiorectal fossae and a coronal section of the rectum and anal canal.

vaginal deviation anteriorly towards contralateral side
- Such haemorrhage can be exceedingly difficult to identify and staunch, and vaginal packing and/or embolization may be needed
- As these spaces are essentially full of fat they are vulnerable to infection which can pass from one side to the other.

Pudendal neurovascular bundle

The pudendal neurovascular bundle supplies the pelvic floor and perineum. The pudendal nerve (S2–4) lies medial to the internal pudendal artery as they exit the pelvis through the greater sciatic foramen, curving round the sacrospinous ligament to re-enter the pelvis through the lesser sciatic foramen, and thence run medial to the ischial tuberosity on the fascial thickening over obturator internus (the pudendal canal) to the deep perineal pouch. The inferior rectal nerve and artery branch off at the posterior end of the canal to travel through the ischiorectal fossa to supply the exter-

nal anal sphincter, anal canal and perianal skin. Thence, the neurovascular bundle continues anteriorly to pass superficially into the urogenital region giving off:
- Perineal branches (supplying skin of the posterior two-thirds of vulva (scrotum) and mucous membranes of urethra and vagina and supplying the perineal muscles of the deep and superficial perineal pouches)
- Dorsal nerve and dorsal and deep artery to the clitoris (penis).

Clinical application

- Pudendal nerve block is carried out by guiding a protected needle through the vagina and palpating the ischial spine. The needle is then inserted just behind the spine and withdrawn to check a vessel has not been entered before injecting the local anaesthetic. A good test of efficacy is loss of the anal reflex, relaxation of the pelvic floor and loss of sensation to the vulva and lower third of the vagina (Fig. 5.26).

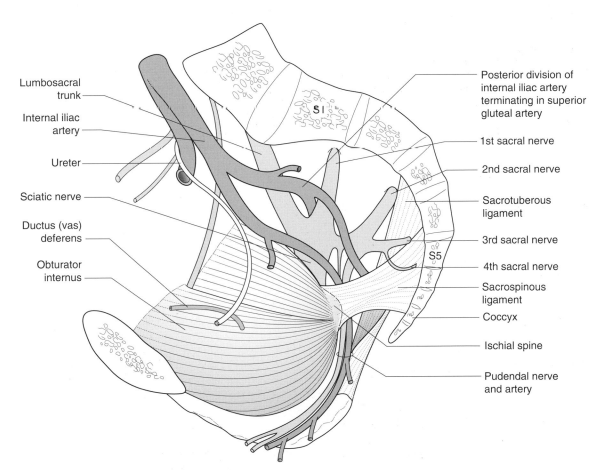

Figure 5.26 • The side wall of the pelvis showing the relative positions of nerves and vessels, and highlighting the course of the pudendal neurovascular bundle.

- Sacrospinous fixation for recurrent vault prolapse secures the vaginal vault to either one or both sacrospinous processes. The ligament is identified after reflecting the rectum away and burrowing across the ischiorectal fossa digitally. It is then grasped approximately 2 cm posteromedially from the spine to avoid damage to the neurovascular bundle.

Nerve supply to the pelvic floor

This is largely the pudendal nerve (S2–4) as described above but also includes:

- Perineal branch of S4 (passes through between coccygeus and iliococcygeus to supply the skin over the ischiorectal fossa)
- Obturator nerve (L2–4) L3 fibres supply the pelvic peritoneum explaining referred pain to the thigh.

Lateral pelvic wall

Pelvic ureter

The pelvic ureter crosses over the common iliac bifurcation to enter the pelvis and passes round the lateral wall anterior to the internal iliac artery crossing the superior vesical vessels, lying in close proximity to the obturator nerve, and passing just lateral to the base of the infundibulopelvic fold (suspensory ligament of the ovary). Once it reaches the ischial spine it turns anteromedially to pass above the lateral fornix of the vagina, lateral to the cervix and below the broad ligament and the uterine vessels, to enter the bladder. In either sex, the ureter is crossed by only one structure through its course in the pelvis: the vas in the male, and the uterine artery in the female (Figs 5.22, 5.26 and Tables 5.6, 5.7).

Pelvic organs

Ovary

Each oval gland is approximately $2 \times 3 \times 4$ cm weighing approximately 8 g during adult reproductive life. The long axis lies vertically with the infundibulopelvic fold suspended off the upper pole with the ovarian ligament connecting the lower pole to the uterine cornu. The mesovarium from the posterior aspect of the broad ligament supplies the ovary anteriorly and its posterior border lies free. Laterally, the peritoneum lines the ovarian fossa on the lateral pelvic wall adjacent to (Fig. 5.27):

- The bifurcation of the common iliac artery above
- The ureter and the internal iliac artery and vein behind

Table 5.6 Relations of the ureters

Right ureter	Left ureter
Lies behind the second part of the duodenum	
In the abdomen is crossed by:	
• Ovarian (or testicular) vessels • Right colic vessels • Ileocolic vessels	• Ovarian (or testicular) vessels • Left colic vessels • Mesosigmoid
In the pelvis is crossed by:	
• Vas deferens in the male • Uterine vessels in the female	• Vas deferens in the male • Uterine vessels in the female

Table 5.7 The relations of the ductus deferens and ureter on the pelvic side wall

Ductus deferens crosses:	Ureter crosses:
External iliac artery	External iliac artery
External iliac vein	External iliac vein
Obliterated umbilical artery	Obturator nerve
Obturator nerve	Superior vesical artery
Obturator artery	Obturator artery
Obturator vein	Obturator vein

- The obturator vessels and nerve laterally
- The ampulla of the uterine tube (curls round the top of the ovary so the ostium and fimbriae come to lie on its medial surface)
- Coils of ileum and, on the right side, the appendix.

Histology

This varies with age and the time in the sexual cycle, but the ovary has an inner medulla of loose connective tissue (blood vessels, lymphatics and nerves), while the outer cortex contains richly nucleated connective tissue stroma and follicles. The germinal epithelium covers the cortex and the dense collagenous tunica albuginea lies underneath.

At birth, there are about 2 million primordial follicles, each containing an oocyte, but follicular degeneration continues throughout life (approximately

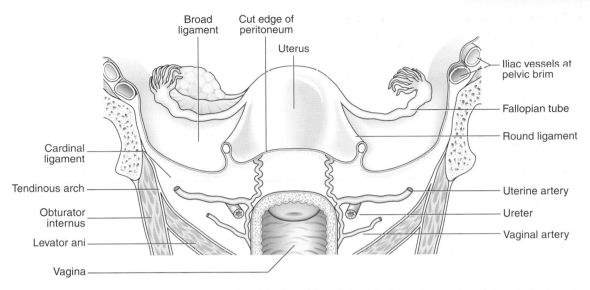

Figure 5.27 • Coronal section through the female pelvis viewed from in front illustrating the ovarian relations to the broad ligament and tube, and highlighting the relations of the uterine and vaginal vessels with the ureter lateral to the upper vagina and cervix.

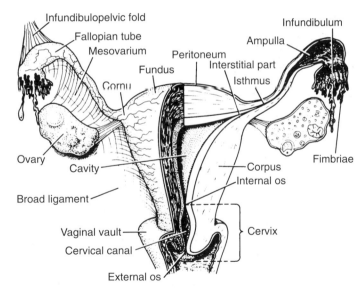

Figure 5.28 • Posterior view of the uterus and its relations.

300 000 follicles exist in a pre-pubertal girl) until the menopause, by which time no follicles remain. Each month throughout sexual life a follicle matures to become a Graafian or vesicular follicle reaching up to 2 cm in diameter. Following ovulation the follicle collapses, the granulosa cells enlarge and multiply taking on a yellow pigment, lutein and fatty material, to form the corpus luteum which persists in the event of fertilization for a few months. In the absence of fertilization, the corpus luteum functions for just under 2 weeks before degenerating to form a pale corpus albicans.

Fallopian tube (oviduct)

These fibromuscular cylinders suspend the broad ligament which forms their mesentery (mesosalpinx). Medially they open into the uterus at the uterine ostia and the thin intramural portion of the tube passing through the uterine wall continues for approximately 3 cm before expanding a little into the isthmus of the tube which is a similar length. Then the tube expands into a wide and long ampulla which becomes the infundibulum opening into the peritoneal cavity at the abdominal ostia surrounded by finger-like fimbria (Fig. 5.28).

Histology

A muscular coat (inner circular and outer longitudinal smooth muscle) surrounds a folded mucous membrane. The epithelial lining cells are low columnar but they are increasingly ciliated laterally (Fig. 5.29).

Uterus

This pear-shaped organ weighs approximately 50 g and measures approximately 8 × 5 × 3 cm in adulthood (Figs 5.27, 5.28). Its walls are 1–2 cm thick surrounding the triangular endometrial cavity whose anterior and posterior walls lie in close apposition. The whole uterus grows in pregnancy but a notable development occurs in the second half of pregnancy where the upper portion of the cervix expands upwards to accommodate the growing pregnancy and becomes the lower segment of the uterus, while the body of the uterus becomes the upper segment.

Relations of the uterus (Fig. 5.15) are:

- Anteriorly the peritoneum is reflected from the bladder to the front of the uterus at the level of the isthmus (the junction of the cervix and uterine body) to form the uterovesical pouch. It is loosely attached to the uterus inferiorly for about 1 cm, but above this level, as with serosal peritoneum elsewhere, it is firmly adherent to the underlying organ
- Laterally the double layer of peritoneum raised by the uterine covering bilaterally produces the broad ligaments which extend to the pelvic side walls each containing a fallopian tube, round ligament and ovarian ligament. At the base of the broad ligaments the extraperitoneal adipose tissue (the pelvic cellular tissue) lying lateral to the vaginal vault and cervix forms the parametrium
- Posteriorly the peritoneum remains adherent as it passes down to cover the back of the cervix and the posterior aspect of the upper quarter of the vagina. It is then reflected onto the anterior aspect of the rectum, forming the recto-uterine pouch of Douglas.

Blood supply to the uterus comes from the uterine arteries while venous drainage is by means of a plexus of uterine veins which pass below the artery in the base of each broad ligament to communicate with the vesical and rectal venous plexuses before passing into the internal iliac veins.

Lymphatic drainage from the cervix and lower uterus passes to external and internal iliac and obturator nodes, the upper uterus drains to the para-aortic nodes, and the region of the cornua and round ligament drain to the superficial inguinal nodes (Fig. 5.30).

The nerve supply to the uterus is sympathetic vasoconstrictor (T10–11) from the inferior hypogastric plexus. Pain fibres from the upper cervix and body of the uterus pass with these while pain from the cervix passes with the pelvic splanchnics.

Uterine supports

The normal uterus is anteverted (tilted forwards on the vagina) and anteflexed (bent forwards at the isthmus) but mobile with its axis at right angles to the vagina and the cervix at the level of the ischial spines.

The round ligament

The round ligament arises from the body of the uterus anteroinferior to the cornua and runs laterally between

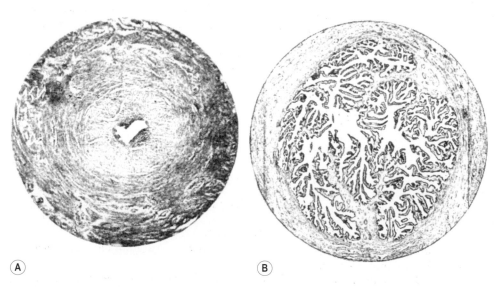

(A) (B)

Figure 5.29 • Sections through the fallopian tube: (A) through the isthmus, (B) through the ampulla.

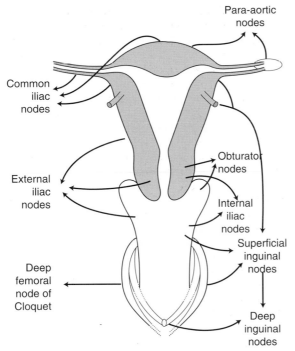

Figure 5.30 • Diagrammatic illustration of the lymphatic drainage patterns of the female genital organs.

Para-aortic nodes

Common iliac nodes

External iliac nodes

Obturator nodes

Internal iliac nodes

Superficial inguinal nodes

Deep femoral node of Cloquet

Deep inguinal nodes

Clinical applications

- The upper limit of freely mobile peritoneum on the anterior surface of the uterus is a good reliable landmark identifying the junction of lower and upper segments of the uterus at caesarean section
- Lateral to the inferior portion of the cervix, the ureter lies under the uterine vessels as it passes forwards and medially to enter the bladder. As it is within 1–2 cm of the lateral vaginal fornix, care must be taken to identify, reflect and avoid damage to it at hysterectomy (Fig. 5.27)
- In the fetus, the round ligament is surrounded by a tube of peritoneum, the processus vaginalis, which is usually obliterated at birth, but may remain patent as the canal of Nuck, the rare indirect inguinal hernia in females.

Histology

The uterus may be divided into the body of the uterus and the uterine cervix. In the body of the uterus the myometrium consists of smooth muscle fibres held together by connective tissue with blood vessels and lymphatics throughout. In pregnancy there is hyperplasia and hypertrophy of the muscle fibres but as the pregnancy grows the uterus stretches and the wall actually gets thinner.

The endometrium is in constant flux:

- Permanent thin basement membrane left after menstruation
- Regeneration by proliferation due to the influence of oestrogen
- By midcycle, endometrium thickness is 2–3 mm (columnar epithelial cells invaginate into the endometrial stroma forming tubules or glands which reach the myometrium and remain after menstruation giving rise to a basal layer from which re-epithelialization may occur)
- The secretory phase follows under the influence of progesterone (from the corpus luteum), which thickens the endometrium further (approx. 6 mm). The glands become increasingly elongated, tortuous and sacculated and the spiral arterioles are in abundance
- Ischaemia followed by necrosis results in the endometrium shedding
- If pregnancy occurs, menstruation does not take place and the endometrium continues to thicken (10–12 mm). The secretory changes continue and stroma cells are converted into large glycogen-laden decidual cells
- After the menopause the endometrium is thin and atrophic.

The cervix is largely fibrous but there is smooth muscle encircling the cervix with an outer longitudinal layer.

the layers of the broad ligament across psoas and the external iliac vessels to pass through the deep inguinal ring and the inguinal canal to the labium majus. It is largely fibrous but has some smooth muscle fibres medially (from the uterus) and some striated fibres laterally (from the internal oblique and transversalis muscles). These latter fibres correspond to the cremaster muscle in the male.

Ligaments formed from pelvic fascia

Musculofibrous bands form from condensed connective tissue over the levator ani muscles and insert into the cervix and upper vagina to form important supports to the bladder, uterus, vagina and rectum.

- The pubocervical ligament arises from fascia over the pubic bones and passes around the bladder neck
- The transverse cervical (cardinal) ligaments arise from the arcuate line on the pelvic side wall
- The uterosacral ligaments, which arise from the second sacral vertebra, are almost vertical when the woman is standing upright. As such, they pull the cervix backwards which not only supports the uterus and vagina but maintains the uterus in an anteverted position.

The mucosa is of tall columnar cells which meet the stratified squamous epithelium at the external os.

The vagina

This fibromuscular tube passes up and back from the vestibule to the cervix and lies at right angles to the axis of the uterus. Like the endometrial cavity, its anterior and posterior walls lie in apposition, with the posterior wall being slightly longer. As the cervix projects into the apex of the vagina, the resultant pockets produce the anterior, posterior and two lateral fornices.

Relations

The anterior vaginal wall lies adjacent to the bladder base, the termination of the ureters and, in its lower two-thirds, to the urethra. The posterior wall is covered by peritoneum in its upper portion, its middle third is separated from the rectum by the rectovaginal septum, while its lower third is separated from the anal canal by the perineal body. At the junction of the middle and lower third of the vagina the levator ani muscles blend with the lateral vaginal walls.

Blood supply to the upper two-thirds is supplied by the uterine and vaginal branches of the internal iliac arteries while the lower one-third is supplied by the perineal artery and dorsal artery of the clitoris which are both branches of the pudendal artery.

The venous drainage consists of an interconnecting venous plexus which follows the course of the arteries draining back into the internal iliac veins.

Lymphatic drainage occurs in three ways: its upper third drains with the cervix (to internal and external iliacs and obturator), its middle third drains to the internal iliac nodes, and its lower third drains with the vulva and perineum to the superficial inguinal nodes (Fig. 5.30).

Histology

The vagina is lined by a non-keratinized stratified squamous epithelium which is surrounded by smooth muscle and then fibrous tissue containing erectile venous plexuses, nerves and lymphatics. There are no muscularis mucosae and no glands.

The vulva

The vulva (Fig. 5.31) is comprised of fatty folds covered by skin: the labia majora lie externally and contain hair follicles, sebaceous and apocrine (modified sweat) glands, while the smaller labia minora are similar (except they are devoid of adipose tissue and contain no hair follicles) and meet anteriorly to form a prepuce over the clitoris.

The vestibule describes the area between the clitoris anteriorly, the labia minora laterally, the fourchette

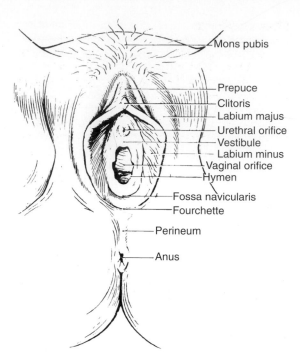

Figure 5.31 • Diagrammatic representation of the vulva.

posteriorly and the hymen superiorly. The urethra opens into its anterior portion with the para- and peri-urethral ducts of Skene. Posteriorly is the vaginal introitus with the ducts of the greater vestibular glands of Bartholin opening at 5 and 7 o'clock posterolaterally. These mucoid alkaline secreting glands of Bartholin are arranged as lobules and consist of alveoli lined by cuboidal or columnar epithelium.

The clitoris consists of two small erectile corpora cavernosa which terminate in the sensitive glans. They are attached to the medial aspects of the ischiopubic rami. The bulbospongiosus muscles lie deep to the labia and insert into the dorsum of the clitoris. They are surrounded by erectile tissue at the sides of the vestibule (the bulb of the vestibule).

The blood supply is via the internal and external pudendal arteries, while venous drainage is from an extensive plexus draining to surrounding areas.

The lymphatic drainage includes superficial and anterior areas draining to the superficial inguinal nodes and the lymph node of Cloquet, and posterior and deeper areas draining via the inferior rectal plexus to the internal iliacs (Fig. 5.30). *The nerve supply* is from the iliohypogastric and ilioinguinal nerves (mons and labia majora) and branches of the pudendal nerve.

The nerve supply is from the iliohypogastric and ilioinguinal nerves (mons and labia majora) and branches of the pudendal nerve.

The rectum

This segment of large bowel continues on from the sigmoid colon in front of the third sacral vertebrae and ends in the anal canal being approximately 15 cm long. The rectum descends following the sacral curve, but has an acute angulation in its midportion produced by the muscle sling of puborectalis, which divides it into two anteroposterior curves, and it also has three lateral curves producing small folds in the canal (valves of Houston). It lies behind the middle third of the vagina from which it is separated by the rectovaginal septum. Like the large bowel, it is lined by columnar mucosa and has an outer longitudinal and an inner circular layer of smooth muscle but, unlike the rest of the large intestine, has no taeniae or appendices epiploicae.

The rectum is largely retroperitoneal: in its upper third it is covered with peritoneum anterolaterally, in its middle third it is covered anteriorly, while in its lower third it lies below the level of the peritoneum (Fig. 5.25).

Relations of the rectum

- Posteriorly lie the sacrum and coccyx with the middle sacral vessels and lower sacral nerves
- Anterosuperiorly the pouch of Douglas usually contains loops of small bowel or sigmoid colon
- Anteroinferiorly the fascia of Denonvilliers separates it from the vagina (or prostate and bladder in the male)
- Laterally it is supported by the levator ani.

Blood supply and venous drainage are via the superior (inferior mesenteric), middle (internal iliac) and inferior (internal pudendal) rectal vessels which all anastomose freely.

Lymphatic drainage is mostly upwards via the pararectal nodes and thence along the inferior mesenteric vessels to the pre-aortic nodes, but the lower rectum drains to the internal iliac nodes (via the middle and inferior rectal vessels).

Clinical application

In obstetric injury when a fourth-degree perineal tear has occurred, the important feature to distinguish is whether the height of the anorectal mucosa tear extends above the pelvic floor. Puborectalis is the obvious sling that can normally be felt on rectal examination, which causes the acute angulation of the rectoanal junction, but this can be disrupted during parturition, or the pelvic floor can be relaxed by regional anaesthesia, making assessment more difficult. If the damage extends beyond this level, peritoneal contamination may occur and a coloproctologist should be called in for help as a defunctioning colostomy may be needed.

The anal canal

The anal canal (Fig. 5.25) is the terminal part of the alimentary canal and is 4 cm long. Its internal sphincter is an expanded portion of the circular layer of smooth muscle of rectum and involuntary while the external sphincter is a continuation of the striated voluntary levator ani muscle. The puborectalis sling produced by the levator ani which produces an acute angle in the rectum is important in continence.

The conjoint longitudinal coat is a continuation of longitudinal smooth muscle which becomes fibrous and separates external from internal sphincter attaching to the intersphincteric groove (Hilton's white line)

The upper third of the anal canal is occupied by:
- Anal columns (ridges of mucous membrane covering venous channels)
- Anal valves (connect columns of anastomosing veins)
- Anal sinuses where mucous glands open.

The pectinate line is level with the anal valves, while the pecten is the smooth part of the anal canal. The mucosa below this gradually changes from columnar to squamous epithelium which becomes keratinized and pigmented at the anal orifice, where it also contains hairs, sebaceous and sweat glands.

Arterial blood supply to the anus is from the superior rectal artery above and down to the level of the intersphincteric groove, and from the inferior rectal artery (from the pudendal artery) below this. The middle rectal and the median sacral arteries supply muscle layers.

Venous drainage follows the arterial pattern but unlike the arterial supply communicates widely, together providing portosystemic communications.

Lymphatic drainage above the intersphincteric groove is to the rectum; below the groove drainage is to the superficial inguinal nodes.

Nerve supply to the external (voluntary) sphincter is via the inferior rectal branch of pudendal nerve. The internal sphincter (involuntary smooth muscle) has a sympathetic nerve supply from the inferior hypogastric plexus (contracting the internal sphincter) and has a parasympathetic supply from nervi erigentes (relaxing it).

The bladder

This acts as a reservoir for urine (normal capacity 500 mL) and is best visualized as the bow of a boat (Fig. 5.22). It has inferolateral surfaces, is relatively sharp anteriorly (with the urachus attached from it – medial umbilical ligament), a superior surface (closely adherent to parietal peritoneum), and a flat posterior vertical surface referred to as its base. The lowest portion of the base is the trigone which is a smooth triangular area whose three points include the two ureters superiorly and the urethral orifice inferiorly. The ureters enter at an angle after tunnelling a small way through the bladder and their orifices are approximately 2–3 cm apart. The bladder is retroperitoneal and as it fills and enters the abdomen it strips off the peritoneum from the anterior abdominal wall.

Blood supply

- Two vesical (superior and inferior)
- Two visceral (vaginal and uterine)
- Two parietal (internal pudendal and obturator).

Venous drainage

Via vesico (prostatic) plexus to the internal iliacs.

The lymphatic channels

Follow the arteries draining to internal iliac nodes.

Nerve supply

- Parasympathetic supply via the pelvic splanchnics (S234) is motor to the detrusor (*para p*ees) and inhibitory to the sphincter, and these also carry pain fibres and sensory fibres relaying bladder fullness
- Sympathetic (T11–L2) is motor to the internal sphincter, inhibitory to the detrusor.

Histology

The bladder is lined by transitional epithelium surrounded by elastic areolar tissue (except at the trigone) to accommodate bladder expansion during filling. The smooth involuntary detrusor muscle becomes organized at the bladder outlet to form outer and inner longitudinal and a middle circular layer.

The urethra

This musculoelastic tube which drains the bladder originates from the pelvic portion of the urogenital sinus and is endodermal in origin. It is 3–4 cm long in the adult female and is lined by transitional epithelium proximally and stratified squamous epithelium distally. This distal portion contains small mucous glands (Skene's glands). There is an inner longitudinal urethral smooth muscle (which shortens during micturition) and an outer voluntary striated circular muscle which has a role in urinary continence.

Blood supply

- Inferior vesical artery and the internal pudendal artery.

Venous drainage

- Vesical plexus.

Lymphatics

- To the internal iliac nodes
- External urethral meatus drains to the superficial inguinal nodes.

Nerve supply

- The smooth muscle of the urethra is predominantly innervated by the parasympathetic splanchnic nerves, which cause a rise in intraurethral pressure on stimulation
- The striated voluntary urethral muscle is innervated by the somatic fibres of S2–3 via the perineal branch of the pudendal nerve.

The breast

The breast is a modified apocrine sweat gland (exocrine compound gland).

Pre-pubertal

Fully formed areola and small nipple. Composed of ducts embedded in fibrous tissue (no alveoli).

Development of the breast at puberty

- Commences between 9 and 12 years of age (thelarche)
- General maturation is promoted by growth hormone, parathyroid hormone, thyroid hormone, cortisol and insulin
- Duct growth is stimulated by oestrogen
- Alveolar (glandular) development is stimulated by progesterone
- Nipple grows, areola stays the same (no fat under either)
- Increased size due to fat deposition
- Few alveoli
- 15–20 main (lactiferous) ducts:
  - Each drains directly onto nipple surface
  - Each has dilatation or 'ampulla' under the areola
  - Each drains a lobe
  - Divided into approx. 30 lobules by fibrous septae
  - Each lobule drains 10–100 alveoli.

Changes with pregnancy

The weight of the breast and its blood supply doubles. In the first trimester alveoli bud off the duct system (progesterone stimulates glandular development/oestrogen stimulates duct growth). From the second trimester prolactin secretion increases four-fold and this with human placental lactogen stimulates colostrum formation. In the third trimester colostrum production increases and fat droplets accumulate in the alveolar cells. Postpartum, the fall in sex steroids releases the inhibition on prolactin which results in milk synthesis within a few days. This causes the breast to increase further in weight and volume as lactation establishes.

Exocrine gland milk production:

* Merocrine secretions, i.e. exocytosis – proteins
* Apocrine secretion, i.e. membrane-bound droplets – lipids.

Position

The base of the breast lies over the second to sixth rib in the mid-clavicular line extending to the parasternal margin medially and the mid-axillary line laterally. It gains its support from the ligaments of Astley Cooper (fibrous tissue connecting deep fascia to the dermis).

Blood supply

Arterial supply

* Medially: perforating branches of the internal mammary artery
* Laterally: the lateral thoracic artery (from the axillary artery)
* Inferiorly: the anterior and lateral branches of the intercostal arteries.

Other supplies include

* The pectoral branch of the acromiothoracic artery
* The external mammary artery
* The superior thoracic artery.

Venous drainage

An anastomotic circle of veins expands from the base of the nipple draining mainly to the internal mammary and axillary veins.

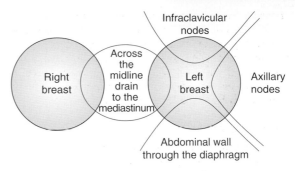

Figure 5.32 • Lymphatic drainage patterns of the breast.

Lymphatic drainage

* Lateral two-thirds to the axilla
* Medial one-third via internal thoracic to lymph trunk in root of neck and across midline draining to the mediastinum
* Superiorly drains into the infraclavicular nodes
* Inferiorly drains through the diaphragm to the mediastinum.

Free communication exists between the drainage channels but essentially:

* Superficial to subareolar plexus thence largely to axillary nodes
* Deep to submammary plexus which can go to the axillary nodes but also to the internal mammary and subdiaphragmatic nodes (Fig. 5.32).

Nerve supply

* Supraclavicular nerves (C3 and C4)
* Medial and lateral cutaneous branches of the intercostal nerves (T4–T6).

Chapter Six

Pathology

Neil Sebire

General pathological principles

Adequate understanding of the underlying pathophysiological disease processes associated with the range of obstetric and gynaecological presentations is essential for the rational evaluation of appropriate investigations, therapies and outcomes. Huge volumes of literature are available on almost all of the topics covered in this chapter but the most important essential points are summarized in the sections below. A basic understanding of general pathological principles is covered in the first section of the chapter, with the pathologies of some important examples of obstetric and gynaecological entities described later.

Cellular injury and death

There is a limited cellular repertoire of response to injury from a variety of causes including hypoxia (lack of oxygen supply), ischaemia (lack of blood supply), metabolic insults, mechanical trauma, immunological reactions, infections and toxins. Such insults may cause either a temporary impairment of cellular function followed by complete recovery, structural cellular damage with survival but ongoing impairment or, if severe or prolonged, may result in widespread cell death. Control of cellular proliferation and death is also essential for normal tissue turnover regulation and all aspects of embryonic development. The maintenance of normal tissue architecture, whether normal or neoplastic, is dependent upon the balance between cellular proliferation and cell death. At the basic cellular level there are two major types of cell death which may occur in association with the type, severity and timing of insult, namely necrosis and apoptosis.

Necrosis essentially represents a process of severe widespread cellular damage with marked cell swelling and rupture of the membrane. It usually affects sheets of adjacent cells causing disruption of normal tissue architecture with release of mediators and associated inflammation; necrosis is always pathological. Apoptosis, in contrast, essentially represents the controlled or selective death of individual or selected cells within tissues, without significant tissue destruction or associated inflammatory response, and is an essential process in both embryonic development and normal tissue turnover. The process of necrosis is mediated within the cell by rising intracellular calcium concentration, with massive cellular swelling and uncontrolled activation of intracellular enzymes, whereas apoptosis is mediated by controlled activation of specific intracellular enzyme pathways (caspases, transglutaminases and endonucleases) which result in a controlled destruction of the cell and its subsequent phagocytosis and removal.

Response to tissue injury

Following injury due to any mechanism, at a tissue, rather than cellular, level, there are three basic tissue responses which may be stimulated depending on the type and severity of the insult: acute inflammation, wound healing and chronic inflammation.

Acute inflammation

Acute inflammation is the common and stereotyped tissue response to injury from a wide range of insults. Five classical clinical features are described including redness, heat, swelling, pain and loss of function. The acute inflammatory response is mediated by the activation of a range of vasoactive and chemotactic pathways which result in local vasodilatation, with increased blood flow to the affected area resulting in redness and heat, increased vascular permeability, resulting in exudation of fluid into the interstitial tissue and swelling, and release of numerous mediators which recruit further inflammatory cells to the site and cause pain and loss of function. The primary inflammatory cell mediator of acute inflammation is the neutrophil in the early stage, followed by the macrophage with resolution. Huge numbers of mediators have now been described in association with acute inflammation including histamine, prostaglandins, leukotrienes, bradykinins and complement components in addition to an ever-expanding list of cytokines produced by the inflammatory cells themselves such as interleukin and tumour necrosis factor families. With removal or reduction of the inciting agent, the later stages of acute inflammation merge imperceptibly with the process of tissue repair and wound healing described below. Figure 6.1 shows acute inflammation in fetal membranes in a pregnancy complicated by chorioamnionitis.

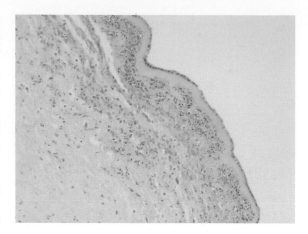

Figure 6.1 • Photomicrograph of fetal membranes from a pregnancy delivered spontaneously at 25 weeks of gestation demonstrating numerous polymorphs infiltrating the fetal membranes (chorioamnionitis); an example of acute inflammation (H&E, ×100).

Tissue repair and wound healing

The process of tissue repair or healing may involve either regeneration of the tissue to its original state by replacement of dead or damaged cells by proliferation of cells of the same type, or repair and organization, in which new connective or scar tissue replaces the original tissue. The type of process to occur depends upon the timing, severity and extent of the insult, in addition to the underlying characteristics of the tissues involved.

An example of this process is the healing of skin wounds. In wounds with closely opposed edges, healing can occur by first intention, in which an initial blood clot forms followed by cellular proliferation and migration of the marginal epidermis across the clot to bridge the defect with proliferation of blood vessels and fibroblasts into the wound edges in the underlying connective tissue to form loose granulation-type tissue which is then remodelled over time. In skin wounds in which the edges are widely separated (healing by secondary intention), there is similar, but more extensive, formation of granulation tissue but since the epithelial proliferation cannot rapidly bridge the defect, there is ongoing remodelling, with wound contraction secondary to the presence of myofibroblasts and replacement of the original tissue by scarring. The process of wound healing is further influenced by additional factors such as the local blood supply, the presence of infection or foreign bodies, excessive movement at the site or other systemic factors such as metabolic abnormalities. Defective wound healing may therefore result in either inadequate union and wound dehiscence or excessive production of scar tissue such as hypertrophic scars or keloid formation. It is clear that the control of the process of wound healing is complex and dependent upon large numbers of mediators such as transforming growth factor beta and epidermal growth factor, the manipulation of which may allow novel interventions in future. It should also be noted that there are marked differences in the potential responses to injury between different tissues and at different stages in development, with fetal wound healing and remodelling, for example, occurring very rapidly.

Chronic inflammation

Histologically, chronic inflammation is defined as an inflammatory process that is occurring simultaneously with attempted healing, rather than a simple sequential process following acute inflammation. It should therefore be noted that it may often be clinically impossible to distinguish between ongoing acute and chronic inflammation, the two potential mechanisms being persistence of a low-grade inflammatory stimulus that initially induced an acute inflammatory response, or a process involving chronic inflammation from its outset. The characteristic histopathological features of chronic inflammation are the presence of predominant mononuclear inflammatory cells, in particular lymphocytes, plasma cells and macrophages, in association with fibroblast proliferation. Many immunological diseases are associated with such chronic inflammatory responses from their outset. A specific type of chronic inflammation is termed granulomatous inflammation, which represents prominent collections of epithelioid macrophages within tissues as a consequence of either an immunological reaction or the presence of foreign organisms or material which cannot be digested and removed by macrophages (Fig. 6.2). It should be noted

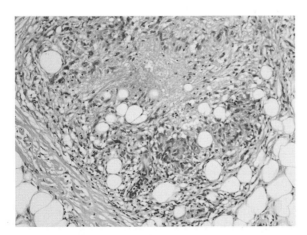

Figure 6.2 • Photomicrograph of a subcutaneous lesion demonstrating granulomatous inflammation with numerous epithelioid macrophages surrounding an area of necrosis, with numerous mononuclear inflammatory cells in the surrounding tissue (H&E, ×250).

that granulomatous inflammation and granulation tissue are entirely different processes.

Control of cell and tissue growth or differentiation

In normal tissue there is very strict control of cellular growth, proliferation, death and differentiation. Several types of abnormal tissue response may occur.

- Hyperplasia represents an increase in the number of cells in a tissue or organ, which may be physiological, such as during pregnancy, or pathological, such as with oestrogen-induced endometrial hyperplasia
- Hypoplasia is a reduction in cell number within an organ or tissue, which may also be physiological or pathological
- Atrophy represents a potentially reversible reduction in mass of the tissue, with atrophic cells usually being smaller than normal. This may also be physiological, such as in postmenopausal endometrial atrophy, or pathological, such as tissue atrophy following damaged nerve or blood supply
- Hypertrophy represents a potentially reversible increase in cell size, which may be physiological, such as the uterus in pregnancy, or pathological, such as myocardial hypertrophy in hypertension
- Metaplasia represents the change in cellular phenotype from one fully differentiated state to another, and usually occurs from stem cells in epithelia, the most common example being columnar to squamous metaplasia of the transformation zone of the cervix (see later)
- Epithelial dysplasia represents the presence of cytological changes associated with malignancy but in the absence of abnormalities of underlying tissue architecture with an intact basement membrane. For many tumours, there is thought to be a clear pathway of progression from low-grade to high-grade dysplasia through to invasive carcinoma, the primary example of which being cervical intraepithelial neoplasia as a forerunner of invasive squamous cell carcinoma of the cervix (see later)
- Neoplasia represents the process of new growth of cells
- Tumour represents a distinct mass lesion, and hence not all tumours are neoplasms
- Tumours may be simply classified as benign or malignant, and primary (arising at the site) or secondary (metastatic from another site), with specific subtyping, grading and staging on the basis of clinical and histopathological features.

Neoplasms may be benign or malignant. In general terms, benign neoplasms are usually localized, do not exhibit local destructive infiltration, do not metastasize and are often composed of relatively well differentiated cells. Malignant neoplasms demonstrate local destructive invasion of the surrounding normal tissue and the ability to metastasize (grow at sites distant from the site of origin). Despite these apparently clearcut definitions, in a range of clinical situations, the precise distinction between a benign and malignant neoplasm may be extremely difficult, although most of these are not of significance to the obstetrician and gynaecologist.

The terminology commonly used for many neoplasms implies their benign or malignant nature from the nomenclature. For example, benign mesenchymal neoplasms usually have the suffix 'oma', such as a leiomyoma, whereas malignant mesenchymal neoplasms usually have the suffix 'sarcoma', such as a leiomyosarcoma. Malignant epithelial neoplasms are termed carcinomas and many paediatric malignancies that mimic embryonal tissues are termed blastomas. Malignant neoplasms of haematological stem cells in the bone marrow are termed leukaemias, whereas other malignancies of lymphoid tissue are termed lymphomas. There are well described specific and detailed classification systems and staging systems (extent of spread) for all described malignancies from the World Health Organization (WHO) and, in the context of gynaecological malignancies, the International Federation of Gynecology and Obstetrics (FIGO).

Malignancies are defined histopathologically on the basis of abnormalities of tissue architecture and cytological features. There is loss of the normal well defined microarchitecture, with destruction of the underlying basement membrane in the case of carcinomas, and invasion of the surrounding tissue by malignant cells. Cytological features of malignancy in general include abnormal nuclear shape and size, abnormal mitoses and an increased nuclear to cytoplasmic ratio. In addition, many malignant cells demonstrate reduced or abnormal differentiation. (It should be noted here that the cell of origin of a tumour is not necessarily the same as the phenotype to which it is differentiating.) Neoplasms are a consequence of abnormalities in the normal cellular proliferation and differentiation control mechanisms, the majority of which are associated with either activation of oncogenes or loss of function of tumour suppressor genes.

Pathology of gynaecological tumours

The basic principles of neoplasia, tumorigenesis and benign versus malignant tumours have been introduced above. A wide variety of examples of such pathologies may be encountered in the female genital tract and the characteristic pathological features of some common examples are described below. Similar to most tumours in adults, by far the commonest group of malignant lesions are epithelial derived (carcinomas), the specific subtypes of which are primarily dependent on the type of epithelium normally present at that site, although it should be noted that, since the majority of the female genital tract is derived from Müllerian structures, carcinomas developing at any point may essentially recapitulate any type of Müllerian derived epithelium. Mesenchymal malignancies are rare at these sites but many of the benign neoplasms commonly encountered are derived from connective tissue components such as uterine fibroids (leiomyoma) arising from the myometrium.

Vulva

The vulva is covered by squamous epithelium and squamous cell carcinoma accounts for more than 90% of malignancies at this site, and about 5% of all female genital tract cancers. This is primarily a disease of elderly women and presents with an ulcerated or thickened area on the vulva. There is local invasion and lymphatic spread, first to the inguinal lymph nodes. In an analogous manner to the cervix (see below), preinvasive epithelial changes have now been recognized, and gradings described, termed vulval intraepithelial neoplasia (VIN). In this condition, there are mitoses, often abnormal, above the normal basal layers in association with other features of cytological atypia such as nuclear pleomorphism and a high nuclear to cytoplasmic ratio, but with an intact basement membrane.

Vagina

The vagina is normally lined by non-keratinizing squamous epithelium, and neoplasms of the vagina are rare, when they do occur most being squamous cell carcinomas in elderly women, which usually present as an ulcerating or fungating mass lesion in the upper third, with local and lymphatic spread. In a similar manner to the cervix and vulva, vaginal intraepithelial neoplasia (VAIN) has also now been described, often in women with previous cervical malignancy, the process probably representing a premalignant 'field change'. Glandular structures may sometimes be present in the subepithelial stroma of the vagina, termed vaginal adenosis, occurring either sporadically or in association with females exposed prenatally to diethylstilbestrol. Such adenosis is usually asymptomatic but may predispose to the development of clear cell adenocarcinoma of the vagina. In young girls, usually in the first 5 years of life, the vagina may also be a relatively common site of embryonal rhabdomyosarcoma, which develops in the subepithelial stroma and may present as a polypoid lesion with discharge.

Cervix

The normal ectocervix is covered by non-keratinizing squamous epithelium whereas the endocervix and endocervical canal is lined by columnar type epithelium. During puberty, the squamocolumnar junction may become situated onto the anatomical ectocervix and the exposed endocervical epithelium undergoes squamous metaplasia forming the transformation zone. Due to this mixture of epithelial types present, squamous cell carcinoma, adenocarcinoma and sarcoma may all occur in the cervix, although the commonest neoplasm by far is squamous cell carcinoma affecting the area of the transformation zone. It is hypothesized that during the process of metaplasia the epithelium at this site shows increased susceptibility to oncogenic agents such as smoking and human papilloma virus (HPV) infection, and it is increasingly clear that infection with certain subtypes of HPV is a significant risk factor for the subsequent development of cervical carcinoma.

Abnormal changes in the epithelium of the cervix are often apparent many years before the development of invasive carcinoma, i.e. there are cytological abnormalities but the changes are confined to the epithelium and have not breached the basement membrane. These preinvasive changes are termed cervical intraepithelial neoplasia (CIN), which may be graded according to increased severity of architectural and cytological changes, from grade 1 to grade 3. Invasive carcinoma of the cervix may follow high-grade CIN and initially spreads locally, often presenting as a fungating or ulcerated lesion, and then by lymphatic spread. The peak age for development of invasive squamous cell carcinoma of the cervix is around 60 years, with CIN developing around 20 years earlier.

Endometrium

The endometrium is composed of numerous glands set within a background stroma, the structure of which varies with age and throughout the menstrual cycle due to the sensitivity of the endometrium to the steroid hormones oestrogen and progesterone. Oestrogen, in the absence of progesterone, leads to proliferation of the endometrial epithelium, a normal finding in the first half of the menstrual cycle. Metaplasia of endometrial epithelium may occur but is extremely uncommon compared with metaplasia occurring in the cervix, and is not required for the development of endometrial malignancy. As expected from the nature of its normal structure, the commonest malignancy at this site is endometrial adenocarcinoma, which again, due to its derivation from Müllerian epithelium, may differentiate towards various epithelial phenotypes. The proposed precursor lesion of endometrial adenocarcinoma is endometrial hyperplasia which may occur in high oestrogen states, the risk being greatest for atypical complex hyperplasia in which there are both architectural and cytological abnormalities. Endometrial adenocarcinoma usually presents with abnormal vaginal bleeding in a peri or postmenopausal woman and often remains confined to the uterus at presentation, although may spread locally or by lymphatics. Histologically, endometrial adenocarcinoma demonstrates abnormal, closely packed glandular structures with cytological abnormalities including nuclear enlargement, hyperchromasia and abnormal mitoses. Rarely, endometrial stromal sarcomas or malignant mixed Müllerian tumours may occur with a malignant component derived from the stroma.

Myometrium

The connective tissue elements of the female genital tract only rarely give rise to neoplasms, the commonest by far being benign smooth muscle tumours of the myometrium (leiomyomata or fibroids). These occur as single or multiple intramyometrial lesions composed of interlacing bland spindle cells, which may show secondary changes such as infarction or myxoid degeneration. The other lesion that may commonly present as intramyometrial pathology, although not a true neoplasm, is adenomyosis, characterized by nests or nodules of endometrium within the myometrium (or at other extrauterine sites).

Ovary

The pathology of the ovary varies somewhat from the remainder of the female genital tract since, in addition to being covered with Müllerian derived surface epithelium and containing a stromal component, the ovary also contains germ cells. The three major groups of primary tumour of the ovary may therefore be classified into those derived from epithelium, sex cord stromal tumours and germ cell tumours.

About 90% of malignant ovarian tumours are derived from the surface epithelium and are therefore carcinomas. Analogous to carcinomas from other sites in the female genital tract, ovarian carcinomas may differentiate along various pathways normally taken by Müllerian epithelia, and hence may be serous, mucinous or endometrioid adenocarcinomas, although other rare types may of course also occur. Ovarian adenocarcinoma generally affects elderly women and, due to the lack of direct communication with a lumen, presentation is often with non-specific features, the disease being of advanced stage at diagnosis. Benign epithelial tumours may also occur (cystadenomas), and a group of epithelial tumours of intermediate malignancy have also been described (borderline tumours).

Sex cord stromal tumours represent neoplasms of specialized stromal cells such as granulosa cells, Sertoli cells, theca cells, Leydig cells or specialized fibroblasts. Since these cells are often hormone-producing, such tumours may present with the consequences of abnormal hormone levels.

Germ cell tumours are relatively common in the ovary, especially in younger patients and represent a diverse group which may show minimal phenotypic differentiation, such as dysgerminomas, or extreme degrees of differentiation along all three embryonic pathways, such as mature teratomas. In addition, differentiation may be towards extraembryonic developmental elements such as trophoblast in choriocarcinoma (see Fig. 6.3) or yolk sac structures in yolk sac tumour. Teratomas are the commonest ovarian neoplasms, most being mature teratomas in which a wide range of well differentiated histological tissue types are present with associated generally benign behaviour. Some teratomas may contain immature elements such as neuroepithelial tubules, with an increased risk of malignant behaviour, and other teratomas may contain frankly malignant elements such as embryonal carcinoma or yolk sac

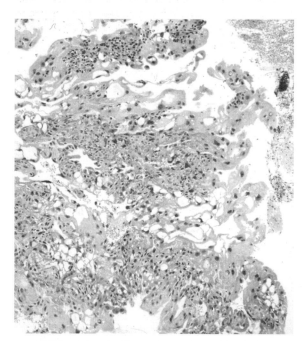

Figure 6.3 • Photomicrograph of fragments of choriocarcinoma demonstrating abnormal trophoblast with biphasic architecture and cellular features of malignancy such as nuclear pleomorphism, nuclear hyperchromasia and apoptotic debris (H&E, ×250).

tumour. Pure malignant germ cell tumours of the ovary, such as pure yolk sac tumour, may also occur, and are the commonest ovarian malignancies in young children.

Pathology of miscarriage and gestational trophoblastic disease

For the purposes of this chapter, miscarriage will be defined as the loss of the conception prior to viability. This is a relatively common event, occurring in around 15% of clinically recognized pregnancies. The underlying causes of miscarriage are varied and, although epidemiological studies have shed light on possible associated underlying categories of factors, the cause often cannot be determined with certainty in an individual case.

Chromosomal abnormalities

The commonest demonstrable underlying abnormality in first- and early second-trimester miscarriage is fetal chromosomal abnormality, including trisomies, polyploidy and other abnormalities such as monosomy. In cases in which karyotyping has been carried out, up to 50% of first-trimester miscarriages may be chromosomally abnormal, varying with underlying predisposing factors such as maternal age.

Infection

Obstetric and pathological literature from several decades ago suggested that infection was a common and important underlying cause of miscarriage. More recent data suggest that, although some infections may be teratogenic or cause miscarriage in early pregnancy, underlying infection is in reality an uncommon cause of first-trimester pregnancy loss. In contrast, ascending genital tract infection with either localized inflammation overlying the cervical os or frank chorioamnionitis is the commonest cause of late second-trimester spontaneous miscarriage.

Maternal disease

Miscarriage has been reported in association with a wide range of underlying maternal diseases or exposure to external agents such as drugs or radiation. However, documented and identifiable maternal disease represents the underlying cause of only a tiny proportion of spontaneous miscarriages.

Other factors

It will be clear from the above discussion that the underlying aetiology in many miscarriages cannot be determined with certainty, despite appropriate investigation. Pathological examination of the miscarriage specimen may be of use in identifying certain specific underlying causes, such as molar pregnancies (see below), or to suggest an underlying fetal abnormality or chromosomal defect, in a minority of cases. However, data from various sources, including pathological examination, have demonstrated that a relatively common mechanism involved in first-trimester pregnancy loss is defective trophoblastic invasion of the decidual and uterine vasculature with subsequent excessive blood flow to the developing conceptus in early pregnancy and secondary mechanical or oxidative damage. It is likely that such defective trophoblastic invasion represents a final common pathway of many conditions that may be associated with miscarriage, such as the presence of thrombophilic maternal conditions (e.g. antiphospholipid antibody syndrome) or other proposed maternal immunological factors.

The causes of second-trimester miscarriage and intrauterine death in the third trimester are similarly varied, with the major underlying aetiological categories being fetal abnormality, ascending genital tract infection and defects of uteroplacental and intervillous flow secondary to impaired trophoblastic invasion (see below).

Gestational trophoblastic neoplasia

A related group of abnormalities characterized by abnormal trophoblast proliferation are encompassed by the term gestational trophoblastic neoplasia (GTN), and include partial and complete hydatidiform mole, invasive mole, choriocarcinoma (Fig. 6.3) and placental site trophoblastic tumour. The commonest of these entities, partial and complete hydatidiform moles, occur in 1 in 500–1000 pregnancies and usually present with first-trimester miscarriage, the diagnosis of mole being suspected at ultrasound examination or following routine pathological examination of the evacuated products of conception. Both partial and complete hydatidiform moles are characterized by abnormal trophoblastic proliferation in association with abnormal fetal development due to defective imprinting as a consequence of an abnormal chromosomal constitution with an excess of paternal genomic material. Complete hydatidiform moles are diploid, but with both sets of chromosomes derived from the father following fertilization of an anucleate oocyte, whereas partial hydatidiform moles are triploid, with the extra set of chromosomes derived from the father following fertilization of a normal oocyte by two sperm. In both cases, the relative excess of paternal chromosomal material results in overgrowth of the trophoblast of the placenta and impaired embryonic development.

In addition to presenting clinically as miscarriage, the main clinical consequence of partial and complete hydatidiform moles is the possibility of their developing into persistent gestational trophoblastic neoplasia, occurring in around 0.5% and 15% of cases, respectively. Should it occur, such persistent disease may represent localized invasive mole, malignant and often metastatic choriocarcinoma, or the rare placental site trophoblastic tumour. Cases of hydatidiform mole should therefore undergo surveillance by measurement of maternal serum hCG concentrations (produced by the proliferating trophoblast) in order to detect persistent disease at an early stage when it is highly responsive to chemotherapy. The malignant forms of gestational trophoblastic neoplasia, choriocarcinoma and placental site trophoblastic tumour, although orders of magnitude more common following molar pregnancies, may also rarely complicate non-molar pregnancies, and even those resulting in live birth require specialist management.

Pathology of common congenital abnormalities

A huge range of congenital abnormalities is now described with a corresponding entire subspecialty dedicated to their pathogenesis and management. An understanding of the appropriate terminology makes their classification more intuitive and improves understanding of the literature in this field.

- An anomaly is defined as any deviation from the expected normal type of structure, form or function which is interpreted as abnormal
- A malformation is a morphological defect of an organ or region of the body as a consequence of an intrinsically abnormal developmental process
- Dysplasia, in the context of congenital abnormality, is defined as an abnormal organization of a tissue, or defective histogenesis
- A disruption represents a morphological abnormality of an organ or region of the body resulting from extrinsic interference with an originally normal developmental process
- A deformation is defined as an abnormality in shape or position of part of the body due to mechanical forces
- A sequence is a term used for a pattern of multiple abnormalities derived from a single presumed prior factor
- A syndrome represents multiple associated abnormalities thought to be pathogenically related but not representing a sequence
- An association is a non-random occurrence of multiple morphological abnormalities not identified as a sequence or syndrome

- A developmental field defect is a combination of abnormalities as a result of disturbed development of an embryonic morphogenic field.

It will be apparent from the above terms that a wide range of underlying aetiological factors may therefore result in the phenotype of congenital abnormality, the most common of which include chromosomal abnormalities, single gene defects, polygenic defects, mitochondrial defects, imprinting abnormalities, triplet repeat sequence defects and a large number of disruptions due to teratogens, metabolic diseases, immunological reactions and infections. The recurrence risk may therefore theoretically range from essentially 0% to 100% depending on the underlying aetiology. It should however be noted that the vast majority of human congenital abnormalities appear to be sporadic, with low empirical recurrence risks, presumably the cause of an interaction of genetic factors and environmental factors (so-called multifactorial defects) which do not fit neatly into the other categories listed above.

Congenital abnormalities can also be classified according to the presumed stage of human development which is primarily affected to lead to the phenotype. These include abnormalities of pregenesis, blastogenesis, embryogenesis or phenogenesis, examples of each being fetal aneuploidy such as trisomy 18, holoprosencephaly, isolated limb defects and deformations such as talipes secondary to oligohydramnios, respectively.

Pathology of the placenta

In order to understand the pathology which may affect the placenta, an understanding of normal placental development, anatomy and physiology is required, which is covered in other parts of the text. In summary, however, the human placenta is a discoid, haemomonochorial, multivillous organ in which fetal blood perfuses the vascular bed within the branching chorionic villous tree, whereas maternal blood directly enters the intervillous space to surround the villi. In later pregnancy, focally only a single layer of trophoblast and basement membrane separates the maternal and fetal circulations, which in normal circumstances never come into direct contact. The anatomy and physiology of the placenta changes throughout gestation and both developmental and acquired disease processes may occur.

A potentially wide range of pathologies may affect the placenta, just as any other organ, including neoplastic (choriocarcinoma), infective (chorioamnionitis) and inflammatory (autoimmune) processes; however, the vast majority of the important conditions in which there are specific placental pathological features represent either ascending genital tract infection leading to preterm delivery or abnormalities in uteroplacental,

intervillous or fetal blood flow through the organ. Such abnormalities may simply be classified as those affecting primarily the fetal circulation, such as fetal stem vessel thrombosis, and those affecting primarily the uteroplacental or intervillous flow, such as uteroplacental vascular disease (see below) or massive perivillous fibrin deposition. Although the human placenta has moderate functional reserve capacity, a significant reduction in uteroplacental or intervillous flow can result in reduced oxygen delivery and hence reduced oxygen transfer, with concomitant reduction in the delivery or transport of other substances in addition to secondary consequences on fetoplacental flow.

Intrauterine growth restriction and pre-eclampsia

It is now clear that the underlying pathophysiological basis for a wide range of pregnancy complications such as miscarriage, intrauterine growth restriction and pre-eclampsia is related to abnormal, defective trophoblastic invasion of decidual and uterine vessels, with consequent significant reduction in uteroplacental blood flow and therefore perfusion of the intervillous space, as pregnancy advances. In normal pregnancies, there is early trophoblastic invasion of the decidua with coordinated invasion of the decidual arterial branches which are completely or partially occluded by trophoblastic 'plugs' in early pregnancy. With advancing gestation into the second trimester and beyond, the interstitial and endovascular trophoblastic invasion progresses to involve deeper uterine vessels with conversion of the muscular uterine artery branches into the relatively flaccid and low-resistance uteroplacental vessels normally encountered in later pregnancy. Such physiological changes are thought to prevent excessive blood flow during the implantation period but allow a dramatic increase in uteroplacental blood flow with advancing gestation in association with significant reductions in the vascular reactivity of these uteroplacental vessels.

Pathological studies have clearly demonstrated that defective trophoblastic invasion and conversion of uterine arteries to uteroplacental vessels is the common underlying mechanism in cases of severe asymmetrical intrauterine growth restriction (IUGR) and pre-eclampsia, with or without superimposed acute vascular changes such as atherosis or thrombosis with infarction (Figs 6.4, 6.5). More recently, this defective haemodynamic process has been identified by Doppler ultrasound imaging of the uterine arteries in midgestation, manifest by the presence of a notch in the Doppler flow velocity waveform or increased resistance indices. Although the underlying defect is a marked reduction in uteroplacental blood flow, there are autoregulatory and compensatory mechanisms within the fetal part of

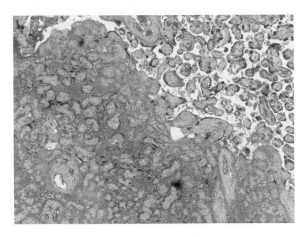

Figure 6.4 • Photomicrograph of placenta from a case of severe intrauterine growth restriction demonstrating an area of evolving villous infarction, indicating severe reduction in uteroplacental blood flow (H&E, ×40).

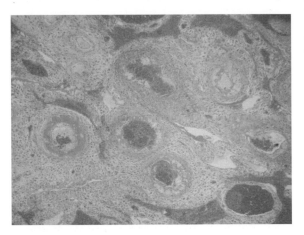

Figure 6.5 • Photomicrograph of the decidual basal plate from a patient with severe pre-eclampsia demonstrating numerous abnormal vessels, many of which exhibit foam cells within their walls (atherosis), indicating severely impaired trophoblastic invasion (H&E, ×25).

the placenta which allow a degree of fetal compensation, but when severe may lead to characteristic pathological changes within the structure of the placenta, such as vasoconstriction of the fetal stem vessels in association with the presence of small, poorly branched and poorly vascularized chorionic villi. Such changes lead to secondary abnormalities of fetoplacental flow with high fetoplacental resistance, which can be identified antenatally by Doppler ultrasound imaging of the umbilical arteries, manifest as increased pulsatility index and absent or reversed end-diastolic frequencies. It should be noted that, although this mechanism is the

presumed underlying pathophysiological mechanism for the majority of cases of asymmetrical intrauterine growth restriction, other mechanisms for growth restriction also exist in specific circumstances.

Although the underlying pathophysiological changes in the placenta appear to be similar in cases of classical intrauterine growth restriction and pre-eclampsia, the difference in maternal phenotype is probably a consequence of the maternal response to the haemodynamic changes, which appears to be related to both fetal and maternal characteristics. The underlying concept central to the development of pre-eclampsia is probable release of an, as yet unidentified, vasoactive substance by the placental tissue which leads to widespread maternal vasoconstriction and abnormal vascular permeability.

In response to a severe reduction in uteroplacental flow, and hence oxygen and nutrient delivery, the fetus demonstrates several haemodynamic compensatory responses, together commonly known as 'fetal brain sparing' or 'redistribution'. This response is characterized by reduced flow resistance and increased blood flow to the brain in association with reduced blood flow to the abdominal viscera and limbs. Such fetal redistribution of blood flow is mediated by vasoactive responses to fetal hypoxia and acidosis. In association with severe and long-standing uteroplacental IUGR, secondary haemodynamic changes occur in the fetal venous system, which probably represent cardiac dysfunction, and are indicators of advanced stages of the condition, preceding intrauterine fetal death. Determination of a combination of these haemodynamic fetal factors using Doppler sonography can allow optimal management and timing of delivery in fetuses with severe IUGR.

Ascending genital tract infection

Although bacteria are always present within the vagina, the uterine cavity is usually sterile during pregnancy. Infection may be transmitted to the placenta and fetus by several potential mechanisms, including direct inoculation (e.g. at the time of amniocentesis), haematogenous spread, or infection ascending along the cervical canal. The cervix is normally plugged by mucus and is closed anatomically. Development of ascending genital tract infection probably requires a combination of factors including the type of bacteria present in the vagina, loss of the normal cervical mucous plug and cervical shortening and dilatation. Once it occurs, ascending infection causes a supracervical inflammatory reaction with local production of mediators such as prostaglandins and cytokines which can initiate the cascade of events leading to delivery. Hence, depending on the timing, ascending genital tract infection may lead to spontaneous miscarriage or extremely pre-term delivery. Furthermore, the infection may pass into the amniotic cavity with resulting fetal infection, further compromising the prematurely delivered infant. Finally, due to the inflammatory mediators associated with infection combined with the complications of preterm delivery, chorioamnionitis has been suggested as a significant risk factor for the development of cerebral palsy.

Only a minority of cases of ascending genital tract infection will manifest with maternal systemic symptoms and signs of sepsis, the majority leading to the onset of labour without systemic upset. Histologically, ascending genital tract infection is characterized by infiltration of the fetal membranes with neutrophil polymorphs, most marked in the area overlying the cervix.

Chapter Seven

7

Microbiology and virology

Geoffrey Ridgway & Paul Taylor

Bacteriology, mycology and parasitology

Introduction

Bacteria are the smallest organisms capable of a free-living existence. That is, with the exception of a few highly evolved examples, they are able to take up nutrients from the environment, grow and self-replicate independently of other living cells. Their biochemical pathways are similar to those of other organisms, but they are morphologically less complex than the cells of higher organisms. The adjective 'prokaryotic' distinguishes the absence of membrane-bound organelles characteristic of bacteria from the 'eukaryotic' cell characterized by the presence of a nuclear membrane.

Morphology and structure

Most bacteria are 1 μm in diameter or larger, which means that they are readily visible by light microscopy and conventional bright-field illumination. However, to visualize the internal structures of the cell, the resolv-

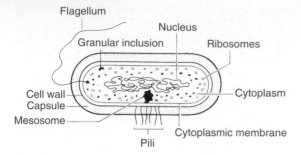

Figure 7.1 • Prototype bacterial cell.

ing power of an electron microscope is required. Figure 7.1 is a diagrammatic representation of the internal structures of the prokaryotic cell.

Many bacteria have a capsule or loose slime around the cell wall. This is an important protective mechanism. The ability of organisms such as *Staphylococcus epidermidis* to produce slime (glycocalyx) on the surfaces of cannulae results in the protection of the organism from the action of antimicrobial agents, and difficulty in eradicating the organism in catheter-associated sepsis.

The cell wall of bacteria is unique. It consists of a backbone of *N*-acetyl-glucosamine and *N*-acetyl-muramic acid residues linked to polypeptides, polysaccharides and lipids, called 'peptidoglycan'. Peptidoglycan is responsible for the rigidity of the cell wall, and maintenance of the characteristic shape of an organism. Gram's stain differentiates bacteria into those that take up and retain a complex of crystal violet and iodine, and those that do not. This ability is a function of the cell wall. Gram-positive organisms (stained blue/black) have a cell wall consisting largely of peptidoglycan linked to teichoic acids. In contrast, the cell wall of Gram-negative organisms (usually counterstained pink) is far more complex with an outer membrane of lipoprotein and lipopolysaccharide (also unique to bacteria), separated from the peptidoglycan layer by the periplasmic space. This arrangement has important consequences for the ability of Gram-negative bacteria to neutralize the activity of certain antimicrobial agents such as the cell wall active β-lactams (penicillins and cephalosporins). Peptidoglycan is synthesized with the assistance of transpeptidases, also known as penicillin-binding proteins (PBPs), which are a target for β-lactams. This group of antibacterial agents is thus acting against a metabolic pathway unique to bacteria, with consequent low toxicity to eukaryotic cells. The presence of β-lactamases in the periplasmic space may result in the bacteria being resistant to these agents. Mycoplasmas are unique among bacteria in not having a rigid cell wall, while the chlamydiae lack peptidoglycan. Not surprisingly, these bacteria are essentially resistant to β-lactams.

The cell wall of acid-fast bacteria such as the mycobacteria and *Nocardia* spp. contains a high lipid content. They are difficult to stain by most stains, but a solution of hot phenolic carbol fuchsin, or the fluorochrome auramine, which binds to the lipid, will resist decoloration with sulphuric acid, and stain the organism.

The nucleus is a tightly coiled circular double strand of DNA, which replicates by simple fission. Other units of straight or circular DNA termed 'plasmids' may occur loosely in the cytoplasm. These may code for non-essential features such as antibiotic resistance or ability to ferment certain sugars such as lactose. The ability of bacteria to transfer plasmid DNA between bacteria of the same or different species may result in the spread of antimicrobial resistance (plasmid mediated). Bacteria may also transfer genetic material from the nucleus (the so-called 'jumping gene'), leading to stable, chromosomally mediated resistance.

Projecting through the cell wall may be flagellae, fimbriae or pili. Flagellae are long whip-like structures associated with motility. Fimbriae form a fringe around bacteria allowing gliding movement. Pili are longer than fimbriae, and more numerous than flagellae. They are associated with conjugation between bacteria of the same or different species, during which the exchange of genetic material, and hence transferable antibiotic resistance, can occur.

The majority of bacteria are either rod-shaped (bacilli) or spherical (cocci). Cocci may be in chains, e.g. streptococci, or in clusters, e.g. staphylococci. Comma-shaped bacteria called 'vibrios' and the spirochaetes are examples of spirally coiled bacteria. The actinomycetes are the only genus-forming branching filaments. However, in smears, lactobacilli which are morphologically similar may appear to branch, leading to confusion in the evaluation of cervical specimens for actinomycosis.

A few bacteria will produce endospores, a highly resistant resting phase. This is a particular feature of the genera *Bacillus* spp. and *Clostridium* spp.

Classification and typing

The classification of bacteria is complicated by the lack of clearcut evolutionary relationships between different members. Although the familiar hierarchy of species, genus, family, order, etc. is preserved, it often represents a grouping of organisms with shared characteristics rather than evolutionary relatedness. Knowledge of a simple classification is however important for a number of reasons. It enables communication between scientists, gives a broad picture of how the organism may behave *in vitro* and *in vivo*, and may give some indication of the likely efficacy of proposed antimicrobial chemotherapy. Properties used in the classification of bacteria include: morphology, staining reaction, need for oxygen, utilization or production of various chemicals, chemical constitution and, increasingly, genomic make-up. The latter includes genome size, guanosine and cytosine ratio (GC ratio) and DNA relatedness as determined by hybridization and sequencing techniques.

The naming of bacteria follows the conventional Latin binomial system which is overseen by an international body that applies strict rules. The genus is always written with a capitalized first letter, and followed by the specific epithet commencing with a lower-case letter. Both components are written in italics – thus, *Staphylococcus* spp. and *Staphylococcus aureus*. The generic name may be abbreviated after first use, thus *S. aureus*, or if confusion is likely to *Staph. aureus*. All other references to specific bacteria are not italicized, including family names such as 'Enterobacteriaceae', trivial names such as 'coliform', or adjectives such as 'staphylococcal'. Table 7.1 is a simple classification of medically important bacteria based on these characteristics.

In addition to a need to classify bacteria, it is often necessary to distinguish between infecting organisms of the same species, for example when trying to trace the source of a staphylococcal outbreak, or confirming the chain of infection in a case of alleged sexual abuse. A variety of methods are available; some more applicable to some species than others. It is always much easier for bacteriologists to prove that two organisms are different, than the converse.

The protein and polysaccharide components of the bacterial cell are highly antigenic. Differences in the structure of lipopolysaccharides in the cell wall of Enterobacteriaceae (see Table 7.2) are the basis for somatic or O typing of strains. Capsular polysaccharide antigens are used for K typing and flagella antigens provide the H antigens. Typing using antibodies to H and O antigens is of particular importance in 'speciating' *Salmonella* spp. The Vi antigen is a further virulence marker particularly associated with *S. typhi*. *Shigella* spp. and enteropathogenic *Escherichia coli* isolates are also typed using antibodies to the O antigens.

Staphylococci are infected with highly host-specific viruses called 'phages'. These phages may transfer genetic material between different staphylococci in a way analogous to plasmid transfer in other bacteria. The pattern of phages infecting a staphylococcus can also be used to demonstrate that the same strain of staphylococcus is responsible for an outbreak. Other methods include biotyping on biochemical features, serotyping based on specific antibodies, antibiograms based on antimicrobial resistance, protein composition (e.g. gel electrophoresis and isoelectric focusing) and plasmid typing. Application of molecular technology has produced highly specific techniques based on

Table 7.1 A simple classification of medically important bacteria

Free living organisms

Gram-positive cocci
  Aerobic
    Staphylococcus spp.
    Streptococcus spp., *Enterococcus* spp.
  Anaerobic
    Peptostreptococcus
Gram-positive bacilli
  Aerobic
    Spore forming
      Bacillus spp.
    Non-spore forming
      Lactobacillus spp.
      Corynebacterium spp., *Listeria* spp.
  Anaerobic
    Clostridium spp.
Gram-negative cocci
  Aerobic
    Neisseria spp., *Moraxella* spp.
  Anaerobic
    Veillonella spp.
Gram-negative bacilli
  Aerobic or facultative anaerobic
    Small rod-shaped
      Legionella spp., *Haemophilus* spp.
      Bordetella spp., *Brucella* spp.
      Pasteurella spp., *Bartonella* spp.
    Comma-shaped
      Vibrio spp.
    Helically curved
      Campylobacter spp., *Helicobacter* spp.
    Large rod-shaped
    Fermentative
      Escherichia spp., *Klebsiella* spp.
      Enterobacter spp.
      Salmonella spp., *Shigella* spp., *Yersinia* spp.
    Non-fermentative
      Pseudomonas spp., *Stenotrophomonas* spp.
  Anaerobic
    Bacteroides spp.
    Prevotella spp.
Gram-variable cocco-bacilli
  Mobiluncus spp., *Gardnerella* spp.
Stain with acid-fast stains (e.g. Ziehl–Neelsen)
  Mycobacterium spp., *Nocardia* spp.

Obligate intracellular organisms

  Chlamydia spp., *Rickettsia* spp., *Coxiella* spp.

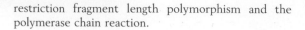

restriction fragment length polymorphism and the polymerase chain reaction.

Pathogenesis

The distinction between commensal and pathogenic organisms is far from clearcut. Indeed, many of the organisms associated with common infections are part of the normal or transient flora of the body. Mere isolation of the organism from a specimen does not necessarily equate with disease, rather it is isolation of the organism in a site normally sterile. The presence of *E. coli* in the bowel reflects its normal habitat, but its presence in bladder urine indicates urinary tract infection. *Haemophilus influenzae*, *Streptococcus pneumoniae* and *Moraxella catarrhalis* are all on the one hand normal inhabitants of the upper respiratory tract, and on the other capable of causing lower respiratory tract infection.

Some organisms are always pathogenic to humans. Examples include the plague bacillus, *Brucella* spp. and *Treponema pallidum*. At the other extreme are organisms that are usually quite innocuous unless the host's defences are markedly impaired. These are the 'opportunistic' organisms, such as *Pseudomonas aeruginosa*, often associated with sepsis in the immunosuppressed. These organisms are much more at home in the environment than growing on or in the patient. It is not possible to maintain a biological surface as sterile. The surface (e.g. an initially sterile burn) will soon become colonized with whatever organisms are around. If in addition the biological surface has become selective because of antibiotic administration, the colonizing organism is likely to be resistant to that antibiotic. The concept of creating the selective medium is important; it is, after all, what the laboratory does to select a single organism from a mixture – merely an *in-vitro* version of what the clinician may unwittingly be doing *in vivo*.

While a breakdown in the host immune system may lead to commensal organisms causing disease, bacteria have evolved a number of mechanisms to enhance their disease-causing potential, and allow them to evade the immune system. Resistance to lysis by serum is a feature of the Enterobacteriaceae, associated with the presence of lipopolysaccharide at the cell surface. Initial contact with the host may be facilitated by a variety of adhesions. Once attached, the next obstacle will be the host's immune system. The presence of a capsule, with or without antigenic similarity to the host, or the production of a protective biofilm may protect the organism. More sophisticated evasive mechanisms include the production of proteases that cleave IgA, a feature of pathogens invading via mucosal surfaces such as *Neisseria* spp., or coating with host proteins, such as fibronectin as found in *T. pallidum*. *Chlamydia trachomatis* is able to prevent the fusion of lysosomes to the intracellular phagosome containing the infectious elementary body; thus the host protects the invading organism from destruction.

In order to initiate an infection of a clean wound with *Staph. aureus*, some 10^5 organisms are required. However, the presence of a foreign body, be it traumatic or a medically inserted cannula, reduces the required inoculum by 99% to 10^3. Such numbers are small by microbiological standards.

Iron is an important growth factor for some bacteria, and they are able to fix iron-binding proteins either by having specific receptors for lactoferrin or transferrin (e.g. *Staph. aureus*), or by producing extracellular chelators (e.g. some coliforms). Other extracellular products such as hyaluronidase and the ureases of *Proteus* spp. and *Helicobacter pylori* may contribute to pathogenesis.

Toxin production is important for the ability of many pathogens to cause disease (virulence). These toxins may be found extracellularly as exotoxins, or released on cell death as endotoxins. Exotoxins are a feature of Gram-positive and Gram-negative organisms. Examples of the action of exotoxins include the neuromuscular effects of *Clostridium botulinum* and *Cl. tetani* toxins, gastrointestinal symptoms of cholera, *E. coli*, *Shigella* spp. and *Staph. aureus*, and skin necrosis from *Staph. aureus*. Some toxins require the infection of the bacteria with a phage for expression, for example diphtheria toxin which affects the heart and lungs, and the erythrogenic toxin of *Str. pyogenes* (Group A streptococcus). Staphylococcal toxic shock syndrome toxin is a potent pyrogen. Some exotoxins can be formalin fixed to produce toxoids, which are used as vaccines, e.g. tetanus toxoid.

Endotoxin is a feature of the Gram-negative cell wall. It is otherwise known as lipopolysaccharide (LPS). The important component is lipid A, which links the LPS to the outer membrane. Lipid A seems to be responsible for the inflammatory responses associated with the endotoxic shock found in severe Gram-negative septicaemia.

Laboratory identification

Specimen collection

The quality of the specimen is particularly important in microbiology. There is little point in taking a poor specimen and transporting it to the laboratory under less than ideal conditions. At best, the result will be unhelpful, and, at worse, highly misleading. In general, specimens from sites thought to be infected will be collected for microscopy, culture and antigen or genome detection. In addition, serum samples may be sent for antibody determination. While the pressures on a clinician are appreciated, it is important that full clinical details including any current or intended anti-microbial therapy are given. The laboratory will be putting up tests, and interpreting the results in the light of the clinical information supplied.

Specimens should almost always be taken before treatment is commenced. Sensitive bacteria will not survive in the presence of antibiotics, and even if clinically resistant may not be recoverable on artificial media. The correct transport medium should always be used for swabs, to maintain the balance of organisms as similar to the clinical situation as possible, and to ensure the likely survival of pathogens. Because organisms will continue to divide at ambient temperature, specimens should be kept at +4°C and transported to the laboratory as soon as feasible. Some organisms, for example chlamydiae and viruses, survive better at −70°C. The use of a conventional deep freeze at −20°C is satisfactory for preserving bacteria and storing serum samples, but is lethal to chlamydiae. Exceptions to these rules are fastidious organisms such as the gono-coccus, which do not survive well out of the clinical situation and should be either direct plated at the bedside or rapidly transported to the laboratory. To increase the likelihood of a positive result, liquid pus should always be preferred to a swab dipped in the pus; gas liquid chromatography which in skilled hands can rapidly discriminate different anaerobes is now rarely used in practice. Different antigen or genome tests require different collection media, even where the same organism is being detected. It is therefore necessary to check with the laboratory before sending these specimens. If the possibility of sexual abuse arises, it is vital to set up a formal chain of evidence with the laboratory, or the evidence may not be admissible in court.

Culture

The majority of bacteria are still identified by culture on solid agar media. This means that a minimum of 18 h will elapse before even presumptive results are available. Microscopy will assist in some cases, but where there is a heavy normal flora, such as in the respiratory tract, identification of potential pathogens may be impossible. It is never possible to speciate organisms on microscopy. Thus intracellular Gram-negative cocci are not necessarily synonymous with *N. gonorrhoeae*, and should never be reported as such until confirmatory results are available. Culture of organisms is necessary in most circumstances to define a full picture of the organisms colonizing or infecting a particular site. Sites that are normally sterile, such as blood and cerebrospinal fluid, should present little problem to the laboratory as any organism ought to be significant. However, the possibility of contamination of the specimen during collection, even under optimal conditions, may make interpretation difficult. The problem is much greater with specimens from a site with normal flora, because, as previously stated, many potentially pathogenic organisms may also be part of the normal flora. Further, it is not yet routinely possible to predict sensitivity to antibiotics without exposure of actively dividing organisms to them.

Antigen detection

No microbiological test is 100% sensitive, but the specificity of culture approaches 100%. The same may not be true of antigen-detection systems, although even here the tendency is to concentrate on good specificity over sensitivity. This is because a false-positive diagnosis is more likely to mislead than a false-negative one. In the latter situation clinical impression will override the negative report from the laboratory. Non-culture detection tests provide two useful functions. First, they may be used in situations where rapid diagnosis has important therapeutic and public health consequences, e.g. in meningitis. Second, the tests are useful to diagnose pathogens that are difficult or slow to isolate in the laboratory. The best example of this group is in the diagnosis of chlamydial infection. Because of the need for cell culture to isolate the organism, the development of non culture detection tests has served to highlight the prevalence and importance of the organism, and also to make diagnostic facilities more widely available. The disadvantage is that the tests are of variable sensitivity, and in some hands specificity is less than optimal. Direct immunofluorescence tests are of good sensitivity, but are subjective; in contrast enzyme-immunoassay systems are of high specificity, but generally of lower sensitivity. The importance of this discussion is that, in low prevalence populations, a low sensitivity (around 90%) may lead to a positive predictive value of under 50%. That is, one in two positive results may be a false positive.

Nucleic acid detection

Molecular technology is revolutionizing diagnostic microbiology. Tests based on the polymerase chain reaction (PCR) and the closely related ligase chain reaction (LCR) are now established in the routine diagnosis of certain pathogens such as *Neisseria meningitidis* and *C. trachomatis*. These techniques are extremely powerful, and as such are subject to contamination problems. Only validated tests should ever be used for routine diagnostic purposes. Biological inhibitors may reduce the sensitivity of these tests in practice.

Antibody detection

Antibody detection tests have the theoretical advantage that all that is required is a sample of clotted blood. Unfortunately, in practice, it is unusual for a definitive diagnosis to be made on a single sample of serum. The antibody rise takes a minimum of 10–14 days, and in some infections, e.g. chlamydial infections, more than 3 weeks may elapse. The safest criterion for the diagnosis of infection using serology is a greater than four-fold rise in specific antibody titre in at least a pair of sera. The exceptions are diseases where antibodies to the organism in question are rare in the normal population, or the organism cannot be cultured. An example of the former is plague, and of the latter syphilis. In the case of syphilis, several different tests are carried out on a single specimen in an attempt to confirm the treponemal infection, and also to define the stage of the disease.

Bacteria and disease

Normal flora

The relationship between humans and their microbes is complex. Products synthesized by one organism may assist the growth of another organism, which may in turn produce factors which will protect the host from invasion by extraneous organisms. Constant stimulation of the host immune system by resident bacteria will lead to early recognition and elimination of related but potentially pathogenic organisms, as well as contributing to the control of potentially neoplastic host cells by virtue of antigens similar to aberrant host ones. Bowel organisms are capable of synthesizing vitamins. The interactions of the various species of organism found on the skin are important for maintaining a healthy integument by production of fatty acids and other substances that inhibit the growth of potential pathogens. Disruption of this delicate balance will result in symptoms; for example antibiotics that affect the normal gut flora will result in a change in the proportion of different bacterial species, with overgrowth of some at the expense of others. This imbalance is manifest by diarrhoea. A more sinister consequence may be the proliferation of *Cl. difficile*, an anaerobic rod usually present in small amounts, leading to toxin-mediated pseudomembranous colitis.

The interaction of aerobic organisms with anaerobic organisms is particularly intriguing. The aerobes serve to consume oxygen, thus lowering the oxygen tension (eH) to very low levels, and allowing the proliferation of strictly anaerobic organisms. The anaerobes outnumber the aerobes by 10 : 1 to 100 : 1 on the skin, rising to over 1000-fold excess in the large intestine. One gram of faeces contains some 10^8 aerobic organisms and 10^{11} anaerobic organisms. Maintenance of the anaerobic gut flora is essential for health, and the use of anaerobe-sparing antibiotics (e.g. ciprofloxacin) where indicated is less likely to lead to diarrhoea as a side-effect.

The predominantly Gram-positive resident flora of the skin is supplemented by transient organisms, usually from the environment, and often Gram-negative. They are unable to establish themselves, but may survive for several hours. This is long enough for transfer to occur to susceptible individuals via the examining fingers.

Normal genital tract flora of women

The normal flora of the vagina changes under the influence of circulating oestrogens. The presence of oestrogen leads to an environment rich in glycogen, which favours the growth of lactobacilli and other acid-tolerant organisms. The metabolism of glycogen to lactic acid results in a pH < 4.5. Other bacteria commonly present include anaerobic cocci, diphtheroids, coagulase-negative staphylococci and α-haemolytic streptococci. In addition, a number of organisms that are also potential pathogens may colonize. These include β-haemolytic streptococci including *Str. agalactiae*, and *Actinomyces* spp. The balance between health and disease in the vagina is delicate. Factors leading to alteration of this balance will lead to overgrowth of organisms at the expense of the lactobacilli leading to bacterial vaginosis. Specific disease is caused by yeast-like fungi (e.g. *Candida* spp.), or infection with the protozoon *Trichomonas vaginalis*. Gonococcal and chlamydial infections affect the cervix, causing upper genital discharge. Bacterial vaginosis, gonococcal and chlamydial infections all predispose to ascending infection resulting in endometritis and salpingitis, with the attendant sequelae of ectopic pregnancy or infertility. Bacterial vaginosis also appears to be a factor in the pathogenesis of pre-term labour.

Gram-positive and Gram-negative bacteria

Table 7.2 lists some of the more medically important bacteria. *Staph. aureus* is distinguished from other staphylococci by production of coagulase. Increasingly, these organisms are proving to be resistant to the anti-staphylococcal β-lactam antibiotics (penicillins and cephalosporins). Such strains are designated methicillin-resistant *Staph. aureus* (MRSA) after the now obsolete antibiotic used as a laboratory test to detect them. Strains are frequently also multi-resistant, and some are able to spread easily through clinical areas (epidemic MRSA – EMRSA). MRSA are usually no more virulent than other coagulase-positive staphylococci, and frequently colonize wounds and carrier sites.

Table 7.2 Bacterial species of medical importance

Group or genus	Important species	Diseases caused, comments
Gram-positive cocci		
Staphylococci	Staphylococcus aureus	Wound infections, abscess, bacteraemia/septicaemia, osteomyelitis, tampon-associated toxic shock syndrome, food poisoning
	S. epidermidis	Vascular cannula-associated infection
	Staph. saprophyticus	Urinary tract infections
Streptococci (α-haemolytic)	Streptococcus milleri	Normal mouth flora, deep-seated abscesses, endocarditis
	S. pneumoniae	Lobar pneumonia
	Enterococcus (Streptococcus) faecalis	Normal bowel flora, urinary tract infection, opportunistic wound infection
Streptococci (β-haemolytic)	S. pyogenes (Group A)	Bacterial upper respiratory tract infection, wound infection, abscesses, bacteraemia/septicaemia, puerperal sepsis, necrotizing fasciitis, scarlet fever, septic arthritis
	S. agalactiae (Group B)	Normal vaginal flora, neonatal bacteraemia/septicaemia and meningitis
Peptostreptococcus	P. anaerobius	Anaerobic abscesses
Gram-positive bacilli		
Bacillus spp.	B. anthracis	Anthrax
	B. cereus	Normal flora of air, food poisoning with diarrhoea and vomiting
Lactobacilli	Lactobacillus casei	Normal vaginal flora
Corynebacteria	Corynebacterium diphtheriae	Diphtheria
	C. jeikeium	Skin flora, line- (cannula/vascular) associated bacteraemia/septicaemia
Listeria	L. monocytogenes	Maternal and neonatal listeriosis
Clostridium spp.	C. perfringens	Gas gangrene
	C. tetani	Tetanus
Actinomycetes	Actinomyces israelii	Pelvic actinomycosis
Nocardia	N. asteroides	Chronic infection in transplant patients
Gram-negative cocci		
Neisseriae	Neisseria gonorrhoeae	Gonorrhoea, pelvic inflammatory disease, arthritis, bacteraemia/septicaemia, infertility, neonatal ocular infection
	N. meningitidis	Meningitis
Moraxellae	Moraxella (Branhamella) catarrhalis	Respiratory flora, exacerbations of chronic bronchitis
Veillonella	Veillonella spp.	Normal oropharyngeal flora

Table 7.2 Bacterial species of medical importance (cont'd)

Group or genus	Important species	Diseases caused, comments
Gram-negative bacilli		
Haemophilus spp.	*H. influenzae*	Respiratory flora, exacerbations of chronic bronchitis
Legionella spp.	*L. pneumophila*	Atypical pneumonia
Pasteurella spp.	*P. multocida*	Animal bites
Yersinia	*Y. pestis*	Plague
	Y. enterocolitica	Mesenteric adenitis
Comma-shaped	*Vibrio cholerae*	Cholera
Helically curved	*Campylobacter fetus*	Normal flora of chickens, food poisoning with diarrhoea
	Helicobacter spp.	Gastritis and peptic ulcers
Bartonellae	*Bartonella henselae*	Cat-scratch disease, bacillary peliosis, bacillary angiomatosis
Enterobacteriaceae	*Escherichia coli, Klebsiella pneumoniae, Enterobacter cloacae*	Urinary tract infection, abdominal sepsis, wound infection, bacteraemia/septicaemia, nosocomial respiratory infection
	Proteus mirabilis	Enteric fever
	Salmonella typhi, Salmonella enteritidis	Food poisoning with diarrhoea
	Shigella dysenteriae	Dysentery
Pseudomonads	*Pseudomonas aeruginosa*	Nosocomial urinary tract infection and respiratory infection, opportunistic wound infection, bacteraemia/septicaemia
	Stenotrophomonas maltophilia	
Anaerobic Gram-negative bacteria	*Bacteroides fragilis*	Normal gut flora, abdominal sepsis, pelvic inflammatory disease
	Prevotella melaninogenica	Respiratory tract infection
	P. bivia	Normal vaginal flora, abdominal sepsis, pelvic inflammatory disease
	Fusobacterium nucleatum	Severe oral sepsis
Others		
Gram-variable coccobacilli	*Mobiluncus curtisii*	Normal vaginal flora, but predominant in bacterial vaginosis
	Gardnerella vaginalis	Associated with clue cells
Mycobacteria	*Mycobacterium tuberculosis*	Tuberculosis
	M. avium-intracellulare	Chronic respiratory infection and bacteraemia in severely immunosuppressed patients

Table 7.2 Bacterial species of medical importance (cont'd)

Group or genus	Important species	Diseases caused, comments
Spirochaetes	*Treponema pallidum*	Syphilis
	T. pertenue	Yaws
	Leptospira interrogans	Leptospirosis
	Borrelia recurrentis	Relapsing fever
Mycoplasmas	*Mycoplasma pneumoniae*	Atypical pneumonia
	M. hominis	Normal vaginal flora, pyelonephritis, pelvic inflammatory disease
	Ureaplasma urealyticum	Normal vaginal flora, non-gonococcal non-chlamydial urethritis, neonatal respiratory infection
Chlamydiae	*Chlamydia trachomatis*	Non-gonococcal urethritis, cervicitis, endometritis, pelvic inflammatory disease, infertility, neonatal ocular and respiratory infection
	C. pneumoniae	Atypical pneumonia, possible association with coronary heart disease
	C. psittaci	Animal pathogen, atypical pneumonia in humans
Rickettsiae and *Coxiella* spp.	*Rickettsia prowazekii*	Typhus
	Coxiella burnetii	Q fever

However, when they do cause infection the antibiotic choice is considerably limited compared with methicillin-sensitive strains.

Streptococci are divided into three broad groups based on their haemolysis of horse blood agar. Strains producing partial haemolysis (resulting in a greenish pigmentation of the agar) are termed α-haemolytic. This group comprises a number of commensal strains found particularly on the skin and in the mouth ('viridans' streptococci), but they are also important pathogens in deep-seated abscesses and endocarditis. The pneumococcus and enterococci (*Enterococcus (Streptococcus) faecalis* and *Ent. faecium*) are also important members of this group. Pneumococci are showing increasing resistance to penicillin. The enterococci are frequent super-infecting organisms, particularly associated with cephalosporin therapy. Glycopeptides (vancomycin and teicoplanin) are often required to treat enterococcal infection; consequently the emergence of vancomycin- and teicoplanin-resistant strains (VRE) is a major worry. Complete haemolysis is termed β-haemolysis. Organisms in this group are further subdivided into the Lancefield Groups A to O. Some α-haemolytic strains also have Lancefield antigens, e.g. the enterococcus is Lancefield Group D. The major human pathogens are in Groups A, B, C and G. However, members of these four groups may also occur as normal human flora. The Group A streptococcus is the most important pathogen (*Str. pyogenes*) and remains fully sensitive to penicillin. The third broad group is the non-haemolytic streptococci, which are commensal organisms, although anaerobic streptococci may cause wound infections.

The corynebacteria are Gram-positive rods widely distributed over the skin and upper respiratory tract. It is important to differentiate rapidly the pathogenic *C. diphtheriae* strains from the commensals, and to determine whether the former are toxin-producing strains. *C. jeikeium* strains have achieved some notoriety by their ability to colonize intravenous cannulae, particularly in the immunosuppressed. Strains are frequently multiply resistant, and may require glycopeptide therapy, or removal of the cannula.

Listeria monocytogenes is of particular importance in obstetrics. It is a motile Gram-positive rod widely distributed in nature. The organism is capable of active division at low temperatures, e.g. in display refrigerators. Depending on regional, occupational and animal exposure, between 5% and 70% of the population carry the organism in the bowel, and strains can be isolated from soil, vegetables, salads and dairy products, and uncooked or partly cooked chicken. Of the 13 serovars, only two are of importance in human disease. Infection in adults is an important cause of meningitis. Maternal infection usually occurs late in pregnancy, and symptoms range from mild 'flu-like' to chills, fever and back pain and bacteraemia. Neonates infected during pregnancy are ill at or soon after birth. Symptoms are non-specific, but respiratory distress is common, with bradycardia, jaundice and hepatosplenomegaly; neurological symptoms and skin rashes are also found. The characteristic lesions found in the placenta, and at post-mortem examination of infected neonates are miliary granulomata with focal necrosis. Routine macroscopic inspection of the placenta to exclude these macroscopic lesions should be encouraged. Intrapartum neonatal infection will lead to predominantly meningitic symptoms with an incubation period of 5–7 days.

The only bacteria to show branching are the actinomycetes. These are regarded as higher bacteria, with some characteristics similar to those of fungi. The organism occurs in the mouth, gut and female genital tract. The organism may also colonize intrauterine devices. Pelvic actinomycosis is a rare chronic granulomatous disease. The diagnosis can be made by observing the yellow mycelial masses (sulphur granules) in tissue. Symptoms may mimic pelvic neoplasia, and the distinction is important because actinomycosis may be treated with extended courses of appropriate antibiotics such as amoxicillin or co-trimoxazole. Cytologists frequently report *Actinomyces*-like organisms seen on cervical smears. This statement is not synonymous with actinomycosis. The organisms seen are usually commensal lactobacilli, which are also long Gram-positive rods and may appear to show branching in smears.

Clostridium perfringens is a component of normal bowel flora. Resistant spores are produced under certain conditions, which may survive inadequate disinfection or sterilization. The organism will proliferate in necrotic or poorly perfused tissue, giving rise to gas gangrene. The source is almost always the patient's own flora. *Cl. difficile* is also found in the normal bowel, in small numbers. Antibiotics may lead to overgrowth of this organism, and production of an exotoxin which gives rise to pseudomembranous colitis. Practically all antimicrobials may lead to this condition, but it is particularly associated with clindamycin, cephalosporins and more recently ciprofloxacin. Neonatal tetanus may be encountered in areas of poor hygiene, acquired via the umbilical stump wound. *Cl. botulinum* produces a powerful neurotoxin. The disease in adults results from ingestion of the pre-formed toxin, but neonatal botulism may develop from bacteria growing in the gut.

The Gram-negative cocci of medical importance are contained within the genus *Neisseria*. Both *N. gonorrhoeae* and *N. meningitidis* are fastidious organisms, and care is necessary with specimen collection to ensure that the organisms remain viable. The organisms are usually found within inflammatory exudate cells. *N. meningitidis* is a common nasopharyngeal commensal, and the

commonest bacterial cause of meningitis. Both organisms are capable of causing genital infection. *N. gonorrhoeae* infects columnar cells; it is therefore a parasite of the cervix, not the vagina. *Moraxella catarrhalis* strains are usually resistant to penicillins, which may compromise treatment of exacerbations of chronic bronchitis.

The enteric Gram-negative rods comprise a large group of morphologically identical organisms. All are to be found in the gut. The simplest classification divides them into those that ferment lactose, and those that do not. The lactose fermenters include *Escherichia coli*, *Enterobacter* spp. and *Klebsiella pneumoniae*. The non-lactose fermenters include the enteric pathogens such as *Shigella* spp. and the salmonellae. There are over 2000 types of salmonella, including enteric fever-causing typhoid and paratyphoid, and the common species associated with food poisoning such as *Sal. typhimurium* and *Sal. enteritidis*. Other important Gram-negative aerobic bacilli include *Pseudomonas* spp. and *Acinetobacter* spp. These are predominantly environmental organisms that will colonize and infect wounds opportunistically – that is, wounds in patients who are debilitated, immunosuppressed or on long-term inappropriate broad-spectrum antibiotics.

The anaerobic Gram-negative bacilli are non-sporing. Although their growth requirements are very precise, they are widely distributed in the body, colonizing bowel, oropharynx and vagina. They may contribute to the formation of abscesses in association either with other anaerobes, or with aerobic organisms.

The precise cause of bacterial vaginosis is unknown. However, the effect is a change in the balance of the bacterial species making up the normal flora. The normally predominant Gram-positive lactobacilli are replaced by Gram-variable coccobacilli. These organisms characteristically adhere to the squamous cells and are called 'clue cells' when seen in vaginal smears. The organisms include the anaerobic *Mobiluncus* spp. and the microaerophilic *Gardnerella vaginalis*. The term 'vaginosis' implies that there is no inflammation of the vaginal wall, but a fishy smelling, watery vaginal discharge is produced with a pH > 5.0.

Spirochaetes, mycoplasmas, chlamydiae and other bacteria

T. pallidum, the spirochaete that causes syphilis, cannot be cultivated in the laboratory. It is also serologically indistinguishable from the spirochaetes that cause yaws and pinta. In consequence, the laboratory can only provide evidence of current or past treponemal infection. It cannot diagnose syphilis. This unsatisfactory state means that, if there is any doubt as to the cause of serum treponemal antibodies, the patient must be assumed to have active syphilis and be treated accordingly. Syphilis in pregnancy will affect the fetus, resulting in a number of characteristic clinical features such as rashes, snuffles, teeth abnormalities, hepatosplenomegaly, proceeding over months and years to osteochondritis and gummata. Specific treatment at any time in pregnancy will result in a healthy neonate.

Mycoplasmas are widely distributed throughout plants and animals. There are more than a dozen species colonizing humans, in the oropharynx, bowel and genital tract. The majority of these strains are commensal, and their role in disease is controversial. *Mycoplasma pneumoniae* is an important cause of atypical pneumonia. *Mycoplasma hominis* is found in some 20% of sexually active women, and may be associated with bacterial vaginosis and PID; it causes some cases of pyelonephritis. *Ureaplasma urealyticum* is present in up to 80% of sexually active women. Its role in disease is less clear. Both *U. urealyticum* and *M. hominis* have been isolated from chorioamnionitis. Mycoplasma should be considered as a cause of postpartum pyrexia and treatment with tetracyclines considered if the fever does not settle. *M. hominis* differs from other mycoplasmas infecting humans by being resistant to macrolides (e.g. erythromycin) but sensitive to clindamycin. *Mycoplasma genitalium* is difficult to isolate in the laboratory for routine purposes, but there is evidence from molecular studies that it plays a role in pelvic inflammatory disease.

The chlamydiae are among the most sophisticated bacteria known. They are obligate intracellular parasites with a unique lifecycle involving an extracellular transport phase – the elementary body (EB) – and an intracellular phase – the reticulate body (RB). The lifecycle is about 48 h, during which the EB is taken up into a phagosome within the host cell, and transforms into a RB. Division of the RB leads to an inclusion full of daughter RBs, which condense to form the much smaller EBs. Release of the EBs by rupture of the host cell allows infection of further cells. The organisms cannot be cultured on artificial media, requiring living cells. This makes their laboratory isolation inconvenient. Culture has for routine purposes been superseded by antigen detection, e.g. direct immunofluorescence or enzyme immunoassay, or by molecular technology using PCR. Serology is of limited use in the diagnosis of acute chlamydial genital infection owing to cross-reaction of C. trachomatis with the commoner respiratory species C. pneumoniae. As with N. gonorrhoeae, C. trachomatis also infects columnar epithelium, and so is found in cervical cells.

Killing bacteria

Action of antibiotics

The unique structure of the bacterial cell wall has led to the development of chemotherapeutic agents with specific antibacterial activity and low host toxicity (see also Ch. 12). The β-lactam antibiotics comprise two main groups – the penicillins and cephalosporins – each of which contains a large number of members giving an antibacterial spectrum, at least in theory, spanning the bacterial genera of medical importance. Other members of the class include the monobactams and carbapenems (e.g. imipenem). All act selectively on the penicillin-binding proteins unique to the region of the bacterial cell wall. Glycopeptides such as vancomycin and teicoplanin are also important inhibitors of the cell wall construction, preventing incorporation of new units.

The cell membrane structure of all living organisms is very similar, so polymyxins, which are active at the bacterial cell membrane, are toxic to humans and rarely used systemically. The antifungal agents, nystatin and amphotericin B, act on the unique sterol-containing membrane of fungi, but are in themselves also toxic to animals. The azole antifungals block sterol synthesis and are less toxic.

Similarities of the basic metabolic and nucleic acid synthesizing pathways of plants, animals, fungi and bacteria also causes problems of selective toxicity. Consequently, it is necessary to exploit differing enzyme affinities or alternative pathways to kill infecting organisms selectively with minimal adverse effects on the host. The 70S ribosomes of bacteria are different to the 80S ribosomes of mammals, so that antibiotics affecting bacterial protein synthesis are likely to be ineffective against the host's mechanism. Examples include the macrolides (e.g. erythromycin) and lincosamides (e.g. clindamycin), tetracyclines, aminoglycosides (e.g. gentamicin), fusidic acid and chloramphenicol.

Antibiotics can also affect nucleic acid synthesis. Differing enzyme affinities ensure that toxicity to humans is minimized. The quinolones inhibit the α-subunit of bacterial DNA gyrase, preventing supercoiling of the DNA. The ansamycins (e.g. rifampicin) inhibit bacterial DNA-dependent RNA polymerase. Bacteria need to synthesize folic acid in the same way as other organisms. Sulphonamides and trimethoprim act at different points along the folic acid pathway. Bacteria must synthesize folic acid, while mammalian cells require pre-formed folate, and hence are not affected by sulphonamides, which inhibit folic acid formation. Further along the pathway, the reduction of dihydrofolate to tetrahydrofolate requires the action of dihydrofolate reductase. Trimethoprim, the antiprotozoal pyrimethamine and the anti-cancer drug methotrexate all act at this site. Selective toxicity reflects selective affinity for the relevant enzyme.

The actual site of action of nitroimidazole drugs such as metronidazole is unknown. However, the active compound is known to be a reduced form of the drug which is produced only at the very low oxygen tension (eH) produced in the cells of anaerobic bacteria. The action of this active form is thought to be against the nucleus.

Bacterial resistance may be mediated by one of four mechanisms:

1. The antibiotic may not get into cells, e.g. vancomycin and Gram-negative organisms.
2. It may be rapidly eliminated by efflux mechanisms, e.g. tetracycline resistance.
3. Enzymes may destroy the antibiotic, such as β-lactamases and aminoglycoside-modifying enzymes.
4. The target site may be altered or blocked, such as by rifampicin or quinolone resistance.

What is apparent is that the ingenuity of the bacterial cell knows no bounds when it comes to the battle for survival. The antibiotic that has no resistance to it has not yet been discovered. Multi-resistant bacteria are becoming more common, and more difficult or even impossible to treat with currently available drugs.

Physical methods

The technological advances in medicine have resulted in a vast array of different materials being used to manufacture devices for insertion into the body for therapeutic purposes. Ever since antisepsis was first demonstrated to reduce postoperative sepsis by Joseph Lister in 1867, it has been axiomatic that devices should be pathogen free. Antisepsis was replaced by asepsis at the turn of the century, but the comment that is ascribed to the surgeon Berkeley Moyhnihan (1865–1936) that 'every operation in surgery is an experiment in bacteriology' remains as true today as in the 1920s.

Sterilization/disinfection

Sterilization is the removal of all microorganisms including spores, and is defined internationally as a viable organism count of less than 10^{-6}. That is, a single viable organism in one of a batch of 1 million surgical packs would mean that sterile conditions had not been achieved. Disinfection is the removal of all actively dividing organisms, and may not necessarily include spores of fungi or bacteria, nor viruses or prions (such as the spongiform encephalopathy agents). It equates to a reduction in bacterial load in excess of 10^5. The difference between the two concepts is crucial. Sterilization is not easy to obtain reliably and disinfection may be adequate in some circumstances if done properly. Sterilization is always preceded by disinfection, in order to reduce the bioburden. The three components of disinfection are: (1) cleaning, (2) heat and (3) chemicals.

Heat

Heat results in coagulation of proteins and loss of viability. Heat can be in the form of dry heat, which penetrates surfaces poorly, or moist heat in the form of pure steam. The process of sterilization by heat requires a heating-up period, a sterilizing time at the correct sterilizing temperature, a further safety period at this temperature, to give a total holding time at the sterilizing temperature, and a cooling period. The entire process time is the cycle time, and will depend on the method of sterilization and the type of load, e.g. an open tray of instruments or a wrapped operative pack containing metal and other materials.

Dry heat is of limited use in surgical practice because it requires a holding time of 1 h at 160°C, giving a cycle time of over 2 h. At this temperature, materials other than metal may char. The use of pure steam is considerably more efficient, requiring lower temperatures for shorter holding times. The basic time/temperature used in the UK is 134–137°C held for 3 min. This equates to a cycle time of some 10 min, and should not be confused with the American standard of 137°C with a holding time of 10 min. Two basic forms of steam sterilizer are in use. The downward displacement autoclave relies on the incoming steam to displace air from the load. Any combination of air and steam will result in sterilizing conditions not being achieved. Therefore a downward displacement autoclave using the UK cycle cannot be used to sterilize wrapped loads or loads with narrow lumens, such as liposuction cannulae. To achieve reliable air removal and steam penetration, a vacuum autoclave is required, which draws a high pre-vacuum before steam is introduced to the autoclave chamber. It is important that the instruments placed in a downward displacement autoclave are packed loosely, not placed within impervious containers. In contrast a high vacuum autoclave is packed tightly to physically remove the bulk of air in the chamber. Recently, benchtop vacuum autoclaves have been developed. These allow small wrapped loads or a few items with lumens to be processed away from sterile service departments. These machines must not be overloaded. The quality of water used to generate the steam is also important. Water for irrigation should be used in benchtop autoclaves and changed at least daily; this prevents the build-up of pyrogens such as endotoxin, which may remain despite the organisms being killed. It is important that autoclaves are properly maintained, with daily, weekly, quarterly and annual checks being performed relevant to the machine and type of cycle and an audit loop of recording these checks.

Disinfection by heat usually involves the use of machines called washer disinfectors. These are in use for disinfection of crockery, as bedpan washers, and for processing instruments before sterilization. The key is obtaining a temperature of at least 80°C for 1 min. The load is usually heat-dried to avoid the use of drying cloths.

Chemicals

The inappropriate use of chemicals is a potential source of infection. Chemicals are incapable of reliable sterilization, except under very carefully controlled circumstances, seldom reached in clinical practice. The term 'high-grade disinfection' describes attempts to achieve chemical sterilization of articles that cannot be sterilized by conventional means. Chemicals are markedly affected by a number of factors, including:

- Spectrum of activity
- Temperature of use
- Presence of organic debris
- Contact time and penetrability
- Dilution
- Stability at in-use dilution
- Inactivators (such as plastics and hard water).

Many disinfectants are odourless and have the 'disinfectant' smell added. 'Pine fluid' has practically no disinfectant action. Cetrimide is widely used in the laboratory as a selective medium for growing *P. aeruginosa*. It is vital that the correct disinfection process is used for the proposed task. Prior cleaning must always occur. For the processing of endoscopes, this should involve a mechanical washer because cleaning is likely to be more efficient than manually, reducing the chances of biofilm build up in the lumens. All disinfectants are toxic to humans and require care in use. Many disinfectants are corrosive, and it is prudent to ensure that the manufacturer has confirmed that the intended process will not damage the instrument and will be effective in decontamination. The machines used to clean scopes must also be fully maintained to avoid their becoming colonized and recontaminating the scopes at the end of the process.

Other

Ethylene oxide gas may be used to sterilize heat-sensitive devices. The process is difficult to control, and requires a prolonged aeration phase after sterilization. More recently, gas plasma has become practical. Thoroughly cleaned and dried instruments are placed in a chamber with hydrogen peroxide. Low-frequency radio waves are used to generate a plasma, which converts the hydrogen peroxide to lethal superoxide and superhydroxyl ions. The process is suitable for heat-sensitive items. Radiation is used to sterilize single-use items such as syringes after manufacture. It has little practical role in medical practice.

Mycology

Fungi are generally larger than bacteria and are commonly multicellular. Fungal cell walls do not contain peptidoglycan but owe their rigidity to fibrils of chitin embedded in a matrix of protein and the polysaccharides mannan or glucan.

Most fungi that infect humans grow at a wide range of temperatures, although the optimal temperature for the majority is between 25°C and 30°C. The dermatophytes responsible for skin infections, such as ringworm, grow best between 28° and 30°C, while organisms such as *C. albicans* or *Aspergillus fumigatus*, which are responsible for systemic infections, grow best at 37°C. Fungi are predominantly aerobic, but many yeasts can produce alcohol by fermentation as an end-product of anaerobic metabolism. Virtually all fungi have the potential to reproduce by production of asexual spores. These may be conidia, produced in large numbers by moulds, such as aspergillus or the dermatophytes, or the chlamydospores produced in small numbers for survival in extreme conditions by fungi such as *C. albicans*.

The majority of fungi pathogenic to humans were thought to lack a sexual phase in their lifecycle and were therefore classified as 'fungi imperfecti'. A sexual phase has now been demonstrated in the laboratory for many of these pathogenic fungi, allowing them to be more accurately classified; however, it is convenient in the medical context to leave them under a single grouping of 'fungi imperfecti'.

Pathogenic fungi

There are four main groups of pathogenic fungi:

1. Moulds (filamentous fungi)
2. True yeasts
3. Yeast-like fungi
4. Dimorphic fungi.

Most pathogenic fungi are easily cultured in the laboratory, using Sabouraud's dextrose agar, with and without supplements. *Candida* spp. and many other pathogenic fungi will also grow on blood agar.

Moulds

These grow as long, branching filaments called 'hyphae', which intertwine to form a 'mycelium'. Reproduction is by spores, including sexual spores, which are characteristic and are important in identification. The fungi often appear as powdery colonies on culture owing to the presence of abundant spores. Included in this group are the dermatophytes, responsible for common superficial skin, nail and hair infections, and belonging to the genera *Trichophyton*, *Microsporum* and *Epidermophyton*, and also the moulds causing systemic infections in the immunocompromised, for example *Aspergillus fumigatus* or *Mucor* spp.

True yeasts

These are unicellular, round or oval fungi. Reproduction is by budding from the parent cell. Characteristically, cultures show creamy colonies. The major pathogen in this group is *Cryptococcus neoformans*, which has a large polysaccharide capsule. Encapsulated yeasts seen in biological fluids are diagnostic of cryptococcal infection.

Yeast-like fungi

Like yeasts, these appear as round or oval cells and reproduce by budding. They also form long branching filaments known as 'pseudohyphae'. *Candida* is the characteristic genus in this group with C. *albicans* being the major pathogen. Formation of germ tubes in serum broth distinguishes C. *albicans* from other members of the genus for practical purposes. C. *albicans* may be normal flora of the gastrointestinal tract, vagina or skin. Vaginal carriage is increased in pregnancy. Vaginal candidosis (thrush) is a common cause of vaginal discharge. Systemic candidal infection is a feature of the immunosuppressed, or severely ill patient on broad-spectrum antibacterial therapy.

Dimorphic fungi

These grow as yeast forms in the body and at 37°C on culture media, and in a mycelial form in the environment or on culture media at 22°C. *Histoplasma capsulatum* is a well-known member of this group. Infection is usually asymptomatic, but may produce calcified lung lesions. Chronic infection may lead to lung cavities, but a rare acute progressive disease involving widespread infection of the reticuloendothelial cells is usually fatal.

Pneumocystis carinii was originally considered to be an uncommon parasite until, as a result of DNA analysis, it was re-classified in 1988 as an unusual fungus which is very difficult to culture. The human form of *Pneumocystis* was named *P. jiroveci* in 2002, although the acronym PCP for the respiratory disease caused has been retained.

Parasites

Protozoa

These are unicellular eucaryotic organisms. They are able to reproduce by simple asexual binary fission, or by a more complex sexual cycle with the formation of cystic forms. Among the parasitic protozoa, both forms may occur in a single host.

The protozoa of medical importance are usefully classified into three groups: the sporozoa (containing the non-flagellate blood and tissue parasites), the amoebae, and the flagellates (containing the trypanosomes that cause sleeping sickness, *Giardia lamblia* and *T. vaginalis*). A list of some medically important species is given in Table 7.3. The two protozoa of importance in obstetrics and gynaecology are *T. vaginalis* and *Toxoplasma gondii*.

Table 7.3 Some protozoal parasites of humans

Protozoa	Site of infection
Entamoeba spp., *Giardia lamblia*, *Cryptosporidium parvum*	Intestine
Trichomonas vaginalis	Vagina
Plasmodium spp.	Blood
Trypanosoma spp.	Blood and tissue
Toxoplasma gondii	Tissues

T. vaginalis infects the vagina. The organism is sexually transmitted, and although men may become colonized they generally clear the organism from the urethra within a few days. The organism is similar in size to a white blood cell (10–20 µm), and readily identified by flagella movement in wet preparations under a ×40 microscope objective. The organism has three free flagella, and a fourth is embedded in an undulating membrane along the anterior two-thirds of the cell. The organism may cause an irritant, purulent vaginal discharge, with a pH > 5.0. The vaginal wall may be erythematous. In the USA, some 5–10% of men with a non-gonococcal urethritis (NGU) are infected with *T. vaginalis*. Treatment is with metronidazole.

T. gondii is an intracellular protozoon with a worldwide distribution, causing infection in humans and a wide range of animals. The asexual phase of the organism (bradyzoite) is able to develop in the tissues of a wide variety of vertebrate hosts, including humans. The definitive host is the cat, both domestic and wild cats, in which the sexual cycle occurs in the intestine. Human infection rates may be as high as 90% in some populations. Infection is most often acquired by ingesting bradyzoites in undercooked meat. It may also follow ingestion of oocysts containing tachyzoites resulting from the sexual cycle in the intestine of a cat, which are then excreted in its faeces. Cat litter trays and garden soil contaminated with cat faeces are a likely source to be avoided in pregnancy. After ingestion, the tachyzoites are distributed to many organs and tissues via the bloodstream and invade nucleated cells in all parts of the body and fetus. They multiply within the host cells, disrupting them by producing tissue cysts containing large numbers of slowly metabolizing bradyzoites. Focal areas of necrosis occur in many organs, particularly the muscles, brain and eye. Human infection is usually subclinical but may produce a glandular fever-like syndrome or choroidoretinitis. Transplacental infection may occur during an acute infection in the mother, which may not be diagnosed but may result in serious disease in the fetus. Infection early in pregnancy may result in a stillbirth, or the birth of a live baby with disseminated infection. Features include: choroidoretinitis, microcephaly or hydrocephalus, intracranial calcification, hepatosplenomegaly and thrombocytopenia. Maternal infection during the third trimester can also be transmitted to the fetus, but at this stage of development it usually causes no damage. Controversy surrounds the benefits of antenatal screening. Maternal infection may go undetected unless serological screening is carried out, but a single estimation of antibody may give rise to unnecessary anxiety because of infection before pregnancy began, which carries no risk to the fetus. A rise in the mother's toxoplasma antibody titre during pregnancy or the finding that she has IgM antibodies, indicating recent infection, raises the question of whether to treat the infection, given that treatment does not guarantee the infant will be unaffected, or to terminate the pregnancy even though it is not certain that the fetus has been damaged. Spiramycin (a macrolide) is the drug of choice for treatment of the mother and her fetus.

Helminths (worms)

The helminth parasites of humans belong to three zoologically distinct groups: trematodes (flukes), cestodes (tapeworms) and nematodes (roundworms, e.g. hookworm, *Ascaris lumbricoides*). None of the infections has particular significance during pregnancy other than as a cause of chronic anaemia with intestinal infection.

Virology

Introduction

The layperson (and some doctors) think of viruses as being 'small germs'. Although it is true that most viruses are indeed very small, size is not a distinguishing feature since some of the larger viruses (e.g. pox viruses) are larger than small bacteria. Some idea of the size of viruses may be obtained by comparing the size of an animal cell to a lecture theatre seating about 200 people; in such circumstances, a polio virus would be about the size of a squash ball, rubella virus the size of a tennis ball, and measles virus the size of a football.

Viruses are distinguished from other microorganisms by their nucleic acid content and method of replication. Microorganisms other than viruses are really cells; they contain both forms of nucleic acid but DNA is their repository of genetic information. They have their own machinery for producing energy and can synthesize their own macro-molecular constituents, i.e. nucleic acid, proteins, carbohydrates and lipids. They all multiply by binary fission. Viruses contain no ribosomes, mitochondria or other organelles; they are dependent on the host cell machinery for protein synthesis and energy metabolism. Consequently, they are totally dissimilar from other microorganisms; they can reproduce themselves from a single nucleic acid molecule.

Viral nucleic acid

Viruses contain either DNA or RNA as their genetic material, usually as single molecules but never both. In contrast, all other microorganisms contain both forms of nucleic acid. Viral nucleic acid may be either single-stranded (ss) or double-stranded (ds) and the nucleic acid may be in the form of a single piece or it may be segmented, as in influenza and rotaviruses. The nucleic acid content of viruses is very small when compared with that of the cell. For example, influenza viruses have about one-hundredth of the nucleic acid of the cells they infect. RNA viruses (riboviruses) represent the only form of 'life' utilizing RNA as genetic material.

Replication

Viruses can only replicate in living cells, which may be of plant, bacterial (infecting viruses being termed phage) or animal origin. The result of infection of a cell is two-fold: first, and most usually, the formation of new virus particles and, second, some change in the cell (often but not always resulting in its destruction). Thus, viruses may establish latent infection in the cells they infect (e.g. the herpes group of viruses, papovaviruses and some adenoviruses). Alternatively, some viruses (e.g. papillomaviruses and the Epstein–Barr virus) may induce malignant transformation in the cells they infect.

The host cell provides the source of all the machinery required for viral reproduction; the invading virus introduces specific information relating to its own structure and constitution, as well as that required to divert cellular mechanisms to viral ends and for the construction of enzymes needed to manufacture viral products. This information is contained, in coded form, in the sequence of bases in the viral nucleic acid. Thus, infection with the virus results in the introduction into the living cell of an infective and foreign nucleic acid with specific biological properties. Once the virus particle has been taken into the cell, the virus merges its identity with it and the whole entity becomes a new and different cell which may be considered as 'a virus–cell complex'.

Details of the method by which different viruses replicate can be found in standard textbooks. In simple terms for DNA viruses, viral messenger RNA is transcribed from the parental virus DNA within the host cell, and codes for the formation of virus-specific proteins. For RNA viruses, the viral genome acts as a template for the synthesis of new viral RNA. Single-stranded RNA viruses are classified as positive or negative strand according to the way in which coding information is stored in the viral genome. With positive-strand RNA viruses, the viral genome is of the same polarity as messenger RNA, and may itself act as messenger RNA, being translated into code for virus-specific proteins. With negative-strand viruses, a complementary RNA copy of the viral genome, or part of it, acts as messenger RNA. One further group of RNA viruses known as reversi viruses replicates by reverse transcription of viral genomic RNA to form a DNA intermediate, from which both messenger RNA and progeny viral genomes are transcribed. This group includes retroviruses, such as the human immunodeficiency virus (HIV), and hepadnaviruses, such as hepatitis B virus (HBV).

Structure of viruses

Even before negative staining techniques by electron microscopy were available to determine the fine structure of viruses, X-ray diffraction studies indicated that viruses displayed distinct symmetry properties. Because of the limited genetic information available and for reasons of economy, Crick and Watson postulated that the nucleic acid of viruses would code for a virus coat (capsid) consisting of identical subunits arranged in a single repetitive form; negative staining techniques have confirmed these findings. There are two main types of symmetry: cubic and helical. Helical symmetry is generally associated with rod-shaped viruses and cubic symmetry with the more spherical ones.

In its simplest form, a virus consists of nucleic acid and a protein coat, and it is this protein coat which contains the regular assembly of protein molecules. Some viruses, e.g. viruses of the herpes group and myxoviruses (e.g. influenza), are surrounded by an envelope, which is derived from the host cell membrane during release of the virus particles. The capsid consists of numerous identical smaller units, designated capsomeres, which are constant in number and identical in shape. Figure 7.2 illustrates cubic symmetry and Figure 7.3 helical symmetry. The nucleic acid and capsid (nucleocapsid) of viruses exhibiting helical symmetry bear a resemblance to a spiral staircase. Each step bears a constant relationship to its neighbours around a central axis which could be represented by the well of the staircase. Cubic symmetry is more complex and describes a group of regular units which have symmetry properties in common with a cube. Specifically for viruses, it includes the tetrahedron, octahedron and icosahedron. Most viruses exhibiting cubic symmetry that infect humans have icosahedral symmetry (Fig. 7.4). The particle is three-dimensional with 20 identical faces with 12 vertices; each face is in

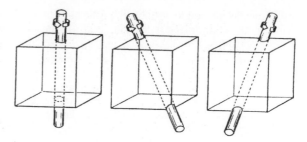

Figure 7.2 • Axes of symmetry of a cube: 4-fold, 3-fold, 2-fold.

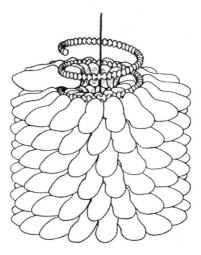

Figure 7.3 • Capsomeres arranged helically around central nucleic acid. Model of tobacco mosaic virus. (Reproduced from Advances in Virus Research 1960; 7:274.)

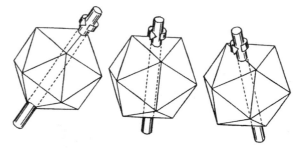

Figure 7.4 • Axes of symmetry of a icosahedron: 5-fold, 3-fold, 2-fold.

the form of an equilateral triangle. Figure 7.5 illustrates the fine structure of some of the viruses discussed in this chapter. No satisfactory electron micrographs of the hepatitis C virus have been published to date and, although an electron micrograph of Japanese B virus is not included, it is somewhat similar in its fine structure to the rubella virus.

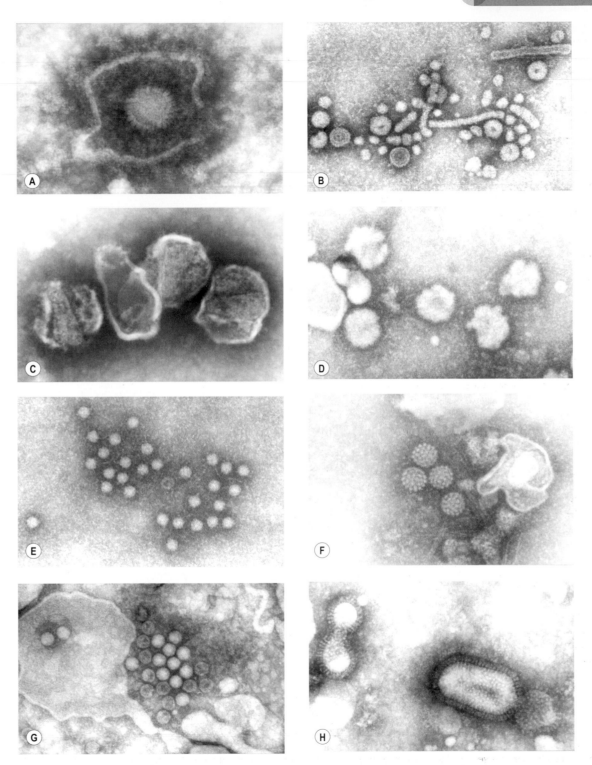

Figure 7.5 • Electron micrographs of common viral types. (A) Herpes simplex virus from a vesicular lesion from a patient with herpes simplex. (B) Hepatitis B virus showing 42 nm virions – the 'Dane' particles – and 22 nm HBsAg spheres and filaments. The serum sample was from an HIV-positive male, hence the large proportion of intact virions. (C) Human immunodeficiency virus. (D) Rubella virus. (E) Human parvovirus. The serum sample was from an HIV-positive male. (F) Human papillomavirus. (G) Enterovirus. (H) Influenza virus.

Diagnosis of viral infections

An understanding of the nature, including the structure, of viruses is of importance in the diagnosis of viral infections. Viruses may be identified by demonstrating the effect they induce in living cells (cell culture), which can be visualized by low-power light microscopy. Different viruses induce different changes (cytopathic effects) in different cell lines and the virus may be identified by neutralizing the virus infectivity in cell culture by specific antisera.

Whole virus may also be visualized by electron microscopy but high virus concentrations are necessary and electron microscopy cannot distinguish viruses which are morphologically identical within a single group, e.g. different members of the herpesvirus group. Nevertheless, electron microscopy may rapidly identify a herpesvirus from a vesicular lesion, which may be all that is necessary for clinical purposes. Another virus belonging to the herpes group (cytomegalovirus) may be visualized in the urine of congenitally infected infants.

Using specific antibodies, most usefully monoclonal antibodies, the presence of viral antigens may be identified directly from clinical samples. Alternatively, non-structural proteins may also be identified in clinical samples. Such techniques are used for the identification of respiratory syncytial virus in children with respiratory infections, and cytomegalovirus in the blood and urine of patients with suspected cytomegalovirus infection.

More recently, techniques of considerable sensitivity and specificity have been employed to identify viral nucleic acid. Thus, nucleic acid hybridization and gene amplification techniques (particularly polymerase chain reaction) are now frequently used in diagnosis to identify a number of viral infections, including infections by the herpes group of viruses, enteroviruses, hepatitis C, hepatitis B and HIV viruses. These methods can also be used to quantify the amount of virus in specimens. This is useful for monitoring virus infections in patients who are immunosuppressed or receiving antiviral therapy.

Serological techniques can be used to determine evidence of immunity to viruses, usually by detecting the presence of virus-specific IgG responses. Diagnostically, a significant rise in antibody titre (> 4-fold) between acute and convalescent sera is significant for determination of recent infection. However, more frequently, evidence of current, recent or persistent infection may be detected by a virus-specific IgM response directed towards viral capsid proteins. Such responses are useful in the diagnosis of intrauterine and some perinatal infections, e.g. rubella, cytomegalovirus and parvovirus B19 infections.

Viruses of importance in obstetrics and gynaecology

Rather than provide basic information on different groups of viruses, attention will be focused on the importance of viruses which may induce severe infections in pregnancy, as well as intrauterine, perinatal and gynaecological infections. The classification and properties of these viruses is shown in Table 7.4. Some of these viruses, such as the influenza virus, cause classical acute infections, characterized by a rapid onset of symptoms and a brief period of viral replication, followed by clearance of the virus and resolution of symptoms. Naturally acquired infection with a particular strain of influenza A or B results in long-term immunity to that strain, but not those influenza strains which have exhibited major antigenic changes (antigenic shift) or even minor degrees of variation (antigenic drift). Others cause persistent infections, in which the patient often remains infected for life. Persistent infections may be characterized by an acute phase of infection, which may or may not be symptomatic, followed by life-long latency, where the virus persists in a non-replicative form with restricted viral gene expression. Subsequent reactivations of infection may occur, although in the immunocompetent person reactivated infection is usually more limited than primary infection, and may be asymptomatic. This pattern of persistence is typical of herpesviruses such as herpes simplex virus (HSV) and varicella-zoster virus (VZV). Other persistent viral infections such as HIV and hepatitis B and C viruses (HBV and HCV) are characterized by ongoing virus replication and chronic, evolving disease.

Viruses which may induce severe infection in pregnancy

The features of these viral infections, together with preventive measures where applicable, are listed in Table 7.5. Some infections may be prevented by immunization, e.g. influenza A and B, and poliomyelitis, and recombinant-derived vaccines are under trial for the hepatitis E virus, which carries a high mortality rate among pregnant patients in developing countries. Although there is some doubt as to whether varicella is more severe in pregnancy, infection is often severe and occasionally fatal among adults generally, particularly those who smoke. Thus, pregnant women who give no history of varicella, or in whom screening tests for VZV antibodies indicate susceptibility, should be protected by the administration of varicella-zoster immune globulin (VZIG) within 72 h of an exposure. Aciclovir treatment should also be used for pregnant women with established infection as they are at

Table 7.4 Classification and characteristics of viruses of significance in pregnancy

Virus	Maternal, intrauterine or perinatal infection	Classification	Properties of virus			
			Genome	Symmetry	Diameter	Envelope
Herpes simplex virus types 1 and 2	Perinatal	Herpesvirus[a]	dsDNA	Cubic	120–300 nm	Yes
Varicella-zoster virus	Maternal, intrauterine	Herpesvirus[a]	dsDNA	Cubic	180–200 nm	Yes
Cytomegalovirus	Intrauterine	Herpesvirus[b]	dsDNA	Cubic	150–200 nm	Yes
Hepatitis B virus	Perinatal	Hepadnavirus	dsDNA	Cubic	40–42 nm	Yes
Hepatitis C virus	Perinatal	Hepacivirus	(+) ssRNA	Cubic	Not known	Yes
Hepatitis E virus	Maternal	Uncertain	(+) ssRNA	Cubic	27–34 nm	No
Human immunodeficiency virus types 1 and 2	Intrauterine, perinatal	Retrovirus	(+) ssRNA	Cubic	110 nm	Yes
Human T cell lymphotropic virus type 1	Perinatal (breastfeeding)	Retrovirus	(+) ssRNA	Cubic	110 nm	Yes
Rubella virus	Intrauterine	Rubivirus	(+) ssRNA	Cubic	58 nm	Yes
Human parvovirus B19	Intrauterine	Parvovirus	(+) or (−) ssDNA	Cubic	18–26 nm	No
Human papillomavirus	Perinatal	Papovavirus	dsDNA	Cubic	55 nm	No
Enteroviruses	Intrauterine, perinatal	Picornavirus	(+) ssRNA	Cubic	24–30 nm	No
Influenza virus A and B	Maternal	Orthomyxovirus	(−) ssRNA	Helical	120 nm	Yes
Japanese B virus	Maternal	Flavivirus	(+) ssRNA	Cubic	40–60 nm	Yes
Lassa fever virus	Maternal	Arenavirus	Ambisense ssRNA	Cubic	90–110 nm	Yes

[a]Herpes simplex viruses and varicella-zoster viruses are subclassified as alphaherpesviruses. These herpesviruses have a variable host range, grow rapidly in cell culture, destroy infected cells efficiently, and establish latency *in vivo* in primarily sensory ganglia.
[b]Cytomegalovirus is subclassified as a betaherpesvirus. These herpesviruses usually have a restricted host range and grow slowly in cell culture; infected cells often show cytomegalic inclusions both *in vivo* and *in vitro*. They establish latency in a variety of tissues including secretory glands, the kidney and lymphoreticular cells.

Table 7.5 Virus infections that may be severe or fatal in pregnancy

Virus infection	Comments	Prevention
Influenza A (B)	Increased mortality in 1918 and 1957 associated with chronic heart disease	Influenza vaccine (inactivated)
Varicella	Mortality associated with pneumonia among adults. Possibly more severe in pregnancy	Varicella-zoster immune globulin preferably within 72 h of contact (treat established infections if severe with aciclovir systemically) Varicella vaccine for specific at-risk groups
Poliomyelitis	Spinal paralysis increases with gestational age	Polio vaccine (attenuated or inactivated) for travellers to any remaining endemic areas
Measles	Increased mortality and complications in pregnancy	In the absence of previous vaccination or history of measles give normal human immunoglobulin
Hepatitis E	12–18% mortality rate with fetal death in last trimester. Endemic in many developing countries	Trials in progress with recombinant-derived vaccines
Lassa fever	70–90% mortality rate with fetal death in last trimester. Endemic in West Africa	? Prophylactic ribavirin to pregnant household contacts (treat patient with ribavirin systemically)
Japanese B encephalitis	20–40% mortality rate; higher in pregnancy with fetal death. Widely distributed in South-East Asia and the Far East	Vaccine available on named-patient basis for travellers to endemic areas

increased risk of varicella pneumonia, and this has a high mortality rate. Japanese B encephalitis is one of the more widely distributed arbovirus infections, being present in Asia. Although subclinical infection is common, those exhibiting clinical features may experience a mortality rate of up to 20% in outbreaks. Fetal death is common. An inactivated vaccine is available on a 'named-patient basis', but since it may be reactogenic is not recommended in pregnancy. Lassa fever may be particularly severe in the latter stages of pregnancy, and the fetal death rate is high.

SARS and other coronaviruses

Severe acute respiratory syndrome (SARS) is caused by a coronavirus that first emerged in the southern Chinese province of Guangdong in November 2002. Pregnant women with SARS appear to have a worse prognosis and a higher mortality rate. Therefore early delivery or termination of pregnancy should be considered in those who are seriously ill. The following criteria for early delivery have been proposed by Wong et al (2003).

- Maternal rapid deterioration
- Failure to maintain adequate blood oxygenation

- Difficulty with mechanical ventilation due to the gravid uterus
- Multi-organ failure
- Fetal compromise
- Other obstetric indications.

There seems to be no reason for elective pre-term delivery in those women who are relatively well with SARS infection. Pregnant women should be treated empirically since a laboratory diagnosis may be prolonged. It has been suggested that the treatment of pregnant women with SARS should be without the use of ribavirin.

Infections due to other coronaviruses are relatively mild and have not been reported as causing problems during pregnancy.

Intrauterine infections

Viruses which may damage the fetus are shown in Table 7.6. The rubella virus, and two viruses belonging to the herpesvirus group – cytomegalovirus (CMV) and varicella-zoster virus (VZV) – as well as human parvovirus B19 may induce persistent infections in the fetus.

Table 7.6 Viruses which may infect or damage the fetus

Virus infection	Birth defects	Persistent infection	Fetal death
Rubella	Yes	Yes	Yes
CMV	Yes	Yes	Yes
Varicella	Yes	Possible	Yes
Parvovirus B19	No	Yes	Yes
HIV-1 and -2	No	Yes	Yes
Hepatitis C	No	Yes	Unknown
Hepatitis E	No	? Yes	Yes
Poliomyelitis	No	No	Yes
Coxsackie B virus	No	No	Yes
Japanese B encephalitis	Unknown	Unknown	Yes
Lassa fever	No	No	Yes

Rubella

As a result of immunization programmes against rubella, now being directed against pre-school children of both sexes and rubella-susceptible adult women, only about 2% of women of childbearing age born and brought up in Britain are susceptible to infection. However, susceptibility rates equivalent to or higher than those observed in developed countries during the pre-vaccination era are present in many developing countries. Congenitally acquired rubella is now rare in Britain and most industrialized countries, although rubella-induced defects have been reported with varying frequencies in other parts of the world.

Rubella virus produces an anti-mitotic protein and consequently, if infection occurs during the critical phase of organogenesis (i.e. during the first 8 weeks of pregnancy), severe and multiple defects are likely to occur. If infection occurs during the first trimester, fetal infection is almost invariable, and 75–80% of conceptuses are damaged. After the first trimester, the incidence and spectrum of defects is much less. Although congenital heart disease, eye defects (particularly cataracts) and deafness are the commonest manifestations of congenitally acquired infection if maternal infection is acquired in early pregnancy, rubella induces a generalized and persistent infection with multi-organ involvement, and a wide spectrum of defects may be present at birth or evolve in infancy.

CMV

About 40–50% of women of childbearing age in Britain have no serological evidence of previous CMV infec-tion. In contrast with rubella, primary maternal CMV infection is often asymptomatic, but may result in fetal infection and damage throughout pregnancy. The viral transmission rate to the fetus is of the order of 30–40%, but fetal damage occurs in only about 10% of infected conceptuses. Nevertheless, the burden induced by congenitally acquired CMV infection is considerable; it has been estimated that somewhere in the order of 300–400 CMV-damaged babies are born in the UK each year. CMV is the commonest microbial cause of psychomotor retardation, although deafness may be the sole manifestation of congenitally acquired disease. Recurrent CMV infection or reactivation is rarely associated with fetal damage.

Varicella

Although very few indigenous adult women born in the UK are susceptible to varicella, the proportion may be considerably higher – up to 35% – among those born and brought up in rural areas of developing countries. The overall risk of congenitally acquired disease follow-ing maternal varicella is restricted to the first 20 weeks of gestation, but, in contrast to rubella and CMV, the risks are low (about 1% overall); the incidence is greater between 13 and 20 weeks of gestation (2%) than between 1 and 12 weeks (0.4%). Defects involve the CNS and musculoskeletal system; limb hypoplasia and cicatricial scarring may be present.

If acquired towards term, the infant may develop varicella after delivery. If maternal varicella occurs 8 days or more before delivery, neonatal varicella is usually mild. In contrast, maternal varicella infection that occurs less than 1 week before delivery may be severe and, without treatment, occasionally fatal. VZIG should therefore be given to infants whose mothers develop varicella 8 days or less before delivery; aciclovir may be given if neonatal infection is severe, despite administration of VZIG. Varicella-susceptible pregnant women exposed to infection during the last 3 weeks of pregnancy should be given prophylactic VZIG.

Parvovirus B19

About 40% of women of childbearing age in Britain are susceptible to parvovirus B19 infection. Human parvovirus may induce a rubella-like rash, sometimes accompanied by arthralgia, although infection may also be asymptomatic. The fetus is infected in about 33% of cases, and in about 10% of these spontaneous abortion may occur, usually in the second trimester. Parvovirus B19 binds to a globoside (P antigen) expressed on the membrane of erythrocytes and fetal heart, and this results in a reduction of fetal erythroid progenitor cells, which may result in a severe fetal anaemia, leading to heart failure and development of hydrops fetalis. Heart failure may also result from viral myocarditis. However, developmental defects have not been recorded. Parvovirus infection is therefore not a reason for therapeutic abortion. Fetal anaemia and hydrops may be 'rescued' by fetal blood transfusion.

HIV-1 and -2

WHO estimates that, globally, 38.0 million adults and 2.3 million children were living with HIV at the end of 2005. In developing countries, infection is usually contracted heterosexually. In Britain, HIV infection tends to be concentrated in London. In its inner-city areas, up to 0.5% of pregnant women are now HIV-1 positive. In the absence of treatment with a combination of antiretroviral drugs, HIV-1 is transmitted to the fetus of infected mothers in about 12–15% of cases. Combination antiretroviral therapy has reduced the HIV transmission rate, and studies suggest that chemotherapy together with delivery by caesarean section further reduces the risk of transmission to 1–2%. Infection may be transmitted *in utero* but occurs more frequently during delivery, or when breastfeeding. In contrast to HIV-1, HIV-2 is transmitted in only about 1% of cases, and this is almost certainly a manifestation of the much lower maternal viral load present. If HIV infection occurs *in utero*, it is usually possible to establish a diagnosis during the first few weeks of life. If infection occurs during delivery or via breastfeeding, or in infants born to mothers on antiretroviral treatment, it may take considerably longer to establish a diagnosis of HIV infection in infancy. Diagnosis of HIV infection in infancy is usually made by detecting the virus by

molecular techniques; serological techniques are of limited value since maternal antibody may persist for up to 18 months.

Enteroviruses (polioviruses, coxsackie A and B viruses, echoviruses)

Most developed countries are now free of poliomyelitis, and the WHO Expanded Programme of Immunization has resulted in a marked decline in poliomyelitis cases in developing countries. Very occasionally, maternal poliomyelitis results in the delivery of infants with limb paralysis. Maternal infection by other enteroviruses may result in the delivery of infants with severe generalized infections in which myocarditis and central nervous system (CNS) disease are prominent features. Scandinavian studies suggest that enterovirus infection, if acquired *in utero*, may be associated with the subsequent development of insulin-dependent diabetes mellitus (type 1 diabetes) in childhood. Infection may also be acquired during delivery, transmission occurring via contamination with enterically shed maternal virus. Infected babies may also transmit infection nosocomially.

Perinatal infections

Viruses which may cause severe infection if acquired perinatally or during the neonatal period are listed in Table 7.7. A range of diagnostic methods may need to be employed to confirm viral infection in such cases including qualitative and quantitative molecular techniques.

HSV

About 75% of genital infections are caused by HSV-2 and about 25% by HSV-1. Infants may be infected by maternal genital lesions, fetal scalp monitoring, maternal non-genital lesions or contact with HSV-infected nursery staff or visitors. Primary maternal lesions carry a much higher risk of infection than recurrent lesions,

Table 7.7 Perinatal infections

Herpes simplex virus (HSV)
Varicella-zoster virus (VZV)
Cytomegalovirus (CMV)
Hepatitis B
HIV
Enteroviruses
Papillomaviruses
Human T cell leukaemia virus (HTLV-1)

since primary infections are associated with high concentrations of virus over a long period.

The incidence of neonatal herpes in Britain is estimated to be of the order of 1.6 per 100 000 deliveries, whereas in Sweden and USA it is considerably higher (5 and 7 per 100 000, respectively). The presence of maternal lesions at or within 6 weeks of birth is an indication for caesarean section provided membranes are intact, or ruptured less than 6 h before delivery. Infants delivered via an infected birth canal should be given prophylactic aciclovir intravenously. Although it is recommended that women with evidence of a recurrent lesion at delivery should deliver by caesarean section, transmission is rare; studies from the Netherlands have shown that the risks of acquiring neonatal HSV following caesarean section and vaginal delivery are not significantly different. Testing mothers with a history of recurrent herpes, or whose partners give a history, is no longer recommended, since virus shedding in late pregnancy does not correlate with transmission to the neonate. There is some evidence to suggest that treatment of mothers with oral aciclovir who have a history of recurrent genital herpes during the last month of pregnancy may reduce the incidence of lesions at delivery and consequently the necessity for caesarean section.

Clinical manifestations may be delayed until 10–14 days after birth. Infants may present with lesions of the skin and mucous membranes (60% will disseminate), CNS involvement or generalized infection.

Hepatitis B

There are 350–400 million HBV carriers worldwide, the highest rates being in South-East Asia (~15%) and sub-Saharan Africa (~10%). In some inner-city areas in Britain, the HBV carrier rate among pregnant women is about 1%. Pregnant women with acute HBV infection are likely to transmit infection to newborn infants perinatally. Infants delivered of mothers who are HBV surface antigen (HBsAg) and 'e' antigen (HBeAg) positive should be protected by the administration of hepatitis B immune globulin (HBIG) and HBV vaccine (active/passive immunization) at birth. Provided a full course of vaccine is given (three doses and a booster), this procedure will effectively reduce the risk of persistent HBV infection in the infant by about 95%, thereby reducing the risk of long-term chronic liver damage and primary hepatocellular carcinoma. Infants delivered of mothers who have antibody to HBeAg (anti-HBe) should be given HBV vaccine without HBIG. Infants whose mothers are HBsAg positive without 'e' markers, or where the 'e' marker status has not been determined, or whose mothers had acute hepatitis B during pregnancy, should be given active/passive immunization. There is currently a debate on whether using molecular methods to detect HBV DNA in mothers with anti-HBe may detect those with high levels of viraemia, whose children should be given active/passive vaccination.

Hepatitis C

It is estimated that there are about 170 million HCV carriers worldwide, relatively high carrier rates (2.5–5%) occurring in some developing countries, particularly in sub-Saharan Africa, Asia and Latin America. In Britain, infection is common among multi-transfused persons, injecting drug users, and those from countries with a high prevalence. The prevalence among pregnant women in some inner-city areas in London is about 0.25%. Infection may be transmitted *in utero* if acute maternal infection occurs in the last trimester of pregnancy, but mothers who are carriers may also occasionally transmit *in utero* since HCV RNA has been detected in neonates at birth, and caesarean section may not prevent transmission. Neonatal infection occurs in about 6% of infants delivered of mothers who are HCV carriers and who are HCV RNA positive, but in mothers co-infected with HIV the transmission rate is 30–35%. Mothers who are HCV antibody positive but HCV RNA negative are very unlikely to transmit infection. HCV-infected infants are likely to develop persistent HCV infection which may in due course result in chronic liver damage.

Human papillomavirus (HPV)

About 100 different genotypes have been identified, of which at least 30 are found in the genital tract. HPV types 6 and 11 cause genital warts, and are known as 'low risk' types as they are rarely found in cancers. HPV types 16, 18, 31 and a few other types are designated as 'high risk' as they are associated with pre-malignant and malignant cervical disease; viral DNA can be detected in ~95% of cancers, often integrated into host cell chromosomes, and virus-encoded oncoproteins, which bind to and inactivate the p53 and pRB tumour suppresser proteins, are expressed.

HPV 6 and 11 may be transmitted from mother to infant at delivery and may cause juvenile laryngeal or genital warts, but this is rare. High-risk types may also be transmitted at birth and may persist in infancy, but they are not associated with obvious disease and the consequence of these infections is unknown. Girls aged 12–13 years are now vaccinated with HPV vaccine to protect against cervical cancer.

Human T cell lymphotrophic virus type 1 (HTLV-1)

This virus is endemic in South West Japan, the South Pacific, parts of West Africa, the Caribbean basin, southern USA and parts of South America. Persons who have emigrated from these areas may also be carriers. The prevalence of antibodies among antenatal patients in London and Birmingham is 0.14–0.26%. Studies in Japan and the Caribbean have shown that this virus is transmitted via breast milk. Of the carriers of this retrovirus, 2.5–4.0% who have not acquired infection through blood transfusion may develop adult T cell leukaemia or tropical spastic paraparesis 10–30 years after infection.

References

Wong S F, Chow K M, de Swiet M 2003 Severe acute respiratory syndrome and pregnancy. BJOG: An International Journal of Obstetrics and Gynaecology 110:641–642

Chapter Eight

Immunology

Andrew George

Introduction

The immune system exists to protect the organism from the consequences of infectious disease and, to a lesser extent, neoplasia. It does this by having a complex system of organs, cells and molecules that are distributed throughout the body. Most of the cells involved are highly motile, adding to the complexity of the system. The importance of the immune system in health and disease is highlighted by rare congenital abnormalities of components of the system, which in many cases result in early death due to uncontrollable infections.

The immune system plays an important role in a number of conditions of pregnancy including spontaneous abortion, pre-eclampsia and hypersensitivity reactions that damage the fetus. Pregnancy can also result in changes in the severity of autoimmune diseases. In addition, one of the most interesting questions in immunology is why a fetus is not recognized by the immune system and destroyed; if an equivalent organ were transplanted into a woman without massive immunosuppression it would be rapidly rejected. This might seem an academic question, of little practical importance. However, new strategies for preventing graft rejection are being developed based on our knowledge of how the fetus/placenta blocks rejection.

The immune system

Frequently, the immune system is characterized as differentiating between 'self' (anything originating from the organism) and 'foreign' (anything that is not self), and destroying anything it recognizes as foreign. However, this is a gross simplification. When the immune system is first introduced to a foreign molecule or organism, it needs to decide whether to respond or not. Frequently it does not – we normally fail to produce immune responses to the large amounts of foreign antigen that we ingest as food or are present as commensal organisms in our gut. Having decided to mount an immune response, there is a secondary decision – what sort of response should be initiated? Different pathogens need to be dealt with in different ways, and an inappropriate immune response will not only be ineffective, but may also damage the organism.

The decision-making is vital because there are important consequences to mistakes. The failure to mount an immune response when needed may cause uncontrolled infection or malignancy. However, mounting an immune response to foreign material when it is not needed can result in pathology, for example allergies. Immune responses against self can result in autoimmunity. Choice of inappropriate types of response will result in damage. Even appropriate immune responses frequently damage the organism; the necessary immune responses against tuberculosis mycobacteria result in scarring and granuloma formation in the lung. In the context of pregnancy, the immune response against an infection may result in abortion of the fetus, although the consequences of failing to respond would be more serious.

There are two main parts to the immune system: the innate and the adaptive immune systems. The innate immune system contains both cells and soluble molecules, and is often thought of as the first line of defence against pathogens. Unlike the adaptive immune system (see below), it does not recognize specific antigens on the pathogens, but rather responds to general common features of pathogens (for example sugar molecules expressed on the surface of bacteria but not mammalian cells).

The innate immune system is always present and ready to recognize and destroy pathogens (though it can be upregulated during inflammation). The adaptive immune system, in comparison, recognizes specific antigens using receptors (antibody and T cell receptors). When first faced with a pathogen, the adaptive immune response must first select and then amplify cells bearing the appropriate receptors (clonal selection; see below). Only then can it produce a specific immune response, resulting in a delay of several days before it is effective.

The adaptive immune response is characterized by its memory; once it has responded to an antigen it will mount a rapid and vigorous secondary immune response if it is re-exposed to the antigen (Fig. 8.1). This is the basis of both immunization and protection by prior infection.

However, the divide between the adaptive and innate immune system masks the considerable interactions that occur. This is both at the level of regulation of the immune response (the innate immune system is

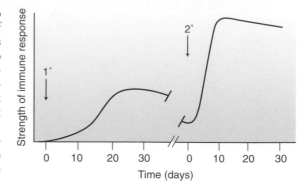

Figure 8.1 • Immunological memory. A cardinal feature of the adaptive immune system is its memory. When the immune system is first exposed to antigen (1° exposure, indicated by arrow) it takes a number of days for the immune response to get going. However, a secondary exposure (2°) to the same antigen results in a more rapid and stronger immune response. This is the basis of protection found following immunization or a primary infection.

essential in instructing the adaptive response), and at the level of effectors where components of the adaptive response amplify and focus the effector mechanisms of the innate system onto their targets.

In looking at the immune system, we will look first at the cells and molecules of the adaptive and innate systems. We will then go on to consider some examples of how they interact to control immune responses. Finally, we will turn to look at areas of particular interest to reproductive immunology.

Adaptive immune systems

The main cells of the adaptive immune system are the bone marrow-derived lymphocytes. There are two main categories of lymphocyte: the B lymphocyte (or B cell) and the T lymphocyte (T cell). B cells are responsible for producing the soluble antigen-specific effector molecule of the immune system, the antibody. T cells have two roles; one is to regulate the immune system (T helper cells and T regulatory cells) and the other is to kill virally infected or neoplastically transformed cells (cytotoxic T cells).

Antibody molecules

The main role of the B cell is to produce antibody molecules, or immunoglobulins (Fig. 8.2). Immunoglobulins have a basic structure consisting of four polypeptide chains: two identical heavy chains and two identical light chains. When different antibody molecules are compared, most of the antibody is similar.

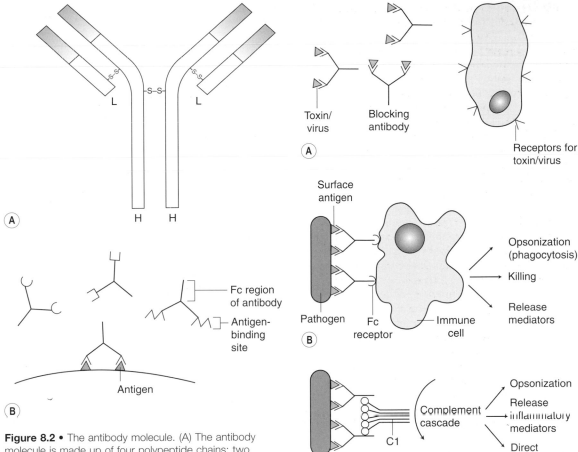

Figure 8.2 • The antibody molecule. (A) The antibody molecule is made up of four polypeptide chains: two identical heavy chains (H) and two identical light chains (L), held together with disulphide bonds. Within any one antibody class or subclass the sequence of most of the antibody is the same. However, the N-terminal parts of the molecule (shaded) vary between antibodies. The result is that every antibody molecule has a unique antigen binding site, as shown in cartoon form in (B), where the antibodies are depicted as a simple Y-shaped molecule with each antibody having a different antigen binding site. Where the antibody has a complementary structure to the antigen (for example of the surface of a pathogen), it can bind to the molecule.

Figure 8.3 • Antibody function. Antibodies can serve to block the binding of toxins and viruses to receptors on the surface of cells (A). They can also direct immune cells bearing Fc receptors to antibody-coated cells, the result of which depends on which cells are targeted but can include opsonization of the pathogen (preparing it for phagocytosis), killing, or the release of soluble mediators (B). In addition, the first component of the complement cascade (C1) can bind to the Fc regions, activating the complement cascade. This results in opsonization of the coated target, release of inflammatory mediators and direct killing of the target cell (C).

However, the N-terminal regions of the heavy and light chains are variable in sequence. These come together to form, for each antibody, a unique three-dimensional shape. It is this part of the antibody that binds to the antigen. Because each antibody has a different antigen binding site, it binds to a different antigen.

The antibody molecule has three main functions (Fig. 8.3). One of these is to act as the B cell receptor for antigen. The second is to bind directly to toxins, viruses and other molecules and block their ability to bind to a target cell. This is how anti-toxin (diphtheria/tetanus) antibodies work. The third function of anti-bodies is to recruit effector mechanisms to the target cell. It does this with the part of the molecule that does not vary (the constant region – in particular the upright 'stalk' of the molecule, called the Fc region). The Fc region binds to receptors (Fc receptors) on cells of the innate system, such as macrophages, neutrophils and eosinophils, and focuses them onto the target that carries the antigen recognized by the antibody.

In addition to targeting cells, the antibodies can also target a system of soluble molecules that are present

133

in the circulation, termed the 'complement system'. This consists of a large number of components that are organized in a cascade such that activation of one molecule leads to activation of the next molecule in the cascade (similar in many respects to the blood clotting system). Activation of the complement cascade results in the production of inflammatory proteins that cause increased vascular permeability, vasodilatation and recruitment of inflammatory cells. In addition, components of the complement cascade are coated onto the target cell. There they can act as recognition elements for cells of the immune system (phagocytes such as macrophages) and can also directly kill some pathogens. Complement can be activated in several manners, including innate recognition of pathogens. However, antibody will also activate the complement system by binding of the first component of the cascade to the Fc region of antibodies.

There are five different classes of antibody: IgM, IgG, IgD, IgA, IgE (in addition, there are subclasses of IgG and IgA). The different antibody classes have different functions. Thus, the different Fc regions recruit different effector responses – IgE, for example, binds strongly to mast cells and basophils and is important in allergic responses seen in asthma. IgA is found in mucosal secretions and provides protection for mucosal surfaces. IgM, which, consisting of five basic antibody units joined together, is important early in the immune response where the ability to bind to 10 antigen molecules simultaneously increases the strength of binding.

B cells

The adaptive immune response controls the production of antibody by a mechanism termed clonal selection (Fig. 8.4). During development, a large number (10^8 in the mouse, 10–100 times more in the human) of B cells are generated, each of which makes a unique antibody molecule. These early (termed naive or virgin) B cells do not secrete their antibody molecules, but express them on the surface of the cell as a receptor for antigen. These B cells are resident in the lymph nodes and spleen. When an antigen is introduced into the system (following infection or immunization), it is 'shown' to the different B cells there. Most B cells will not recognize the antigen, but, given the vast number of different antibody molecules, there will by chance be some that do bind to the antigen. The cells bearing these

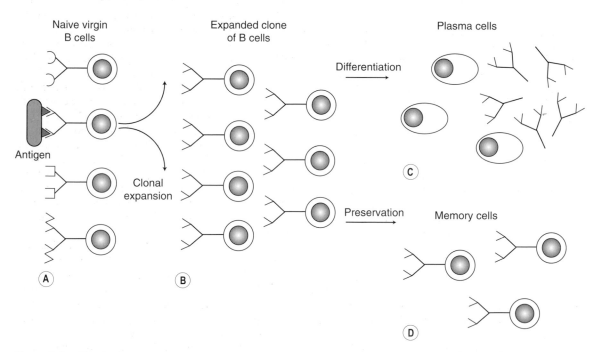

Figure 8.4 • Clonal selection theory. The clonal selection theory states that there are a large number of virgin, naive B cells, each of which expresses a different antibody on its surface – four are shown in (A). If antigen is introduced into the system, any B cell that has an antibody receptor that binds the antigen is activated and undergoes clonal expansion, resulting in a large number of B cells, all with the same antibody molecule (B). Some of these cells then differentiate into plasma cells, which secrete soluble antibody that can act as an effector molecule (C), while others persist to act as memory cells and form the basis of a rapid response upon re-exposure to antigen (D). Clonal selection also operates on T cells.

antibodies will start to divide, forming a clone of B cells recognizing the antigen, resulting in a swelling of the lymph node. After a period of clonal expansion, the B cells start to differentiate, no longer expressing the antibody on their surface but secreting it. In addition some of the B cells become memory cells, so that the next time the system encounters the antigen there is an increased pool of cells capable of recognizing the antigen, providing the basis for the memory of the immune response.

In addition, the B cell will, under control of the T helper cell (see below), change the class of antibody that it makes. Initially all the antibodies are IgM, but if, for example, the antibody is needed on a mucosal surface, then the class will switch to IgA.

During the course of a response, the immune system will also mutate the sequence of the antigen binding site of the antibody, selecting molecules that bind better to the antigen. This process is known as affinity maturation and improves the ability of the antibody to recognize the antigen.

T cells

Antigen recognition

The T cells are so called because they mature in the thymus. They recognize antigen through the T cell receptor (TCR). Like the antibody molecule, the TCR has a variable region that binds to antigen. In a similar manner to the B cell, the T cell with an appropriate TCR specificity undergoes clonal selection during an immune response. However, unlike the antibody, the TCR is only a cell surface receptor and is never secreted by a cell.

The way in which the TCR recognizes antigen is more complex. The TCR does not bind directly to pathogen-derived antigens, but rather recognizes the antigen in association with molecules of the major histocompatibility complex (MHC, also known as HLA in human). There are two types of MHC molecule involved in TCR recognition: class I molecules that are expressed on all nucleated cells and class II molecules that, under normal conditions, are expressed only on B cells and specialized antigen presenting cells (such as macrophages and dendritic cells, see below). Both MHC class I and class II molecules have a structure which allows them to bind to short peptides derived from the antigens (Fig. 8.5), and the TCR recognizes a combination of the foreign peptide and the MHC molecule, and is unable to recognize either individually.

The two MHC molecules present their peptides to different types of T cell, and also vary in how the peptide gets into the binding groove of the MHC molecule. Thus MHC class I molecules present peptide to cytotoxic T cells (Fig. 8.6A). The peptide is derived

from within the cell, and may result from a viral infection or be an antigen associated with neoplastic transformation of the cells (e.g. a mutated oncogene). These proteins are made in the cytoplasm, where they are chopped into small peptides by a molecular complex termed the proteosome. The peptides are then pumped into the endoplasmic reticulum by the T cell-activating protein (TAP) molecule, where they are loaded into the MHC class I peptide binding groove. The complex is then exported to the surface of the cell.

The T cells capable of recognizing antigen in the context of MHC class II are the helper and the regulatory T cells (see below) (Fig. 8.6B). In this case, the antigens are acquired from outside the cell, and are taken up by the antigen presenting cell. They are then degraded into peptides that are loaded onto MHC class II molecules before being exported to the cell surface.

Function of T cells

T cells can be differentiated in terms of both their function and markers expressed on their surface. Cytotoxic T cells express the molecule CD8 on their surface. Helper and regulatory T cells express CD4.

The role of CD8 cytotoxic T cells is to kill the target cells expressing the appropriate peptide in the context of MHC class I. In most cases this peptide will be derived from a virus or be a mutated oncogene.

CD4 T cells recognize peptide in the presence of MHC class II, which is only expressed on the surface of antigen presenting cells. There are two main roles of CD4 cells. The majority of CD4 cells are helper cells that serve to amplify the responses of other cells, both of the adaptive and innate immune systems. Indeed, in general the action of cytotoxic T cells and B cells are dependent upon such help. The T helper cells operate both by cell surface contact and, more generally, by secreting molecules termed cytokines that act on nearby cells. Thus secretion of cytokines such as tumour necrosis factor (TNF) by helper cells can activate macrophages, neutrophils and other cells to generate inflammatory responses.

The action of T helper cells is more subtle than just turning on immune responses. Different types of helper cell can be induced under different conditions, which by secreting different cytokines can determine the nature of the immune response. The two main types of helper cell characterized are Th1 and Th2 cells. The Th1 cells secrete interleukin (IL) 2, INFγ, TNFα and, in general, help inflammatory responses. Th2 cells secrete IL4, IL5, IL10 and IL13, which help antibody-mediated responses. The cytokines secreted by helper cells can also modify the nature of the antibody response, for example IL4 instructs B cells to switch antibody class to IgE production. More recently, a new T helper cell subset has been defined, the Th17

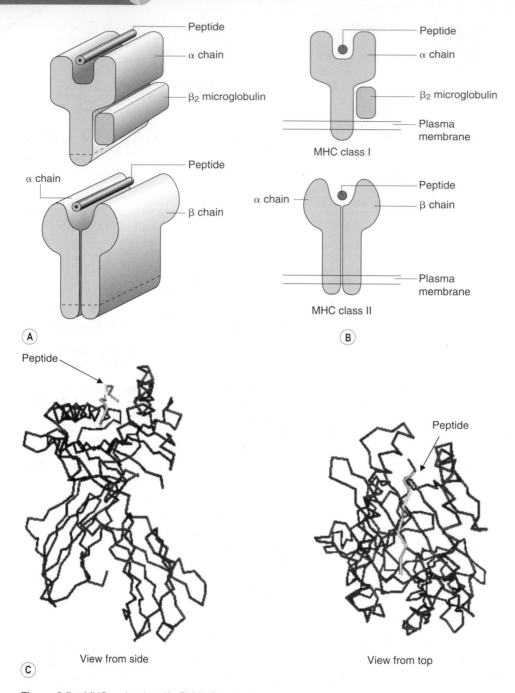

Figure 8.5 • MHC molecules. (A, B) MHC molecules are transmembrane molecules that bind peptide. The MHC class I molecule consists of one transmembrane chain (α chain) complexed to β_2 microglobulin. The MHC class II molecule contains two transmembrane chains, α and β. In both class I and class II molecules there is a similar binding site, or groove, which holds short linear peptides. The TCR 'recognizes' the combination of MHC and peptide. (C) The MHC molecules act to hold short linear antigenic peptides in a peptide binding groove of the molecule. The figure shows the structure of a MHC class I molecule binding a virus-derived peptide. The peptide is shown in light colour and the backbone of the MHC molecule in black. The left-hand figure shows a side view, with the peptide binding groove at the top. The right-hand figure shows a view from the top of the molecule, as would be 'seen' by a TCR docking – the TCR would 'recognize' both the MHC and the peptide together. The structure of the MHC class II peptide binding groove is similar.

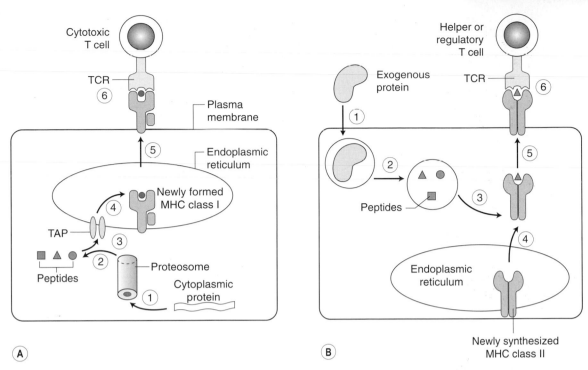

Figure 8.6 • Loading of peptides onto MHC molecules. (A) The MHC class I molecule binds peptides derived from cytoplasmic proteins. These are degraded by the proteosome (1) to form peptides (2), which are then transported by the TAP protein into the endoplasmic reticulum (3) and loaded onto newly formed MHC class I molecules (4), which are then transported to the cell surface (5) for recognition by cytotoxic T cells (6). (B) The MHC class II molecule binds peptides derived from extracellular (exogenous) proteins. The proteins are taken up and internalized by the antigen presenting cell (1), before being chopped up into peptides (2) and then associating (3) with MHC class II molecules that have been newly synthesized in the endoplasmic reticulum (4). The complex of peptide and MHC class II is then exported to the plasma cell membrane (5) where it can be recognized by T helper or regulatory cells (6).

cell. This subset of T helper cells is characterized by production of IL17, and is important in the pathogenesis of some autoimmune diseases.

The other type of CD4 cell is a regulatory T cell. These cells damp down immune responses, and have been shown to be responsible, in part, for blocking the action of T cells that recognize self-antigen, thus preventing autoimmunity. As with the helper cells, T regulatory cells operate by secreting cytokines (such as IL10 and TGFβ) and by self surface contact. As we shall discuss later, T regulatory cells have a role in preserving the fetus from immunological rejection.

Cells of the innate immune system

There are many cell types in the innate immune system, and we shall discuss only the most central. Indeed, many cells in the body that are not normally thought of as being immune cells can participate in immune responses by secreting cytokines and altering the expression of cell surface molecules. Thus, endothelial cells are involved in the recruitment of inflammatory cells, and many parenchymal cells can secrete cytokines that modify the immune cells in their locality.

NK cells

The natural killer (NK) cell is a lymphocyte; however, unlike T and B cells, it does not have receptors for specific antigens. Its main role is to kill target cells, in a manner similar to cytotoxic T cells. The NK cell recognizes its targets either by virtue of their being coated by an antibody (NK cells carry Fc receptors that allow them to recognize the antigen), or by receptors that recognize alterations in the cell surface molecules of the target cell. The most notable of these are receptors that recognize MHC class I molecules, expressed on all nucleated cells. If a cell downregulates its MHC class I expression then the absence of the class I molecules is detected by the NK cell, which kills it. This is an important mechanism because an obvious way for a virally infected or malignant T cell to escape from being killed by a cytotoxic T cell would be to downregulate expression of MHC class I molecules – preventing recognition of the antigenic peptide. However, NK cells circumvent this strategy as they wipe out class I-negative cells.

Macrophages

Macrophages are mononuclear phagocytic cells that take up and ingest foreign material and damaged cells. They recognize their targets either by general receptors on the surface (e.g. against carbohydrates expressed on bacteria), or because they are coated with antibody or complement components. Macrophages also express MHC class II, and so are capable of presenting antigen derived from the phagocytosed material to T helper cells, which in turn can secrete cytokines that activate the macrophages – an example of the intimate cooperation between adaptive and innate immune systems.

Macrophages are members of the monocyte family. Other closely related members of the family include the Kupffer cells that line the sinusoids of the liver and phagocytose circulating antibody-coated antigens.

Granulocytes

The granulocytes, so called because they have granules in their cytoplasm, include the neutrophil, eosinophil and basophil. These are capable of recognizing foreign material directly, but also can be focused by antibody and complement components. All granulocytes are capable of killing target cells by secreting toxic molecules present in granules and the production of reactive oxygen species, and also of inducing and amplifying inflammation by secreting soluble cytokines and other molecules. The most common is the neutrophil, which is important in controlling bacterial infections and is recruited in large numbers in inflammatory sites. The other cells have more specialized roles; for example the eosinophil kills parasites.

The dendritic cell

The dendritic cells are responsible for initiating adaptive immune response, because they are the only cells that stimulate naive T cells. Dendritic cells, in the form of Langerhans cells, are present in most tissues, such as the skin. In their resting state, they continually take antigens up from their surroundings and process them to present them on MHC class II molecules. In this state, the dendritic cell is known as an immature dendritic cell. However, if the dendritic cell is activated (by a pathogen or danger signal, see below) then it stops taking up antigen and moves rapidly to the lymph nodes where it can stimulate the response of an antigen-specific T cell.

Regulation of the immune system

The danger theory

As indicated above, the immune system has considerable control mechanisms. However, one control system, popularized as the 'danger theory', is fundamental to our understanding of immune responses. This suggests that the most important decision the immune system has to make is when to respond, and that questions about specificity (i.e. about what antibodies and TCRs recognize) are secondary. The immune system is activated to respond only where there is evidence that there is a damaging event happening, as indicated by the presence of 'danger signals'. These signals are caused by the presence of tissue damage and dead cells, as well as by the presence of some components derived from pathogens. If these signals are not present, then the immune system does not respond, even in the presence of foreign antigen.

The central interaction that mediates the danger signal is that involving the dendritic cell and the T cell (Fig. 8.7). The immature dendritic cell, which as described above expresses low levels of MHC class II, is resident in the tissues and traffics only slowly to the draining lymph nodes. When it reaches the lymph nodes, it is incapable of stimulating T cell proliferation (indeed it 'turns off' or anergizes T cells – see below), because it does not express a series of molecules called co-stimulatory molecules. However, if there are danger signals, for example tissue damage caused by a pathogen infection, a surgeon's scalpel or stepping on a rusty nail, then receptors on the dendritic cell are engaged by the resulting danger signals. The dendritic cell is then activated into a mature dendritic cell and upregulates expression of both MHC class II and co-stimulatory molecules, and rapidly moves to the lymph node where it can activate T cells specific for any foreign antigen that it has picked up.

The importance of the danger theory is that it allows us to understand when the immune system responds. It also explains why in some circumstances damage to tissues by infection or trauma can initiate immune responses in settings where normally there would be no such response.

Tolerance

While the danger theory can explain when the immune system responds, it is not enough to prevent autoimmunity, when there is an immune response against

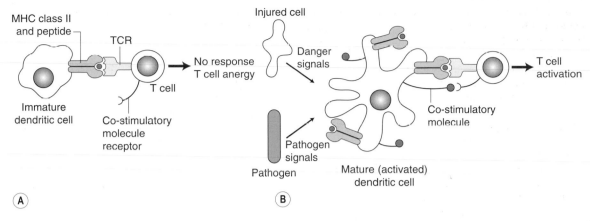

Figure 8.7 • Dendritic cell–T cell interactions and the danger signal. (A) Immature dendritic cells express low levels of MHC class II and co-stimulatory molecules. If T cells interact with these antigen presenting cells they are not activated, but rather are rendered anergic (refractory to further stimulation). This is because a T cell needs signals both from the TCR engagement of MHC and peptide, and from engagement of co-stimulatory molecules. (B) However, if the dendritic cell is activated either by danger signals from injured cells or by pathogen-derived signals then it undergoes a shape change, upregulated expression of MHC class II and co-stimulatory molecules, and rapidly migrates to the lymph node. Now if an antigen-specific T cell encounters the dendritic cell it is activated, as it receives signals both through the TCR and by binding co-stimulatory molecules.

self. If the danger theory was the only control process, then every time we cut ourselves with a kitchen knife, causing danger signals, we would initiate an auto-immune response against skin antigens. There are many mechanisms that prevent autoimmunity, the most fundamental of which is deletion of autoreactive cells.

The main time in which autoreactive lymphocytes are deleted is soon after they are formed. There is a window after the generation of a new B cell in the bone marrow when, if it recognizes antigen, it is killed. T cells develop in the thymus, where the same process of deletion occurs.

However, some autoreactive cells escape from the bone marrow or thymus, either by chance or because the antigen that they recognize is not found there (e.g. tissue-specific molecules). These cells are controlled by several additional mechanisms. One is the presence of regulatory T cells which turn off cell responses. These regulatory cells can be generated in the thymus, but also can be made in lymph nodes and other tissues.

Autoreactive T cells can also be turned off when they encounter antigen presented in particular ways. The most important example is when autoreactive T cells encounter an immature dendritic cell presenting a self-antigen (e.g. a tissue-specific antigen) and they become anergic (unresponsive to future stimulation). This means that an encounter with antigen in the absence of a danger signal will turn off an immune response.

The fetus as an allograft

One major focus of immunological research is in transplantation. It is important to understand some of the issues of transplantation when considering reproductive immunology because, from an immuno-logical point of view, the fetus is a form of transplanted tissue.

If an organ is transplanted from one individual to another without any drug treatment, it is rapidly rec-ognized by the immune system and destroyed. This alloresponse (between different members of the same species) is very strong because MHC molecules are highly polymorphic, showing considerable variability between individuals. These differences are recognized by a high frequency of T cells, termed alloreactive T cells.

Clinically, the rejection of allografts is minimized by attempting to match the MHC types of the donor and recipient (HLA matching). While it is realistically impossible (except in the case of twins) to obtain a perfect match, the better the match, the weaker the rejection response. The second approach is to immuno-suppress the recipient, using drugs, antibody or (not commonly in the clinical setting) irradiation. In the experimental laboratory setting, it is also possible to 're-educate' the immune system not to recognize the donor tissue, and to be tolerant of the transplanted organ. These strategies are being moved into the exper-imental clinical setting.

The fetus is a semi-allogeneic graft; half of its MHC molecules come from the mother and half from the father. It therefore presents a major target for the immune system. It is thus interesting to understand why the fetus is not normally rejected. It is now recognized that there are active processes by which fetal tissues (in particular at the placental interface between the mother and fetus) prevent cells of the maternal immune system from rejected the tissue.

Systemic control mechanisms

These processes have both a systemic and local action. At the systemic level, there is an increase in regulatory T cells during pregnancy, as well as a shift in the responses from a Th1 to a non-inflammatory Th2 type. The absence of regulatory T cells in animals leads to failure of gestation in mothers carrying allogeneic but not syngeneic (MHC identical) fetuses, indicating their role in preventing rejection. The presence of a Th1 type response in the placenta is associated with miscarriages, and can be caused by infection or stress. The factors responsible for Th2 bias in the immune responses include hormones and cytokines secreted by the placenta, including progesterone. The increase in the number of regulatory cells and the alteration in the Th1/Th2 balance are likely to be important reasons why several autoimmune diseases (including rheumatoid arthritis) are mitigated during pregnancy, with the symptoms getting worse after delivery. However, patients with some autoimmune diseases, such as systemic lupus erythematosus, can undergo mild to moderate 'flares' during pregnancy or immediately after, possibly because Th2 responses are important in the pathogenesis of this disease.

When the fetus is rejected by the immune system, it need not involve direct killing mechanisms. Thus, Th1 cytokines can act on trophoblastic cells to induce a procoagulant phenotype in the placental circulation, clotting off the maternal circulation.

Local immunomodulation

More local immunomodulation may be the result of expression of molecules by cells at the interface between the mother and fetus. A key cell is the syncytiotrophoblast, which forms the fetal-derived boundary between the mother and fetal cells. These cells have no or little expression of MHC molecules. As such, they might be a target for attack by NK cells. However, they express an alternative MHC molecule (HLA-G in the human) that binds to NK cells, giving them a negative signal that prevents activation (Fig. 8.8). The cells also express an enzyme, indoleamine 2,3-dioxygenase (IDO), that catabolizes tryptophan. This is an essential amino acid, and T cell responses are inhibited by both low concentrations of tryptophan and by the metabolites (kynurenines) generated by IDO breakdown of tryptophan (Fig. 8.8). Syncytiotrophoblasts also express CD95-ligand (CD95L, also known as FasL). This is the receptor for CD95 (Fas) which is expressed by activated leukocytes. Engagement of CD95 on the leukocytes by CD95L induces apoptosis in any alloreactive T cells (Fig. 8.8).

Antibodies and pregnancy

Antibodies are important in pregnancy. In some cases this is because of the damage that they cause, for example in rhesus incompatibility and anti-phospholipid syndrome. Importantly, antibodies are actively transported from the maternal circulation into the fetal circulation, where they are responsible for much of the immunity of the infant post partum.

Maternal anti-fetal antibodies can be induced during pregnancy or may be pre-existing (such as the ABO blood group antibodies). In order to prevent damage to placental cells that bind these antibodies, there are high levels of complement regulatory molecules expressed on trophoblastic cells, which prevent activation of complement by antibody coating these cells.

Anti-phospholipid syndrome, in which there are circulating antibodies against molecules such as cardiolipin or phosphatidylserine, is associated with early and late fetal loss, as well as intrauterine growth retardation and other fetal morbidities. While there is still debate about how the antibodies cause disease, the anti-phospholipid antibodies may have a direct effect on trophoblast development, with a failure to establish a good feto-placental circulation being responsible for early pregnancy losses. In later pregnancy the proinflammatory and prothrombotic effects of the antibody on the endothelial cells (probably in combination with complement) may be responsible for the pathologies associated with this syndrome.

At birth the neonate has almost no endogenous antibodies. One of the roles of the placenta is to transport maternal immunoglobulin into the fetus. Following birth, this maternal antibody provides temporary immunity while the infant's own immune system matures. In many other mammals, the maternal antibody is predominantly provided through milk rather than via the placenta (in the human IgA antibodies in the maternal milk are important in protecting the infant's gut). The maternal antibody is transported through the syncytiotrophoblast layer, probably via the neonatal Fc receptor (FcRn), which binds to the Fc region of the antibody, internalizes it in an endosome and deposits it on the other side of the cell. Immune complexes between antibodies and antigens and antibodies reactive with paternal HLA molecules are

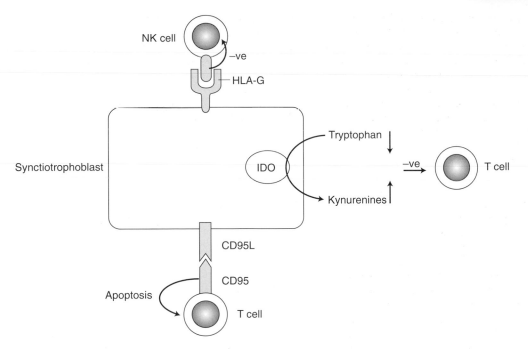

Figure 8.8 • Local immunomodulation by syncytiotrophoblasts. Syncytiotrophoblasts are capable of modulating immune responses in a variety of ways. The expression of HLA-G inhibits NK cell activity. Expression of the enzyme IDO catabolizes tryptophan, and both deprivation of tryptophan and the production of metabolites (kynurenines) inhibit T cell activation. Finally, expression of CD95L (FasL) results in apoptosis of inflammatory cells that express CD95 (Fas).

absorbed in the stroma, and the antibody then crosses the fetal endothelial cells.

Maternal antibodies can damage the fetus and/or newborn infant. This is seen when the mother has an antibody-mediated autoimmune disease, such as Grave's disease or myasthenia gravis, where transfer of autoantibody results in disease in the infant (which remits as the maternal antibody is cleared).

The classic case of maternally derived antibodies damaging the infant is haemolytic disease of the newborn, resulting in general from incompatibilities in the rhesus blood group antigen. RhD-negative women carrying a RhD-positive fetus have no problems with their first pregnancy. However, at birth the passage of fetal blood to the mother can immunize her, resulting in an anti-RhD antibody response. In subsequent pregnancies the anti-RhD antibodies can cross into the fetal circulation prior to birth, leading to lysis of red blood cells. This can be treated by intrauterine blood transfusions, or prevented by administration to RhD-negative women of anti-RhD antisera at the time of each birth (or invasive procedure). These antibodies mop up the fetal blood, preventing maternal immunization.

Other immunological interactions with the fetus

In addition to killing pathogens, the immune system is important in tissue repair and remodelling. Many of the immune system's pathophysiological roles in pregnancy do not involve killing of the fetal allograft, and that active involvement of the immune system is important for successful gestation.

One such example is the interaction between maternal NK cells and fetal cytotrophoblasts that penetrate the maternal decidua and are necessary for the remodelling of the spiral arteries. The NK cells in this process do not have a cytotoxic role, but their recognition, in particular of MHC antigens (HLA-C, -E and -G in the human) on the cytotrophoblasts, results in the secretion of cytokines that are necessary for the action of the cytotrophoblasts. Failure of this recognition can result in poor remodelling of the spiral arteries and inadequate placentation – leading ultimately to pre-eclampsia or intrauterine growth retardation. The importance of this pathway is supported by genetic findings demonstrating that pre-eclampsia is more common when the receptors on the maternal NK cells are poor at being stimulated by the fetal MHC molecules. The immunological component may also explain why pre-eclampsia is more common in first pregnancies.

Conclusion

The immune system is a complex network of cells and molecules that are tightly controlled. In pregnancy, this control ensures that the fetus is not destroyed or damaged. While the main role of the immune system may be to protect the organism against pathogens, it is also involved in tissue remodelling and repair, and these functions may be crucial in pregnancy.

Chapter Nine

9

Biochemistry

Fiona Lyall

CHAPTER CONTENTS

Structure and function of the normal cell

The human body consists of cells and intercellular matrices.

Cells

All cells possess certain basic structural features, regardless of their location, type and function (Fig. 9.1). The major division is into nucleus and cytoplasm.

Nucleus

This is surrounded by a bilaminar nuclear membrane or envelope with occasional pores and contains the chromosomes, made from molecules of deoxyribonucleic acid (DNA), responsible for genetic coding and

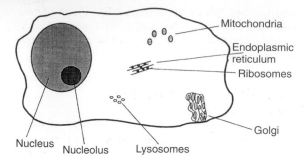

Figure 9.1 • Structure of a cell.

Organelle	Function
Nucleus	Contains chromosomal material and apparatus for cell division
Nucleolus	RNA and ribsosome production
Lysosomes	Degradation of macromolecules
Golgi apparatus	Modification of proteins and their secretion and re-cycling
Endoplasmic reticulum	Membrane system for protein synthesis
Ribosomes	Catalyse peptide bond formation in protein synthesis
Mitochondria	Contain many enzymes involved in metabolism and energy production

inheritance. Within the nucleus, one or more mobile nucleoli are present; they contain ribonucleic acid (RNA), and are involved in cell protein synthesis. Nuclear RNA is a precursor of cytoplasmic ribosomal RNA (see Ch. 1).

Cytoplasm

This comprises the remainder of the cell. It is enclosed within a trilaminar cell membrane, which has a very complex biochemical structure, including many proteins and lipids; it is not rigid, but can alter its shape in response to various stimuli. The major function of the cell membrane is control and maintenance of the appropriate intracellular electrolyte and biochemical environment by energy-requiring active transport mechanisms (e.g. sodium removal by the sodium pump). It also provides adhesion between adjacent cells, and bears the individual's major histocompatibility (transplant or HLA) antigens. In some cells (e.g. polymorphs), it determines motility and phagocytosis.

The cytoplasm contains many organelles:

1. *Mitochondria* are elongated, enzyme-rich bodies; each has a continuous external limiting membrane and an inner membrane folded into septa (cristae), which create partial subdivisions of the matrix. Mitochondria oxidize proteins, carbohydrates and fats into energy, store it as adenosine triphosphate (ATP) and subsequently release it when required by the cell.

2. *Ribosomes* are small granules containing RNA, the molecular structure of which is determined by nuclear DNA. They control synthesis of proteins required for intracellular metabolism. Aggregates of ribosomes are designated polysomes or polyribosomes.

3. *The endoplasmic reticulum* is a complex network of intercommunicating narrow tubules and vesicles (cisternae) mainly responsible for synthesizing proteins subsequently secreted outside the cell. Two continuous types exist: rough endoplasmic reticulum, where ribosomes are attached to the outer surface, and smooth endoplasmic reticulum where ribosomes are absent.

4. *The centrosome* is a relatively clear area, usually near the cell centre, containing two centrioles.

5. *Centrioles* are hollow cylindrical bodies, 0.3–0.7 μm in length, which replicate before mitosis and orientate the mitotic spindle.

6. *The Golgi complex* is usually near the centrosome, and comprises numerous, small, irregular sacs, vacuoles and vesicles. It probably collects, modifies, packages and transports secretions from the rough endoplasmic reticulum to the cell membrane and, when necessary, adds carbohydrate residues.

7. *Lysosomes* are round or oval membrane-bound bodies containing proteolytic enzymes (acid hydrolases) for digesting unwanted endogenous and phagocytosed exogenous material.

8. *Phagosomes* are membrane-bound bodies containing material ingested by phagocytosis. To effect digestion, phagosomes combine with lysosomes to produce phagolysosomes. When indigestible material remains, residual or dense bodies are formed.

9. *Microtubules*, 20–27 nm in diameter, are found throughout the cytoplasm. They constitute the mitotic spindle filaments, and may also facilitate intracytoplasmic transport and maintain cell shape.

10. *Microfilaments*, 4–12 nm in diameter, are of indefinite length. Some (tonofibrils) converge on intercellular junctions (desmosomes) to promote cell adhesion; functions of microfilaments elsewhere are unknown.

Specific structures are unique to, and characteristic of, specialized cells, e.g. myofilaments in muscle cells and melanosomes in melanocytes. Several other structures may also be seen, including glycogen granules, lipofuscin granules, myelinoid bodies, siderosomes and lipid droplets.

Cell types

All cells are classified as one of two types: (1) epithelial or (2) connective tissue.

Epithelial cells cover or line body surfaces and internal cavities; in addition, most glands are epithelial, being derived embryologically from body surfaces. Epithelial cells therefore act as selective and protective barriers and synthesize most secretions.

Connective tissue cells are derived largely from the embryonic mesoderm. Connective tissue exists in many types, and its composition varies in different parts of the body, depending on local requirements. Its main function is to provide structural support, generally as fibrous tissue and specifically as bone, cartilage, muscle and tendon. It is probably also responsible for body defences, since leucocytes and mononuclear phagocyte (reticuloendothelial) system cells are usually considered connective tissue in origin.

Intercellular matrix

This varies considerably in amount; very little is seen between epithelial cells, whereas connective tissue cells are often quite widely separated by matrix, the exact nature of which may provide the unique connective tissue structure (e.g. bone and cartilage). Interstitial extracellular fluid is located in the intercellular matrix.

The epithelial intercellular matrix is a narrow, mucopolysaccharide-rich layer traversed by intercellular junctions. Formerly a designated cement substance, it is now thought, in some instances, to be an integral component of the cell membrane's external surface (glycocalyx).

Connective tissue intercellular matrix contains ground substance and fibres. The ground substance is a gel of variable consistency and viscosity, containing mucoproteins, glycoproteins and mucopolysaccharides; it is probably mainly secreted by fibroblasts. Of the fibres, collagen is the most important, being virtually ubiquitous and providing much structural rigidity. It is a tri-helical structure derived from a soluble precursor (procollagen), secreted by fibroblasts and osteoblasts via an insoluble intermediate (tropocollagen). Four biochemical types, controlled by different structural genes, are described: types I (mature collagen in dermis, bone and tendon), II (unique to cartilage) and III (as 'reticulin' in early scar tissue, cardiovascular tissue and synovium) possess the triple helix and have a banded structure electron-optically; in contrast, type IV (in basement membranes) is probably not helical and appears amorphous ultrastructurally. Elastic fibres, comprising protein (elastin) and polysaccharide, provide resilience and are produced by smooth muscle cells and fibroblasts.

Proteins, peptides and amino acids

Each of the many cell types in the body makes a unique set of proteins. There is considerable variation in the types of protein made by each cell type and a particular cell synthesizes only a fraction of the total human protein repertoire. For example, despite the large amount of albumin present in blood plasma, it is only the hepatocytes in the liver that synthesize albumin; no other cell type does so in the adult. This is despite the fact that every cell contains within its nucleus a copy of the gene for albumin along with a copy of every other human gene. This concept is referred to as 'totipotency'; every cell has a copy of every gene, even though only a fraction are expressed. During development and differentiation, the DNA within each cell type comes under a regulatory mechanism such that some genes are expressed and others are completely repressed. In the case of some proteins, expression does not occur all the time but does so in response to a specific signal such as a hormone. The control of protein expression is aberrant in many tumours and inappropriate proteins are produced.

The proteins synthesized by a cell play a number of different roles. Some proteins have a structural role. This can be intracellular and there are proteins that provide the structural basis for the membrane around the cell and the membranes around the nucleus, mitochondria and the other discrete subcellular organelles. Figure 9.1 is a diagrammatic representation of a cell; each of the subcellular organelles contains structural proteins. Other proteins are secreted by a cell and are then used to support an extracellular structure. An example here is collagen. There are a number of forms of collagen which are encoded by discrete genes. The different collagens play specific roles; for example, collagen type I is the form found in bone, collagen type II is found in cartilage and collagen type IV is found in the basement membranes of epithelia. Collagen type III is found in the tissues of the fetus but this is replaced by type I following birth. Adults have little type III, although it does reappear during the wound response. Collagen type I is a major component of bones, skin and a number of other tissues and this single protein comprises more than 50% of the total protein in the body.

Another role of proteins is enzymic function. The human genome encodes many hundreds of proteins which act as enzymes for specific reactions; these include synthetic reactions, degradative reactions, energy-producing reactions and energy-storing reactions. Very few biochemical reactions occur in the absence of enzymes and thus this catalysis is essential for life.

Some proteins are synthesized and then secreted to carry out a particular function that is non-structural. Hormones and neurotransmitters fall into this category as do the large number of proteins that play a role in transport and are found in plasma. One of the functions of albumin is to transport free fatty acids, and the plasma protein transferrin carries iron from the gut to tissues. In blood, there are different classes of lipoprotein that carry lipids in circulation; chylomicrons carry triglycerides from the gut to adipose tissue and the liver. Low-density lipoproteins carry much of the cholesterol that is required by tissues; some of the cholesterol comes from dietary sources but most has been synthesized in the liver.

Some proteins in plasma play a hormone-binding role. Other major constituents of plasma are the immunoglobulins (antibodies) and complement proteins that are part of the immune system.

Amino acids

There are 20 amino acids used in the synthesis of proteins. The generalized structure of an amino acid in Figures 9.2 and 9.3 shows the chemical structure of the amino acids used by humans along with the two notations that are used to denote them. One has a three-letter code, but as there are so many protein sequences now available, a one-letter code has become the preferred notation.

Not all amino acids can be synthesized *in vivo*. Those that can be synthesized are referred to as the 'non-essential amino acids' and comprise the following:

- Alanine
- Aspartic acid
- Asparagine
- Glutamine
- Cysteine
- Glutamic acid
- Glycine

- Proline
- Serine
- Tyrosine.

The essential amino acids are:

- Arginine
- Histidine
- Isoleucine
- Leucine
- Lysine
- Valine
- Methionine
- Phenylalanine
- Threonine
- Tryptophan.

The situation is slightly more complex than this since cysteine can be synthesized if there is sufficient methionine present; similarly, tyrosine can be synthesized if there is sufficient phenylalanine present. Histidine and arginine are not strictly essential but are required for normal growth. The essential amino acids are required in the diet. A simple estimate of total protein will not indicate sufficiency. For example, if the diet contained insufficient valine, then the total protein content would be immaterial since protein synthesis cannot continue in the absence of valine. This leads to the concept of qualitative and quantitative dietary sufficiency. A diet is only satisfactory if it contains adequate concentrations of the essential amino acids. Because amino acids provide the source of all nitrogen, an individual is said to be in nitrogen balance if intake is exactly equivalent to loss resulting from turnover. Positive nitrogen balance exists when intake is in excess of loss. An individual in negative nitrogen balance will begin to show weight loss even if the total nitrogen, carbohydrate and other dietary requirements are in excess.

A protein is a sequence of amino acids that are chemically coupled by enzymes. The sequence of events that occurs in the synthesis of a protein is depicted in Figure 9.4. The sequence of amino acids for a protein is encoded in the gene for that protein. This genetic information is stored in the form of DNA. The structure of DNA is that of a helix of two long chains. Each chain is a phosphodiester backbone carrying a covalently linked sequence of the bases that make up the genetic code. There are four bases, namely, adenine, cytosine, guanine and thymine. The strands of DNA are held together tightly by interaction between bases on each strand. The base adenine binds to thymine and cytosine binds to guanine. This complementarity provides accurate and strong pairing.

A gene is a sequence of DNA on one of the strands of a chromosome and there are many hundreds of genes on each chromosome. The first stage in the

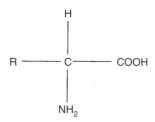

Figure 9.2 • General structure of an amino acid. R is an organic group (see also Fig. 9.5).

AMINO ACID	STRUCTURE	SYMBOL
Basic amino acids		

Arginine	H—N—CH_2—CH_2—CH_2—CH—COO^-
	     | |
	    C=$_4NH_2$ $_4NH_3$
	     |
	    NH_2
		Arg (R)

Lysine	CH_2—CH_2—CH_2—CH_2—CH—COO^- | | $_4NH_3$ $_4NH_3$	Lys (K)
Histidine	⬠—CH_2—CH—COO^- HN $_4NH$ | $_4NH_3$	His (H)
Acidic amino acids		

Aspartic acid	^-OOC—CH_2—CH—COO^-
	                  |
	                $_4NH_3$
		Asp (D)

Glutamic acid	^-OOC—CH_2—CH_2—CH—COO^-
	                         |
	                       $_4NH_3$
		Glu (E)

Asparagine	H_2N—C—CH_2—CH—COO^-
	         || |
	         O $_4NH_3$
		Asn (N)

Glutamine	H_2N—C—CH_2—CH_2—CH—COO^-
	         || |
	         O $_4NH_3$
		Glu (Q)

Aromatic amino acids		

Phenylalanine	⬡—CH_2—CH—COO^-
	              |
	            $_4NH_3$
		Phe (F)

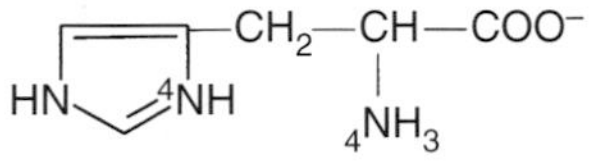

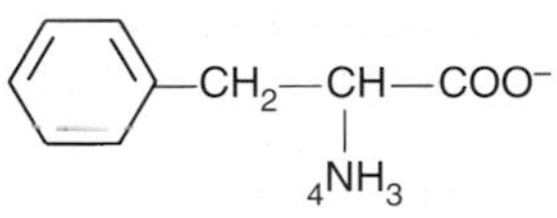

Figure 9.3 • Structures of the amino acids.

AMINO ACID	STRUCTURE	SYMBOL
	Aromatic amino acids	
Tyrosine	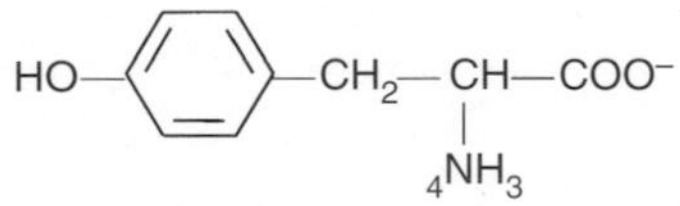	Tyr (Y)
Tryptophan	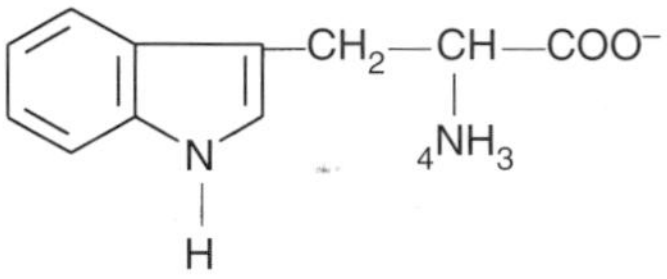	Try (W)
	Amino acids with aliphatic chains	
Glycine	$H{-}\underset{_4NH_3}{\underset{\vert}{CH}}{-}COO^-$	Gly (G)
Alanine	$CH_3{-}\underset{_4NH_3}{\underset{\vert}{CH}}{-}COO^-$	Ala (A)
Valine	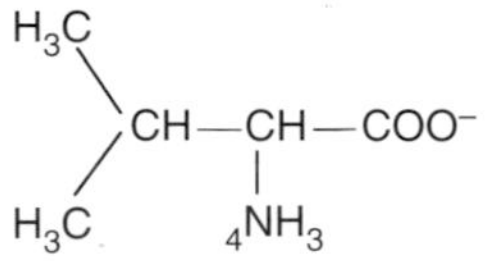	Val (V)
Leucine	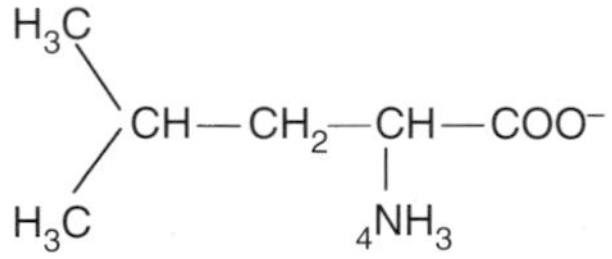	Leu (L)
Isoleucine	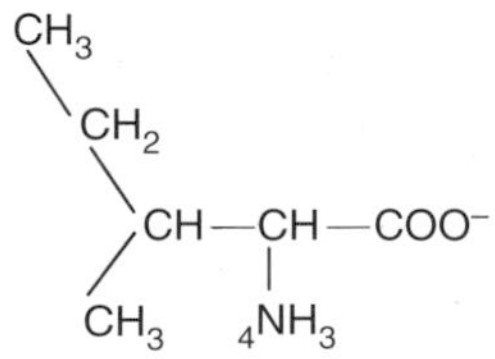	Iso (I)

Figure 9.3 • (cont'd)

AMINO ACID	STRUCTURE	SYMBOL
Amino acids with hydroxyl groups		
Serine	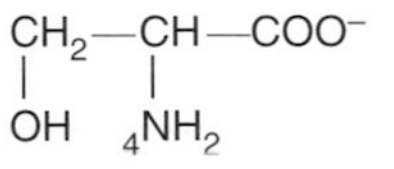 CH_2—CH—COO^- $\mid$ $\mid$ OH $_4NH_2$	Ser (S)

Threonine	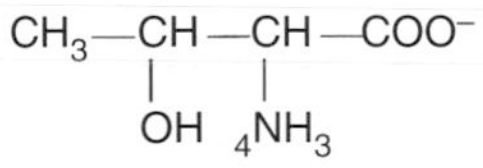 CH_3—CH—CH—COO^-
	     $\mid$ $\mid$
	     OH $_4NH_3$
		Thr (T)

Amino acids with sulphydryl groups		
Cysteine	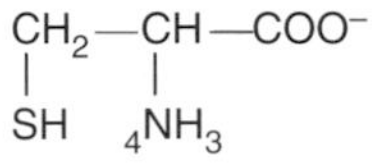 CH_2—CH—COO^- $\mid$ $\mid$ SH $_4NH_3$	Cys (C)
Methionine	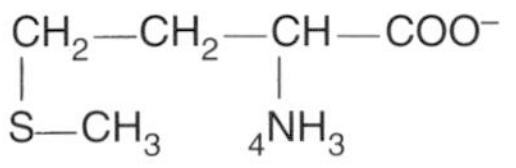 CH_2—CH_2—CH—COO^- $\mid$ $\mid$ S—CH_3 $_4NH_3$	Met (M)
Imino acids		
Proline	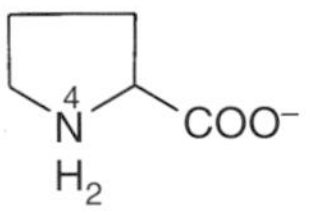 (ring structure) $_4$N COO^- H_2	Pro (P)

Figure 9.3 • (cont'd)

production of a protein is transcription; this is the term used to denote the process in which a complementary copy of the gene is made. The product is messenger ribonucleic acid (mRNA), which is a single-stranded nucleic acid. RNA has ribose rather than deoxyribose in the phosphodiester backbone. Like DNA it contains the bases cytosine, guanine and adenine but, in contrast to DNA, contains uracil rather than thymine. (The terminology of the bases is complex. The terms 'adenine', 'cytosine', 'guanine', 'thymine' and 'uracil' are used to describe the bases. When these are linked to the sugar ribose they are called 'adenosine', 'cytidine', 'guanosine', 'uridine' and 'thymidine'. If they are linked to deoxyribose, the prefix 'deoxy' is used.)

The mRNA becomes attached to ribosomes. Each functional ribosome is composed of two subunits, each of which contains a number of different proteins and RNA species. The function of the RNA is not understood but the proteins are responsible for the recognition of all the substrates and factors that are required for protein synthesis. One of these proteins is the enzyme that couples together successive pairs of amino acids in the fashion shown in Figure 9.5.

Structure of proteins

Proteins vary greatly in size. Small proteins are referred to as 'peptides' and some of these have fewer than 10

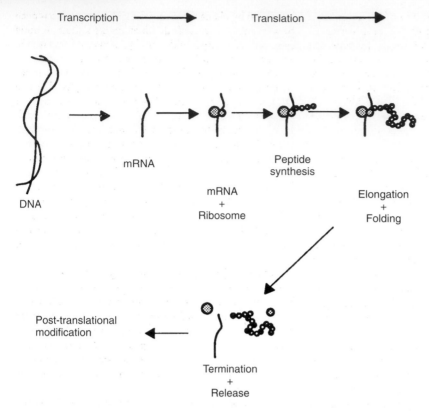

Figure 9.4 • Sequence of events in protein synthesis.

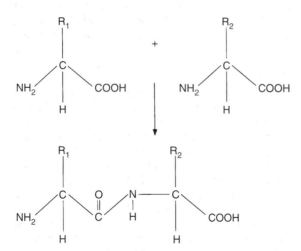

Figure 9.5 • Formation of a peptide bond.

amino acids in their sequence and have molecular weights of about 1000 Da. Examples would be the hormones oxytocin and vasopressin. At the other end of the spectrum, some proteins are close to 1 million daltons in molecular weight and have hundreds of amino acids in their sequence. Examples of larger proteins would be α_2-macroglobulin, an important anti-

protease found in plasma, and the IgM class of immunoglobulins, which play a role in the early defence reaction against infecting organisms.

Proteins fold up into complex three-dimensional structures. Peptide bonds are free to adopt a number of conformational states and the three-dimensional structure of the protein is held together by a large number of interactions. Hydrogen bonding is a relatively weak interaction but can be widespread. Any hydrogen atom can interact with a nucleus that has a small negative charge. This sort of interaction is important in maintaining the helical and pleated sheet structures within proteins. Hydrophilic interactions are essentially charge–charge interactions. They are referred to as hydrophilic since water molecules are usually involved and most commonly they will bond together negatively and positively charged amino acids. Hydrophobic interactions occur when the non-charged side chains of amino acids are in close apposition.

The primary structure of a protein is its simplest description, and relates to the linear sequence of amino acids which has been encoded by the gene for that protein. The primary sequence usually begins with an amino acid with a free amino terminal (N-terminus) and will conclude with the last amino acid which will have a free carboxyl group (C-terminus). All the intervening amino acids will have lost their free amino and carboxyl groups since these will have been involved in the formation of the peptide bonds. Some proteins are modified at the N-terminus. For example, some of the proteins involved in the blood-clotting cascade have the N-terminal glutamic acid modified to become a γ-carboxyglutamic acid residue. The blocking of the N-terminus in this case involves an enzyme cascade that requires vitamin K. Warfarin acts by inhibiting this pathway.

The secondary structure of a protein describes the parts of the sequence that have folded into helical or pleated sheet structures. The nature of the peptide bond is such that the formation of these helices and sheets is thermodynamically favoured and hence these regions are found in most proteins.

The tertiary structure of a protein is the complete three-dimensional arrangement of a single protein subunit. This can only be determined using techniques such as X-ray crystallography and, in the case of smaller proteins, nuclear magnetic resonance. These approaches are now allowing an understanding of the complex manner in which protein function is controlled.

Many proteins are composed of subunits. These can be identical or dissimilar. The subunits are held together by non-covalent forces which are most commonly charge–charge interactions. The three-dimensional structure of all the subunits comprising a protein is referred to as its quaternary structure.

Purification and analysis of proteins

There are several techniques available for the separation of proteins. Most can be used preparatively for the purification of a single protein to homogeneity as well as analytically in order to determine the degree of purity of a protein.

Some methods separate proteins on the basis of size. Thus, gel permeation chromatography involves the use of beds of resin beads that contain pores of a predetermined size. Some proteins will diffuse into these pores while other proteins are too large and are excluded. Large proteins are eluted from the bed before the smaller ones. A second method involving size is gel electrophoresis. A support of agarose or polyacrylamide is used and the protein solution is exposed to an electric field. In the absence of detergent the proteins will move according to their mass/charge ratio. If a detergent such as sodium dodecyl sulphate is added to the system, the proteins move at a rate proportional to their size alone.

Ion-exchange chromatography involves the use of resins that contain at their surface positively or negatively charged groups. Proteins contain negatively charged carboxyl groups and positively charged amino groups. The proteins will bind to the resin and can then be eluted by changing either the pH or the salt strength of the buffers used. Individual proteins have unique patterns of charge and can be separated from one another if gradients of buffer strengths are used.

One technique that has been developed more recently is that of affinity chromatography. Here a chemical moiety is chemically coupled to a bed of support beads. The agent that is coupled binds with high specificity to the protein that is to be purified. When a mixture of proteins in solution is passed through the bed, only the protein in question binds to the beads and, after washing off all non-specifically bound material, a high salt concentration or change of pH is used to elute the protein. The types of ligand that can be coupled to the beads are antibodies or substrate for an enzyme. The technique is very powerful and complete purity can be achieved in a single step.

Modification of protein structure

Very few proteins are composed purely of amino acid chains and most have carbohydrate chains covalently attached. This is referred to as post-translational modification because, after the protein has been synthesized on the ribosomes, the peptide passes to the Golgi apparatus, where enzymes assemble chains of sugars onto the protein.

The carbohydrate is always linked to specific amino acids in the protein chains, namely serine, threonine or asparagine. In the case of serine or threonine, the carbohydrate is linked via the oxygen of the hydroxyl groups and is hence referred to as O-linked carbohydrate. In the case of asparagine, it is linked to the nitrogen of the amino group and is referred to as N-linked carbohydrate.

There is considerable diversity in terms of the size and nature of the carbohydrate that is attached to protein and it appears to serve different functions. Proteins that are part of membranes are heavily glycosylated (the term used to denote the attachment of sugar residues) and the oligosaccharide chains play a role in maintaining the proteins in the correct orientation within the membrane. The proteins found in plasma are glycosylated and in this case the sugar plays a regulatory role in controlling turnover. While sugar chains remain intact, the protein continues to circulate in plasma. When the sugar chains become cleaved or modified, then the proteins are removed from circulation and degraded. The liver has a most efficient mechanism for detecting altered circulating proteins. There are in the newly formed proteins no terminal galactose residues; there is a sialic acid residue after the galactose. If the galactosyl groups are revealed following damage to the protein, it is immediately removed from circulation by hepatocytes which contain at their surface a receptor for the terminal galactose.

Metabolism

Overall energy metabolism

Every cell has to maintain an adequate supply of energy. There are several sources of energy and each is metabolized to produce adenosine triphosphate (ATP). The ATP is essential for cellular processes such as protein synthesis, and transport and maintenance of ionic gradients across the plasma membrane. Carbohydrate and fatty acids are the normal energy sources but under certain circumstances amino acids can also be used. Which particular energy source is used depends upon a number of parameters such as dietary status, circadian rhythm, etc. In this section the individual metabolic pathways will be described followed by the controls that operate and the interrelationships between the pathways.

The metabolism of carbohydrates (sugars), fats (fatty acids) and amino acids begins with pathways that are specific for each energy source. The products from these pathways then feed into common pathways. The overall interaction of the pathways is shown in Figure 9.6.

Sugars, fatty acids and amino acids are metabolized to produce acetate in the form of acetyl coenzyme A (acetyl-CoA). The acetyl group has to be covalently linked to CoA for stabilization.

The acetyl-CoA then enters the tricarboxylic acid (TCA) cycle, which is also known as the 'citric acid cycle' or the 'Krebs cycle', after the biochemist who was involved in its discovery. The TCA cycle results in the complete degradation of acetyl groups. The products are carbon dioxide and hydrogen in the form of nicotinamide adenine dinucleotide (NADH); the role of this co-factor will be described later. The NADH feeds into the respiratory chain inside the mitochondrion and the energy of the NADH is used to drive oxidative phosphorylation to produce ATP from adenosine diphosphate (ADP). This reaction within the respiratory chain requires molecular oxygen, hence the name 'respiratory chain'.

Molecules such as glucose and fatty acids are sources of energy because there is an intrinsic energy within the bonds of the molecule and this energy is released when the molecule is broken into smaller parts. What nature has done is to evolve a mechanism by which this energy can be harnessed to produce ATP, which acts in turn as the energy source to drive most biological reactions. Looking at the sequence of events for a molecule of glucose, the glycolytic pathway converts glucose to three acetate groups:

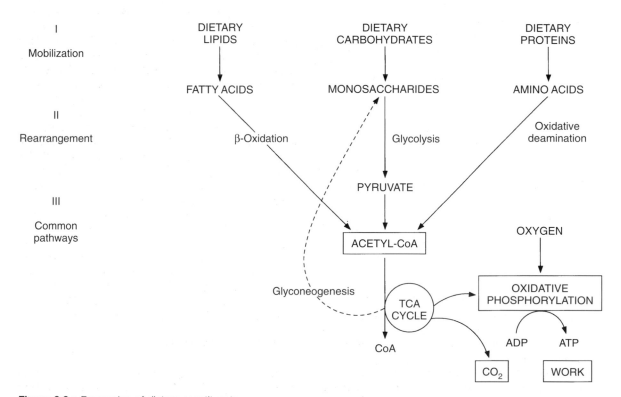

Figure 9.6 • Processing of dietary constituents.

$$C_6H_{12}O_6 \rightarrow 3C_2H_4O_2$$

The three molecules of acetate enter the TCA cycle in the form of acetyl-CoA and are converted to six molecules of carbon dioxide and 24 atoms of hydrogen in the form of NADH:

$$(3C_2H_4O_2) + (6\,H_2O) \rightarrow 6\,CO_2 + 24\,H$$

The carbon dioxide diffuses out of the cell and is expired by the lungs. The NADH enters the respiratory chain in the mitochondrion and, with the consumption of oxygen, is converted to water:

$$24\,H + 6\,O_2 \rightarrow 12\,H_2O$$

This part of the reaction brings about the conversion of ADP to ATP.

The overall reaction has been:

$$C_6H_{12}O_6 \rightarrow 6\,CO_2 + 6\,H_2O$$

i.e. the complete oxidation of a molecule of glucose to carbon dioxide and water. Nature has evolved an efficient sequence of reactions and most of the energy within the glucose molecule is utilized in the production of ATP from ADP. A single molecule of glucose can result in the formation of 38 ATP molecules. The chemical combustion of glucose in the presence of excess oxygen would yield 686 000 cal/mol. Each time an ADP molecule is converted to one of ATP, 7300 cal are required. Thus, since there is a net profit of about 36 molecules of ATP, this indicates that the process is approximately 40% efficient. The remaining energy is released as heat.

Glycolysis

The enzymes of the glycolytic pathway are found in the cytoplasm of the cell. The pathway converts a molecule of glucose that contains six carbon atoms to two molecules of pyruvic acid, each containing three carbon atoms. The pathway for glycolysis is shown in Figure 9.7 and it can be seen that in the first few steps the glucose becomes doubly phosphorylated; this consumes ATP and is thus energy dependent. Glucose is converted to glucose 6-phosphate, which is in turn isomerized to fructose 6-phosphate. (Here, isomerization is the rotation of two bonds around a carbon atom.) The fructose 6-phosphate is then phosphorylated to fructose 1,6-diphosphate and this is then hydrolysed to produce one molecule of 3-phosphoglyceraldehyde and one of dihydroxyacetone phosphate.

The next step is the conversion of the dihydroxyacetone phosphate into 3-phosphoglyceraldehyde. Thus, two molecules of 3-phosphoglyceraldehyde have been generated from one molecule of glucose. These two molecules are then converted to pyruvic acid via the intermediate stages 1,3-diphosphoglyceric acid, 3-phosphoglyceraldehyde and phosphoenolpyruvic acid. The two steps involving the metabolism of 1,3-diphosphoglyceric acid and phosphoenolpyruvic acid are worthy of note. In both cases, the phosphate group that is transferred is of a 'high-energy' type (this means that the phosphate bonding has high internal energy). These groups are transferred to ADP to generate ATP.

Although more ATP is formed during glycolysis than ATP expended, there is a net production of only two molecules of ATP. Unlike the respiratory chain which is where the bulk of cellular ATP is produced, the glycolytic pathway does not require oxygen. Thus, for short periods of time the cell can survive without consuming oxygen by generating ATP via glycolysis.

Citric acid cycle

The enzymes that carry out the citric acid cycle are located inside the mitochondria. Pyruvate ions diffuse into the mitochondrion and become covalently attached to CoA, which acts as a carrier. Nicotinamide adenine dinucleotide (NAD^+) plays a role in these reactions and it is necessary to know some molecular details.

Hydrogen can exist in a molecular form in which two atoms are bonded together. Although this molecular hydrogen (H_2) is highly reactive, under some conditions it is quite stable. Hydrogen never exists in an atomic state under normal conditions. Hydrogen is the simplest element and in theory consists of a nucleus with one proton and a single electron orbiting this nucleus. The reason molecular hydrogen can exist is that there are two electrons surrounding the two nuclei, which is a more stable electronic structure. When hydrogen is part of a more complex molecule, ionization can occur and the proton of hydrogen can leave the original molecule and bind to water. If this happens to an appreciable extent, then the resulting solution is an acid because free protons or, rather, hydrated protons are what constitutes an acid.

NAD^+ contains a positive charge because it is protonated, i.e. the nucleus of a hydrogen atom is part of the NAD molecule, while the electron from the hydrogen has gone somewhere else. During the citric acid cycle it will be seen later that a number of metabolic steps involve NAD^+, and as part of the enzymic reaction a hydrogen atom is transferred to NAD^+ and a proton is released. The reaction can be viewed as:

$$NAD^+ + H \rightarrow NADH + H^+$$

NADH can be viewed as a molecule containing high intrinsic energy. The NADH feeds into the respiratory chain and in the presence of oxygen will provide the

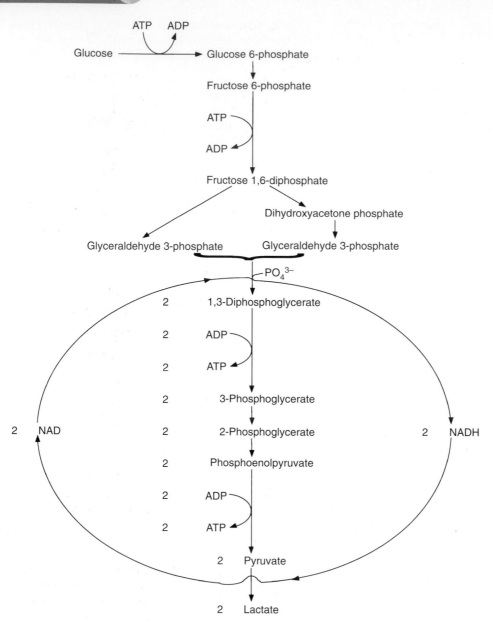

Figure 9.7 • Glycolysis, a metabolic rearrangement in which hexose sugars are converted to pyruvate or lactate. The major attack is the cleavage of fructose 1,6-diphosphate to two trioses. *Note* that two molecules of ATP are used up in the phosphorylation reactions in the first half of glycolysis, while two pairs of ATP molecules are produced in the second half, for an overall gain of two ATP molecules. The two NAD molecules reduced in oxidative phosphorylation of glyceraldehyde 3-phosphate are used in the anaerobic reduction of pyruvate to lactate.

energy for production of most of the ATP that is produced by any cell.

Figure 9.8 shows how the cycle operates and which steps are those that produce NADH; the structures of the substrates are shown separately for clarity.

The pyruvate is supplied into the cycle in the form of acetyl-CoA, but should be viewed as a two-carbon moiety, which is combined with oxaloacetate (four-carbon structure) to yield the six-carbon citric acid. After a rearrangement to isocitric acid, α-ketoglutaric acid is produced with the formation of carbon dioxide and NADH. The next step also generates a molecule of carbon dioxide and of NADH when succinic acid is formed. There is then a series of rearrangements to

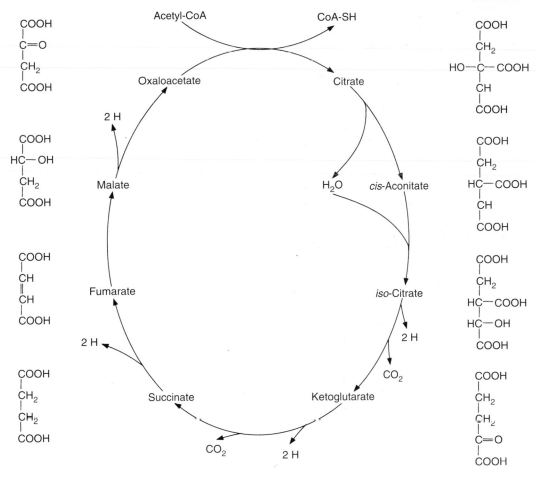

Figure 9.8 • Tricarboxylic acid cycle. For each turn of the cycle, at four points, two hydrogen atoms become available. At two points, carbon dioxide is released; this accounts for the complete combustion of the acetyl group of acetyl-CoA, while acetoacetate is again ready to accept another molecule of acetyl-CoA.

fumaric and then to malic acid. In the final part of the citric acid cycle, a further molecule of NADH is produced as malic acid is converted to oxaloacetate. Thus, the starting substrate has been regenerated and another molecule of pyruvate (acetyl-CoA) can now react to initiate another round of the cycle.

Respiratory chain

The respiratory chain, otherwise known as the electron transport chain, resides in the mitochondria. A single molecule of NADH has sufficient energy to generate three ATP molecules from ADP. The function of the chain can therefore be considered to be a mechanism by which this energy is drawn off in a controlled fashion. The chain consists of a series of electron carriers which can accept and then donate electrons, while the resulting production of energy is used to stimulate

the formation of ATP via oxidative phosphorylation. Figure 9.9 shows an outline of the respiratory chain and the points where energy is produced for ATP production. There is a linear change in the redox potential of the carriers in the chain.

Fatty acid oxidation

Many tissues produce most of their energy by the oxidation of fatty acids. Tissues such as the heart and other muscles only derive limited energy from glucose and rely on circulating free fatty acids. Parts of the kidney are completely unable to utilize glucose or other carbohydrates as energy sources and therefore depend upon a source of fatty acids.

Triacylglycerols (triglycerides) are stored in adipose tissue and, in response to one of a variety of signals, a lipase enzyme becomes activated that cleaves the three

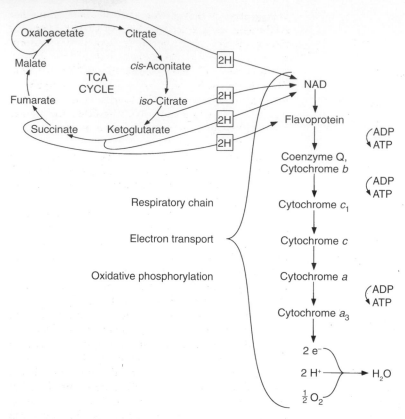

Figure 9.9 • Relationship between the tricarboxylic acid cycle and electron transport and oxidative phosphorylation. Three pairs of hydrogen atoms are needed to reduce NAD, the fourth reduces a flavoprotein. Each pair of hydrogens ultimately reduces one atom of oxygen, and in the process three molecules of ATP are produced. Each turn of the cycle thus yields 12 ATP molecules. Respiratory oxygen is linked via the respiratory chain and the tricarboxylic acid cycle to the combustion of acetyl-CoA and the production of the carbon dioxide that is breathed out.

fatty acids from the glycerol. The free fatty acids then travel to other tissues bound to albumin; fatty acids are insoluble in water and therefore have to be transported by albumin. The glycerol that is formed as a result of triglyceride hydrolysis does not travel to other tissues. It is either used to resynthesize new triglycerides, or, alternatively, it is phosphorylated to 3-phosphoglycerate, which is a component of the glycolytic pathway.

Once a free fatty acid has reached the cell in which it is going to be used, it is subjected to a pathway called β-oxidation. Figure 9.10 shows the sequence of reactions involved. The fatty acid is activated by combination with CoA. There are then four enzymic steps in which the fatty acyl-CoA is reduced, hydrolysed, reduced again and finally hydrolysed to yield a molecule of acetyl-CoA and a molecule of acyl-CoA where the acyl group is now two carbon atoms shorter than the original. The acetyl-CoA feeds into the citric acid cycle and the acyl-CoA goes through the process repeatedly until it is completely degraded. Thus, a molecule of palmitic acid which has 18 carbon atoms

will be degraded to nine molecules of acetyl-CoA, which will be further metabolized to produce ATP.

The metabolism described earlier refers to saturated fatty acids only, i.e. those with no unsaturated double bonds. There are three polyunsaturated fatty acids which are essential for health. Linoleic acid has 18 carbon atoms and two double bonds, while linolenic acid has 18 carbon atoms and three double bonds. Arachidonic acid is 20 carbon atoms long with four double bonds. Although all three are required by cells, since humans can synthesize linolenic and arachidonic acids from linoleic acid, an adequate dietary supply of linoleic acid is sufficient. There are a number of biochemical pathways that require the essential unsaturated fatty acids, and the production of leukotrienes and prostaglandins has been especially well studied.

Regulation of metabolic pathways

In an adult, there is turnover within tissues and so the diet has to provide the nutrients for replacement as

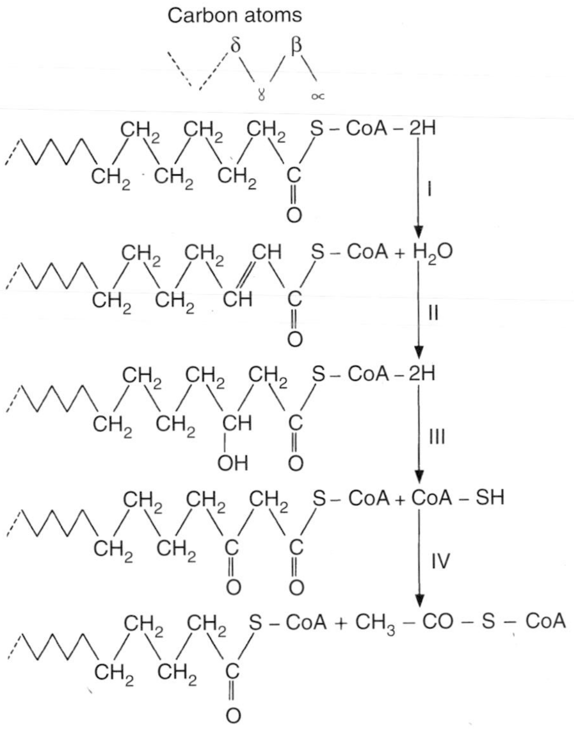

Carbon atoms

Figure 9.10 • β-Oxidation of even-numbered long-chain fatty acids. Reaction I, the initial attack on the α- and β-carbon atoms, with removal of a hydrogen atom from each and the formation of a double bond between them, is catalysed by fatty acyl-CoA dehydrogenases with an electron-transferring flavoprotein as co-factor. Next (reaction II) comes hydration of this double bond, followed by reaction III, oxidation of the secondary alcoholic group to a keto group on the β-carbon atom, catalysed by a β-hydroxy fatty acyl-CoA dehydrogenase. The final step (reaction IV) is cleavage with CoA, catalysed by β-thiolase, to give acetyl-CoA. The resulting fatty acyl-CoA is in the same form as the starting material, and can undergo reaction I again, but is two carbon atoms shorter. Ultimately, the fatty acid is completely disassembled to two carbon acetyl-CoA units.

well as energy utilization. The nutritional requirement includes amino acids, vitamins, salts and trace elements. There are considerable differences in the rates at which tissues turn over. Thus a tissue such as bone has a very slow rate of turnover and the macromolecules in the matrix will be degraded and renewed with half-times measured in weeks if not months. At the other end of the range, the surface of the gut has a high rate of turnover and renewal. Like most epithelia, there is a constant movement and desquamation of cells. This must be balanced by replacement within the germinal layers.

An individual exists in different metabolic states throughout the day, and while at one point in time energy may be derived from carbohydrate, at another ATP might be produced exclusively from oxidation of fatty acids. Following a meal, the body is in an absorptive state and there will be high levels of free glucose, triglycerides and amino acids in the bloodstream. The tissues will use some of these components but most will be stored. The liver becomes active and will take up glucose and convert some to the storage polymer glycogen. Some glucose can be converted to triglyceride.

Triglyceride travels in the circulation in the form of chylomicrons, which are aggregates of lipid and a small amount of protein. Some of the triglyceride in chylomicrons is taken up directly into adipose tissue, while some is taken up in the liver, where the triglycerides are used to make other species of lipoprotein. Very low-density lipoprotein and low-density lipoprotein contain different proportions of triglyceride, phospholipid, cholesterol and protein. Both forms of lipoprotein are secreted from the liver and then circulate to all the tissues where they supply lipids.

As all the circulating products from digestion are taken up into cells, the body turns to a postabsorptive state. Most tissues cannot store adequate amounts of carbohydrate and lipid for their energetic needs and so during the postabsorptive state, the liver and adipose tissue release glucose and triglyceride for use by other tissues. It is often not appreciated that the glycogen in the liver is only able to provide glucose for a matter of 1–2 hours and (apart from the brain) most tissues use fat in the form of free fatty acids as their energy source for most of the day. The liver can also produce ketone bodies such as β-hydroxybutyrate and acetoacetic acid. Ketone bodies can be used as an energy source by a number of tissues, and even the central nervous system, after an adaptation period, can metabolize ketone bodies to provide ATP.

There are very effective control processes that ensure adequate levels of ATP and that the ATP is derived from the most suitable energy source. In general, a cell will not be deriving ATP from carbohydrate and lipid at the same time.

Most of the regulation of and between the metabolic pathways occurs via a mechanism known as allosteric control. Some key enzymes in each pathway have, in addition to the binding sites for substrate, sites at which other components of the metabolic pathways can bind. When these other components bind to the enzyme, its activity is altered. For example, the enzyme phosphofructokinase is part of the glycolytic pathway and is very sensitive to cellular concentrations of ATP, ADP and AMP. When concentrations of ATP are high, then the activity of the enzyme is downregulated, since glycolysis should be slowed down in order to conserve carbohydrate stores. Phosphofructokinase is also regulated by the concentration of citrate and this provides a mechanism for regulation between different metabolic pathways. If there are high concentrations of acetyl-CoA which have been derived from fatty acid oxidation, then this will result in high levels of citrate formation. High concentrations of citrate downregulate phosphofructokinase, and thus the use of fat for energy production will have a conserving effect on carbohydrate stores.

It is now known that many metabolic enzymes can be regulated. In addition to allosteric control, the concentrations of co-factors will also regulate enzyme activity. The status of the respiratory chain will influence NAD/NADH ratios. Since the sum of NAD and NADH concentrations is held fairly constant, if there are high levels of NADH then there will be insufficient substrate for several enzymes in the citric acid cycle and it will consequently be downregulated.

An example of a control that operates in a metabolic cycle, which is important in the neonate, follows. The enzyme ATP-citrate lyase hydrolyses citrate and reverses the first step of the citric acid cycle. Although energy is consumed in this reaction, the step is important for the neonate since it ensures levels of acetyl-CoA are maintained. During growth, cellular proliferation requires adequate lipid for membrane biosynthesis. ATP-citrate lyase ensures that, at a time in development when dietary lipid can be low, fatty acids are not used too extensively as an energy source. This maintains adequate supplies for growth.

Catabolism

Haemoglobin

All the red cells, white cells and platelets in circulation originate in the bone marrow. The stem cells within the marrow divide and differentiate to form the different cellular elements of blood. The process is regulated by a series of peptide growth factors. Erythropoietin, for example, is the peptide that promotes the formation of erythrocytes; it is synthesized and secreted by the juxtaglomerular apparatus of the kidney and it circulates to the bone marrow where it promotes proliferation.

Erythrocytes have a half-life of about 125 days before they are removed from circulation by the spleen. In order for constant replacement of these lost cells to occur, the bone marrow is very active in erythropoiesis. As well as cellular proliferation, there has to be synthesis of haemoglobin. This oxygen-binding molecule is composed of two pairs of globin chains and a haem ring. The haem ring is synthesized in the mitochondria and needs a sufficient supply of iron, which can frequently become the rate-limiting step. The uptake of iron across the gut is not an efficient process and, even in the presence of sufficient dietary iron, the plasma concentration can become limiting.

Unless there is sufficient iron available, the production of the globin peptide chains is redundant. For this reason, there is a sophisticated control mechanism that operates. Only in the presence of sufficient haem does the synthesis of globin chains proceed. Protein synthesis involves a number of elongation factors whose activity is controlled by phosphorylation and dephosphorylation, and the enzymes responsible are regulated by haem levels.

When erythrocytes are degraded in the spleen (or indeed at the site of a wound response following tissue trauma), the haemoglobin is catabolized. The globin chains are degraded to amino acids, which are re-utilized. Haem cannot be re-used and is catabolized in a number of enzyme steps, which finally produce bilirubin. This all occurs at the site of erythrocyte breakdown. The bilirubin is then transferred to the liver; because it is highly insoluble, it travels to the liver bound to albumin. After diffusion into the hepatocytes, bilirubin is solubilized and detoxified by the coupling of two glucuronic acid residues. The conjugated bilirubin is then excreted into the bile.

Urea cycle

In the developed world, most individuals have a diet that is far in excess of requirement. Thus, an individual consumes an amount of protein, which when hydrolysed to amino acids is considerably more than will be required for normal cellular turnover. Like most chemicals with free amino groups, these amino acids will become toxic if allowed to accumulate. There is an efficient detoxification mechanism which results in more than 95% of the nitrogen being excreted via the urine in the form of urea.

Figure 9.11 shows a sequence of metabolic reactions which constitute the urea cycle. The detoxification of amino acids begins before the urea cycle, when a transaminase enzyme results in the transfer of the amino group from the acid onto α-ketoglutaric acid. The product, glutamic acid, is itself one of the amino acids, but it is through this intermediate that all amino groups are metabolized. The glutamate is oxidatively deaminated to produce ammonia, which immediately becomes an ammonium ion.

In a reaction requiring ATP, carbon dioxide and ammonium ions form carbamoyl phosphate and it is this that feeds into the urea cycle. The first step is the formation of citrulline from ornithine and carbamoyl-phosphate. Then, in another ATP-dependent reaction, a molecule of aspartic acid combines with citrulline to generate arginosuccinate. This is next hydrolysed to yield fumarate and arginine and, in the final reaction,

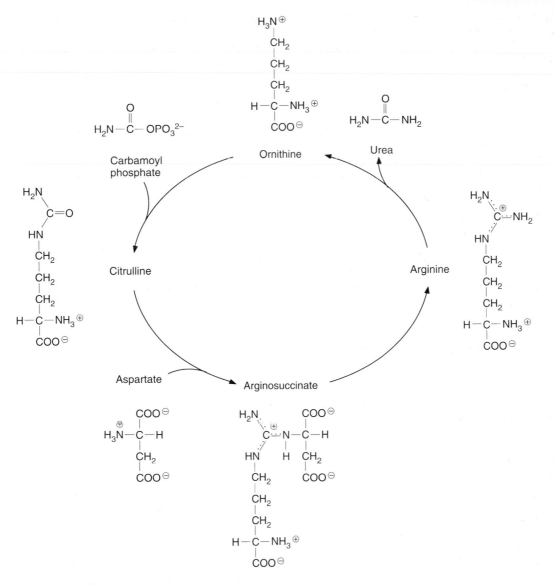

Figure 9.11 • The urea cycle.

arginase releases urea from arginine, leaving ornithine. Thus the cycle is completed.

Most amino acid detoxification in humans occurs in the liver, although small levels of the urea cycle enzymes are found in other tissues. The first few reactions occur in the mitochondria, while the latter part of the cycle takes place in the cytoplasm. The urea diffuses out of the liver into the systemic circulation. Like all small molecules, urea is filtered through the glomerulus of the kidney but, while nutrients such as glucose and amino acids are reabsorbed by the kidney tubules, urea is not and passes quantitatively into the urine. This excretory process is vital and, in chronic kidney failure, accumulation of urea can become a life-threatening process.

Enzymes

Enzymes are proteins that act as catalysts. They bring about the enormous range of sophisticated chemical reactions that are necessary for life. In strict thermodynamic terms, it is incorrect to state that enzymes make reactions occur. Rather, an enzyme shifts the equilibrium of a reaction so that it is more favourable for it to proceed. This is accomplished by reducing the activation energy that is needed to promote the reaction. The catalysis occurs on a part of the enzyme called the active site.

The three-dimensional conformation of an enzyme is crucial to activity and the ability to act as a catalyst can be lost if the three-dimensional shape is altered. A change of shape and resulting loss of activity is referred to as 'denaturation' and can be brought about in a number of ways. Heating an enzyme usually results in complete loss of activity. The three-dimensional structure of the protein is maintained in part by hydrogen bonds. These are fairly weak in nature and can be readily disrupted by heat. Most enzymes are destroyed at 50–60°C.

Organic solvents will usually destroy enzymic activity. The solvent disrupts the internal bonding of the protein, in particular the interactions of the hydrophobic amino acids. Even after removal of the solvent, it is rare that the protein can re-fold in such a way as to regenerate enzyme activity.

Changes in pH will also affect enzyme activity. Because amino acids are zwitterions and partially charged, the local pH will influence the degree to which they are charged. Changes in pH can thus affect the charge of amino acid residues, which in turn affects the interactions between the amino acids and can result in denaturation. Some proteins are extremely sensitive and lose activity with small pH changes; others are less sensitive.

Enzyme kinetics

Enzymes are usually present at low concentrations inside the cell. The substrate binds to the enzyme and, by reducing the activation energy for the reaction, the enzyme brings about a shift in equilibrium and this allows formation of product. If the reaction involves only a single substrate then this can be described by:

Enzyme + Substrate
  → Enzyme–Substrate complex
  → Enzyme + Product

The rate of reaction is dependent upon the concentrations of enzyme and substrate, but at high concentrations of substrate the enzyme will become saturated. At this point the rate of the reaction is maximal (and is depicted as V_{max}). In order to describe the activity of an enzyme, the Michaelis constant (K_m) is used and this is the concentration of substrate at which the velocity of the reaction is half-maximal. K_m is a measure of how tightly a substrate binds to the enzyme. The lower the value of K_m, the more tightly the substrate can bind. Values for the Michaelis constant are commonly in the micromolar range.

Values for K_m and V_{max} can be calculated by measuring enzyme rates of reaction at a number of substrate concentrations and plotting the reciprocals of both parameters against one another. This is called a Lineweaver–Burk plot and normally produces a straight line.

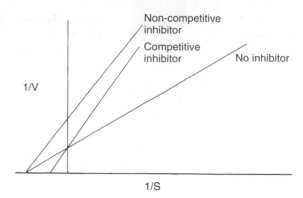

Figure 9.12 • Lineweaver–Burk plots for enzyme inhibitor. V is the reaction rate and S is the substrate concentration.

Enzyme inhibitors can act in a competitive or non-competitive manner. In the case of competitive inhibitors, there is direct competition between the substrate and inhibitor for binding to the active site of the enzyme: K_m is increased but V_{max} is unaltered. In the case of a non-competitive inhibitor, K_m remains the same, while V_{max} is reduced because the inhibitor binds at a location away from the active site but brings about a reduction in activity of the enzyme without affecting substrate binding. Figure 9.12 shows a Lineweaver–Burk plot for the two types of inhibitor.

Vitamins

Many enzymes require a co-factor in order to operate. The co-factors are small in comparison to the enzyme but play an essential role in the binding and activation of the substrate. Most of the co-factors cannot be synthesized by humans and the factor or its precursor have to be supplied in the diet. The dietary components are known as vitamins. To give an example, pyridoxine (also known as vitamin B_6) is a vital dietary requirement. Once it has been absorbed across the gut and transported to a tissue, it is converted enzymically inside the cell by enzymes to pyridoxal phosphate, which is then in turn used as a co-factor for transaminase enzymes.

Vitamins are classified as water or fat soluble. The water-soluble vitamins are the B series and vitamin C, which are all used in a large number of enzymic reactions that concern intermediary metabolism. The four fat-soluble vitamins – A, D, E and K – take part in diverse unrelated reactions ranging from formation of blood-clotting proteins (vitamin K) to formation of visual pigments (vitamin A).

The bacteria in the colon produce some of the vitamins required by humans and this can act as a limited source. Some vitamins turn over fairly rapidly and so a deficiency state can arise soon after withdrawal. In the case of other vitamins, such as vitamin B_{12}, the body maintains significant reserves of material and humans can survive for months without this particular vitamin in the diet.

Role of enzymes in digestion

The diet contains proteins, fats and complex carbohydrates. None of these can be absorbed by the gastro-intestinal tract and enzymic digestion has to occur in order to generate products that can be absorbed into the bloodstream or lymphatic circulation.

Protein
Digestion of protein begins in the stomach. The 'chief' cells secrete pepsinogen. The parietal (oxyntic) cells secrete hydrochloric acid and the resulting low pH causes the hydrolysis of pepsinogen into pepsin, which is a proteolytic enzyme. Pepsin shows specificity and causes peptide bond hydrolysis only next to three particular amino acids, namely tryptophan, phenylalanine and tyrosine; these are all amino acids with aromatic side chains. Pepsin therefore generates peptide fragments from large proteins.

The pancreas synthesizes three protease enzymes in inactive precursor form. These are trypsinogen, pro-carboxypeptidase and chymotrypsinogen. These are secreted in inactive forms and released into the gut via the pancreatic duct. The mucosa of the proximal part of the small intestine secretes an enzyme called entero kinase, which cleaves trypsinogen, converting it to trypsin. Trypsin in turn cleaves and activates pro-carboxypeptidase and chymotrypsinogen. In all these cases the release of a small peptide fragment generates active enzyme.

Chymotrypsinogen is like pepsin and cleaves next to amino acids with aromatic side chains. Trypsin cleaves next to the basic amino acids lysine and arginine, while carboxypeptidase cleaves sequential amino acids starting at the carboxyl terminus. The action of these enzymes is to convert proteins to either amino acids or very small peptides with two or three amino acids.

In the small intestine, the single amino acids are transported by the enterocytes into the systemic circulation. The microvilli of the intestinal mucosa contain peptidases that cleave the di- and tripeptides into single amino acids, which are then also transported into the bloodstream. The small intestine is highly efficient and most of the amino acids are absorbed across the wall of the duodenum and jejunum.

Carbohydrate
Most of the carbohydrate in the diet is starch, which is a large polymer of glucose. The diet will also contain some sucrose and lactose, which are both disaccharides. Sucrose is composed of glucose and fructose while lactose is composed of glucose and galactose.

The salivary glands and the pancreas both secrete amylases, which break down starch into the disaccharides maltose and isomaltose. These two carbohydrates, along with lactose and sucrose, are then taken up by a similar mechanism. The mucosal villi contain the four enzymes maltase, isomaltase, lactase and sucrase and these break down the relevant disaccharide into monosaccharides, which are transported into the bloodstream. The transport of glucose and galactose is an active process and ATP is required; the transport of fructose is passive.

Glucose is the most utilized carbohydrate energy source. Most cells take up glucose from the circulation, and the insulin released from the pancreas following a meal stimulates this process. The glucose can be used immediately for energy production or it can be stored in the form of glycogen, which is a branched polymer of glucose. When the cell requires the use of glucose stored as glycogen, then the enzyme phosphorylase is activated by the cyclic adenosine monophosphate (cAMP) pathway (Fig. 9.13) and glucose 6-phosphate is produced. When glucose is transported into the cell it is also phosphorylated by the enzyme hexokinase or glucokinase. In either case, it is glucose 6-phosphate that enters the metabolic pathway.

Fat
The predominant dietary fat is triglyceride, i.e. three fatty acids esterified to a single molecule of glycerol. It is not until the small intestine that digestion of fat begins. The first stage is the emulsification of the fats with the bile salts. The liver synthesizes bile salts and acids but they are stored in the gall bladder. In response to cholecystokinin, bile is ejected into the small intestine and causes dispersal of dietary fat into small droplets. This has the effect of increasing the surface area, thereby increasing the rate of action of the lipase enzymes secreted by the pancreas. The products are fatty acids and monoacylglycerol, and these diffuse into the epithelial cells lining the gastrointestinal tract. Inside the cell, the monoacylglycerols are broken down to fatty acid and glycerol. The epithelial cells then resynthesize triglycerides and then, along with a small amount of phospholipid, cholesterol and specific protein are assembled into chylomicron particles, which diffuse into the lacteals of the lymphatic system. The process of fat digestion in the healthy individual is also very efficient and is completed in the duodenum and jejunum.

The chylomicrons diffuse into the lymphatic lacteals and then travel along the lymphatic vessels. Ultimately, they enter the bloodstream when the lymph in the thoracic duct flows into the left subclavian vein. The triglycerides in the chylomicrons are taken up and stored by adipose tissue. When there is demand, this fat can be used by a number of organs and tissues. Free

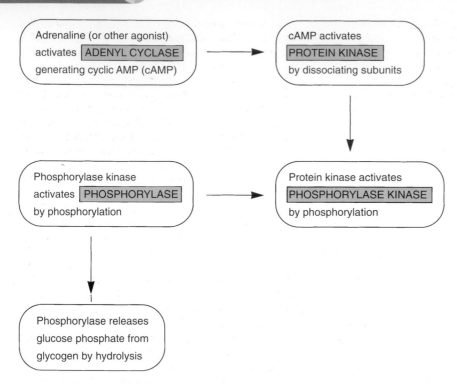

Figure 9.13 • Activation of phosphorylase by the cyclic AMP-dependent pathway.

fatty acids are transported to the site of utilization. Lipases within the adipose tissue will hydrolyse the triglycerides and the resulting fatty acids diffuse out of the adipocytes and become bound to albumin in the bloodstream.

Cell signalling and second messaging

General overview

Communication between cells is essential to regulate their development, to organize them into tissues and organs, and to allow normal physiological processes to take place. There are many methods that cells use to communicate. This chapter reviews some of the most common methods used in mammals and the basic mechanisms involved. In particular, the major signalling mechanisms and second messengers activated within a cell when it receives an external signal (often released from another cell) are highlighted. The three main methods of communication by cells are by the cells secreting chemicals which act at a distance, by forming gap junctions which join the cytoplasm of the cells, or by a cell's expression of plasma membrane-bound molecules, which can affect other cells. Most cells secrete one or more chemical mediators, which only act locally because they are either rapidly taken up again or destroyed. Specialized endocrine cells secrete hormones which can travel throughout the body or can have their effects on cells locally (paracrine effects). Some even secrete hormones which bind back to the same cells' surface receptors (autocrine effects). Nerve cells form specialized junctions known as synapses and secrete short-range, short-lived neurotransmitters. Information is clearly conveyed much faster by nerve cells than hormonal methods since, while nerves use electrical impulses to carry information, hormones rely on diffusion or blood flow. Hormones usually act at very low concentrations ($<10^{-8}$ M) since they become diluted in blood. Neurotransmitters are less diluted and work at much higher concentrations, for example acetylcholine in synaptic clefts acts at 5×10^{-4} M. In most other respects hormones and neurotransmitters have similar cell signalling mechanisms.

Most animal cells have a characteristic of specific high-affinity receptors, allowing a range of responses. Some signalling molecules can have different effects depending on the cell type they encounter. For example, acetylcholine contracts skeletal muscle but decreases heart rate force and contraction. Cells can also modulate their response by altering the number of receptors on the cell surface for a particular ligand. Some chemical signalling mechanisms are rapid and transient, such as insulin secretion in response to raised blood sugar levels; some are even faster, such as neuro-transmission. Some are slow in onset and long-lasting such as oestradiol production by the ovaries at the onset of puberty. Cells require many signalling molecules just to survive and additional signalling molecules to proliferate. When deprived of survival signalling molecules, cells may undergo programmed cell death (apoptosis).

Eicosanoid synthesis

Eicosanoids are signalling molecules which are continuously made in the plasma membrane of all mammalian tissues. They are synthesized from 20-carbon fatty acid chains (mainly arachidonic acid), which in turn are cleaved from membrane phospholipids by phospholipases. There are four major groups of eicosanoid: prostaglandins, prostacyclins, thromboxanes and leukotrienes. Prostaglandins are important stimulators of myometrium. They are formed from arachidonic acid released from membrane phospholipids (Fig. 9.14). The key enzymes in this step are phospholipase A_2 and phospholipase C; the latter releases diacylglycerol (see later), which eventually leads to arachidonic acid release. The free arachidonate is the substrate for prostaglandin H_2 (PGH$_2$) synthase or cyclooxygenase (COX), an enzyme with two activities. PGH$_2$ synthase has both COX activity, which converts arachidonic acid to prostaglandin G_2 (PGG$_2$), and a peroxidase activity which converts prostaglandin G_2 to PGH$_2$. PGH$_2$ is then converted to a range of prostaglandins including PGF$_{2\alpha}$ and PGE$_2$.

Until recently, there were two recognized forms of PGH$_2$ synthase or COX, now known as COX-1 and COX-2. These two enzymes function similarly but are the products of two distinct and different genes. The gene which encodes COX-1 is large, with large introns, and a promoter that contains transcription factor binding domains which suggest that it is generally a constitutively expressed gene. The gene for COX-2 is far smaller, with only small introns, and its promoter contains transcription factor binding domains which suggest that it is a gene which is inducible. In general, COX-1 is found in tissues which produce prostaglandins constantly, such as the stomach mucosa, whereas COX-2 is only expressed at sites of inflammation. Older non-steroidal anti-inflammatory drugs (NSAIDs) such as indometacin, inhibit both COX-1 and COX-2. More recent NSAIDs are selective for COX-2. In general, the more COX-2 selective an NSAID is, the better its side-effect profile. More recently, a COX-3 form was identified and is formed by alternative splicing of the COX-1 gene.

Aspirin inhibits both COX-1 and COX-2 (it is actually much more active against COX-1 than COX-2, hence its poor side-effect profile). Unlike most

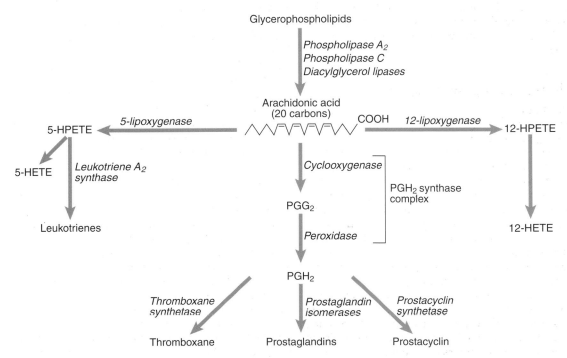

Figure 9.14 • The synthesis of eicosanoids. There are four major classes of eicosanoid: prostaglandins, prostacyclins, thromboxanes and leukotrienes, and most are made from arachidonic acid.

NSAIDs, which are competitive antagonists, aspirin functions by permanently acetylating the active site of the COX enzyme. It can be used at a low dose to inhibit platelet thromboxane synthesis with little effect upon vascular endothelial prostacyclin synthesis. This may be of value in thromboprophylaxis, and in the management of pre-eclampsia. A low dose of aspirin permanently disables platelet COX as the platelets pass through the hepatic portal system. Since the platelet has no nucleus it cannot synthesize new COX and so platelet thromboxane synthesis is permanently inhibited. Most of the aspirin is then inactivated within the liver. The small amount of aspirin which then passes into the general circulation may acetylate vascular endothelial COX but, since these cells have a nucleus, they can synthesize the new COX enzyme and maintain prostacyclin synthesis. High concentrations of prostanoids have been reported during normal menstruation and in particular with menorrhagia, dysmenorrhoea and endometriosis; all correlate with painful menstruation. COX-2-selective inhibitors are just as effective as NSAIDs but have fewer gastrointestinal side effects. During labour, the fetal membranes are the main source of prostaglandins. The increase in prostaglandins is thought to be due to induction of COX-2 in the fetal membranes. Bacterial products and pro-inflammatory cytokines can increase expression of COX-2 and hence prostaglandin synthesis. It is known that women with intra-amniotic infection have raised pro-inflammatory cytokines in the amniotic fluid and fetal membranes, although cytokines are also elevated in spontaneous term labour in the amniotic fluid and membranes.

In addition to the prostaglandin synthetic pathway, a 5-lipoxygenase pathway converts arachidonate to 5-hydroperoxyeicosatetraenoic acid (5-HPETE), which leads to formation of leukotrienes. A 12-lipoxygenase pathway leads to formation of 12-HPETE and a 15-lipoxygenase pathway to 15-HPETE. These lipoxygenase compounds have a direct stimulatory effect on the myometrium. Prostacyclin and thromboxanes are also formed through a cyclo-oxygenase pathway which utilizes prostacyclin synthetase and thromboxane synthetase, respectively. The synthetic pathways of eicosanoids can be targeted by therapeutic drugs. For example, corticosteroid drugs such as cortisone inhibit phospholipase and are used to treat inflammatory conditions such as arthritis. NSAIDs including aspirin and ibuprofen block the first oxidation step of the fatty acid, which is catalysed by cyclooxygenase.

Gap junctions

Gap junctions are specialized cell–cell junctions which form from a mirror image of protein units (connexons) between plasma membranes of cells. The cytoplasms of the cells are connected by narrow water-filled channels. These channels allow passage of small signalling molecules such as calcium and cyclic AMP, but not of large molecules such as proteins. In the myometrium, gap junctions provide low-resistance pathways between the smooth muscle cells, thereby increasing their electrical coupling to allow increased coordination of myometrial contractility. During pregnancy, gap junctions are present at very low numbers in the myometrium; however labour is associated with increased numbers and size of gap junctions. This has led to the idea that gap junctions are essential, but not sufficient, for effective labour and delivery.

Nitric oxide is an important signalling molecule

Although most signalling molecules are hydrophilic molecules, some are small enough to pass straight into the cell where they can directly exert their effects. One such example is the gas nitric oxide (NO). NO is produced from L-arginine by the enzyme NO synthase in the presence of co-factors and oxygen. The by-product is L-citrulline. There are three main forms of this enzyme, each the product of separate genes and sharing about 50–60% sequence homology. One of these enzyme isoforms was first described in endothelial cells and thus is commonly known as eNOS. It is constitutively expressed and is calcium–calmodulin dependent (see later). NO has a very short half-life (5–10 s) and is converted to nitrates and nitrites in the blood. However, when released from endothelial cells on blood vessels in response to increased shear stress or agents such as acetylcholine, NO diffuses to the underlying smooth muscle, where it reacts with iron in the active site of the enzyme guanylate cyclase to produce the intracellular mediator cGMP (see later). The effects of this enzyme are rapid and result in muscle relaxation. Thus continual release of NO from blood vessels is one of the main mechanisms for keeping blood pressure at its normal level. In pregnancy, blood pressure falls and it is thought that the vasodilatation is partly mediated by increased NO release. In contrast, evidence for reduced NO release as a cause of increased vascular resistance and hence hypertension in pregnancy or pre-eclampsia is controversial. NO is also important in regulating blood flow within the placenta and eNOS expressed on the entire syncytiotrophoblast surface is thought, just like that on blood vessels, to inhibit aggregation of neutrophils and platelets present in maternal blood in the intervillous space. In contrast the expression of another NO synthase enzyme is induced in response to inflammatory signals such as bacterial cell wall products which include lipopolysaccharides and cytokines such as γ-interferon or tumour necrosis factor-α. This enzyme is commonly known as iNOS. The activity of iNOS is calmodulin independent and is induced in activated macrophages and neutrophils. NO released from these cells helps them to kill invading microorganisms. This third nitric oxide synthase was first described in the brain and is known as bNOS. Like eNOS it is constitutively expressed and is also dependent on calcium–calmodulin for activity. NO is released by many types of nerve cell to signal neighbouring cells, for example NO released by autonomic nerves in the penis causes the local blood vessel dilatation that is responsible for penile erection. It is emerging that the distribution of nitric oxide synthase enzymes is not simple with many cells expressing more than one form. In reproductive biology, NO has also been implicated in the control of myometrial quiescence, in the onset of labour and in cervical ripening, although the evidence for some of these is certainly not conclusive. The effects of NO on blood vessels also explain the mechanism of action of nitroglycerine, which has been used for nearly 100 years to treat angina. Nitroglycerine is converted to NO, which relaxes blood vessels in the heart. Other chemicals such as GTN, which breaks down to NO, have also been used in an attempt to prevent pre-term labour by relaxing myometrial smooth muscle and in ripening the cervix. These studies have met with mixed success rates. Carbon monoxide (CO) is another gas which also stimulates guanylate cyclase. CO is produced by the action of the enzymes haemoxygenase (HO) 1 and HO-2. HO-1 is inducible while HO-2 is constitutively expressed. The functions of CO are only now being unravelled.

Calcium as an intracellular messenger

Cells maintain low concentrations of free calcium (10^{-7} M) despite much higher extracellular concentrations in the extracellular fluid (10^{-3} M) and endoplasmic reticulum. Increases in intracellular calcium concentrations are one way in which extracellular signals are transmitted across the plasma membrane. When calcium channels are transiently opened in the plasma membrane or endoplasmic reticulum membranes, intracellular calcium concentrations rise to about 5×10^{-6} M and activate calcium-responsive proteins in the cell. Resting calcium concentrations are kept very low by several means. Calcium-ATPases in the plasma membrane pump calcium out of the cell while cells such as nerve and muscle, which use calcium much more for signalling, have an additional calcium pump (sodium calcium antiporter) in the plasma membrane which couples Na$^+$ influx to calcium efflux. In the endoplasmic reticulum there is also a pump (Ca^{2+}-ATPase) that also takes up calcium from the cytosol. Mitochondria can also pump calcium inside; a low-affinity high-capacity calcium pump in the inner mito-

chondrial membrane uses the electrochemical gradient generated across the membrane during electron transport in oxidative phosphorylation. This pump only operates when calcium levels are extremely high, usually as a consequence of cell damage.

These transport mechanisms are represented in Figure 9.15. Calmodulin is a calcium-binding protein found in all eukaryotic cells. It mediates many calcium-regulated processes and undergoes a conformational change when bound to calcium. When this happens the calcium–calmodulin complex can bind to various target proteins and alter their activity. Among the calcium–calmodulin targets are various enzymes (such as eNOS and bNOS) and membrane transport proteins. Most effects of calcium–calmodulin are, however, indirect and are mediated by calcium–calmodulin-dependent protein kinases; an example of this is myosin light chain kinase, which activates smooth muscle contraction. Two pathways of calcium signalling have been well defined. One is used mainly by excitable cells; when nerve cell membranes are depolarized by an action potential, voltage-gated calcium channels open and calcium enters the cell leading to secretion of the neurotransmitter. In the other pathway, binding of extracellular signalling molecules to cell surface receptors ultimately leads to the opening of channels in the endoplasmic reticulum and a rise in intracellular calcium. The opening of these channels is brought about by an intermediate molecule known as inositol trisphosphate (see later).

Signals acting on intracellular receptors

While all neurotransmitters and most hormones are water soluble, steroid hormones such as cortisol, oestrogen and progesterone, retinoids, vitamin D and thyroid hormones are not; they are small hydrophobic molecules. The latter are made water soluble for transport within the body by being transported in the blood by specific carrier proteins. Steroid hormones are released from their carrier proteins and pass through the plasma membrane where they exert their effects. Because water-soluble proteins are hydrophilic, they cannot pass directly through the lipid layer of the plasma membrane and instead bind to specific receptors on the cell surface. In addition, water-soluble molecules are usually broken down within minutes of entering the blood. Neurotransmitters are broken down even faster, within seconds or milliseconds. In contrast, steroid hormones persist in the blood for hours, thyroid hormone for days.

On reaching their target cell, steroid hormones, thyroid hormones, retinoids and vitamin D diffuse across the plasma membrane and bind to intracellular receptor proteins. These intracellular receptor proteins

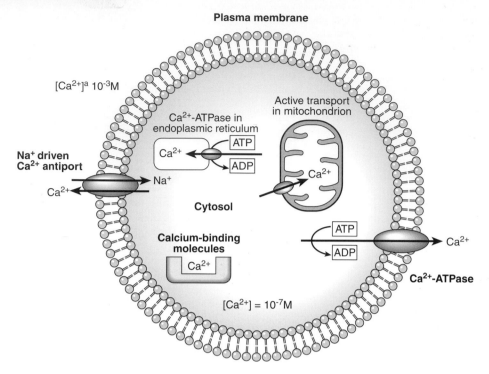

Figure 9.15 • Schematic representation of the main methods used by cells to maintain low levels of cytosolic calcium concentrations in the face of much higher concentrations of calcium outside.

are held in an inactive state by being complexed with an inhibitory protein. When the ligand binds to the receptor, it causes the inhibitory protein to dissociate (Fig. 9.16). This activates the receptor by exposing its DNA-binding site and causes a conformational change. The end result is activation, or sometimes suppression, of gene transcription. This often occurs in two steps. First, there is the direct induction of transcription of a small number of specific genes within 30 min, and this is known as the primary response. Some of the primary response proteins can then turn on secondary response genes, while other primary response proteins can turn off primary response genes (Fig. 9.16). Even when different cell types have the same intracellular receptor, the response in each cell is different. This is because a combination of gene regulatory proteins must bind to the DNA and some of these are cell specific.

As stated earlier, all water-soluble signalling molecules bind to specific receptors on their target cell. Cell surface receptors act as signal transducers, i.e. binding to the receptor by the ligand leads to intracellular signals which modulate the response of the cell. There are three main classes of cell surface receptor: (1) those which are ion channel linked, (2) those which are G-protein linked and (3) those which are enzyme linked.

Ion channels

Ion channels are not open all the time but have 'gates' that open in response to specific stimuli. The main types of stimuli which open ion channels are changes in voltage across the plasma membrane (voltage-gated channels), mechanical stress (mechanical-gated channels), or the binding of a ligand (ligand-gated channels). The activity of many channels is additionally regulated by protein phosphorylation and dephosphorylation.

G-protein-linked receptors which increase cyclic AMP

The interaction between a receptor and a target protein (enzyme or ion channel) can be mediated by a trimeric GTP-binding regulatory protein (G-protein). Receptors linked to G-proteins are the largest (>100) family of cell surface receptors. Many hormones, neurotransmitters and local mediators signal through G-protein-linked receptors. All G-protein-linked receptors have a similar structure consisting of a polypeptide chain that threads back and forth through the plasma membrane seven times. Most G-proteins regulate the concentrations of the intracellular signalling molecules cyclic AMP or calcium.

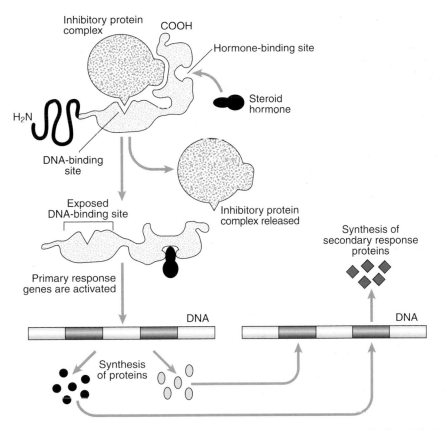

Figure 9.16 • Model of intracellular receptor activation by steroid hormone. Binding of the ligand to the receptor results in dissociation of the inhibitory complex, thus activating the receptor by exposing its DNA-binding site. The steroid hormone–receptor complex activates primary response genes, leading to the synthesis of different proteins. Some of these proteins turn off primary response genes, while others turn on secondary response genes. Thus one hormone can lead to a complex change in gene expression.

Cyclic AMP (cAMP) is synthesized from ATP by a plasma membrane-bound enzyme, adenylate (adenylyl) cyclase. cAMP is rapidly and continually destroyed by cyclic AMP phosphodiesterases. Adenylate cyclase is an example of an enzyme, the activity of which is regulated by a trimeric G-protein. Since in this case the enzyme is activated by the G-protein, the G-protein is called a stimulatory G-protein (G_s). Some of the best studied receptors linked to adenylate cyclase are the β-adrenergic receptors.

Trimeric G-proteins are so called because they are made up of an α and a βγ subunit. In its inactive state Gs exists as a trimer with GDP bound to the α subunit. When a ligand binds to the receptor, the conformation of the receptor is altered, exposing a binding site for the G_s protein complex. Association of the ligand-receptor–G_s complex is brought about by diffusion of the subunits within the membrane and results in the α-subunit changing its affinity for GDP to GTP. This causes the α-subunit to dissociate from the β- and γ-subunits and, in doing so, exposes the α-subunit's

binding site for adenylate cyclase. The α-subunit then binds to and activates adenylate cyclase, which then produces cAMP. When the ligand dissociates, the receptor returns to its original conformation. The GTP is then hydrolysed to GDP by the α-subunit's GTPase activity, brought about by its binding to adenylate cyclase. This is shown schematically in Figure 9.17. This causes it to dissociate from the adenylate cyclase and the system returns to the original inactivated state. Cholera toxin is an enzyme which alters the α-subunit so that it can no longer hydrolyse its bound GTP. The prolonged production of cAMP in intestinal epithelial cells causes a large efflux of Na^+ and water leading to severe diarrhoea characteristic of cholera.

Inhibitory G-proteins

The same signalling molecule can increase or decrease cAMP depending on the receptor it binds to. For example when adrenaline binds to α-adrenergic receptors, it activates adenylate cyclase, whereas when it

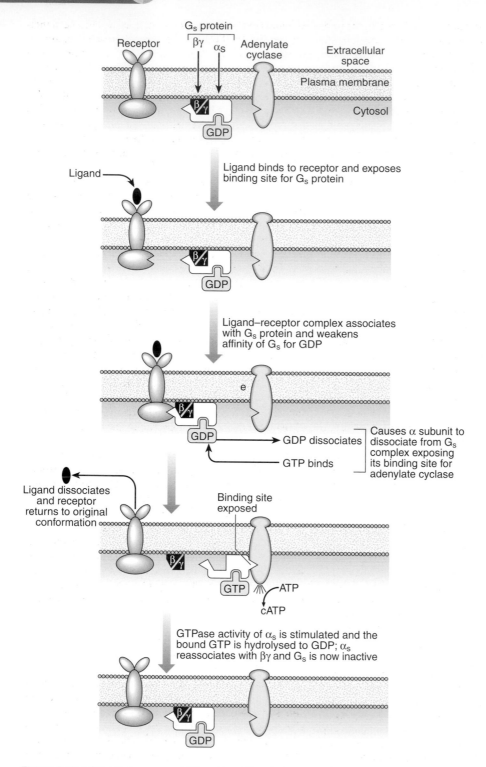

Figure 9.17 • Schematic representation of how G_s couples receptor activation to adenylate cyclase activation. As long as the ligand is bound to the receptor, the receptor can continually activate the G-protein.

binds to β_2-adrenergic receptors it inhibits the enzyme. The reason for this is that these receptors are coupled by different G-proteins. An inhibitory G-protein (G_i) has a different subunit (α_i rather than α_s). When activated, these receptors bind to G_i, causing α_i to bind to GTP and dissociate from the α-complex. Both the released α-complex and the α_i contribute to the inhibition of adenylate cyclase. G_i also has a role in opening K^+ channels in the plasma membrane. Pertussis toxin, made by the bacterium which causes whooping cough, alters α_i to prevent it from interacting with receptors, so that it cannot inhibit adenylate cyclase or open K^+ channels.

cAMP-dependent protein kinase (protein kinase A)

cAMP mediates its effects mainly by activating the enzyme known as cAMP-dependent protein kinase (protein kinase A). Protein kinase A catalyses the transfer of the terminal phosphate group from ATP to specific serine or threonines of particular proteins. This in turn regulates the activity of the target protein. In some cells, cAMP can also regulate gene transcription. Some genes contain a sequence known as the 'cyclic AMP response element' (CRE), which is recognized by a gene regulatory protein known as CRE-binding protein. When this protein is phosphorylated on a single serine residue, it is activated to turn on gene transcription. In order to control the effects of cAMP in cells, it must be able to dephosphorylate proteins which have been phosphorylated by protein kinase A. This is achieved by a group of enzymes known as serine/threonine phosphoprotein phosphatases.

Inositol phosphate and diacylglycerol second messengers

Inositol phosphate (IP_3) is produced as a result of the hydrolysis of inositol phospholipids (phosphoinositides) located mainly in the inner half of the plasma membrane. It is the breakdown of one class of these inositol phospholipids known as phosphatidyl bisphosphate (PIP_2) which is most important, even though it only accounts for less than 10% of the total inositol lipids and less than 1% of all the phospholipids in the cell membrane. The breakdown of PIP_2 starts with a signalling molecule binding to its receptor in the plasma membrane. The activated receptor stimulates a G-protein, known as G_q, which in turn activates an inositide-specific phospholipase C, known as phospholipase C-β. The enzyme cleaves PIP_2 to produce two products: IP_3 and diacylglycerol (Fig. 9.18). Each of these molecules has a separate role, as will be discussed.

IP_3 is small and water soluble. It diffuses into the cytosol where it binds to IP_3-gated calcium release channels in the endoplasmic reticulum. These channels are similar to those in the sarcoplasmic reticulum of muscle cells (ryanodine receptors) which trigger muscle contraction on calcium release. In many cell types, both forms of calcium receptor are present. To end the calcium response, calcium is pumped back out of the cytosol and IP_3 is broken down by phosphatases within the cell. Some of the IP_3 is also phosphorylated to form IP_4, which may promote the refilling of the intracellular calcium stores and/or mediate slower or longer-lived responses within the cell.

Diacylglycerol has two potential fates. It can be cleaved to give arachidonic acid, which can act as a messenger or can be used in the synthesis of eicosanoids. Its more important role is to activate a serine/threonine protein kinase (a protein kinase phosphorylates serine/threonine residues in target proteins within the cell and changes their properties). This protein is named 'protein kinase C', so called because it is calcium dependent. It is the initial rise in calcium brought about by IP_3 which causes the protein kinase C to move from the cytosol to the plasma membrane, where it is activated. At least four of the eight types of protein kinase C in animals are activated by diacylglycerol. Because diacylglycerol is rapidly metabolized, sustained protein kinase C activation for longer-term responses depends on a second wave of diacylglycerol production released this time by phospholipases which cleave phosphatidyl choline, the major phospholipid in the cell.

Protein kinase C can also alter the transcription of specific genes. In one pathway, it leads to the phosphorylation of a protein kinase called MAP kinase, which in turn phosphorylates and activates the gene regulatory protein Elk-1; this is then bound along with another protein (serum response factor) to a short DNA sequence (called the serum response element). This leads to transcription of the gene. In another pathway, activation of protein kinase results in the release of a gene regulatory protein NF-κB, which then moves into the nucleus and activates the transcription of specific genes.

Enzyme-linked receptors

Unlike G-protein-linked receptors, enzyme-linked receptors are single-pass transmembrane proteins with (like G-proteins) the ligand-binding site outside the cell and the catalytic unit inside the cell. Instead of the cytosolic domain interacting with a G-protein, the cytosolic domain has its own enzyme activity or associates directly with an enzyme. There are five known classes of enzyme-linked linked receptor:

1. *Receptor guanylate (sometimes called guanylyl) cyclases* catalyse the production of cyclic GMP. An example of this group is the atrial natriuretic

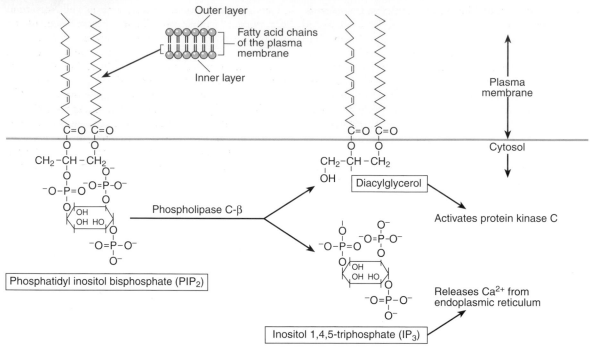

Figure 9.18 • Schematic representation of the inositol phosphate pathway. The activated receptor binds to a specific trimeric G-protein (G_q) causing the α-subunit to dissociate and activate phospholipase C-β (PLC-β). PLC-β hydrolyses PIP_2 to release IP_3 and diacylglycerol. IP_3 diffuses through the cytoplasm and releases Ca^{2+} from the endoplasmic reticulum while diacylglycerol remains within the membrane and activates protein kinase C. PLC-β is one of three classes of phospholipase (PLC-β, γ and δ). This class is activated by G-protein-linked receptors.

peptide (ANP) receptor. ANP is secreted by the atrium of the heart when blood pressure rises and stimulates the kidney to secrete Na^+ and water, and also induces the smooth muscle of vessel walls to relax. The binding of ANP activates the intracellular catalytic domain (guanylate cyclase) to produce cyclic GMP, which in turn binds to and activates a G-kinase; this phosphorylates serine and threonine residues on specific proteins. There are few members in this family.

2. Many receptors are *tyrosine kinases*, which phosphorylate specific tyrosine residues on a small set of signalling proteins. Members of this family include receptors for the epidermal growth factor, fibroblast growth factor, platelet-derived growth factor, vascular endothelial growth factor, nerve growth factor and insulin-like growth factor-1.

3. *Tyrosine kinase-associated receptors* associate with proteins which have tyrosine kinase activity.

4. *Receptor tyrosine phosphatases* remove phosphate groups from signalling molecules.

5. *Receptor serine/threonine kinases* phosphorylate specific serine or threonine residues on particular proteins. Receptors for the transforming growth factor-β superfamily receptors, which are important in development, are a member of this group.

Vascular endothelial growth factors

Vascular endothelial growth factors (VEGFs) are important regulators of vascular development during embryogenesis (vasculogenesis) as well as during blood vessel formation (angiogenesis) in the adult. VEGFs have been studied intensively in reproduction. VEGFs are thought to play important roles in many aspects of reproductive biology. They are active during menstruation, during placental development and in implantation. The concentration of circulating VEGF falls during pregnancy and falls even more in pre-eclampsia. This is due to the free circulating VEGF being 'mopped up' by being bound to a circulating VEGF receptor. In mammals, five VEGF ligands (differently spliced variants and processed forms) have been identified to date.

The VEGF ligands bind in an overlapping fashion to three receptor tyrosine kinases (RTKs), known as VEGF receptor-1, -2 and -3 (VEGFR-1–3), as well as to co-receptors that lack established VEGF-induced catalytic function, such as heparan sulphate proteoglycans (HSPGs) and neuropilins. VEGFs share some regulatory mechanisms with other well-characterized RTKs, such as the platelet-derived growth factor receptors (PDGFRs) and the epidermal growth factor receptors (EGFRs). These mechanisms include receptor dimerization and activation of the tyrosine kinase, as well as creation of docking sites for signal transducers. VEGFRs induce cellular events that are common to many growth factor receptors, such as cell migration, survival and proliferation. Tumour growth depends on new angiogenesis and, recently, tumour therapies that are based on neutralizing anti-VEGF antibodies and small-molecular-weight tyrosine kinase inhibitors that target the VEGFRs have been developed. These new treatments for cancer show the importance of understanding signal transduction pathways and their clinical relevance. It is important, when treating cancer and other diseases that are associated with pathological angiogenesis, to select therapy that preserves pathways that are important for the survival of blood vessels in healthy tissues.

Chapter Ten

10

Physiology

David Williams, Anna Kenyon & Dawn Adamson

CHAPTER CONTENTS

Biophysical definitions

Molecular weight

One mole of an element or compound is the atomic weight or molecular weight, respectively, in grams. For example, 1 mol of sodium is 23 g (atomic weight Na = 23) and 1 mol of sodium chloride is 58.5 g (atomic weight Cl = 35.5; 35.5 + 23 = 58.5). A 'normal' (molar) solution contains 1 mol/L of solution. Therefore a 'normal' solution of sodium chloride contains 58.5 g and is a 5.85% solution. This is very different from a physiological 'normal' solution of sodium chloride, where the concentration of sodium chloride (0.9%) is adjusted so that the sodium has the same concentration as the total number of cations in plasma (154 mmol/L). The concentrations of biological substances are usually much weaker than molar. However, commonly used intravenous solutions that combine sodium chloride with glucose often contain sodium chloride 0.18% (sodium 30 mmol/L and chloride 30 mmol/L) and glucose 4%. Injudicious use of excessive volumes of this combination with 30 mmol NaCl will quickly lead to hyponatraemia.

The conventional nomenclature for decreasing molar concentrations is given below. The same prefixes may be used for different units of measurement:

1 millimole (mmol) = 1×10^{-3} mol

1 micromole (μmol) = 1×10^{-6} mol

1 nanomole (nmol) = 1×10^{-9} mol

1 picomole (pmol) = 1×10^{-12} mol

1 femtomole (fmol) = 1×10^{-15} mol

1 attomole (amol) = 1×10^{-18} mol

1 equivalent (Eq) = 1 mol divided by the valency. Thus 1 Eq of sodium (valency 1) = 23 g, and 1 mol of sodium = 1 Eq, i.e. 1 mmol = 1 mEq.

However, 1 Eq of calcium (valency 2, mol wt 40) = 20 g. 1 mol of calcium = 2 Eq, and 1 mmol Ca^{2+} = 2 mEq Ca^{2+}.

Measurements in medicine are wherever possible being made in Systeme Internationale (SI) units. Under this system, the concentration of biological materials is expressed in the appropriate molar units (often mmol) per litre (L).

The units used in the measurement of osmotic pressure are considered below.

Distribution of water and electrolytes

A normal 70 kg man is composed of 60% water, 18% protein, 15% fat and 7% minerals. Obese individuals have relatively more fat and less water. Of the 60% (42 L) of water, 28 L (40% of body weight) are intracellular; the remaining 14 L of extracellular water are made up of 10.5 L of interstitial fluid (extracellular and extravascular) and 3.5 L of blood plasma. The total blood volume (red cells and plasma) is 8% of total body weight, or about 5.6 L.

Total body water can be measured by giving a subject deuterium oxide (D_2O), 'heavy water', and measuring how much it is diluted. Extracellular fluid volume can be measured with inulin by the same principle. Intracellular fluid volume = total body water (D_2O space) less extracellular fluid volume (inulin space). Intravascular fluid volume can be measured with Evans blue dye. Total blood volume can be calculated knowing intravascular fluid volume and the haematocrit. Interstitial fluid volume = extracellular fluid volume (inulin space) less intravascular fluid volume.

The distribution of electrolytes and protein in intracellular fluid, interstitial fluid and plasma is given in Figure 10.1. Note that, for reasons of comparability, concentrations are expressed in milliequivalents per litre (mEq/L) of water, not millimoles per litre (mmol/L) of plasma.

The major difference between plasma and interstitial fluid is that interstitial fluid has relatively little protein. As a consequence, the concentration of sodium in the interstitial fluid is less and so is the overall osmotic pressure (see below). There are further major differences between intracellular fluid and extracellular fluid. Sodium is the major extracellular cation, whereas potassium and, to a lesser extent, magnesium are the predominant intracellular cations. Chloride and bicarbonate are the major extracellular anions; protein and phosphate are the predominant intracellular anions.

Anion gap

In considering the composition of plasma for clinical purposes, account is often taken of the 'anion gap'. This is calculated by considering sodium the principal cation, 136 mEq/L, and subtracting from it the concentrations of the principal anions, chloride, 100 mEq/L, and

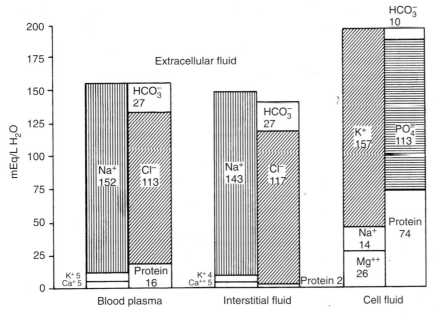

Figure 10.1 • Electrolyte composition of human body fluids.

bicarbonate, 24 mEq/L. This leaves a positive balance of 12 mEq/L. The normal range is 8–16 mEq/L. The gap is considered to exist because of the occurrence of unmeasured anions, such as protein or lactate, which would balance the number of cations. An increase in the anion gap suggests that there are more unmeasured anions present than usual. This occurs in such situations as lactic acidosis, or diabetic ketoacidosis, where the lactate and acetoacetate are balancing the excess sodium ions. A more complete explanation of the anion gap would be to consider both the unmeasured cations as well as the unmeasured anions, as in Table 10.1. Situations where the anion gap is increased include ketoacidosis, lactic acidosis and hyperosmolar acidosis, and poisoning with salicylate, methanol, ethylene glycol and paraldehyde, and hypoalbuminaemia. A decreased anion gap occurs in bromide poisoning and myeloma.

Transport mechanisms

These mechanisms account for the movement of substances within cells and across cell membranes. The transport mechanisms to be considered include diffusion, solvent drag, filtration, osmosis, non-ionic diffusion, carrier-mediated transport and phagocytosis. Not all of these mechanisms will be considered in detail.

Diffusion is the process whereby a gas or substance in solution expands to fill the volume available to it.

Table 10.1   Anion gap (mEq/L)

Cation		Anion	
Na^+	136	Cl^-	100
		HCO_3^-	24
	——		——
	136		124
		Gap	12
	——		——
	136		136
The gap consists of unmeasured cations and anions:			
K^+	4.5	Protein	15
Ca^{2+}	5	PO_4^{3-}	2
Mg^{2+}	1.5	SO_4^{2-}	1
		Organic acids	5
	——		——
	11		23
	——		——
	147		147

Relevant examples of gaseous diffusion are the equilibration of gases within the alveoli of the lung, and of liquid diffusion, the equilibration of substances within the fluid of the renal tubule. An element of diffusion may be involved in all transport across cell membranes because recent research suggests that there is a layer of unstirred water up to 400 μm thick adjacent to biological membranes in animals.

If there is a charged ion that cannot diffuse across a membrane which other charged ions can cross, the diffusible ions distribute themselves as in the following example:

In	Out
K_i^+	K_0^+
Cl_i^-	Cl_0^-
Protein$^-$	

$$\frac{[K_i^+]}{[K_0^+]} = \frac{[Cl_0^-]}{[Cl_i^-]}$$ **Gibbs–Donnan equilibrium**

The cell is permeable to K^+ and Cl^- but not to protein. Since K_i is about 157 mmol/L and K_0 is 4 mmol/L, the Gibbs–Donnan equilibrium would predict that the ratio of chloride concentration outside the cell to that inside should be 157/4, i.e. about 40. In fact, there is almost no intracellular chloride so that the ratio *in vivo* is even greater than 40. This is because there are other factors than simple diffusion affecting both potassium and chloride concentrations.

Solvent drag is the process whereby bulk movement of solvent drags some molecules of solute with it. It is of little importance.

Filtration is the process whereby substances are forced through a membrane by hydrostatic pressure. The degree to which substances pass through the membrane depends on the size of the holes in the membrane. Small molecules pass through the holes, larger molecules do not. In the renal glomerulus the holes are large enough to allow all blood constituents to pass through the filtration membrane, apart from blood cells and the majority of plasma proteins.

Osmosis describes the movement of solvent from a region of low solute concentration, across a semipermeable membrane to one of high solute concentration. The process can be opposed by hydrostatic pressure; the pressure that will stop osmosis occurring is the osmotic pressure of the solution. This is given by the formula:

$$P = nRT/V$$

where, P = osmotic pressure, n = number of osmotically active particles, R = gas constant, T = absolute temperature, V = volume. For an ideal solution of a non-ionized substance, n/V equals the concentration of the solute. In an ideal solution, 1 osmol of a substance is then defined such that:

1 osmol = mol.wt in grams/number of osmotically active particles in solution

So for an ideal solution of glucose:

1 osmol = mol.wt/1 = mol.wt = 180 g

However, sodium chloride dissociates into two ions in solution. Therefore, for sodium chloride:

1 osmol = mol.wt/2 = 58.5/2 = 29.2 g

Calcium chloride dissociates into three ions in solution. Therefore, for calcium chloride,

1 osmol = mol.wt/3 = 111/3 = 37 g

However, the molecules or ions of all solutions aggregate to a certain degree so that interaction occurs between the ions or molecules, and they each do not behave as osmotically independent particles and do not form ideal solutions. Freezing point depression by a solution is also caused by the number of osmotically active particles. The greater the concentration of osmotically active particles, the greater the freezing point depression. In an ideal solution, with no interaction, 1 mol of osmotically active particles per litre depresses the freezing point by 1.86°C. Therefore, an aqueous solution which depresses the freezing point by 1.86°C is defined as containing 1 osmol/L. One which depresses the freezing point by 1.86°C/1000, i.e. 0.00186°C, contains 1 mosmol/L. Plasma (osmotic pressure 300 mosmol/L) has a freezing point of (0 −0.00186 × 300)°C = −0.56°C.

Osmolarity defines osmotic pressure in terms of osmoles per litre of solution. Since volume changes at different temperatures, osmolality which defines osmotic pressure in terms of osmoles per kilogram of solution is preferred, though not always employed. The major osmotic components of plasma are the cations sodium and potassium, and their accompanying anions, together with glucose and urea.

The concentration of sodium is about 140 mmol/L. This, and the accompanying anions, will therefore contribute 280 mosmol/L. The concentration of potassium is about 4 mmol/L, which, with its accompanying anions, will give 8 mosmol/L. Glucose and urea contribute 5 mosmol/L each to a total of 300 mosmol/L in normal plasma. During pregnancy, due to an expansion of plasma volume this falls to below 290 mosmol/L. The mechanism of plasma volume expansion appears to relate to a resetting of the hypothalamic thirst centre, so that in early pregnancy women still feel thirsty at a lower plasma osmolality.

We are now in a position to consider some of the forces acting on water in the capillaries (Fig. 10.2). The capillary membrane behaves as if it is only permeable to water and small solutes. It is impermeable to colloids such as plasma protein. There is a difference of 25 mmHg in osmotic pressure between the interstitial water and the intravascular water due to the intravascular plasma proteins (see above). This force (oncotic pressure) will tend to drive water into the capillary. At the arteriolar end of the capillary, the hydrostatic pressure is 37 mmHg; the interstitial pressure is 1 mmHg. The net force driving water *out* is therefore 37 − 1 − 25 = 11 mmHg, and water tends to pass out of the arteriolar end of the capillary. At the venous end of the capillary, the pressure is only 17 mmHg. The net force driving water *in* the capillary is therefore 25 + 1 − 17 = 9 mmHg. Fluid therefore enters the capillary at the venous end. Factors which would decrease fluid reabsorption and cause clinical oedema are a reduction in plasma proteins, so that the osmotic gradient between the intravascular and interstitial fluids might be only 20 mmHg, not 25 mmHg, or a rise in venous pressure so that the pressure at the venous end of the capillary might be 25 mmHg, rather than 17 mmHg.

Non-ionized diffusion is the process whereby there is preferential transport in a non-ionized form. Cell membranes consist of a lipid bilayer with specific transporter proteins embedded in it. Lipid-soluble drugs,

e.g. propranolol, can cross the lipids of the blood–brain barrier or the placenta by non-ionized diffusion. But small hydrophilic molecules such as O_2 can also diffuse across the lipid bilayer, which is also permeable to water.

Carrier-mediated transport implies transport across a cell membrane using a specific carrier. If the transport is down a concentration gradient from an area of high concentration to one of low concentration, this is known as facilitated transport, e.g. the uptake of glucose by the muscle cell, facilitated by the participation of insulin in the transport process. If the carrier-mediated transport is up a concentration gradient from an area of low concentration to one of high concentration, this is known as active transport, e.g. the removal of sodium from muscle cells by the ATPase-dependent sodium pump. The channel may be ligand gated where binding of external (e.g. insulin as earlier) ligands or an internal ligand opens the channel. Alternatively the channel may be voltage gated, where patency depends on the transmembrane electrical potential; voltage gating is a major feature of the conduction of nervous impulses.

Phagocytosis and pinocytosis involve the incorporation of discrete bodies of solid and liquid substances, respectively, by cell wall growing out and around the particles so that the cell appears to swallow them. If the cell eliminates substances, the process is known as exocytosis; if substances are transported into the cell, the process is endocytosis. In endocytosis, the Golgi apparatus is involved in intracellular transport and processing to varying extents depending on whether exocytosis is via the non-constitutive pathway (extensive processing) or the constitutive pathway (little processing). Similarly, endocytosis may involve specific receptors for substances such as low-density lipoproteins (receptor-mediated endocytosis) or there may be no specific receptors (constitutive endocytosis).

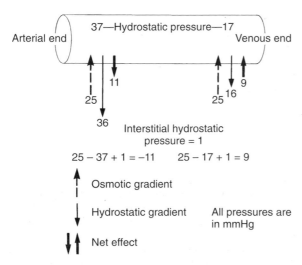

Figure 10.2 • At the arterial end of the capillary the hydrostatic forces acting outwards are greater than the osmotic forces acting inwards. There is a net movement out of the capillary. At the venous end of the capillary, the hydrostatic forces acting outwards are less than the osmotic forces acting inwards. There is a net movement into the capillary.

Acid–base balance

Normal acid–base balance

A simple knowledge of chemistry allows some substances to be easily categorized as acids or bases. For example, hydrochloric acid is clearly an acid and sodium hydroxide is a base. But when describing acid–base balance in physiology, these terms are used rather more obscurely. For example, the chloride ion may be described as a base. A more applicable definition is to define an acid as an ion or molecule which can liberate hydrogen ions. Since hydrogen ions are protons (H^+), acids may also be defined as proton donors. A base is then a substance which can accept hydrogen ions, or a proton acceptor. If we consider the examples below, hydrochloric acid dissociates into hydrogen ions and chloride ions, and is therefore a proton donor (acid). If the chloride ion associates with hydrogen ions to form hydrochloric acid, the chloride ion is a proton acceptor (base). Ammonia is another proton acceptor when it forms the ammonium ion. Carbonic acid is an acid (hydrogen ion donor); bicarbonate is a base (hydrogen ion acceptor). The $H_2PO_4^-$ ion can be both an acid when it dissociates further to HPO_4^{2-} and a base when it associates to form H_3PO_4:

$$HCl \rightleftharpoons H^+ + Cl^-$$
$$NH_3 + H^- \rightleftharpoons NH_4^+$$
$$H_2CO_3 \rightleftharpoons H^+ + HCO_3^-$$
$$H_3PO_4 \rightleftharpoons H_2PO_4^- + H^+$$
$$H_2PO_4^- \rightleftharpoons H_3PO_4^{2-} + H^+$$

pH

The pH is defined as the negative $\log_{10}$ of the hydrogen ion concentration expressed in mol/L. A negative logarithmic scale is used because the numbers are all less than 1, and vary over a wide range. Since the pH is the negative logarithm of the hydrogen ion concentration, low pH numbers, e.g. pH 6.2, indicate relatively high hydrogen ion concentrations, i.e. an acidic solution. High pH numbers, e.g. pH 7.8, represent lower hydrogen ion concentrations, i.e. alkaline solutions. Because the pH scale is logarithmic to the base 10, a 1-unit change in pH represents a 10-fold change in hydrogen ion concentration.

The normal pH range in human tissues is 7.36–7.44. Although a neutral pH (hydrogen ion concentration equals hydroxyl ion concentration) at 20°C has the value 7.4, water dissociates more at physiological temperatures, and a neutral pH at 37°C has the value 6.8. Therefore, body fluids are mildly alkaline (the higher the pH number, the lower the hydrogen ion concentration).

A pH value of 7.4 represents a hydrogen ion concentration of 0.00004 mmol/L as seen in the following example:

$$pH = 7.4$$
$$[H^+] = 10^{-7.4} \text{ mol/L}$$
$$= 10^{-8} \times 10^{0.6} \text{ mol/L}$$
$$= 0.00000001 \times 4 \text{ mol/L}$$
$$= 0.00000004 \text{ mol/L}$$
$$= 0.00004 \text{ mmol/L}$$
$$(1 \text{ mol/L} = 1000 \text{ mmol/L})$$

Partial pressure of carbon dioxide (P_{CO_2})

In arterial blood, the normal value is 4.8–5.9 kPa (36–44 mmHg). It is a fortunate coincidence that the figures expressing P_{CO_2} in mmHg are similar to those expressing the normal range for pH (7.36–7.44).

Henderson–Hasselbalch equation

This equation describes the relationship of hydrogen ion, bicarbonate and carbonic acid concentrations (see Equation (3) below). It can be rewritten in terms of pH, bicarbonate and carbonic acid concentrations, as in Equation (4), but carbonic acid concentrations are not usually measured. However, because of the presence of carbonic anhydrase in red cells, carbonic acid concentration is proportional to P_{CO_2} (Equation (1)). Equation (4) can therefore be rewritten in terms of pH, bicarbonate and P_{CO_2} (Equation (5)). All these data are usually available from blood gas analyses. If we know any two of these variables, the third can be calculated.

Carbonic anhydrase:

$$CO_2 + H_2O \longrightarrow H_2CO_3 \qquad (1)$$

$$[H_2CO_3] \rightleftharpoons H^+ + HCO_3^- \qquad (2)$$

By the Law of Mass Action:

$$[H_2CO_3] = K[H^+][HCO_3^-] \qquad (2)$$

$$\therefore [H^+] = \frac{1}{K}\left(\frac{[H_2CO_3^-]}{[HCO_3^-]}\right) \qquad (3)$$

By taking logarithms of the reciprocal:

$$pH = K' + \log\left(\frac{[HCO_3^-]}{[H_2CO_3]}\right)$$

K' is a constant equal to 6.1:

$$pH = 6.1 + \log\left(\frac{[HCO_3^-]}{[H_2CO_3]}\right) \qquad (4)$$

$$pH = 6.1 + \log\left(\frac{[HCO_3^-]}{P_aCO_2 \times 0.04}\right) \qquad (5)*$$

Control of pH

The Henderson–Hasselbalch equation, expressed in Equation (5), indicates that the variables controlling pH are P_{CO_2} and bicarbonate concentration. Ultimately, P_{CO_2} is controlled by respiration. Short-term changes of pH may therefore be compensated for by changing the depth of respiration. Bicarbonate concentration can be altered by the kidneys, and this is the mechanism involved in the long-term control of pH. Further details of these mechanisms are given on pp 197 and 201.

*For Equation (5), because of the action of carbonic anhydrase, $[H_2CO_3]$ is proportional to P_aCO_2. For the given constants of equation (5), P_{CO_2} is expressed in mmHg.

Buffers

A buffer solution is one to which hydrogen or hydroxyl ions can be added with little change in the pH.

Consider a solution of sodium bicarbonate to which is added hydrochloric acid (Fig. 10.3). The hydrogen ions of the hydrochloric acid react with bicarbonate ions of the sodium bicarbonate to form carbonic acid. Carbonic acid does not dissociate so readily as hydrochloric acid. Therefore the hydrogen ions are buffered. Reading from right to left in Figure 10.3, we have a solution that starts as 100% bicarbonate ions, and becomes 100% carbonic acid, as hydrochloric acid is added. Initially, in the pH range 9–7, a very small change in bicarbonate concentration, requiring the addition of only a few hydrogen ions, is associated with a large change in pH. However, in the steep part of the curve, between pH 5 and 7, a considerable quantity of hydrogen ions can be added, as indicated by a marked fall in the proportion of bicarbonate remaining, with relatively little change in pH. It is in that pH range that the buffering ability of bicarbonate is greatest.

The pH at which 50% of the buffer is changed from its acidic to its basic form (or vice versa) is known as the pK. For bicarbonate the pK is 6.1, making bicarbo-nate rather poor as a buffer for body fluids, since the pK is considerably towards the acidic side of the physiological pH range (7.36–7.44). The buffer value of a buffer (mmol of hydrogen ion per gram per pH unit) is the quantity of hydrogen ions which can be added to a buffer solution to change its pH by 1.0 pH unit from $pK + 0.5$ to $pK - 0.5$.

In blood, the most important buffers are proteins. These are able to absorb hydrogen ions onto free carboxyl radicals, as illustrated in Figure 10.4. Of the proteins available, haemoglobin is more important than plasma protein, partly because its buffer value is greater than that of plasma protein (0.18 mmol of hydrogen per gram of haemoglobin per pH unit, vs 0.11 mmol of hydrogen per gram of plasma protein per pH unit), but also because there is more haemoglobin than plasma protein (15 g haemoglobin per 100 mL vs 3.8 g of plasma protein per 100 mL). These two factors mean that haemoglobin has six times the buffering capacity of plasma protein. In addition, deoxygenated haemoglobin is a weaker acid and a more efficient buffer than oxygenated haemoglobin. This increases the buffering capacity of haemoglobin where it is needed more, after oxygen has been liberated in the peripheral tissues.

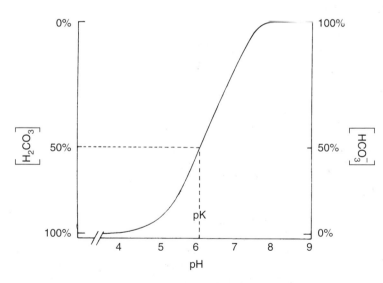

Figure 10.3 • Effect of adding H^+ (as HCl) to an HCO_3^- solution (as $NaHCO_3$). The pH changes from 9.0 when the solution is 100% HCO_3^- and 0% H_2CO_3 to <4 when the solution is 0% HCO_3^- and 100% H_2CO_3. At the pK value when the HCO_3^- is 50% changed to H_2CO_3 the curve is steepest, indicating that there is relatively little change in the pH for a relatively large change in HCO_3^- concentration. The pK is 6.1.

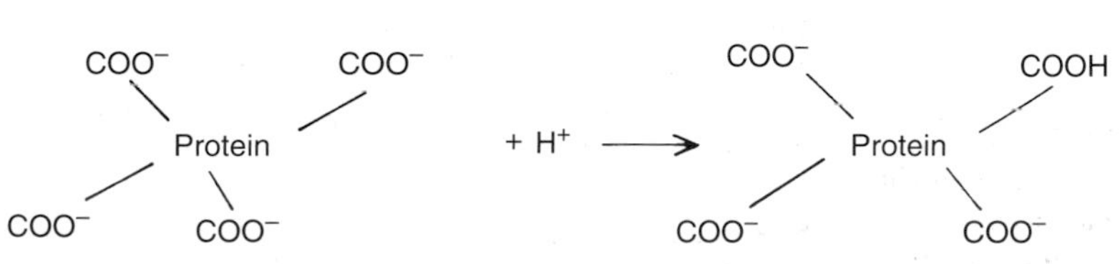

Figure 10.4 • The absorption of hydrogen ions onto free carboxyl radicals.

Buffer base and base excess

The buffer base is the total number of buffer anions (usually 45–50 mEq/L of blood) and consists of bicarbonate, phosphate and protein anions (haemoglobin and plasma protein).

Base excess is the difference between the actual buffer base and the normal value for a given haemoglobin and body temperature. It is negative in acidosis and is then sometimes expressed as a positive base deficit, and positive in alkalosis. It gives an index of the severity of the abnormality of acid–base balance.

Standard bicarbonate

This is the carbon dioxide content of blood equilibrated at a P_{CO_2} of 40 mmHg and a temperature of 37°C when the haemoglobin is fully saturated with oxygen. In general it represents the non-respiratory part of acid–base derangement, and is low in metabolic acidosis and raised in metabolic alkalosis. The normal value for the standard bicarbonate is 27 mmol/L.

Abnormalities of acid–base balance

These are usually divided into acidosis (pH < 7.36) and alkalosis (pH > 7.44). In addition, we consider respiratory acidosis and alkalosis where the primary abnormality is in respiration (carbon dioxide control) and metabolic acidosis and alkalosis, which are best defined as abnormalities that are not respiratory in origin. Only initial, single abnormalities will be considered. For these single uncomplicated abnormalities, respiratory and metabolic acidosis and alkalosis can be defined according to Table 10.2, which gives the values of pH and P_{CO_2} characterizing each abnormality.

Respiratory acidosis

There is a low pH and a high P_{CO_2}. Here the basic abnormality is a failure of carbon dioxide excretion from the lungs. Carbon dioxide dissolves in the blood, and in the presence of carbonic anhydrase, carbonic acid is formed which dissociates into hydrogen ions and bicarbonate (Equations (1) and (2), p. 178). Respiratory acidosis may arise from abnormalities of respiration, which may range from impaired respiratory control due to excessive sedation, to chronic pulmonary disease. In the long term, respiratory acidosis is compensated by bicarbonate retention in the kidneys, which increases pH towards normal values.

Respiratory alkalosis

There is a high pH and a low P_{CO_2}. This is induced by hyperventilation, whatever the cause. Perhaps the commonest clinical presentation is anxiety, where the acute fall in hydrogen ion concentration due to blowing off carbon dioxide may cause paraesthesiae, or even tetany. Tetany occurs because more plasma protein is ionized when the pH is high. This protein binds more calcium, lowering the ionized (metabolically effective) calcium level (see p. 255). However, respiratory alkalosis is also seen in the early stages of exercise, at altitude and in patients who have had a pulmonary embolus. In pregnancy, there is hyperventilation but the kidney excretes sufficient bicarbonate to compensate fully for the fall in carbon dioxide, and there is therefore no change in pH.

Metabolic acidosis

There is a low pH and the P_{CO_2} is not elevated. This may occur because of excessive acid production, impaired acid excretion, or excessive alkali loss. Examples of excess acid production are diabetic ketoacidosis and methanol poisoning, in which methanol is metabolized to formaldehyde, which subsequently forms formic acid.

Failure of acid excretion occurs in chronic renal failure, and more specifically in renal tubular acidosis, where the patients are not initially uraemic but acid excretion by the kidney is impaired. Acetazolamide is a diuretic drug which inhibits ammonia formation within the kidney, and this too causes metabolic acidosis. Excess alkali loss is seen in patients who have a pancreatic fistula or prolonged diarrhoea, since both the bodily fluids lost are alkaline.

Metabolic alkalosis

The pH is high and the P_{CO_2} is not reduced. This may occur due to prolonged vomiting. The mechanism is less to do with the loss of acidic fluid, and move to a loss of fluid volume and a compensatory activation of the renin–angiotensin–aldosterone system. Sodium is reabsorbed at the renal tubules at the expense of potassium and hydrogen ions. Metabolic alkalosis also occurs in excessive alkali ingestion, seen in patients who take antacids for peptic ulceration. Metabolic alkalosis frequently accompanies hypokalaemia.

Table 10.2 Values of pH and P_{CO_2} characterizing acidosis and alkalosis

	pH	P_{CO_2} (kPa)	P_{CO_2} (mmHg)
Normal	7.36–7.44	4.8–5.9	36–44
Respiratory acidosis	<7.36	>5.9	>44
Respiratory alkalosis	>7.44	<4.8	<36
Metabolic acidosis	<7.36	<5.9	<44
Metabolic alkalosis	>7.44	>4.8	>36

Cardiovascular system

This section will detail the physiology of both cardiac output and the conduction system in a normal pregnancy as well as examining normal pregnant haemodynamics and the potential changes that can occur in cardiac disease.

Conduction system of the heart

The heart has its own unique electrical conduction tissue (Figure 10.5) which allows orderly coordinated activity between atria and ventricles to ensure maximum efficiency and cardiac output. The electrical impulse is generated by the sino-atrial (SA) node which is located high in the right atrium at the entry of the superior vena cava. The impulse is then transmitted across both atria by crossing adjoining cardiomyocytes of the smooth muscle via gap junctions resulting in atrial contraction. There is an electrical seal allowing no conduction between the atria and ventricles which in the normal heart is broken only by the atrioventricular (AV) node. The electrical impulse once arrived at the AV node is stored for a few milliseconds to allow maximum ventricular filling from the atria. The AV node, which sits in the atrioventricular ring, conducts the impulse through specialized conduction tissue called the His–Purkinje system. The His bundle divides into a right and left branch which innervate the right and left ventricles respectively. The right bundle is a

relatively narrow group of fibres. The left bundle is a much wider sheet of fibres and divides further into fascicles. Thus right bundle branch block due to damage to the right bundle occurs relatively easily, and is not necessarily of pathological significance. Left bundle branch block implies considerable additional damage to the underlying myocardium to interrupt such a wide sheet of fibres, and is always pathological. Interruption or damage to the normal conduction system can lead to varying degrees of heart block. In the event of failure of the SA or AV node, the ventricular tissue has the ability to contract under its own intrinsic rate, although this is usually at a much slower rate than normal.

Some patients have additional electrical pathways which cross the atrioventricular seal and can conduct impulses antegradely (from atria to ventricles) and retrogradely (vice versa). By having this pathway in addition to the AV node, it allows the impulse to pass from atria to ventricles and return back to the atria in a circuit fashion which leads to the formation of tachyarrhythmias. The most common example of this is Wolff–Parkinson–White (WPW) syndrome.

Factors affecting heart rate

The activity of the SA node is controlled neurogenically by the sympathetic and parasympathetic nervous systems, directed by the vasomotor and cardio-inhibitory centres, respectively (see later). At rest, the dominant tone is parasympathetic, mediated via the vagus nerve (a muscarinic effect; Table 10.3).

In addition, the discharge rate from the SA node and therefore heart rate is increased by the direct actions of thyroxine and high temperature, by β-adrenergic activity, and by atropine, which blocks the dominant parasympathetic tone; it is decreased by hypothyroidism, hypothermia, and β-adrenergic blockade. SA node activity is also decreased in ischaemia, and under these circumstances other pacemakers (AV node, ventricles) can take over the pacemaker activity of the heart at a slower intrinsic rate.

Cardiac chambers

Table 10.4 shows the normal dimensions for the cardiac chambers outside of pregnancy. In pregnancy, the chambers increase to accommodate the increased circulating volume with the largest changes being seen in the left and right atrium (an increase of 5 and 7 mm, respectively) (Campos 1996).

Electrocardiogram (ECG)

Figure 10.6 shoes a normal ECG. The P wave is atrial depolarization which leads to atrial contraction while the QRS complex is ventricular depolarization which leads to ventricular contraction. The T wave is second-

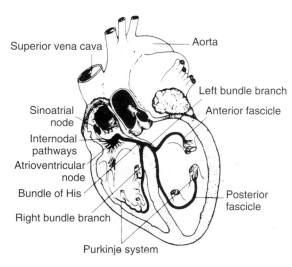

Superior vena cava

Aorta

Sinoatrial node

Internodal pathways

Atrioventricular node

Bundle of His

Right bundle branch

Left bundle branch

Anterior fascicle

Posterior fascicle

Purkinje system

Figure 10.5 • The conducting system of the heart. Internodal pathways in the atria are not specialized conducting tissue in normal individuals. Aberrant pathways have been found in subjects susceptible to dysrhythmias. (Reproduced with permission from Ganong W. Review of medical physiology. Lange Medical, Los Altos, CA.)

ary to ventricular repolarization. Atrial repolarization is not seen on the surface ECG as it occurs at the same time as ventricular depolarization and it is too small an electrical signal to be seen within the QRS. The normal ECG is recorded at a speed of 25 mm/s, so each small square represents 0.04 s and each large square represents 0.2 s. In the vertical axis, the ECG is calibrated so that 1 cm equals 1 mV. In order to calculate the heart rate, divide 300 by N, where N is the number of large squares between successive R waves. In the event of atrial fibrillation, where it is variable, an average is taken.

The normal PR interval is between 0.12 and 0.20 ms. If there is a delay, then there is a delay in conduction between the atria and ventricles and this is known as first-degree heart block. If the PR interval is short, then the electrical impulse is being transmitted between the atria and ventricles through a much faster pathway than normal, which implies aberrant conduction. This is typically seen in WPW syndrome and leads to a rapid inflection on the upstroke of the R wave known as a delta wave.

The normal QRS width should be no greater than 0.12 s (three small squares) and any longer is due to a delay in the impulse travelling along the His–Purkinje system. This is known as bundle branch block and, depending upon which bundle is involved, leads to a different morphology of the QRS seen best in lead V1. The QT interval is between 0.30 and 0.45 s and is dependent upon heart rate. It is increased in hypocalcaemia, hypokalaemia, rheumatic carditis and with a large number of drugs. It is decreased in hypercalcaemia, hyperkalaemia and digoxin.

Table 10.3 Autonomic receptors affecting the heart and blood vessels

Location	Receptor	Comments
Heart muscle and conducting tissue	Cholinergic	↓ Heart rate ↓ Conduction velocity ↓ Contractility
	α-adrenergic	Nil
	β₂-adrenergic	↑ Heart rate ↑ Conduction velocity ↑ Contractility
Blood vessels	Cholinergic (vasodilator)	Muscle Coronary artery Salivary glands
	α-adrenergic (vasoconstrictor)	All tissues
	β₁-adrenergic (vasodilator)	Brain Skeletal muscle Intra-abdominal

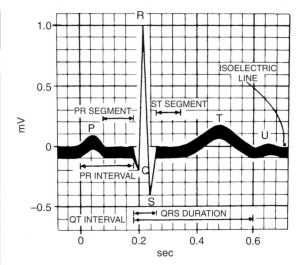

Figure 10.6 • The normal electrocardiogram. (Reproduced with permission from Ganong W. Review of medical physiology. Lange Medical, Los Altos, CA.)

Table 10.4 Cardiac chamber dimensions

	Control	Weeks 8–12	Weeks 20–24	Weeks 30–34	Weeks 36–40	Change cf control
LVEDd	40.1	41.1	42.7	43.0	43.6	3.5
LA	27.9	29.6	31.5	33.1	32.8	4.9
RVEDd	28.5	30.1	31.9	35.5	35.5	4.4
RA	43.7	42.8	47.4	50.8	50.9	7.2

Source: Campos (1996).
LVEDd, left ventricular end-diastolic dimension; RVEDd, right ventricular end-diastolic dimension.

Pressure and saturation in the cardiac chambers

Blood enters the right side of the heart via the inferior and superior vena cava (Fig. 10.7). That which comes from the head is more desaturated than that from the rest of the body due to increased consumption by the brain, and normal mixed venous oxygen saturation in the right atrium is usually around 60%. If there is oxygenated blood abnormally entering the atrium due to a shunt or atrial septal defect, then this will lead to a step up in the saturations if sampled from high to low RA and will lead to an increased mixed venous saturation. True mixed venous blood, however, is best taken from the pulmonary artery (PA) as blood from the coronary sinus enters the right atrium and with streaming, which occurs in the right atrium and ventricle, blood is not fully mixed until it reaches the PA. Blood in the left side of the heart is 96% saturated with oxygen, giving a PCO_2 of 90–100 mmHg (100 mmHg = 13.3 kPa). There is no difference in saturation in blood in the left atrium and ventricle.

All pressures in the circulation should be measured relative to a fixed reference point, ideally the level of the right atrium. The normal ranges are shown in Table 10.5. Using this reference point, the mean right atrial pressure is usually between 1 and 7 mmHg (average 4 mmHg). This is determined indirectly by assessing the jugular venous pressure, and more directly by measurement of central venous pressure. The pressure in the left atrium is approximately 10–15 mmHg, and this can be measured using a Swan–Ganz catheter. The catheter is placed in the pulmonary artery either under direct radiological vision or the balloon tip inflated and the device floated through the right heart via a central vein. Once in the pulmonary artery, the inflated balloon can be wedged into a branch of the distal pulmonary artery. Providing there are no significant reasons for pressure across the lung capillaries to be raised then the pressure reflects that of the left atrium. The same Swan–Ganz catheter can also be used for measuring cardiac output by the thermodilution method which involves injecting a bolus of cold saline into the pulmonary artery and recording the area under the curve of the temperature change over time. Essentially, the higher the cardiac output, the quicker the cold saline is replaced with warm blood and hence the area under the curve will be reduced.

Haemodynamic events in the cardiac cycle and their clinical correlates

This section describes events in the left side of the heart, although the events occurring on the right side of the heart are similar. However, left atrial systole occurs after right atrial systole and left ventricular systole precedes right ventricular systole.

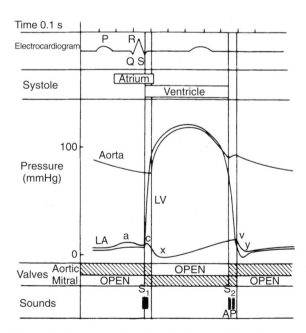

Figure 10.7 • Haemodynamic and electrocardiographic correlates of events in the cardiac cycle. (Reproduced with permission from Passmore R, Robson J (eds) Companion to medical studies. Blackwell Scientific, Oxford.)

Table 10.5   Normal values for cardiac pressure and saturations

	Normal pressure (mmHg)	Normal saturation (%)
Right atrial pressure	2–6	
Right ventricle Systolic End-diastolic	15–25 0–8	Mixed venous saturations
Pulmonary artery Systolic/diastolic Mean	15–25/8–15 10–20	70–75
Pulmonary capillary wedge	6–12	
Left ventricle end-diastolic pressure (EDP)	<12	95–100
Cardiac output (L/min)	4.0–8.0	
Cardiac index (L/min per m²)	2.8–4.2	

At the very beginning of ventricular systole, the mitral valve is open; the pressure in the left atrium is somewhat greater than that in the left ventricle. As ventricular systole continues, the pressure in the left ventricle exceeds that in the left atrium, thus closing the mitral valve. Shortly afterwards, the pressure in the left ventricle exceeds that in the aorta, and this opens the aortic valve; ejection of blood then occurs from the left ventricle. As the ventricle starts to relax, the pressure in the left ventricle falls below that in the aorta; initially, the aortic valve stays open because of the forward kinetic energy of the ejected blood. With a further fall in pressure in the left ventricle, the aortic valve then closes. As the pressure in the left ventricle continues to fall below and becomes lower than that in the left atrium, the mitral valve opens, and blood passes from the atrium to the ventricle.

In the period of rapid passive filling (early in diastole) blood falls from the atria to the ventricles. However, the remaining one-third of ventricular filling is caused by atrial systole (active filling), which, in turn, causes the *a* wave in the jugular venous pressure trace. The *c* wave coincides with the onset of ventricular systole, making the tricuspid valve bulge into the atrium and raising the pressure there. The *v* wave is due to the filling of the atrium while the tricuspid valve is shut, and the upward movement of the tricuspid valve at the end of ventricular systole. Active filling constitutes approximately 5% of cardiac output in a normal heart and is lost in atrial fibrillation (AF). This may not be noticed by women with normal left ventricular function. However, in patients with a fixed cardiac output, e.g. mitral stenosis, it may reduce cardiac output significantly.

During the early part of ventricular systole, both the mitral and aortic valves are closed. The volume of blood within the ventricle must then remain the same. This is therefore known as the period of isovolumetric contraction. As the ventricle relaxes, there is a similar period when both aortic and mitral valves are closed: the period of isovolumetric relaxation.

In those with normal hearts, valve closure is associated with heart sounds, but valve opening is not. The first sound is caused by mitral valve closure, and the second sound by aortic valve closure. Patients with abnormal valves may have an ejection click (aortic stenosis) at aortic valve opening, or an opening snap (mitral stenosis) at mitral valve opening. The third heart sound occurs at the period of rapid ventricular filling; the fourth heart sound is related to atrial systole. The fourth heart sound is therefore absent in patients with atrial fibrillation. Heart sounds, other than the first and second, are usually considered pathological, although the third heart sound in particular is very commonly heard in pregnancy and in young people.

The electrical events of the electrocardiograph precede mechanical ones. Thus, the P wave representing atrial depolarization occurs before the fourth heart sound, and the QRS complex representing ventricular depolarization occurs at the onset of ventricular systole. The T wave (ventricular repolarization) is already occurring at the height of ventricular systole.

Alterations in heart rate are associated with changes in the length of diastole rather than the length of systole. This can be a problem in patients where filling of the ventricles is impaired, as in mitral stenosis; such patients are very intolerant of rapid heart rates.

Since right ventricular systole occurs a little later than left, the second sound is split, the second component being due to the closure of the pulmonary valve. During inspiration, the delay of ejection of blood from the right side of the heart is even greater, so that splitting of the second sound widens.

Control of cardiac output

Cardiac output (CO) is the product of stroke volume (SV) and heart rate (HR), where stroke volume is the volume of blood ejected by the heart per beat and is normally 70 mL.

$$\textbf{CO (L/min) = SV (mL)} \times \textbf{HR (rate/min)}$$

Normal resting cardiac output is 4.5 L/min in females and 5.5 L/min in males. While this can be a useful measurement, it does not take into account the differences between individuals and thus an 80-year-old small woman does not have the same cardiac output as a 90 kg large man. The cardiac index is therefore a measurement which is corrected for surface area and is thus more accurate than cardiac output. It is calculated as the CO divided by the body surface area in square metres, and normal is 3.2 L/min per m^2. CO can therefore be affected by either changes in heart rate or contractility. Starling's law states that the force of contraction is proportional to the initial muscle fibre length. This initial fibre length is in turn dependent upon the degree of stretch of the ventricular muscle, or the amount that the ventricle is dilated in diastole, i.e. the venous return. As end-diastolic volume increases, the force of contraction increases until a maximum is reached and the hearts starts to fail (Fig. 10.8).

Factors affecting end-diastolic volume (also called preload) are those factors that control effective blood volume, i.e. the total blood volume, body position (pooling of blood in the lower limbs in the upright posture) and pumping action of muscles in the leg which encourages the venous return. Venous tone also affects the effective blood volume. The veins are the capacitance vessels of the circulation. If venous tone is

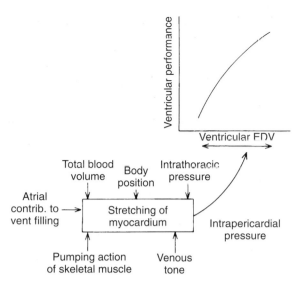

increased, venous return is also increased. Intrathoracic pressure is also important. If intrathoracic pressure is high, as in patients who are being artificially ventilated, blood does not return so effectively to the heart. When patients have a pericardial effusion, intrapericardial pressure may be high, the heart cannot dilate and ventricular filling is impaired, so cardiac output falls. Atrial systole, as described above, contributes to one-third of ventricular filling.

Figure 10.8 shows one curve relating ventricular performance to end-diastolic volume. However, one can also draw a series of such curves (Fig. 10.9) showing how ventricular performance may be increased without change in end-diastolic volume. Such an increase moving from a lower to a higher curve represents an increase in contractility. This is seen in treatment with digoxin and other 'inotropic' agents such as aminophylline, with sympathetic nerve stimulation and with β-adrenergic catecholamines, e.g. adrenaline (epinephrine) and isoprenaline. The reverse is seen with drugs such as β-adrenergic blocking agents (e.g. propranolol) and quinidine which are pharmacological depressants of myocardial activity, in hypoxia, hypercapnia and acidosis, in patients who have lost myocardial tissue as after a myocardial infarction and with increased systemic arterial pressure. Systemic arterial pressure is a major component of afterload, the resistance against which the heart must work to pump out blood.

Figure 10.8 • Relation between ventricular end-diastolic volume (EDV) and ventricular performance (Frank–Starling curve), with a summary of the major factors affecting EDV. Atrial contrib. to vent filling = atrial contribution to ventricular filling. (Reproduced with permission from Braunwald E, Ross J Jr, Sonnenblick E 1967 Mechanisms of contraction of the normal and failing heart. New England Journal of Medicine 277:1012–1022.)

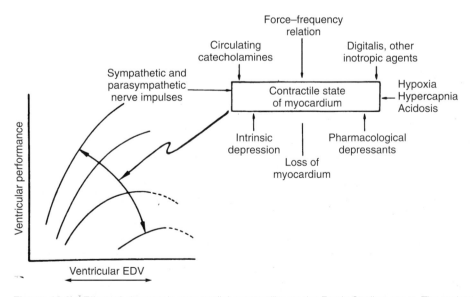

Figure 10.9 • Effect of changes in myocardial contractility on the Frank–Starling curve. The major factors influencing contractility are summarized on the right. EDV = end-diastolic volume. (Reproduced with permission from Braunwald E, Ross J Jr, Sonnenblick E 1967 Mechanisms of contraction of the normal and failing heart. New England Journal of Medicine 277:1012–1022.)

Changes in blood volume and cardiac output during pregnancy

During pregnancy, plasma volume increases from the non-pregnant level of 2600 mL to about 3800 mL (Fig. 10.10). This increase occurs early in pregnancy and there is not much further change after 32 weeks' gestation. The red cell mass also increases steadily until term from a non-pregnant level of 1400 mL to 1650–1800 mL. However, since plasma volume increases proportionately more than red cell mass, the haematocrit and haemoglobin concentration fall during pregnancy. A haemoglobin level of 10.5 g/L would not be unusual in a healthy pregnancy. Cardiac output also rises by about 40% from about 4.5 to 6 L/min. This rise can be seen early in pregnancy, and cardiac output reaches a plateau at 24–30 weeks of gestation. The rise is maintained through labour, and declines to pre-pregnancy levels over a rather variable time course after delivery. If the patient is studied lying supine, the gravid uterus constricts the inferior vena cava, and decreases the venous return, thus falsely decreasing cardiac output. This is also the mechanism of hypotension seen in patients lying flat on their backs at the end of pregnancy (supine hypotensive syndrome) and may be a contributory factor to fetal distress in patients lying in this position during labour.

The vasodilator substance bradykinin is formed from protein precursors (kininogens) in the plasma and tissues under the influence of the kallikrein enzymes. Bradykinin is inactivated by angiotensin-converting enzyme (ACE) (see p. 188).

Cardiac output increases by about 40%, but heart rate increases by only about 10%, from 80 to 90 b.p.m.

during pregnancy. Therefore, there must be an associated increase in stroke volume. The increase in cardiac output is more than is necessary to distribute the extra 30–50 mL of oxygen consumed per minute in pregnancy. Therefore, the arteriovenous oxygen gradient decreases in pregnancy.

Figure 10.11 indicates the distribution of the increase in cardiac output seen in pregnancy. At term, about 400 mL/min goes to the uterus and about 300 mL/min extra goes to the kidneys. The increase in skin blood flow could be as much as 500 mL/min. The remaining 300 mL would be distributed among the gastrointestinal tract, breasts and the other extra metabolic needs of pregnancy, such as respiratory muscle and cardiac muscle. Early in pregnancy, uterine blood flow has not increased, although cardiac output and renal blood flow have. There is therefore a disproportionately higher quantity of extra blood perfusing skin, breasts and other organs at this time.

Blood pressure control

Blood pressure is proportional to cardiac output and peripheral resistance. Cardiac output is controlled by heart rate and stroke volume (see p. 184). Peripheral resistance is controlled neurogenically by the autonomic nervous system, and directly by substances that act on blood vessels: angiotensin II, serotonin, kinins, catecholamines secreted from the adrenal medulla, metabolites such as adenosine, potassium, H^+, P_{CO_2}, P_{O_2} and prostaglandins.

From the Poiseuille formula the flow (f) in a tube of radius (r) and length (L) is governed by the relation:

$$f \propto Pr^4/\eta L$$

where P is the pressure gradient and η the viscosity of the fluid. Flow and peripheral resistance are therefore extremely sensitive to blood vessel radius. A 5%

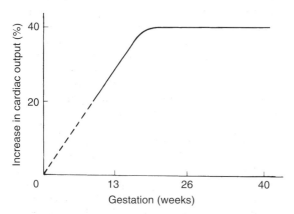

Figure 10.10 • Changes in cardiac output through pregnancy. Note that cardiac output is considerably increased by the end of the first trimester, and the increase is maintained until term. (Reproduced with permission from Hytten F, Chamberlain G. Clinical physiology in obstetrics. Blackwell Scientific, Oxford.)

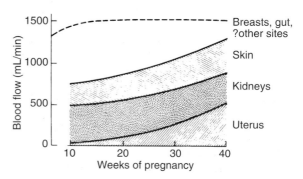

Figure 10.11 • Distribution of increased cardiac output during pregnancy. (Reproduced with permission from Hytten F, Chamberlain G. Clinical physiology in obstetrics. Blackwell Scientific, Oxford.)

increase in vessel radius increases flow and decreases resistance by 21%. In blood, which is not a Newtonian fluid, viscosity rises markedly when the haematocrit rises above 45%. Such a marked increase in viscosity therefore causes a considerable reduction in blood flow.

Autonomic nervous system and blood pressure control

Receptors involved in blood pressure control in blood vessels and the heart are shown in Table 10.3. Both cholinergic and α- and β-adrenergic receptors are involved. The major tonic effect is adrenergic vasoconstriction, and vasodilatation is largely achieved by a reduction in vasoconstrictor tone rather than active vasodilatation.

The action of the autonomic system in controlling blood pressure is governed by the cardioinhibitory and vasomotor centres. The cardioinhibitory centre is the dorsal motor nucleus of the vagus nerve. Impulses pass from the cardioinhibitory centre via the vagus nerve to the heart, causing bradycardia and decreasing contractility. These effects reduce cardiac output and therefore blood pressure. The input to the cardioinhibitory centre is from the baroreceptors (see later). An increase in baroreceptor firing rate stimulates the cardioinhibitory centre and so produces reflex slowing of the heart and a reduction in blood pressure. The cardioinhibitory centre also receives inputs from other centres, so that pain and emotion can both increase vagal tone. If the vagal stimulation caused by pain and/or emotion is severe enough, blood pressure is decreased to the point where cerebral perfusion is impaired and the subject faints.

Sympathetic output to the heart and blood vessels is controlled by the vasomotor centre. The input to the vasomotor centre is from the baroreceptors; a *fall* in baroreceptor activity is associated with increased output from the vasomotor centre, thus increasing blood pressure. The vasomotor centre also receives fibres from the aortic carotid body chemoreceptors so that a fall in the PO_2 or pH or a rise in the PCO_2 will stimulate the vasomotor centre and cause a rise in blood pressure. In addition, baroreceptors in the floor of the fourth ventricle, which are sensitive to cerebrospinal fluid (CSF) pressure, innervate the vasomotor centre. These act so that a rise in CSF pressure causes an equal rise in blood pressure (Cushing reflex). Pain and emotion can also stimulate the vasomotor centre as well as the cardioinhibitory centre. Therefore, these stimuli can cause a rise in blood pressure, as well as a fall in blood pressure.

The carotid sinus baroreceptor is located at the bifurcation of the internal carotid artery. Fibres of the glossopharyngeal nerve carry impulses at frequencies that, within certain limits, are proportional to the instantaneous pressure in the carotid artery. In experimental animals at pressures below 70 mmHg, the receptors do not fire at all. Between 70 and 150 mmHg the receptors fire with increasing frequency as the blood pressure rises. This frequency reaches a maximum at 150 mmHg. Therefore, the carotid sinus baroreceptors can modulate blood pressure between 70 and 150 mmHg, but not outside this range. In patients with hypertension, the baroreceptors adapt and shift upwards the pressures over which they respond.

Local control of blood flow

Metabolites that accumulate during anaerobic metabolism cause vasodilatation. This allows tissues to autoregulate their blood flow; vasodilatation allows an increased blood flow and decreases the tendency for anaerobic metabolism. The metabolites involved are hydrogen ions, potassium, lactate, adenosine (in heart but not skeletal muscle) and carbon dioxide. In addition, hypoxia itself causes vasodilatation.

Another form of autoregulation is the myogenic reflex. If the perfusion pressure in the arteriole decreases, thus tending to decrease local blood flow, the smooth muscle in the arteriole relaxes allowing vasodilatation and an increase in local blood flow. The converse occurs at high perfusion pressures: arteriolar smooth muscle then contracts, causing vasoconstriction, and a reduction in blood flow to offset the high perfusion pressure. Note that these changes induced by the myogenic reflex maintain local blood flow but will exacerbate changes in systemic blood pressure.

Other substances affecting the blood vessels locally are prostaglandins derived enzymatically from fatty acids. The cyclooxygenase pathway creates either prostaglandins or thromboxane from the intermediate phospholipase A2 whereas the lipoxygenase pathway forms leukotrienes. The cyclooxygenases (COX1 and COX2) are located in blood vessels, the kidney and stomach. Technically, prostaglandins are hormones though are rarely classified as such but are known as mediators which have profound physiological effects. Prostaglandins are found in virtually all tissues and act on a variety of cells but most notably endothelium, platelets, uterine and mast cells. Prostaglandin E and prostaglandin A cause a fall in blood pressure by reducing splanchnic vascular resistance. Prostaglandin F causes uterine contraction and bronchoconstriction. Prostacyclin, the levels of which increase considerably in pregnancy and which is produced by blood vessels and the fetoplacental unit, causes a marked vasodilatation, which will cause a fall in blood pressure unless the cardiac output also increases. Thromboxane derived from platelets causes vasoconstriction.

Other locally active substances are the vasodilator endothelium-derived relaxing factor (EDRF), which has been shown to be nitric oxide locally made from L-arginine, and endothelin, a 21-amino-acid peptide that is intensely vasoconstrictive. Another potent vaso-constricting agent is angiotensin II, produced under the influence of renin. Renin is an enzyme largely produced by the juxtaglomerular apparatus of the kidney, but also by the pregnant uterus. It cleaves the peptide bond between the leucine and valine residues of angio-tensinogen forming the decapeptide angiotensin I, which itself has no biological activity. The stimuli to renin secretion are β-adrenergic agonists, hyponatrae-mia, hypovolaemia, whether induced by bleeding or changes in posture, and pregnancy. A similar but smaller rise in renin levels is also seen in patients taking oestrogen-containing contraceptive pills. Angiotensin I is then converted to the intensely vasoconstrictive angiotensin II in the lungs, by angiotensin-converting enzyme, which removes a further two amino acid resi-dues. Angiotensin II has a number of effects through-out the body other than its vasoconstrictive properties. It has prothrombotic potential due to its adhesion and aggregation of platelets and production of PAI-1 and PAI-2. It also affects blood volume in a number of ways. Angiotensin II increases thirst sensation, decreases the response to the baroreceptor reflex and increases the desire for salt. It has a direct effect on the proximal tubules of the kidney to increase Na^+ absorption as well as complex and variable effects on glomerular filtration and renal blood flow. In addition, angiotensin II also stimulates aldosterone production from the zona glomerulosa of the adrenal gland, and this will, in turn, cause a rise in blood volume, and blood pressure over the longer term, by sodium reten-tion. In the luteal phase of the menstrual cycle, ele-vated plasma angiotensin II levels are responsible for the elevated aldosterone levels found.

All three levels of the renin–angiotensin–aldosterone system (RAAS) are now being targeted by drugs in order to reduce blood pressure. The action of angiotensin II is blocked by angiotensin receptor-block-ing drugs (ARB, e.g. irbesartan, losartan) whereas the angiotensin-converting enzyme (ACE) is inhibited by the ACE inhibitors ramipril and other similar drugs. Most recently, direct renin inhibitors, such as aliskeren, are now available for use alone or in direct combination with an ACE or ARB.

Blood pressure changes in pregnancy

The marked rise in cardiac output which occurs in pregnancy does not cause a rise in blood pressure, unless a pathological process such as pre-eclampsia occurs. Therefore, there must be a decrease in total peripheral resistance, and this vasodilatation accom-modates the increased blood flow to the uterus, kidney, skin and other organs (see Fig. 10.11).

The decreased peripheral vascular resistance does not always keep strictly in proportion with the increase

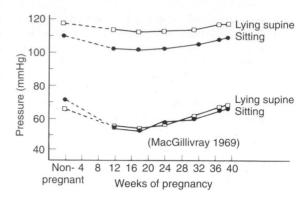

Figure 10.12 • Effect of pregnancy on systolic and diastolic blood pressure as found by MacGillivray. (Reproduced with permission from Hytten F, Chamberlain G. Clinical physiology in obstetrics. Blackwell Scientific, Oxford.)

in cardiac output and during the middle of pregnancy, from, say, 8 to 36 weeks, the systolic blood pressure may fall by up to 5 mmHg, and the diastolic blood pressure by up to 10 mmHg, because the peripheral resistance falls by more than cardiac output rises (Fig. 10.12). Other factors affecting blood pressure are posture and uterine contractions, which act via the changes in cardiac output already described. Uterine contractions expel blood from the uterus, increase cardiac output and increase blood pressure. The supine position, by causing vena caval obstruction, decreases cardiac output and will decrease blood pressure.

Endothelium in pregnancy

The endothelium is a single cell layer that lines the internal surface of all blood vessels and plays a far more important role than that of a barrier between intra- and extravascular spaces. The endothelium controls vascu-lar permeability, it determines vascular tone of the underlying smooth muscle and plays a major role in the inflammatory response. In normal pregnancy, the endothelium undergoes many subtle changes in func-tion which contribute to the maintenance of normal cardiovascular function in mother and fetus. The onset of similar cardiovascular changes during the luteal phase of the menstrual cycle suggests that maternal rather than feto-placental factors initiate the vaso-dilatation associated with early pregnancy. There is now clear evidence that maternal endothelium plays a major role in this adaptation of the cardiovascular system to pregnancy.

Endothelium as a barrier

The endothelium provides a passive barrier between blood and extravascular compartments, and prevents easy passage of erythrocytes and leucocytes. Transduction of fluid and small molecules occurs in accordance with the balance of Starling's forces (see p. 177); hydrostatic (blood) pressure favours fluid transfer out of the vessel and plasma oncotic pressure provides the predominant breaking force which limits outward flow. It is also now accepted that an almost invisible layer positioned above the cells in the lumen, the glycocalyx, provides another 'ultrafilter', which contributes to the molecular selectivity of the endothelium. The high incidence of oedema in normal pregnancy is likely to be the result of increased fluid transfer across the endothelium. It is currently uncertain whether the oedema arises from a simple increase in the balance of transcapillary hydrostatic pressure favouring outward fluid transduction or from a combination of this and increased fluid conductivity.

Endothelium as a modulator of vascular tone

The endothelium (Fig. 10.13) synthesizes a number of potent vasoactive factors that can influence the tone of the underlying vascular smooth muscle. Vasodilators include nitric oxide, prostacyclin and an as yet unidentified endothelium-derived hyperpolarizing factor. Constrictor factors include endothelin, angiotensin and thromboxane. Several of these have been implicated in gestational vasodilatation.

Endothelium-derived vasodilators
Nitric oxide

Nitric oxide (NO) is an inorganic molecule synthesized within the endothelium to relax underlying vascular smooth muscle. Endothelial nitric oxide synthase (eNOS) is one of three NOS isoforms that catalyses the conversion of L-arginine to NO and the co-product L-citrulline. NO evokes relaxation in vascular smooth muscle through activation of soluble guanylate cyclase and subsequent stimulation of cGMP. Although there is much evidence to support increased activity of the L-arginine–NO pathway during animal pregnancy, assessment of the L-arginine–NO pathway in human pregnancy and pre-eclampsia has proved more challenging.

Nitric oxide has a short half-life and cannot easily be measured directly. Other indirect methods have therefore been employed to evaluate its role in pregnancy. In human pregnancy, urinary concentrations of cGMP increase early in pregnancy and remain elevated until term. It is unclear whether plasma cGMP changes during normal pregnancy. A confounding issue is that cGMP is also a second messenger for atrial natriuretic peptide (ANP). However, the circulating concentration of ANP does not rise until the third trimester, long after the increase in urinary cGMP.

Nitric oxide combines with oxygen to produce nitrite (NO_2^-), which itself is rapidly oxidized to a more stable nitrate (NO_3^-). These molecules or their

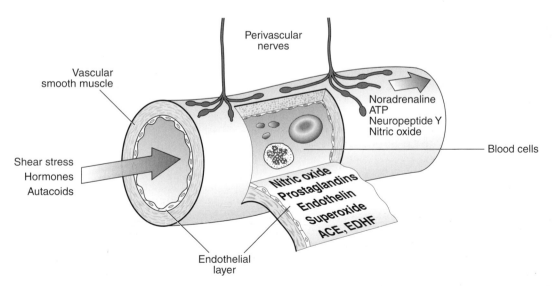

Figure 10.13 • Vascular smooth muscle tone is under the influence of endocrine, autocrine and neuronal factors. The endothelium contributes through the synthesis of locally active vasodilatory factors including nitric oxide, the prostaglandin, prostacyclin, and the uncharacterized endothelium-derived hyperpolarizing factor (EDHF). Under physiological conditions these predominate over the endothelium-derived vasoconstrictors endothelin and the prostanoid, thromboxane. Local activity of angiotensin-converting enzyme (ACE) in the endothelial cell may also contribute to vasoconstrictor activity through angiotensin II synthesis, as may the production of superoxide anions, which act by quenching nitric oxide.

product, NOx, can be measured in plasma or urine as markers of nitric oxide synthase (NOS) activity. However, most studies in human pregnancy have ignored the problem that nitrite is unstable in blood and nitrate is sensitive to dietary nitrogen intake. This has led to conflicting results.

In vivo studies provide the most compelling evidence that NO synthase is upregulated in the maternal peripheral circulation during normal pregnancy. Infusion of the NO synthase inhibitor, L-NMMA, into the brachial artery causes a greater reduction of hand and forearm blood flow in pregnancy compared with that in non-pregnant women. Normal pregnancy is also associated with enhanced endothelium-dependent flow-mediated vasodilatation in the brachial artery and isolated vessels. All of these studies support the view that basal and stimulated NOS activity contributes to the fall in peripheral vascular resistance during a healthy pregnancy. Furthermore, circulating levels of an endogenous inhibitor to NOS, asymmetrical dimethylarginine (ADMA), fall during a healthy pregnancy in association with a gestational fall in blood pressure.

Prostacyclin

Prostacyclin (PGI_2) is a vasodilator derived from the arachidonic acid pathway after conversion by cyclooxygenase. In common with NO, PGI_2 has a short half-life and evaluation of PGI_2 synthesis depends on the measurement of stable metabolites, e.g. 6-oxo-PGF_1. The high circulating concentrations of these metabolites during pregnancy does not necessarily indicate that PGI_2 is the predominant vasodilator in pregnancy. This conclusion is upheld by studies in pregnant animals and women in which infusion of the cyclooxygenase inhibitor indometacin was shown not to affect blood pressure or peripheral vascular resistance. In sheep, PGI_2 biosynthesis seems to be increased preferentially in the uterine circulation during pregnancy, possibly in response to elevated angiotensin II (AII). Pregnancy in the ewe is also associated with a dramatic rise in the expression of COX-1 mRNA and protein in the uterine artery endothelium.

Endothelium-derived hyperpolarizing factor

Nitric oxide and prostacyclin do not account for all agonist-induced endothelium-derived vasodilatation. The residual vasodilatation is abolished by potassium channel blockers or by a depolarizing concentration of potassium ions, so this factor has become known as endothelium-derived hyperpolarizing factor (EDHF). As the name implies, it causes hyperpolarization of the underlying vascular smooth muscle. Hyperpolarization, in turn, provokes relaxation. While the existence of an EDHF is indisputable, its variable nature and mechanisms of action has meant that any singular and distinct chemical identification is not possible. For this reason it is more appropriate to consider EDHF as representing a mechanism of action, rather than a specific factor.

EDHF is most evident in small arteries where it is influential in controlling organ blood flow and blood pressure, especially when NO production is compromised. Intriguingly, there are gender differences with the effects of EDHF. For example, in mice where eNOS and COX-1 have been deleted, blood pressure changes little in females, but males become hypertensive. Due to the nature of its actions, EDHF has not been widely studied in humans. Nitric oxide is, however, undoubtedly the predominant endothelium-derived relaxing factor. Increased synthesis of a vascular EDHF has been described in animal and human pregnancy, and so may play a role in peripheral vasodilatation.

Vascular endothelial growth factor

Vascular endothelial growth factor (VEGF) has potent angiogenic and mitogenic actions. It induces nitric oxide synthase in endothelial cells, and is likely to play a part in decreasing vascular tone and blood pressure in healthy pregnancy. The VEGF family of proteins includes VEGF/VEGF-A, VEGF-B, VEGF-C, VEGF-D and VEGF-E. Vascular endothelial growth factor is a homodimeric 34–42-kDa glycoprotein, which in normal tissues is expressed in a number of cell types, including activated macrophages and smooth muscle cells. VEGF-A is expressed in syncytiotrophoblast cells and, along with VEGF-C, is also present in the cytotrophoblast. Vascular endothelial growth factor interacts through three different receptors: VEGFR-1 (soluble FMS-like tyrosine kinase 1, sFlt-1), VEGFR-2 (KDR/Flk-1) and VEGFR-3 (Flt-4), which mediate different functions within endothelial cells. VEGFR-1 (sFlt-1) is a soluble receptor and has been localized to the placental trophoblast. Soluble Flt-1 is found in high concentrations in early pregnancy in women who go on to develop pre-eclampsia. Both VEGFR-1 and 3 are expressed on invasive cytotrophoblast cells in early pregnancy. VEGFR-1 is present in serum from pregnant women but only in small concentrations in serum from non-pregnant females or males. Anti-VEGFR-1 reactivity has been demonstrated in the first cell layers of the cytotrophoblast column, which indicates a likely autocrine or paracrine effect that activates VEGF receptors in close proximity to the maternal extracellular matrix.

There have been conflicting results relating to changes in VEGF levels in pregnancy, as a consequence of difficulties in measuring free as opposed to bound VEGF. Levels appear to be lower in the vasoconstricted state of pre-eclampsia.

Placental growth factor

Placental growth factor (PlGF) is a member of the VEGF family and is also distantly related to the platelet-derived growth factor (PDGF) family. Placental growth factor is a 149-amino-acid mature protein with a 21-amino-acid signal sequence and a centrally located PDGF-like domain. It shares a 42% sequence homology with VEGF, and the two are structurally similar. Placental growth factor has angiogenic properties, enhancing survival, growth and migration of endothelial cells *in vitro*, and promotes vessel formation in certain *in-vivo* models. It is thus regarded as a central component in regulating vascular function.

Placental growth factor was first identified in the human placenta and is expressed in greatest quantities under normal conditions. It is important in placental development, as it is present in high concentrations within villous cytotrophoblastic tissue and the syncytiotrophoblast. Placental growth factor concentrations increase throughout pregnancy, peaking during the third trimester, and falling thereafter, probably as a consequence of placental maturation.

Thromboxane

Human pregnancy is associated with increased synthesis of the constrictor prostanoid, thromboxane (TXA_2), as assessed by measurement of its stable systemic metabolite 2,3-dinor-TXB_2. Thromboxane, which in pregnancy is mainly derived from platelets, increases 3–5-fold during gestation and remains elevated throughout.

Endothelin

The family of endothelins, of which endothelin-1 (ET-1) plays the predominant physiological role in the control of vascular tone, are highly potent constrictor agonists. ET-1 is cleaved from a larger precursor polypeptide, big-endothelin, by the action of membrane-bound enzymes, the endothelin-converting enzymes. The plasma concentration of ET-1 is very low or undetectable in maternal plasma and not affected by healthy pregnancy. Endothelin may however play a role in constriction of the umbilical circulation at birth. Paradoxically, binding of endothelin to a receptor subtype, the ET_B receptor, in the endothelium can lead to vasodilatation through stimulus of nitric oxide release. Studies in rats have suggested that this mechanism may play a role in the increase in renal blood flow in pregnancy.

Angiotensin II

Angiotensin II (AII) was once considered to be synthesized predominantly in the pulmonary circulation, in which angiotensin-converting enzyme (ACE) activity is high, but it is now known that it is synthesized in the endothelium. In a normal pregnancy, despite a dramatic increase in activity of the renin–angiotensin–aldosterone axis, there is a well-documented blunting of the pressor response to AII, which may contribute to lowering of peripheral vascular resistance.

Oestrogen and the endothelium

High oestrogen levels have far-reaching systemic effects on pregnant women. They include changes to serum lipoprotein concentrations, coagulation factors, antioxidant activity and vascular tone. Oestrogen has two direct effects on blood vessels: rapid vasodilatation (5–20 min after exposure) and chronic (hours to days) protection against vascular injury and atherosclerosis. The rapid vasodilatory effects of oestrogen are nongenomic, i.e. they do not involve changes in gene expression of vasodilator substances. There are two functionally distinct oestrogen receptors (ERs), α and β. ER-α a receptors on the endothelial cell membrane can directly activate NOS. A study of oestrogen receptor (ER) knockout mice has confirmed a role for ERs in NO synthesis. The non-genomic mechanism by which oestrogen rapidly activates NOS has not been fully elucidated. Animal studies suggest that involvement of the endothelium in the vasodilatation induced by longer-term exposure to oestrogen is similar to that seen during pregnancy. Enhanced NO-mediated relaxation in the sheep uterine artery induced by oestrogens is associated with greater NOS enzymatic activity.

Clinical evidence that supports a vasodilatory role for oestrogens has mainly come from studies on postmenopausal women given exogenous oestrogen. For example, 17β-estradiol potentiates endothelium-dependent vasodilatation in the forearm and coronary arteries of postmenopausal women. Oestrogen can also act directly on vascular smooth muscle, independent of the endothelium, by opening calcium-activated potassium channels. Furthermore, 17β-estradiol may also decrease synthesis of the superoxide free radical, and thereby prolong the half-life of pre-existing NO.

Much less is known about the vascular effects of progesterone. Circulating progesterone levels increase by a similar amount to 17β-estradiol and may play a role in reducing pressor responsiveness to AII.

Endothelium and haemostasis

In anticipation of haemorrhage at childbirth, normal pregnancy is characterized by low-grade, chronic activation of coagulation within both the maternal and utero-placental circulations. The endothelium is directly involved in promoting a procoagulant state in healthy pregnancy. During the third trimester, plasma levels of endothelium-derived von Willebrand factor are elevated, promoting coagulation and platelet adhesion. Circulating levels of clotting factors, especially fibrinogen, factor V and factor VIII, are increased, while there is a gestational fall in the level of the endogenous anticoagulant, protein S. Furthermore, endothelial production of both plasminogen activator inhibitor (PAI-1) and tissue plasminogen activator (t-PA) are increased during pregnancy, with the effect of both inhibition and promotion of fibrinolysis, respectively. The procoagulant state of the endothelium therefore is to some extent compensated by upregulation of the fibrinolytic system.

Endothelium and inflammation

A healthy pregnancy stimulates a generalized inflammatory response. Not only do peripheral blood leucocytes develop a more inflammatory phenotype than in non-gravid women, but the expression of leucocyte adhesion molecules on the endothelium also increases. It has recently been shown that these inflammatory changes are even more pronounced during pre-eclampsia. Further details of the complex immune interactions involving many different immune cell types can be found in Chapter 8.

Pre-eclampsia

Relative to the vasodilated, plasma-expanded state of a woman in a healthy pregnancy, pre-eclampsia is a vasoconstricted, plasma-contracted condition with evidence of intravascular coagulation. Whereas healthy maternal endothelium is crucial for the physiological adaptation to normal pregnancy, the multiple organ failure of severe pre-eclampsia is characterized by widespread endothelial cell dysfunction. The endothelium of women destined to develop pre-eclampsia both fails to adapt properly, and can be further damaged during a pre-eclamptic pregnancy. Prior to the onset of clinically identifiable disease, women destined to develop pre-eclampsia show evidence of poor placentation, high uteroplacental resistance and abnormal placental function. This placental dysfunction is associated with endothelial abnormalities in the mother who is more likely to have classical risk factors for cardiovascular disease including hypertension, diabetes mellitus and hyperlipidaemia.

Endothelial dysfunction in pre-eclampsia

Damaged endothelial cells in pre-eclampsia (Fig. 10.14) cause increased capillary permeability, platelet thrombosis and increased vascular tone. Evidence of endothelial cell damage prior to clinical manifestation of pre-eclampsia can be demonstrated by the presence of markers of endothelial cell activation. Specifically, levels of fibronectin and factor VIII-related antigen are elevated. Furthermore, women with endothelial cell damage secondary to pre-existing hypertension or other microvascular disease have a higher incidence of pre-eclampsia than normotensive women.

Nitric oxide in pre-eclampsia

The L-arginine–NO pathway is an expected casualty of endothelial cell damage in pre-eclampsia. However, probably because of methodological limitations, there is no consensus on whether NOS activity is altered by pre-eclampsia. NOS is competively inhibited by an endogenous guanidino-substituted arginine analogue, N^GN^G-dimethylarginine (asymmetrical dimethylarginine, ADMA). During pre-eclampsia, ADMA levels are significantly higher compared with gestation-

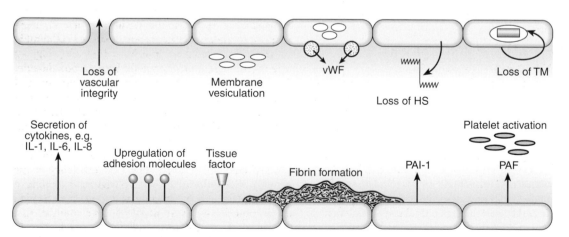

Figure 10.14 • The vascular endothelium in pre-eclampsia shows many of the characteristics of the inflammatory state of 'endothelial cell activation'. Upon stimulation by inflammatory cytokines the endothelium undergoes a series of metabolic changes leading to loss of vascular integrity, prothrombotic changes (loss of heparan sulphate, HS; loss of thrombomodulin, TM; release of plasminogen activator inhibitor, PAI-1, platelet activating factor, PAF, tissue factor and von Willebrand factor, VWF), secretion of cytokines and upregulation of leucocyte adhesion molecules. The cell adhesion molecules promote the adhesion and migration of leucocytes across the endothelium and so contribute to the inflammatory process.

matched, normotensive controls. Consequently, endogenous inhibition of NOS by a specific inhibitor is a possible mechanism whereby NO production could be reduced in pre-eclampsia.

In-vivo studies of forearm blood flow have suggested that a reduction in NO is unlikely to be involved in the vasoconstriction characteristic of pre-eclampsia. In contrast, *in-vitro* studies on isolated arteries from women with pre-eclampsia have generally reported reduced endothelium-dependent relaxation, although the role of NO has not always been identified. One explanation for these differences is that women have a high cardiac output before the onset of clinical pre-eclampsia, suggesting a possible role for increased nitric oxide synthase activity in a hyperdynamic circulation.

Prostanoids in pre-eclampsia

In contrast to a normal pregnancy, pre-eclampsia is associated with relative underproduction of the vasodilatory PGI_2 and overabundance of the vasoconstrictor TXA_2. The imbalance between the synthesis of these prostanoids formed the rationale for investigations of 'low-dose aspirin' therapy for prevention of pre-eclampsia. Low or intermittent doses of aspirin up to 150 mg daily lead to preferential inhibition of TXA_2 biosynthesis, and could redress the imbalance between these prostanoids in pre-eclampsia.

Prothrombotic states

Stimulation of the coagulation cascade in response to endothelial cell damage may be more likely in women who have a predisposition to thrombosis. A number of studies have suggested that patients with inherited thrombophilias are more likely to develop pre-eclampsia compared with women who have normal clotting parameters.

Aetiology of maternal endothelial dysfunction in pre-eclampsia

How poor placentation and the resultant poor uterine blood flow with placental ischaemia leads to the maternal syndrome of pre-eclampsia, characterized by widespread endothelial cell damage, remains uncertain. Several factors appear to be important and are likely to be variably important in individual women. Soluble Flt-1, soluble endoglin and possibly angiotensin II type-1 receptor autoantibodies have all been shown to be elevated in women who go on to develop pre-eclampsia and to have a pathological role. These factors contribute to endothelial dysfunction, inflammation and increased reactive oxygen species. Leucocyte activation, proinflammatory cytokines, trophoblast fragments and prothrombotic states may also increase a woman's risk of pre-eclampsia.

Classical risk factors for cardiovascular disease are evident in women before they develop pre-eclampsia.

It is no surprise therefore that women who have had pre-eclampsia have an increased risk of cardiovascular disease in later life. It seems unlikely that the brief time a woman has pre-eclampsia causes irreparable harm to make her vulnerable to future cardiovascular disease.

Conclusion

In conclusion, the endothelium plays a central role in the maternal adaptation to a healthy human pregnancy. The peripheral circulation of the healthy mother is vasodilated, prothrombotic and proinflammatory. However, endothelial dysfunction is a characteristic of pre-eclampsia as demonstrated by increased capillary permeability, intravascular coagulation, and vasoconstriction leading to multi-organ ischaemia. The ischaemic placenta is the likely source of anti-angiogenic factors that perpetuate this cycle of endothelial damage until delivery of the fetus and placenta rescues the situation. Women who have had pre-eclampsia will be at increased risk of cardiovascular disease in the future.

Respiration

The lungs, ventilation and its control

Respiration is the process whereby the body takes in oxygen and eliminates carbon dioxide. This section will consider the action of the lungs and transport of oxygen and carbon dioxide to peripheral tissues.

Gas composition

Table 10.6 shows the partial pressures of dry air, inspired air, alveolar air and expired air at body temperature and normal atmospheric pressure (760 mmHg or 101.1 kPa, where 100 mmHg = 13.3 kPa). Dry air consists of oxygen, nitrogen and a little carbon dioxide. We do not normally breathe completely dry air, and inspired air usually has some water vapour (partial pressure 5.7 mmHg). Alveolar air is fully saturated with water (47 mmHg) and is in equilibrium with pulmonary venous blood. The small difference in the PO_2 between alveolar air (100 mmHg) and pulmonary venous blood (98 mmHg) shows the efficiency of gas exchange in the healthy lung. Expired air is a mixture of alveolar air and inspired air with regard to oxygen and carbon dioxide concentrations. As a result of this mixture, the partial pressure of nitrogen is less in expired air (570 mmHg) than in inspired air (596 mmHg). The total volume of alveolar air is about 2 L; alveolar ventilation is about 350 mL for each breath. Alveolar ventilation is therefore a small proportion of total alveolar volume, and the alveolar gas remains relatively constant in composition.

Table 10.6 Partial pressures of gases (mmHg)[a] in a resting, healthy human at sea level (barometric pressure = 760 mmHg)

	Dry air		Inspired air	Alveolar air	Expired air
P_{O_2}	159.1	(21%)	158.0	100.0	116.0
P_{CO_2}	0.3	(0.04%)	0.3	40.0	26.8
P_{H_2O}	0.0	(0%)	5.7	47.0	47.0
P_{N_2}[b]	600.6	(79%)	596.0	573.0	569.9
Total	760.0		760.0	760.0	759.7

[a]1 kPa = 7.5 mmHg.
[b]Includes small amounts of rare gases.

Dead space

Although the alveolar ventilation is 350 mL/breath, the tidal volume is 500 mL/breath. The difference, 150 mL, is the anatomic dead space: the volume of air between the mouth or nose and the alveoli that does not participate in gas exchange. The anatomic dead space (mL) approximately equals body weight (in pounds avoirdupois) (1 kg = 2.2 lb). In addition, on occasion, some alveoli, particularly in the upper part of the lungs, are well ventilated, but rather poorly perfused, whereas other alveoli in the dependent lower part of the lungs are well perfused, but poorly ventilated. This mismatching of ventilation and perfusion represents a further source of wasted ventilation which, together with the anatomic dead space, makes up the total or physiological dead space. In healthy, supine individuals, the anatomic dead space nearly equals the physiological dead space. In patients who are sick with lung disease, or heart failure, the physiological dead space considerably exceeds the anatomic dead space.

Oxygen consumption

The normal oxygen consumption at rest is about 250 mL/min. The oxygen capacity of normal blood is about 20 mL/100 mL (200 mL/L). Oxygen consumption of 250 mL/min at rest is achieved by delivering 1 L of oxygen to peripheral tissues (cardiac output, 5 L × 200 mL oxygen per litre = 1 L), of which 25% is extracted and 75% is returned to the heart in venous blood. In extreme exertion, ventilation increases to about 150 L/min. This allows oxygen delivery of 3.2 L/min with a cardiac output of 16 L/min (cardiac output, 16 L/min × oxygen capacity, 200 mL/L = 3.2 L/min). Of this, 75% is extracted and 25% is returned to the heart, giving an oxygen consumption of 2.4 L/min, almost 10 times that at rest.

Lung volumes

The total lung capacity (Fig. 10.15) is approximately 5 L. Of this, 1.5 L, the residual volume, remains at the

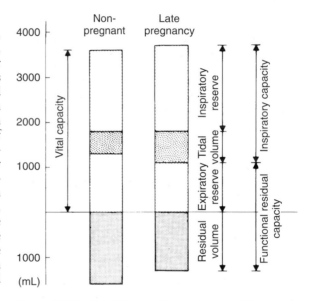

Figure 10.15 • Subdivisions of lung volume and their alterations in pregnancy. (Reproduced with permission from Hytten F, Chamberlain G. Clinical physiology in obstetrics. Blackwell Scientific, Oxford.)

end of forced expiration. The volume of gas, 3.5 L, that can be inhaled from forced expiration to forced inspiration is the vital capacity. The normal tidal volume (500 mL) is a small proportion of the maximum 3.5 L that is possible. The tidal volume is situated in the middle of the vital capacity, so that the inspiratory reserve volume is approximately 1.5 L, as is the expiratory reserve volume.

Mechanics of ventilation

The chest cavity expands by the actions of the intrathoracic musculature, innervated from T1 to T11 and the diaphragm innervated by the phrenic nerve (C3–C5). Thus the cord section below C5 still allows spontaneous ventilation because of the phrenic nerve innervation. Phrenic nerve crush, as used to be performed for the treatment of tuberculosis, still allows spontaneous ventilation because of the action of thoracic musculature. Damage to the spinal cord above the level of C3 needs permanent artificial ventilation, since both the phrenic nerve and thoracic innervation are inactivated.

At rest, the pressure in the potential space between the visceral pleura and the parietal pleura is −3 mmHg, i.e. 3 mmHg less than atmospheric pressure. This pressure can be determined by connecting a balloon catheter with the balloon in the oesophagus at the level of the mediastinum to a pressure transducer. During quiet inspiration, the chest expands and the pressure in the intrapleural space decreases to −6 mmHg. This pressure gradient is sufficient to overcome the elastic recoil of the lung, which therefore expands following the chest wall. In forced inspiration, the pressure in the intrapleural space may fall to as low as 30 mmHg. Expiration is passive; the muscles of the diaphragm and chest wall relax, and the elastic recoil of the lung causes the lung and therefore the chest to contract. Forced expiration may be associated with muscular effort and a positive intrapleural pressure.

Resistance to air flow

The rapidity with which expiration occurs depends on the stiffness of the lungs and the resistance of the bronchi. This is measured clinically, by determining the forced expiratory volume in 1 s (FEV_1). Since this volume depends on the vital capacity, it is most easily expressed as FEV_1/FVC. In normal individuals this ratio exceeds 75%. The ratio decreases with age. In asthma it may be as low as 25%, and the FEV_1, which in healthy individuals is about 3.0 L, is <1 L in patients with severe asthma. An alternative measurement of airway resistance is the peak flow rate, which should be >600 L/min. Both peak flow rate and FEV_1/FVC depend on large airway calibre and the stiffness of the lung. To measure the stiffness of the lungs independently, it is necessary to use more complicated apparatus and to determine lung compliance.

Oxygen transfer

Oxygen is transferred across the 300 million alveoli which have a total surface area of about 70 m^2. Transfer occurs across the type 1 lining cells; apart from the epithelial cells, mast cells, plasma cells, macrophages and lymphocytes, the alveoli also contain type 2 granular pneumocytes, which make surfactant. The granules that these cells contain are thought to be packages of surfactant. Patients who are deficient in surfactant, such as premature infants or adults suffering from the adult respiratory distress syndrome, have type 2 pneumocytes which do not contain granules. Surfactant is necessary to lower the surface tension of alveoli and maintain patency of the alveoli. In the absence of surfactant, the surface tension of the fluid in the alveoli is so high that the alveoli collapse.

Effect of pregnancy

During pregnancy, ventilation is already increased during the first trimester. The total increase is about 40%. A similar, but smaller, effect is seen in women taking contraceptive pills containing progestogens, and in the luteal phase of the menstrual cycle. It is therefore thought to be due to progesterone, which acts partly by stimulating the respiratory centre directly, and partly by increasing its sensitivity to carbon dioxide. Some women are aware of the increase in ventilation and feel breathless, others are not. The increase in ventilation is achieved by increasing the tidal volume, i.e. they breathe more deeply, rather than increase their respiratory rate. This is a more efficient way of increasing ventilation, since an increase in respiratory rate involves more work in shifting the dead space more frequently. The tidal volume therefore expands into the expiratory reserve volume and the inspiratory reserve volume (Fig. 10.15). The consensus of opinion is that the vital capacity does not change. However, the residual volume decreases by about 200 mL, possibly due to the large intra-abdominal swelling. Therefore, the total lung capacity also decreases by about 200 mL. There is no change in FEV_1 or peak flow rate in pregnancy. The increase in ventilation is much greater than the increase in oxygen consumption, which is only about 50 mL extra at term.

The hyperventilation of pregnancy causes a fall in the PCO_2 from a normal value of about 5.3 kPa (40 mmHg) to 4.1 kPa (31 mmHg). The bicarbonate level falls to maintain a normal pH, but, because bicarbonate falls, sodium falls also. There is therefore a decrease in the total number of osmotically active ions and a fall in osmolarity of about 10 mmol/L. Such a fall in osmolarity would normally be associated with profound diuresis, but there is an adaptation of the hypothalamic centres governing vasopressin secretion that permits the reduced osmolarity (p. 202).

During pregnancy, bronchodilator stimuli are progesterone secretion (dilates smooth muscle) and prostaglandin E$_2$. Bronchoconstrictor influences are prostaglandin F$_2$ and the decrease in resting lung volume, which decreases the overall space available for the airways to occupy. These factors balance each other out so that there is no overall change in airway resistance.

Control of respiration

Although several respiratory centres with different functions have been described in the midbrain on the basis of experiments performed in decerebrated or anaesthetized animals, it is not clear to what extent such localization occurs in conscious humans. It is therefore simpler to think of one diffuse medullary respiratory centre. The respiratory centre is responsible for controlling both the depth of respiration and its rhythmicity. Respiratory neurones are of two types: inspiratory and expiratory. When the inspiratory neurones are stimulated at the respiratory centre, the expiratory neurones are inhibited and vice versa. The respiratory centre receives input from higher voluntary centres and pain and emotion will also increase ventilation, but in most healthy patients ventilation is automatic and it is not necessary to be consciously aware of the need to breathe.

The most important input to the respiratory centre comes from chemoreceptors. There are two main groups of these: (1) central chemoreceptors, possibly on the surface of the upper medulla, but separate from the medullary respiratory centre, and (2) peripheral chemoreceptors around the aortic arch and in the carotid body. The aortic arch chemoreceptors are innervated by the vagus nerve and the carotid body chemoreceptors by the glossopharyngeal nerve. The carotid body is highly specialized tissue, which has an exceedingly high blood flow rate. This makes it possible for the chemoreceptors in the carotid body to be sensitive to changes in the P_{O_2}. The carotid body chemoreceptors are the only chemoreceptors sensitive to changes in P_{O_2}. Carotid and aortic body chemoreceptors are also sensitive to changes in P_{CO_2} and pH. The central chemoreceptors are probably only sensitive to changes in the pH; any effect of a change in the P_{CO_2} is mediated by the ensuing pH change.

Response to hypercapnia

If it were not for the activity of the chemoreceptors, a decrease in ventilation would be associated with a rise in the P_{CO_2} (curve A, Fig. 10.16) and an increase in ventilation would be associated with a decrease in the P_{CO_2}. When the P_{CO_2} is <5.3 kPa (40 mmHg) this does occur. However, the activity of the respiratory centre is such that any rise in the P_{CO_2} above 5.3 kPa is associated with a marked increase in ventilation (curve B, Fig. 10.16). The ratio of ventilation observed (b, curve B) to ventilation expected (a, curve A) is the gain of the control system. In normal hyperoxic individuals, this ratio varies between 2 and 5. It is decreased with age and in trained athletes, and it increases in pregnancy to 8, thus increasing the sensitivity of the respiratory centre to carbon dioxide as indicated earlier. Hypoxia also increases respiratory centre sensitivity to carbon dioxide.

Response to hypoxia

This is more subtle than the response to the P_{CO_2}, since the effect of hypoxia is modulated by the effects of ventilation on the P_{CO_2}, and by changes in the buffer-

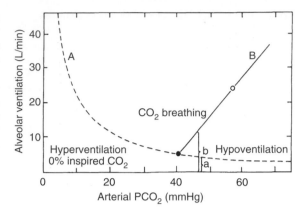

Figure 10.16 • Relations between alveolar ventilation and arterial (alveolar) P_{CO_2} at a constant rate of metabolic carbon dioxide production. See text for information on curves A, B, c, d.

ing ability of haemoglobin. Any increased ventilation associated with hypoxia will also be associated with a decrease in the P_{CO_2}. A decrease in the P_{CO_2} will decrease respiratory drive (Fig. 10.16) and this will therefore decrease the hyperventilation that would otherwise have been caused by falling P_{O_2}; a fall in the P_{O_2} is also associated with increased quantities of deoxygenated haemoglobin. Deoxygenated haemoglobin is a better buffer than oxygenated haemoglobin, and therefore the patient becomes less acidotic. The stimulus to respiration caused by acidosis is therefore also reduced.

For these reasons, ventilation only shows marked increases when the P_{O_2} falls below 8 kPa (60 mmHg) (Fig. 10.17). A fall in oxygen saturation of haemoglobin of 1% is associated with an increase in ventilation of 0.6 L/min. The response is blunted by chronic hypoxia, as occurs in patients living at altitude, with cyanotic congenital heart disease or by hypercapnia due to lung disease.

Effect of changes in hydrogen ion concentration

A rise in hydrogen ion concentration causes an increase in respiration. This is due to peripheral and central stimulation of chemoreceptors. In metabolic acidosis, the increase in ventilation decreases P_{CO_2}, which in turn decreases the hydrogen ion concentration. In metabolic alkalosis, there is a decrease in ventilation which allows the P_{CO_2} to rise with a consequent compensatory increase in hydrogen ion concentration.

Other inputs to the respiratory centre are from proprioceptors in the chest wall, which sense respiratory movements. An absence of respiratory movements causes stimulation of the respiratory centre. There are irritant receptors in the air passages (J receptors) and

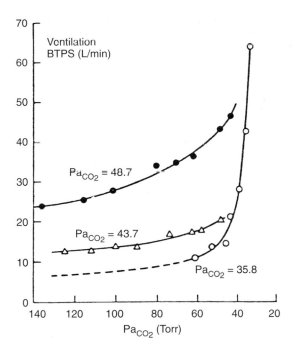

Figure 10.17 • Increase in ventilation due to hypoxia associated with low and high levels of carbon dioxide. (Reproduced with permission from Comroe J. Physiology of respiration. Chicago Year Books.)

lungs which respond to foreign bodies and also stimulate respiration via the respiratory centre. These J receptors are possibly responsible for the increase in ventilation seen in patients with mild respiratory tract infections, where there is no alteration in blood gas composition.

It is not known to what extent the inflation and deflation receptors in the smooth muscle of the airways affect the control of normal respiration.

The baroreceptors have a trivial influence on respiration, in comparison to the profound effect that chemoreceptors have on the circulation. There are also receptors in the pulmonary arteries and coronary circulation, sensitive to *Veratrum* alkaloids, stimulation of which causes decreased respiration and even apnoea. This is the Bezold–Jarisch reflex.

Oxygen and carbon dioxide transport

The lungs maintain an alveolar PO_2 of 13.07 kPa (98 mmHg) and a PCO_2 of 5.3 kPa (40 mmHg), but special transport mechanisms are needed to carry the oxygen absorbed at the lungs to the peripheral tissues and to transport carbon dioxide produced by the metabolism, from peripheral tissues to the lungs.

Oxygen transport

The haemoglobin molecule is specially adapted to transport oxygen. Each molecule has four iron atoms which can combine reversibly with four oxygen atoms. The haemoglobin molecule can alter its shape (quaternary structure) to favour uptake or unloading of oxygen.

However, throughout this molecular adaptation the iron remains in the ferrous state and the association of haemoglobin with oxygen is therefore referred to as oxygenation. If the iron is oxidized to the ferric form, methaemoglobin is formed, which does not act as an oxygen carrier.

Each gram of haemoglobin reacts with 1.34 mL of oxygen. Therefore, 100 mL of blood containing 15 g of haemoglobin can react with 19.5 mL of oxygen. In contrast, 100 mL of blood would only contain 0.3 mL of oxygen in solution at a PO_2 of 13 kPa. Therefore, the presence of haemoglobin increases oxygen-carrying capacity 70-fold. Venous blood at a PCO_2 of 6.1 kPa contains 3.0 mL of carbon dioxide in solution, and 49.7 mL of carbon dioxide as bicarbonate. The formation of bicarbonate (see later) therefore increases carbon dioxide transport 17-fold.

Figure 10.18 shows that the relationship between the PO_2 and oxygen saturation for haemoglobin is hyperbolic. The biggest change in saturation occurs between a PO_2 of 5.3 kPa (40 mmHg) and of 9.3 kPa (70 mmHg), and of course this is the change between the PO_2 in peripheral tissues and the PO_2 in the lungs. There is little change in saturation as the PO_2 falls from 13.3 kPa (100 mmHg) to 9.3 kPa (70 mmHg) and, in this way, haemoglobin compensates for any minor falls in the PO_2 associated with lung disease or a decrease in inspiratory PO_2 which would occur at altitude. However, both acidosis and hyperthermia shift the haemoglobin dissociation curve to the right and decrease the affinity of haemoglobin for oxygen. A fall in the pH to 7.2 or an increase in temperature to 43°C will reduce the oxygen saturation to 90% at a PO_2 of 13.2 kPa, and this can have a significant effect in patients who are ill with acidosis of any cause or high fever. The presence of methaemoglobin or of other abnormal haemoglobins such as haemoglobin S will also shift the dissociation curve to the right, decreasing affinity and decreasing the uptake of oxygen by haemoglobin.

The shape of the dissociation curve is also beneficial when haemoglobin unloads oxygen in peripheral tissues at a low PO_2. Here acidosis (the Bohr effect) and hyperthermia, both of which will occur in metabolically active tissue, are an advantage. They decrease affinity and help haemoglobin to unload oxygen more easily. The formation of carbamino compounds by the combination of carbon dioxide and haemoglobin (see later) also shifts the curve to the right (Haldane effect) and assists unloading in metabolically active tissue. The

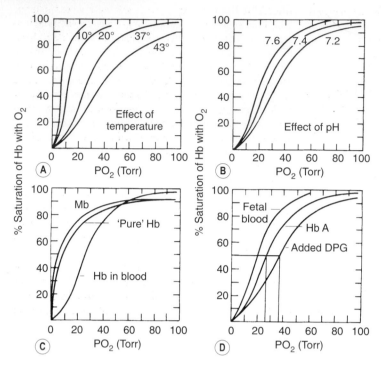

Figure 10.18 • Variations in the haemoglobin (Hb) oxygen dissociation curve. (A) Effect of changes in temperature. (B) Effect of changes in blood pH. (C) Hyperbolic curve of 'purified' haemoglobin A (HbA) (dialysed to be salt free) similar to curve of myoglobin (Mb). (D) The dissociation curve of fetal blood (but not pure HbF) is to the left of adult blood containing HbA; addition of diphosphoglycerate (DPG) shifts curve of blood with HbA to the right and increases P_{50} (decreases affinity of oxygen for Hb and facilitates unloading of oxygen in tissues). (Reproduced with permission from Comroe J. Physiology of respiration. Chicago Year Books.)

position of the haemoglobin dissociation curve can be defined by the P_{50}, the PO_2 at which haemoglobin is 50% desaturated.

2,3-Diphosphoglycerate (2,3-DPG) is formed from 3-phosphoglyceraldehyde, a product of glycolysis via the Embden–Meyerhof pathway. It also affects haemoglobin dissociation in red cells and the presence of 2,3-DPG shifts the dissociation curve to the right. 2,3-DPG levels are decreased in acidosis and banked blood, but increased by androgens, thyroxine, growth hormone, anaemia, exercise and hypoxic conditions (living at altitude and in cardiopulmonary disease). Thus, banked blood does not give up its oxygen very easily but hypoxic individuals do unload oxygen easily, even if their low haemoglobin affinity is less favourable for oxygen uptake.

The fetus clearly needs high-affinity blood since the PO_2 in the fetal umbilical vein is only about 4 kPa (30 mmHg). Different mammalian species have different ways of increasing the affinity of fetal blood. In humans, fetal haemoglobin has a low oxygen affinity, but this is not the mechanism by which fetal red cells increase their affinity for oxygen. Instead, in human fetal red cells the fetal haemoglobin does not interact with 2,3-DPG, and it is this that accounts for the increased affinity of human fetal blood for oxygen.

Carbon monoxide

Carbon monoxide has 210 times greater affinity for haemoglobin than oxygen. Therefore, if the ratio of carbon monoxide to oxygen in inspired air is 1:210, equivalent to a 0.1% concentration of carbon monoxide in air, haemoglobin will be 50% oxygenated and 50% combined with carbon monoxide (*Note* the oxygen concentration is 21%). This effect alone will reduce the oxygen capacity of haemoglobin by 50% and would be the same as giving the patient a haemoglobin concentration of 7.5 g/100 mL. However, the presence of carboxyhaemoglobin also shifts the haemoglobin dissociation curve of oxygen to the left (increased affinity) so that even the oxygen that is combined with haemoglobin is not liberated in peripheral tissues, and this accounts for the profound tissue hypoxia that occurs in carbon monoxide poisoning. It also explains why such patients are not cyanosed, because the oxygen remains combined with haemoglobin. Cyanosis is not seen until the concentration of deoxygenated haemoglobin in the blood is as low as 5 g/100 mL. The cherry-pink colour that these patients have is due to the presence of carboxyhaemoglobin.

The amount of carboxyhaemoglobin associated with smoking (5–8% carboxyhaemoglobin) is sufficient to shift the tissue PO_2 from 6 kPa (45 mmHg) to 5.3 kPa

(40 mmHg). This may account for the deleterious effect of smoking on ischaemic heart disease, and also for the intrauterine growth restriction seen in the fetuses of women who smoke in pregnancy.

Carbon dioxide transport

Carbon dioxide is transported in the plasma, partly in solution, partly by hydration, to form carbonic acid and partly by the formation of carbamino compounds with the N-terminal end of plasma proteins. Hydration is very slow because there is no carbonic anhydrase in the plasma. Hydrogen ions are formed from both reactions, and these are buffered by plasma proteins.

Carbonic anhydrase (red cells only)

$$CO_2 + H_2O \xrightarrow{\hspace{1cm}} H_2CO_3 \rightleftharpoons H^+ + HCO_3^- \quad \textbf{(1)}$$

$$\boxed{Protein} - NH_2 + CO_2 \longrightarrow \boxed{Protein} - N\begin{smallmatrix} H \\ \\ COOH \end{smallmatrix}$$

$$\rightleftharpoons \boxed{Protein} - N\begin{smallmatrix} H \\ \\ COO^- \end{smallmatrix} + H^+ \quad \textbf{(2)}$$

Carbon dioxide also enters the red cells and is again transported in solution, and by hydration. Hydration occurs rapidly in red cells because of the presence of carbonic anhydrase. The products of the reaction are also dealt with; hydrogen ions are buffered by the relatively high levels of deoxygenated haemoglobin (p. 179), and bicarbonate ions are able to diffuse out of the red cells, into the plasma which has a relatively lower bicarbonate concentration. To maintain electrical neutrality, the chloride ions diffuse back into the red cells and this process is known as the chloride shift. The process of hydration is associated with a net increase in the total number of ions that are osmotically active, and therefore water also enters the red cells, which swell. The biconcave disc shape of the red cells allows them to swell without bursting.

In addition, carbon dioxide reacts with haemoglobin to form carbamino compounds. The carbamino compounds are fully ionized, giving a further source of hydrogen ions to be buffered by haemoglobin.

The net effect of these reactions is that two-thirds of carbon dioxide is transported in the plasma as bicarbonate, but that the majority of hydrogen ions produced are buffered in the red cells.

Urinary system

The function of the kidney is to contribute to the homeostasis of the internal environment; in particular, the kidney is concerned with salt and water balance and hence blood volume, long-term adjustments in acid–base balance, and the regulation of the blood level of certain ions, such as calcium and phosphate. The kidney is the main pathway for the elimination of nitrogenous waste products, such as urea, and some drugs, such as salicylate and heparin. It also has a major endocrine role in vitamin D metabolism and the production of renin and erythropoietin. Certain cells in the kidneys secrete prostaglandins, which affect local blood flow and tubular function.

Microanatomy

The functional unit of the kidney is the nephron (45–65 mm long) (Fig. 10.19). Each healthy human kidney contains approximately 1 million nephrons. Blood is filtered at the glomerulus, which is the beginning of the nephron, and the filtrate is subsequently modified by reabsorption or secretion in its passage through the nephron. Urine is the result of all the modifications to the glomerular filtrate after it has left the nephron at

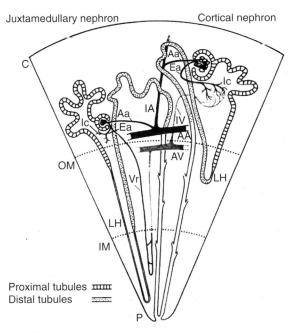

Figure 10.19 • Diagram of nephrons and their blood supply. AA, arcuate artery; AV, arcuate vein; Aa, afferent arteriole; Ea, efferent arteriole; IA, interlobular artery; IV, interlobular vein; Ic, intertubular capillaries; LH, loop of Henle; Vr, vasa recta; P, papilla; C, cortex; OM, outer medulla; IM, inner medulla. (Reproduced with permission from Passmore R, Robson J (eds). Companion to medical studies. Blackwell Scientific, Oxford.)

the collecting duct, although some minor alterations in composition may occur in the bladder.

The glomerulus is an invagination at the closed end of the renal tubule (Bowman's capsule). Blood is brought to the glomerulus by the afferent arteriole that drains into a network of capillaries which fill the glomerulus. The glomerular filtrate has to cross two layers of cells, the capillary endothelium and the tubular epithelium, separated by an amorphous basal lamina, to pass from the blood vessels to the tubule. It is this barrier that is deranged in those forms of kidney disease which affect the glomerulus, such as glomerulonephritis. The filtrate passes out of the glomerular capillaries and across the epithelium of the tubule through epithelial pores, which electron microscopy suggests are 25 nm in diameter, although functionally they appear to be 8 nm in diameter, since molecules larger than 8 nm are not filtered. Therefore the glomerular filtrate contains no red cells (diameter 7.5 μm) and essentially no protein. In addition, the protein around the capillary pores is negatively charged. Therefore, negatively charged substances such as albumin, whose molecules are less than 8 nm in diameter, may not pass through the capillaries. The capillaries of the glomerulus are a portal system since they drain from the afferent arteriole to the efferent arteriole.

The next portion of the tubule after the glomerulus is the proximal convoluted tubule. Here the majority of the reabsorption of ions and water from the glomerular filtrate occurs. The proximal tubule leads to the loop of Henle, which is largely concerned with salt and water concentration. The loop of Henle then leads to the distal convoluted tubule, which in turn leads to the collecting duct. Between the ascending limb of the loop of Henle and the distal convoluted tubule is a portion of the tubule lined by specialized cells, the macula densa. This portion of the tubule is in close apposition to the efferent and afferent arterioles at the glomerulus, and this region is collectively known as the juxtaglomerular apparatus, which is the site of renin secretion. The loop of Henle differs between the tubules located in the cortex (cortical tubules, 85% of the total) and those located near the medulla (juxtamedullary tubules, 15% of the total). The juxtamedullary tubules have much longer loops of Henle and also they alone have a thick portion to the ascending limb of the loop of Henle. This thick portion is thought to be essential for the reabsorption of chloride, an essential part of the mechanism for concentrating urine (see below).

The efferent arteriole leaves the glomerulus to form the blood supply to the tubule. It supplies a network of peritubular capillaries, which then drain into the renal vein. The juxtamedullary nephrons have specialized efferent arterioles, the vasa recta, which supply the loop of Henle (Fig. 10.19).

Renal clearance

Substances such as creatinine or urea which are excreted by the kidney have a lower concentration in the renal vein than the artery; they are therefore said to be cleared by the kidney. But, with few exceptions, most substances are not completely cleared by the kidney. The clearance of a substance such as creatinine is a theoretical concept. Clearance equals the volume of blood that would be totally cleared of creatinine in unit time. Thus, if the creatinine clearance is 120 mL/min and the serum creatinine is 70 μmol/L (0.8 mg/100 mL), the kidney excretes $70 \times 120/1000 = 8.4$ μmol/min (0.1 mg/min). If the renal blood flow is 1.2 L/min, this would reduce the creatinine level by $8.4 \times 1000/1200 = 7.0$ μmol. So a creatinine clearance of 120 mL/min will maintain a renal vein creatinine level of 70 μmol/L if the renal artery creatinine level is 77 μmol/L.

To calculate the clearance of a substance it is best to work from first principles. For example, let us assume we are told that:

> **Serum creatinine = 70 μmol/L**   **(1)**
> **Urine creatinine = 6 mmol/L**
> **24-h urine volume = 2 L/24 h**

Then:

> **24-h urine**
> **creatinine**
> **excretion = 2 × 6 mmol**
>   **= 2 × 6 × 1000 μmol**
>
> **Excretion of**   **(2)**
> **creatinine**
> **in 1 min** $= \dfrac{2 \times 6 \times 1000}{60 \times 24}$ **μmol**
>   **= 8.3 μmol**

From (1), 1 μmol of creatinine occupies

$$\frac{1000}{70} = 14.3 \text{ mL}$$

From (2), with 8.3 μmol excreted per min, creatinine clearance = $8.3 \times 14.3 = 119$ mL/min.

Glomerular filtration rate

The clearance of a substance that is neither reabsorbed from the renal tubule nor secreted into the tubule is equal to the glomerular filtration rate (GFR). The plasma constituent that most closely approaches this is creatinine, and the creatinine clearance is therefore the usual measurement for estimation of the GFR. The normal GFR (both kidneys together) is 120 mL/min. It is proportional to body surface area, but about 10% lower in women than men, even after adjustment for body surface area. Creatinine may be both secreted to and reabsorbed from the renal tubule, but has the great advantage that it is endogenously produced and the blood levels do not fluctuate much. For accurate determination of the GFR the insulin clearance may be used but inulin has to be infused to maintain a steady plasma level. The clearance of radioactive vitamin B_{12} has also been used for measurement of the GFR, but obviously not in pregnancy.

Renal blood flow

Healthy renal blood flow is normally about 1.2 L/min. It varies with body surface and sex in the same way as the GFR. Since only the plasma is relevant to the excretion of most substances, the term renal plasma flow (RPF) is often used, rather than renal blood flow. If the haematocrit is 45%, the RPF is 660 mL/min when the blood flow is 1.2 L/min: 660 = 1200 (100 −45/100) mL/min. Renal blood flow could be measured directly by placing flowmeters on the renal arteries, but this would be a highly invasive procedure. In practice we measure the clearance of substances such as *p*-aminohippuric acid (PAH), which are not metabolized by the kidney, and are assumed to be almost totally excreted through the kidney. Thus the renal vein concentration of PAH is assumed to be zero. Under these circumstances, the secretion of PAH into the renal tubule, PAH clearance, equals renal blood flow.

The renal blood vessels are innervated by the autonomic nervous system via renal nerves. Stimulation of the renal nerves causes vasoconstriction and a decrease in renal blood flow. This occurs via the vasomotor centre in systemic hypotension and also in severe hypoxia. Renal blood flow is also decreased by the direct action of catecholamines and both neural and humoral mechanisms are likely to be involved in the reduction of renal blood flow associated with exercise.

The filtration fraction is the ratio of GFR to RPF. The normal filtration fraction is 120/660 = 0.18. As the RPF falls in hypotension, the filtration fraction increases, thus maintaining the GFR.

Handling of individual substances

Glucose and amino acids

Glucose and amino acids are reabsorbed by active transport at the proximal tubule. If the filtered load of glucose is too great for the proximal tubule to be able to reabsorb all the filtered glucose, it is excreted in the urine. This usually occurs at blood glucose concentra-

tions ≥10 mmol/L. Glycosuria occurs in patients with hyperglycaemia due to diabetes mellitus. Some pregnant women have glycosuria at lower blood glucose concentrations and this does not necessarily indicate gestational diabetes. Patients with aminoaciduria, as occurs in Fanconi syndrome, have a congenital abnormality of the proximal tubules so that they cannot reabsorb amino acids efficiently.

Sodium and chloride

The reabsorption of sodium by the renal tubule is a major feat, which consumes considerable energy. The filtered load of sodium presented to the renal tubules is about 200 000 mmol/day. The vast majority of this is reabsorbed, so that the total quantity of sodium excreted varies between 1 and 400 mmol/day, depending on the salt and water balance of the individual. The chief controlling mechanisms accounting for the variation in the sodium reabsorption are: (1) the levels of aldosterone and other mineralocorticoids, (2) glomerular filtration rate, (3) variations in intrarenal pressure, which affects filtration fraction, and (4) concomitant changes in potassium and hydrogen ion excretion. In addition a peptide secreted by the heart, atrial natriuretic peptide, increases the excretion of sodium but the mechanism of action and precise function of this substance are unclear.

The majority of sodium is reabsorbed actively in the proximal tubule. In addition, sodium is reabsorbed actively in the distal convoluted tubule, collecting duct and bladder under the control of mineralocorticoids. Sodium is also reabsorbed passively in the thick ascending loop of Henle in exchange for chloride ions, which are themselves actively reabsorbed. The anions involved in sodium reabsorption are chloride (80%) and bicarbonate (19%). The remaining 1% of sodium reabsorption takes place in the distal tubule and is accounted for by exchange of potassium (0.5%) and hydrogen (0.5%) ions.

Chloride is usually reabsorbed passively, following sodium and potassium reabsorption in the proximal convoluted tubule. It is also actively reabsorbed in the thick ascending loop of Henle. Chloride reabsorption is decreased when bicarbonate reabsorption is increased, so that the levels of chloride and bicarbonate vary reciprocally in the plasma. Before the measurement of bicarbonate became freely available, it was realized that chloride levels are high in those situations where the bicarbonate level is low, e.g. metabolic acidosis, and much knowledge of acid–base balance was inferred from estimation of the chloride concentration; this is no longer necessary.

Bicarbonate

Bicarbonate is partly reabsorbed passively following sodium reabsorption; it is also reabsorbed by buffering hydrogen ions. Within the renal tubule, hydrogen ions react with bicarbonate to form carbonic acid. The carbonic acid is broken down under the influence of carbonic anhydrase in the brush border of the cells of the proximal convoluted tubule to form carbon dioxide and water. Carbon dioxide is reabsorbed across the tubular cell, and in the proximal tubular cell reacts again with water to form carbonic acid, which subsequently dissociates; bicarbonate is therefore reabsorbed as carbon dioxide, rather than as bicarbonate ions. This mechanism occurs so long as the plasma bicarbonate concentration is less than 28 mmol/L. Once the bicarbonate concentration exceeds this level, bicarbonate appears in the urine, which becomes alkaline.

Potassium

Potassium is reabsorbed actively in the proximal convoluted tubule, in exchange for chloride ions. It is also secreted into the distal convoluted tubule, in exchange for sodium ions, and this is under the control of aldosterone and other mineralocorticoids. High concentrations of aldosterone cause an increase in sodium reabsorption and potassium secretion in the distal tubule, hence the hypokalaemia typical of aldosterone excess, as in Conn's syndrome. The kidney is not nearly as efficient in conserving potassium, as it is at conserving sodium. When there is hypokalaemia, the obligate excretion of potassium is still about 10 mmol/day, whereas in hypovolaemia the kidney can reduce sodium excretion to 1 mmol/day.

Hydrogen ions

Hydrogen ions are actively excreted in the proximal and distal tubules in exchange for sodium. In the tubule the hydrogen ions are buffered by bicarbonate, phosphate and ammonia, which keeps the pH of the tubular fluid >4.5, the minimum for hydrogen ion secretion. Ammonia is produced locally in the kidney tubules by deamination of amino acids, and is secreted into the tubular fluid at the proximal and distal tubules, and collecting duct.

Water

Of the 170 L of water that is filtered per day, all but 1.5 L is reabsorbed under normal circumstances. However, in extreme hydration the total amount of water excreted may be as high as 50% of the glomerular filtration rate. This control of water reabsorption depends on the level of antidiuretic hormone, the glomerular filtration rate and the solute load. The bulk of water reabsorption occurs passively in the proximal tubule, where sodium and chloride are reabsorbed, and water is absorbed isotonically. Concentration of the urine occurs because of the high osmotic pressure achieved by reabsorption of chloride followed by sodium in the thick ascending limb of the loop of Henle in the medulla of the kidney. As the filtrate passes down the collecting duct it becomes exposed to this high osmotic pressure and water is reabsorbed. The permeability of the collecting duct is altered by the level of antidiuretic hormone. High levels of antidiuretic hormone increase the permeability of the cells of the collecting duct, therefore allowing more water to be reabsorbed from tubular fluid, and a lower volume of concentrated urine to be finally secreted. Low levels of antidiuretic hormone decrease permeability of the cells of the collecting duct, so that large quantities of dilute urine are excreted.

Antidiuretic hormone (ADH; arginine vasopressin) is secreted from the posterior pituitary gland, under the influence of the hypothalamus. Its secretion is increased by stress, hypovolaemia, and increase in plasma osmolarity, adrenaline and certain drugs such as morphine. Its secretion is decreased by an increase in circulating blood volume, by a fall in plasma osmolarity and by alcohol. During pregnancy, four times as much ADH is produced in order to counteract the effects of placentally derived vasopressinase. A failure of the mother's pituitary to increase vasopressin production to match placental enzymatic degradation will lead to transient (gestational) diabetes insipidus, until delivery of the placenta.

Urea

Urea accumulates in high concentration in the renal medulla. The kidney tubular cells are freely permeable to urea. When urine flows are low only 10–20% of the filtered urea is excreted, while at high urine flow rates 50–70% is excreted.

Endocrine functions of the kidney

The kidney acts as an endocrine organ to increase production of renin (see above and p. 188), erythropoietin (EPO) and the active hydroxylation of vitamin D. Erythropoietin is a circulating glycoprotein consisting of 165 amino acids. It is normally produced by interstitial fibroblasts in the renal cortex, close to peritubular capillaries. The secretion of EPO is stimulated by a widespread system of oxygen-dependent gene expression, specifically hypoxia-inducible transcription factors (HIFs). It is the degradation of HIF associated with an α subunit (HIF-1α and HIF-2α) that is oxygen dependent and determines EPO production. EPO normally stimulates red cell production by binding to EPO receptors on early erythroid progenitor cells. These primitive cells then mature into red blood cells, rather than undergoing apoptosis. In chronic kidney disease there is a failure of EPO production in response to chronic anaemia.

Vitamin D is either produced in the skin by the action of sunlight or ingested in the diet. In the liver it is converted to 25-dihydroxycholecalciferol. In the kidney this is converted to the active metabolite 1,25-dihydroxycholecalciferol. It is this hormone that increases calcium uptake from the gastrointestinal tract, and mobilizes calcium from bone. Renal rickets is in part due to the failure of the kidney to produce normal quantities of 1,25-hydroxycholecalciferol in renal failure.

Effects of pregnancy

Renal glomerular function during pregnancy

Renal adaptation to pregnancy is anticipated prior to conception, during the luteal phase of each menstrual cycle. Renal blood flow and glomerular filtration rate (GFR) increase by 10–20% before menstruation. If pregnancy is established the corpus luteum persists and these haemodynamic changes continue. By 16 weeks of gestation GFR is 55% above non-pregnant levels (Fig. 10.20). This increment is mediated through an increase in renal blood flow that reaches a maximum of 70–80% above non-pregnant levels by the second trimester, before falling to around 45% above non-pregnant levels, at term. Elegant human studies have confirmed that, unlike the hyperfiltration that precedes diabetic nephropathy, gestational hyperfiltration is not associated with a damaging rise in glomerular capillary blood pressure.

The changes to renal physiology in healthy pregnancy can both hide and mimic renal disease. The increased GFR of pregnancy leads to a fall in serum creatinine concentration (Scr), so that values considered normal in the non-pregnant state may be abnormal during pregnancy. Serum creatinine levels fall from a non-pregnant mean value of 73 µmol/L (0.82 mg/dL) to 60 µmol/L (0.68 mg/dL), 54 µmol/L (0.61 mg/dL) and 64 µmol/L (0.72 mg/dL) in successive trimesters. Serum creatinine is not, however, linearly correlated with creatinine clearance and is influenced by muscle mass, physical exercise, racial differences and dietary intake of meat. As Scr roughly doubles for every 50% reduction in GFR, a more useful parameter by which to monitor serial changes in renal function is the reciprocal of Scr (1/Scr). Estimates of GFR can be further refined using the Cockcroft–Gault equation, which calculates GFR using Scr, maternal age and pre-pregnancy weight. For women the Cockcroft–Gault equation is:

$$GFR\,(mL/min) = 0.8 \times [140 - age\,(years) \times weight\,(kg)]/Scr\,(\mu mol/L)$$

$$(1\,mg/dL\ creatinine = 88.4\,\mu mol/L\ creatinine)$$

The gestational rise in renal blood flow also causes the kidneys to swell so that bipolar renal length increases by approximately 1 cm. During the third trimester renal blood flow falls, leading to a fall in creatinine clearance and a rise in Scr. Serum urea levels, however, continue to fall in the third trimester due to reduced maternal hepatic urea synthesis. This metabolic adaptation ensures that more nitrogen is available for fetal protein synthesis.

The renal pelvicalyceal system and ureters dilate and can appear obstructed to those unaware of these changes, in particular on the right side. The right pelvicalyceal system dilates by a maximum of 0.5 mm each week from 6–32 weeks, reaching a maximum diameter of approximately 20 mm (90th centile), which is maintained until term. The left pelvicalyceal system reaches a maximum diameter of 8 mm (90th centile) at 20 weeks of gestation.

Proteinuria increases as pregnancy progresses, but levels over 200 mg/24 h during the third trimester are above the 95% confidence limit for the normal population. A random urine protein:creatinine ratio is a useful guide to 24-h urinary protein excretion, but is not a substitute for either a 12- or 24-h urine collection, due to the high incidence of both false-positive and false-negative results. A random urine sample that gives a protein (mg):creatinine (mmol) ratio >0.30 is a good predictor of significant proteinuria and is an indication for more accurate assessment of proteinuria with a 12- or 24-h urine collection.

Serum albumin levels fall by 5–10 g/L, serum cholesterol and triglyceride concentrations increase significantly and dependent oedema affects most pregnancies at term. Normal pregnancy therefore simulates the classic features of nephrotic syndrome.

Renal tubular function during pregnancy

Increased alveolar ventilation causes a respiratory alkalosis to which the kidney responds by increased bicarbonaturia and a compensatory metabolic acidosis. Other renal tubular changes include reduced tubular glucose reabsorption, which leads to glycosuria in approximately 10% of healthy pregnant women, a 250–300% increase in urinary calcium excretion and a first trimester increase in urate excretion that decreases towards term, at which time plasma urate levels rise again to non-pregnancy levels.

During healthy pregnancy, a mother gains 6–8 kg of fluid, of which approximately 1.2 L is due to an increase in plasma volume. Plasma osmolality falls by 10 mmol/kg by 5–8 weeks of gestation due to a fall in both the threshold for thirst and for the release of antidiuretic hormone (vasopressin). During pregnancy, vasopressin is metabolized by placental vasopressinase, and at term the maternal posterior pituitary produces four times as much vasopressin to maintain physiological concentrations. Failure of the maternal pituitary to

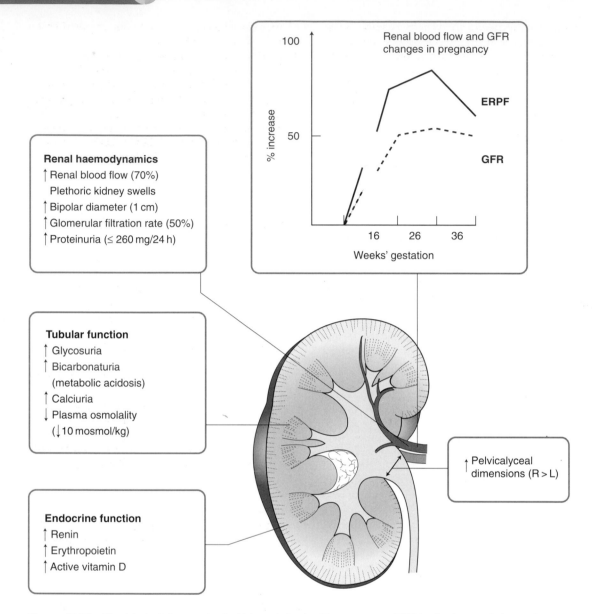

Renal haemodynamics
↑ Renal blood flow (70%)
  Plethoric kidney swells
↑ Bipolar diameter (1 cm)
↑ Glomerular filtration rate (50%)
↑ Proteinuria (≤ 260 mg/24 h)

Tubular function
↑ Glycosuria
↑ Bicarbonaturia
  (metabolic acidosis)
↑ Calciuria
↓ Plasma osmolality
  (↓10 mosmol/kg)

Endocrine function
↑ Renin
↑ Erythropoietin
↑ Active vitamin D

↑ Pelvicalyceal
  dimensions (R > L)

Renal blood flow and GFR
changes in pregnancy

ERPF

GFR

100

50

% increase

16   26   36
Weeks' gestation

Figure 10.20 • Physiological changes to the kidney during healthy pregnancy. ERPF, effective renal plasma flow.

keep up with the increased metabolic clearance of vasopressin leads to a transient polyuric state in the third trimester, which is known as transient diabetes insipidus of pregnancy.

Renal endocrine function during pregnancy

The kidney also acts as an endocrine organ that produces erythropoietin, active vitamin D and renin. The production of all three hormones increases during healthy pregnancy, but their effects are masked by other changes. In early pregnancy, peripheral vasodilatation exceeds renin–aldosterone-mediated plasma volume expansion, so diastolic blood pressure falls by 12 weeks. Conversely, plasma volume expansion exceeds the erythropoietin-mediated increase in red cell mass, causing a 'physiological anaemia', which should not normally lead to an Hb concentration <9.5 g/dL. Similarly, extra active vitamin D produced by the placenta circulates at twice non-gravid levels, but concomitant halving of parathyroid hormone levels, hypercalciuria and increased fetal requirements keep plasma ionized calcium levels unchanged.

Physiology of micturition

Passive phase

The bladder fills with urine at approximately 1 mL/min. Folds of transitional cell epithelium become flattened and the detrusor muscle fibres passively stretch with very little rise of intravesical pressure.

At the same time, the intraurethral pressure caused by the elastic tissue, the arteriovenous shunts and the tone of the smooth and striated muscle components is maintained at a higher level than the intravesical pressure.

Proprioceptive afferent impulses caused by the stretching of the detrusor fibres pass through the pelvic splanchnic nerves to the sacral roots of S2–S4. As urine volume increases, these impulses pass up the lateral spinothalamic tracts to the thalamus and thence to the cerebral cortex, thus bringing the sensation of bladder filling to a conscious level. The act of micturition is initially subconsciously and later consciously postponed by inhibitory impulses blocking the sacral reflex arc.

Active phase

At an appropriate time and place, a suitable posture is adopted through the organization of the frontal lobes of the cerebral cortex and the anterior hypothalamus, and the following sequence of events take place in the act of micturition:

1. The muscles of the pelvic floor are voluntarily relaxed, causing a loss of the posterior urethrovesical angle and funnelling of the bladder neck.
2. At the same time, the voluntary fibres of the external sphincter are relaxed, causing an overall fall of intraurethral pressure by at least 50%.
3. At 5–15 s later, the inhibitory activity of the higher centres on the sacral reflex is lifted, allowing a rapid flow of efferent parasympathetic impulses, mainly from S3, to cause the detrusor to contract. As a result the intravesical pressure rises and can be augmented by the voluntary contraction of the diaphragm and the anterior abdominal wall musculature.
4. Urine flow commences when the intravesical pressure exceeds the intraurethral pressure. The urine flow may also further stimulate the sacral

reflex by the conduction of afferent impulses from its lining to S2–S4.
5. At the end of micturition, the flow rate diminishes, the intravesical pressure falls and the striated musculature of the pelvic floor elevates the bladder neck; the external urethral sphincter interrupts the terminal flow in the region of the midurethra and obliterates the urethral lumen. The inhibitory influence of the higher centres is re-established and the bladder becomes passive once more.

Urodynamic data in the normal adult female

Residual urine	0–10 mL
First sensation of bladder filling	150–200 mL
Voiding volume	220–320 mL
Voiding pressure	45–70 cmH$_2$O
Maximum urine flow rate	20–40 mL/s
Bladder capacity	600 mL
Intravesical pressure rise (0–500 mL)	0–10 cmH$_2$O
	Detrusor contractions do not occur even with rapid filling or at full capacity
Maximal urethral pressure in the absence of micturition	Approx. 50–100 cmH$_2$O, but varies with age and childbearing

Gastrointestinal tract

Mouth

Mechanics

Mastication is accomplished by voluntary muscles innervated by the motor branch of the fifth cranial nerve. Pregnancy results in alteration of microflora in the oral cavity favouring acidophilic organisms and predisposing to development of dental caries which may be exacerbated by calcium deficiency.

Digestive processes

The secretion of the saliva is mediated by autonomic nervous stimulation. Salivary mucus provides lubrication for mastication and swallowing. The salivary glands also produce salivary amylase in the mouth which converts starch and glycogen into maltose and maltotriose. The lingual glands produce lingual lipase (Table 10.7) which converts triglycerides into fatty acids and glycerol.

Table 10.7 Enzymes in the mouth

Enzyme	Substrate	Product
Salivary amylase	Starch	Dextrins, maltose, maltotriose
Lingual lipase	Triglycerides	Fatty acids and glycerol

Oesophagus

Mechanics
Swallowing

There are two stages to this process:

1. *Voluntary stage* – food in the form of a bolus is pressed by the tongue upwards and backwards against the soft palate.
2. *Involuntary stage* – passage of food initially through the pharynx (1–2 s) and then by peristalsis down the oesophagus (4–8 s) to the stomach. The process is controlled by the deglutition centre in medulla and lower pons.

The oesophagus is 25 cm long and consists of an outer layer of longitudinal muscle and an inner circular muscle layer. In the upper part of the oesophagus both layers are comprised of striated muscle, and in the lower part both layers are smooth muscle. The pH of the lower oesophagus is 5–7. At the gastro-oesophageal junction, the squamous epithelium of the oesophagus is replaced by columnar epithelium.

Gastro-oesophageal sphincter

The lower oesophageal sphincter functions as a result of tonic contraction of the circular muscle of the lower end of the oesophagus 2–5 cm above the gastro-oesophageal junction. The sphincter remains contracted at all times other than when swallowing, eructating (belching wind) or vomiting. Sphincter function is enhanced as a result of the angulation at the lower end of the oesophagus by the diaphragm. Closure is therefore promoted on raising the intragastric or intra-abdominal pressure, so creating a shutter or flap-valve effect. Closure is further enhanced by virtue of a portion of the oesophagus resting intra-abdominally. Folding of the mucosa within the oesophageal lumen facilitating occlusion and unimpeded gastric emptying is also important in maintaining the competence of the sphincter.

Gastro-oesophageal reflux

Gastro-oesophageal reflux occurs in 30–50% of all pregnancies and occurs when the lower oesophageal sphincter fails. This results in exposure of the relatively unprotected oesophageal mucosa to the predominantly acidic irritant peptic contents. In pregnancy, gastric relaxation and delayed emptying may predispose to incompetence of the lower oesophageal sphincter. Additional proposed mechanisms include a role for oestrogen and progesterone in reducing lower oesophageal sphincter pressure. Diet and a racial predisposition may also be important, e.g. there is an increased prevalence in white Caucasians compared with Nigerian (9%) or Singaporean (17%) populations. Raised intragastric pressure is a contributory factor in late pregnancy. Simple solutions to reflux in pregnancy include frequent intake of small meals, reduction in fat and alcohol intake and avoidance of manoeuvres that increase intra-abdominal pressure. Drug treatment of gastro-oesophageal reflux is aimed at reducing acid secretion and increasing mucosal resistance to acid.

Gastric pressure and gastric volumes increase in labour and stomach contents are pulmonary irritants if inhaled (aspiration pneumonitis), e.g. during anaesthesia for emergency caesarean section. Foodstuffs of high osmolarity (e.g. glucose) are especially liable to delay emptying. Women should therefore be advised to drink isotonic drinks in labour which prevent ketosis without a concomitant increase in gastric volume. In addition, women considered at risk of caesarean section should be offered antacids to reduce gastric volume and acidity. Non-particulate antacid suspension gels are preferred and seem to mix more effectively with stomach contents and cause less irritation if inhaled.

Stomach

Mechanics

Because a meal is eaten more quickly than the digestive enzymes can break it down, the stomach serves as a holding chamber and mixing device. The stomach is the most distensible part of the gastrointestinal tract and storage of food in quantities of up to 1 L is possible. Mixing and maceration of food with secretions generates chyme by a combination of constrictor waves and peristalsis. Peristalsis forces food towards the pyloric sphincter (which is usually closed) and chyme is forced through. Emptying is promoted by:

1. Increased gastric volume causing antral peristalsis.
2. Release of gastrin (Table 10.8) stimulated by food (especially meat) causing acid secretion. This in turn stimulates the pyloric pump (producing H^+) (see later), while at the same time relaxing the pylorus.

Emptying is inhibited by:

1. Enterogastric reflex from the duodenum to pylorus when there is excess of chyme, acid, hyper- or hypotonic fluids, or excess of protein breakdown products.
2. A possible hormonal reflex from the duodenum to pylorus – especially when chyme contains an excess of fats.

Table 10.8 Gastrointestinal hormones

Hormone	Site of production	Stimulus for release	Gastric acid/gastrin secretion	Gastric emptying	Other effect	Changes in pregnancy
Gastrin	G-cells of gastric antrum	Gastric distension Amino acids in antrum Vagal action (inhibited by pH < 1.5) Calcium, adrenaline (epinephrine)	↑	↑	Secretion of pepsin and intrinsic factor Stimulates pancreatic bicarbonate secretion and secretin	Plasma level unchanged
Cholecystokinin (CCK)	Duodenum & jejunum	Intraluminal fat, amino acids, peptides & some cations (Ca^{++}, Mg^{++})	↓	↓	Pancreatic enzyme and bicarbonate secretion Gall bladder contraction Satiety	
Secretin	Duodenum & jejunum	Intraluminal acid	↓	↓	Stimulates pancreatic bicarbonate secretion Stimulates production and increases the water and HCO_3^- content of bile	
Gastric inhibitory peptide (GIP)	Duodenum & jejunum	Glucose, fats & amino acids	↓	↓	Stimulates insulin secretion	
Motilin	Duodenum & jejunum	Acid in small bowel		↑		
Vasoactive intestinal peptide (VIP)	Small intestine	Neural	↓		Inhibits pepsin secretion Stimulates secretion by intestine and pancreas Splanchnic vasodilatation	
Pancreatic polypeptide	Pancreas	Protein-rich meal			Relaxes gall bladder Inhibits pancreatic enzyme secretion	
Somatostatin			↓	↓	Inhibits secretin and gastrin, most hormones	
Histamine	Histaminocytes in lamina propria		↑			
Glucagon, calcitonin			↓			

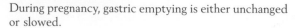

During pregnancy, gastric emptying is either unchanged or slowed.

Digestive processes

Gastric innervation is parasympathetic via the vagus (motor and secretory) and sympathetic via Meissner's and Auerbach's plexus. Blood supply is from the coeliac trunk.

Gastric secretion is initiated reflexly via the vagus and secretions total 3 litres per day. Once food has entered the stomach the hormone gastrin is released from the antral portion, and is carried in the blood to the parietal (oxyntic) cells of the gastric glands. Parietal cells secrete hydrochloric acid and intrinsic factor. The proton pump actively transports H^+ ions (H^+ ATPase) into the gastric lumen in exchange for K^+ ions. K^+ (and Cl^-) then passively diffuse back into the gastric lumen through their own channels. H^+ ions for this purpose are generated within the parietal cell. Water (H_2O) and carbon dioxide (CO_2) form carbonic acid in a reaction catalysed by carbonic anhydrase, which is abundant in parietal cells. The carbonic acid thus formed then dissociates, generating H^+ (and HCO_3^-). The $HCO3^-$ product is then exchanged for Cl^- in the interstitial fluid.

$$H_2O + CO_2 \rightarrow H_2CO_3 \rightarrow H^+ + HCO_3^-$$

Chief cells secrete pepsinogen (Table 10.9) – the only proteolytic enzyme within the stomach. Release of a pro-enzyme (pepsinogen) protects the parietal cell from the proteolytic effect of the enzyme product pepsin. Hydrochloric acid converts pepsinogen into pepsin. Pepsin further acts on pepsinogen in the presence of acid, so enhancing its own production. The low pH (1–2) of the stomach has the additional effect of killing many bacteria in food as well as being the optimum pH for function of pepsin. Gastric pH and gastric acid output are unchanged by pregnancy.

Mucus in the stomach comes from glands around the pylorus and protects the mucosa from the extreme acidity. Gastric lipase and amylase are of little quantitative importance. Indeed gastric lipase splits short-chain triglycerides, as found in milk, although this enzyme functions optimally at pH 5–6 and so has a limited role in the adult stomach. In infants, rennin (chymosin) causes the milk to curdle, so delaying its emptying from the stomach with subsequent early digestion of casein. Intrinsic factor is a glycoprotein which binds cyanocobalamin (vitamin B_{12}). B_{12} is then absorbed in the terminal ileum and intrinsic factor remains in the lumen. The most common cause of B_{12} deficiency is pernicious anaemia where atrophy of the gastric mucosa leads to failure of intrinsic factor production. Pernicious anaemia is seen in the elderly but an association with other auto-immune diseases, e.g. thyroid disease, is observed. Parietal cell antibodies are seen in 90% and intrinsic factor antibodies in 50% of people with pernicious anaemia.

Gall bladder

Mechanics

The gall bladder stores, concentrates and acidifies bile. Emptying into the duodenum is brought about by the presence of fat in the small intestine causing cholecystokinin–pancreozymin (Table 10.8) to be released from the mucosa. Cholecystokinin stimulates the gall bladder to contract and the sphincter of Oddi to relax.

Digestive processes

See under Liver for constituents of bile.

Small intestine

Mechanics

Distension is the main stimulus to peristalsis, by autonomic fibres to the myenteric plexus (Fig. 10.21). The parasympathetic fibres stimulate movement; the sympathetic fibres inhibit movement.

The ileocaecal sphincter and valve allows about 750 mL of chyme/day into the caecum. Both ileal peristalsis and gastrin release relax the ileal sphincter, while increased caecal pressure and irritation of the caecum constrict it.

Digestive processes
Duodenum and pancreas

Pancreatic juice is an alkaline fluid (pH 8) containing enzymes, pro-enzymes and electrolytes for the digestion of carbohydrates, proteins, fats and nucleic acids; 1200–1500 mL/day is secreted from the exocrine acini of epithelial cells, which comprise 98% of the pancreatic mass. The remaining 2% is comprised of the endocrine islets of Langerhans innervated by the coeliac plexus and producing glucagon (alpha cells), insulin (beta cells), somatostatin (delta cells) and pancreatic polypeptide. (The endocrine function of the pancreas is described on p. 248).

Enzyme	Enzyme	Substrate	Product
Pepsinogens	Pro-enzyme converted to pepsin by gastric acid in the lumen	Proteins and polypeptides	Peptides
Gastric lipase		Triglycerides	Fatty acids and glycerol

Table 10.9 Gastric enzymes

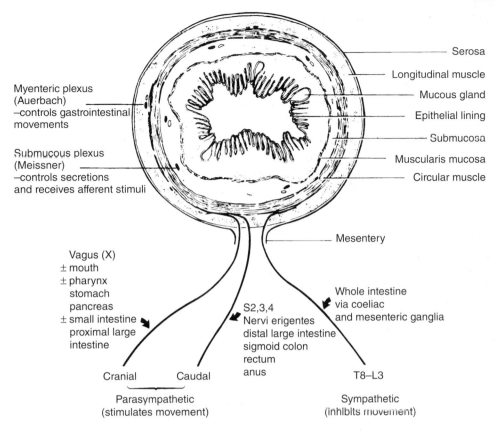

Myenteric plexus
(Auerbach)
–controls gastrointestinal
movements

Submucous plexus
(Meissner)
–controls secretions
and receives afferent stimuli

Serosa

Longitudinal muscle

Mucous gland

Epithelial lining

Submucosa

Muscularis mucosa

Circular muscle

Mesentery

Vagus (X)
± mouth
± pharynx
  stomach
  pancreas
± small intestine
  proximal large
  intestine

S2,3,4
Nervi erigentes
distal large intestine
sigmoid colon
rectum
anus

Whole intestine
via coeliac
and mesenteric ganglia

Cranial   Caudal

T8–L3

Parasympathetic
(stimulates movement)

Sympathetic
(inhibits movement)

Figure 10.21 • Schematic transverse section of the gut showing nerve supply.

Pancreatic juice neutralizes gastric juice to provide optimal pH for enzymes to function. Pancreatic enzyme functions are listed in Table 10.10.

Chyme in the duodenum causes the release of the hormone secretin, which induces the pancreas to produce large volumes of fluid rich in bicarbonate, but lacking in enzymes. A second hormone, cholecystokinin–pancreozymin, has the effect of releasing pancreatic enzymes and inducing the gall bladder to contract. Nervous stimulation of the pancreas occurs to a limited extent. Most fat digestion occurs in the duodenum as a result of the actions of pancreatic lipase. Activity is facilitated when fats are emulsified. Failure of the exocrine portion of the pancreas results in steatorrhoea, i.e. fatty, clay-coloured stools with an increased fat content. Absorption of the fat-soluble vitamins A, D, E and K is deficient if fat absorption is depressed because of lack of pancreatic enzymes or when bile is prevented from entering the intestine.

Small intestine

Digestion and absorption of nutrients, salt and water occur in the small intestine. Some 90% of all water absorption occurs here. Most vitamins are absorbed in the upper small intestine (vitamin B_{12} is absorbed in the terminal ileum). The reactions in the small intestine are shown in Table 10.11.

Small intestinal secretions are mainly induced by reflexes triggered by food stimulating local nerve endings. Brunner's glands secrete mucus, while the crypts of Lieberkühn exude a neutral fluid which is thought to aid absorption of chyle through the epithelial cells of the mucosa, where the constituent substances of chyle are acted on by proteolytic, lipolytic and glycolytic enzymes. Unlike other nutrients, B_{12} and bile salts are not absorbed in the small intestine but have specific receptors in the terminal ileum.

Large intestine (caecum, colon, rectum and anal canal)

Mechanics

In the ascending colon the haustrations propel semi-solid food by combined contractions of circular and longitudinal muscle. In the transverse and sigmoid colon, mass movement drives solid faeces towards the rectum.

Table 10.10 Pancreatic enzymes (exocrine)

Enzyme	Enzyme	Substrate	Product	
Maltase	Enzyme	Maltose	Glucose	
Amylase	Enzyme	Starch	Glucose, maltose and maltotriose	
Lipase	Enzyme	Fats	Free fatty acids and monoglycerides	
Nucleases (ribonuclease and deoxyribonuclease)	Enzyme	RNA & DNA	Nucleotides	
Trypsinogen	Pro-enzyme converted by enteropeptidase to trypsin	Proteins and polypeptides	Polypeptides/ peptides	Cleaves peptide bonds on carboxyl-side basic amino acids (arginine and lysine)
Chymotrypsinogen	Pro-enzyme activated by trypsin	Proteins and polypeptides	Polypeptides/ peptides	Cleaves peptide bonds on carboxyl-side aromatic amino acids
Pro-aminopeptidase	Pro-enzyme	Proteins and polypeptides	Polypeptides/ peptides	
Pro-carboxypeptidase	Pro-enzyme activated by trypsin	Proteins and polypeptides	Polypeptides/ peptides	Cleaves carboxyl terminal amino acids that have aromatic or branched aliphatic side chains
Phospholipase	Activated by trypsin	Phospholipids	Fatty acids	

Table 10.11 Small intestinal mucosal enzymes

Enzyme	Substrate	Product	
Aminopeptidases	Polypeptides	Peptides and amino acids	Cleaves terminal amino acid from peptide
Carboxypeptidase	Polypeptides	Peptides	Cleaves carboxyl terminal amino acid from peptide
Enteropeptidase (enterokinase)	Trypsinogen	Trypsin	
Endopeptidase	Polypeptides	Peptides	Cleaves between residues in mid-portion of peptide
Dipeptidase	Dipeptides	Amino acids	
Lactase	Lactose	Glucose and galactose	
Sucrase	Sucrose	Glucose and fructose	
Maltase	Maltose	Glucose	

Gut transit time is increased in pregnancy. Postulated mechanisms are delayed motility secondary to progesterone or the inhibitory action of motilin.

Digestive processes

Mucus from the goblet cells is produced under normal conditions by the direct contact of food stimulating local myenteric reflexes. No enzymes are secreted. Bacteria ferment any remaining carbohydrates releasing methane, hydrogen and carbon dioxide which is lost as flatus or dissolves to form organic acids rendering the stool slightly acid (pH 5–7). Ammonia is produced and not released if there is liver damage. This may result in raised serum concentrations of ammonia and hepatic encephalopathy. The mucosa of the large intestine facilitates absorption, hence the use of the rectum as a route for administration of drugs. Water, ions and some vitamins are absorbed in the large intestine. Na^+ is actively transported out of the colon and water follows passively along the osmotic gradient generated. Bacteria also decompose bile to give faeces their dark colour. Extreme irritation of the bowel wall, e.g. by infection, will result in the secretion of water and electrolytes, so resulting in diarrhoea. Under conditions of stress, parasympathetic stimulation of the nervi erigentes results in copious mucus secretion, which may also cause frequent bowel actions, but often without any concomitant faecal material.

Defaecation

The rectum is the last 20 cm of the gastrointestinal tract. The terminal 2–3 cm is the anal canal. Faeces entering the rectum stimulate reflex parasympathetic stimuli via the nervi erigentes to contract bowel muscle and relax the internal sphincter. If the external sphincter is not voluntarily contracted, defaecation will occur. Constipation affects up to 40% of pregnancies. The decreased physical activity of pregnancy coupled with iron ingestion contributes to the increased incidence which increases with parity and thus implies mechanical problems in the lower gastrointestinal tract have a contributory role. Constipation may be associated with an exacerbation of haemorrhoids and anal fissures.

Liver

Anatomical considerations

The adult liver weighs around 1.3 kg and contains about 100 000 lobules. The neonatal liver at term weighs around 145 g.

Each liver lobule surrounds a central vein as shown in Figure 10.22. The central vein drains to the hepatic vein.

The sinusoids are lined by Kupffer cells which, together with the endothelial cells, are powerfully phagocytic. Each sinusoid has a rich lymphatic supply.

Metabolic function

The metabolism of carbohydrate and fat is considered in Chapter 9, pp 152–158.

Carbohydrate

Glycogen storage Glycogen is synthesized from glucose and stored in the liver by the following reactions:

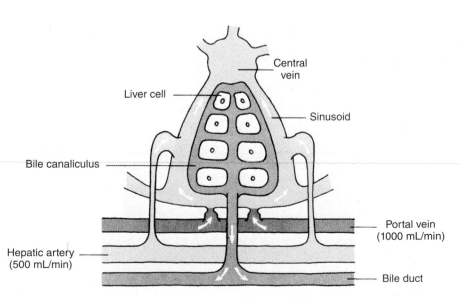

Figure 10.22 • Schematic representation of blood flow through a liver lobule.

1. Glycogen synthetase is activated by high plasma glucose and insulin levels, which thus increase the level of glycogen in the liver and decrease plasma glucose.
2. Phosphorylase is activated by low plasma glucose, adrenaline and glucagon levels, which therefore raise plasma glucose levels by catabolizing glycogen.

Galactose and fructose conversion Galactose and fructose are both converted to glucose in the liver by the following reactions:

Lactose $\xrightarrow[\text{small intestine}]{\text{Hydrolysis in}}$ **Galactose**

$\xrightarrow{\text{Galactokinase}}$ **Glucose**

Fructose $\xrightarrow{\text{Fructokinase}}$ **Glucose**
(**from fruit, sugar, honey**)

Gluconeogenesis Depletion of body stores of carbohydrate causes the liver to form glucose from glucogenic amino acids, which are derived from protein, and also from glycerol, which is derived from fat. Metabolic pathways are shown below:

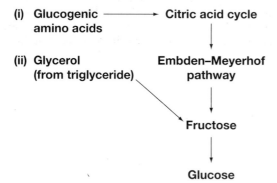

Fat

β-Oxidation and ketosis In states of carbohydrate deprivation or juvenile diabetes mellitus, fatty acids are metabolized to ketones as shown below:

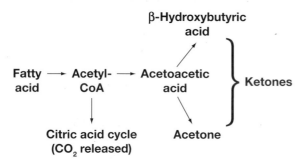

Synthesis of triglyceride (lipogenesis) The liver is able to synthesize triglyceride from fatty acids and glycerol, which are both derived from dietary carbohydrate. Triglyceride (neutral fat) is mainly concerned with energy expenditure:

$$R_1 \atop R_2 \atop R_3 \Bigg\} + {CH_2OH \atop CHOH \atop CH_2OH} \underset{\text{Lipolysis}}{\overset{\text{Esterification}}{\rightleftharpoons}} {CH_2OR_1 \atop CHOR_2 \atop CH_2OR_3}$$

3 fatty acids Glycerol   **Triglyceride**

Synthesis of lipoproteins In particular, the liver synthesizes very low-density lipoproteins (VLDL) and pre-β-lipoproteins, which are carrier proteins for plasma lipids.

Synthesis of phospholipids There are three types: lecithins, cephalins and sphingomyelins. Phospholipids are essentially structural lipids of body tissues. Lecithin is a powerful surface-active agent, reducing surface tension in the lung alveolae.

Synthesis of cholesterol Synthesis is complicated and takes place in several stages whereby acetyl-CoA ($CH_3COS–CoA$) is built up to form the steroid nucleus

and so to cholesterol. About 80% of all cholesterol synthesized is converted into bile acids.

Synthesis of fats This may also occur from excess dietary protein through the conversion of amino acids into acetyl-CoA.

Protein

Deamination of amino acids and urea formation This occurs by the removal of the amino ($–NH_2$) group from the amino acid. The ammonia produced by deamination is removed by combining it with carbon dioxide to form urea.

$$\begin{array}{c} NH_3 \\ \\ NH_3 \end{array} + CO_2 \longrightarrow \begin{array}{c} H_2N \\ \diagdown \\ \diagup \\ H_2N \end{array} C{=}O + H_2O$$

2 molecules of ammonia   **Urea**

Plasma proteins Virtually all albumin and fibrinogen are synthesized in the liver. Seventy per cent of globulin is synthesized in the liver and the remainder is synthesized in the reticuloendothelial system.

Bile

Volumes of the order 250–1100 mL of bile are secreted daily by the liver. The production of bile is increased by stimulation of the vagus nerves and by the hormone secretin. Bile is composed of bile salts, phospholipids, cholesterol, bile pigments (bilirubin and biliverdin) and protein. After reabsorption of the water and electrolytes, the concentrated bile is stored in the gall bladder.

Cholesterol

Cholesterol and triglycerides accumulate in the liver during normal pregnancy. Serum cholesterol levels rise by 25–50% and serum triglycerides by 150% from the fourth month of pregnancy to their peak at term. This, in association with the enlarged gall bladder and super-saturation of bile with cholesterol, contributes to the increased gallstone formation seen in pregnant women. During routine obstetric ultrasound 2–4% of women are found to have asymptomatic gallstones. Symptomatic disease occurs in only 0.5–1%.

Bile acids

Bile acids are transported across hepatocytes by specific transporters. Bile acid concentrations are often elevated in obstetric cholestasis, the cause of which is likely to relate to the interaction between inherited or acquired abnormalities in bile acid transporters and the altered physiology of pregnancy. Since bile contains significant quantities of sodium and potassium and the pH is alkaline, it is assumed that the bile acids and the associated conjugates exist in ionized form, hence

the term bile salts. Bile salts reduce surface tension and in conjunction with phospholipids and monoglycerides emulsify fats into micelles in preparation for their digestion and absorption in the small intestine (see p. 209). Some 95% of bile salts are re-absorbed from the small intestine. The remainder enter the colon and are converted by the action of intestinal microflora to secondary bile acids. A small fraction of these are then re-absorbed and the remainder lost in faeces.

Bilirubin

Bilirubin is one of the main breakdown products of haemoglobin and is excreted by the liver cells, as shown in Figure 10.23. Glucuronyl transferase catalyses conjugation of bilirubin with glucuronide rendering it water soluble for excretion. This enzyme is located in the smooth endoplasmic reticulum. Other compounds compete with bilirubin for the enzyme system, e.g. steroids and some drugs. Barbiturates, antihistamines and anticonvulsants cause proliferation of the smooth endoplasmic reticulum and increase glucuronyl transferase activity.

Hyperbilirubinaemia may occur because of excess production (pre-hepatic) or reduced elimination (hepatic or post-hepatic) of bilirubin. In pre-hepatic jaundice the hyperbilirubinaemia is due to excess production or failure of hepatic uptake and thus bilirubin is unconjugated and insoluble. It does not therefore

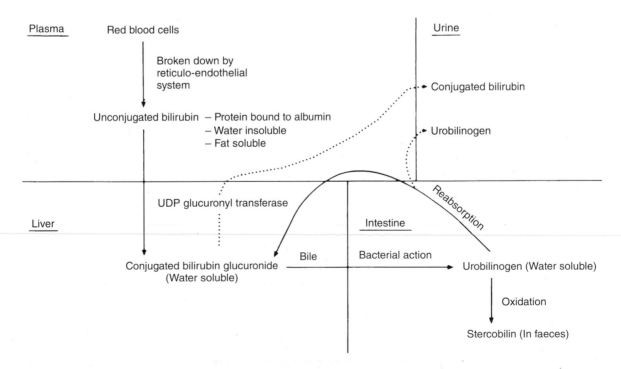

Figure 10.23 • Diagram to illustrate the breakdown and excretion of bilirubin.

appear in the urine. Examples include haemolysis or congenital hyperbilirubinaemia (Gilbert's syndrome). In hepatic jaundice, the defect lies at the level of the hepatocyte whose function is impaired. Both conjugated and unconjugated bilirubin appear in the urine, e.g. viral infection (hepatitis A), drugs (phenothiazines) or cirrhosis. In post-hepatic jaundice, excretion of bilirubin into the biliary system is impaired and conjugated bilirubin in plasma is elevated. Conjugated bilirubin is water soluble and therefore excreted into the urine which is thus dark in colour. Because the bilirubin is not lost to the faeces, the stools are pale. Clinical examples include gallstones, carcinoma of the pancreas, primary biliary cirrhosis or structural abnormalities of the biliary tree.

In the neonate, physiological jaundice results from the inability of the immature liver to conjugate bilirubin. When the unconjugated (fat soluble) bilirubin level exceeds 350 μmol/L, it can no longer be tightly bound to the albumin and so penetrates the blood–brain barrier. This may result in kernicterus where bilirubin staining of the brain occurs producing an encephalopathy with seizures, cerebral palsy and deafness. It is very rare in the term infant but those born prematurely or who are compromised in other ways are at particular risk. Phototherapy alters the shape of the bilirubin molecule in exposed skin, rendering it more water soluble and facilitating secretion.

Cholesterol and alkaline phosphatase are excreted in bile, as are adrenocortical and other steroid hormones. Some of the constituents of bile, e.g. bile acids, are re-absorbed in the terminal ileum and then excreted again by the liver (enterohepatic circulation). This may be interrupted by some drugs (e.g. chelating agents: cholestyramine), ileal disease or bacterial overgrowth causing increased de-conjugation. The latter is of particular relevance as it accounts for the reduced efficacy of the combined oral contraceptive pill during periods of gastrointestinal infection or antibiotic use.

Testing liver function

Laboratory tests of liver function which are widely available for clinical use are bilirubin, albumin, total protein, alanine aminotransferase (ALT), aspartate aminotransferase (AST), gamma glutamyl transpeptidase (GGT) and alkaline phosphatase (ALP). Particular patterns of abnormality in liver function may be helpful in determining the site of damage within the liver, with important exceptions in pregnancy.

Transaminases (AST and ALT) are elevated in hepatocellular damage; ALP and GGT are produced by cells lining the bile canaliculi and are elevated when liver damage occurs at this site. Liver function (rather than liver damage) is reflected by serum albumin and bilirubin which are reduced (reduced synthesis) and elevated (reduced excretion), respectively, in disease.

In pregnancy, serum values for ALT, AST, bilirubin and GGT fall and concentrations are 20% lower than the quoted reference ranges for non-pregnant individuals. Possible mechanisms include a dilutional effect as a result of the expanded plasma volume of pregnancy, an increase in hepatic blood flow or reduced function of the enzymes (and therefore reduced release). Albumin (and total protein) concentrations fall by 20–40% in pregnancy as a result of the increased blood volume. This fall does not reflect reduced synthetic function as it might outside pregnancy. Alkaline phosphatase concentrations rise in the third trimester of pregnancy as the enzyme is produced and released by the placenta. Individual iso-enzyme assays are available; alternatively the proportion of ALP that is placental in origin can be determined by demonstrating the iso-enzyme's instability on heating. Upper limits of normal for pregnancy have been suggested to be three-fold those of non-pregnant individuals, and concentrations in excess of these may suggest disease.

Liver function tests may also be affected by mode of delivery; ALT and AST rise after caesarean section and by a smaller degree after vaginal delivery.

An additional important functional role of the liver is in glucose homeostasis, and hypoglycaemia can occur in disease, e.g. acute fatty liver of pregnancy. The liver is the site of synthesis of blood coagulation substrates such as fibrinogen, prothrombin and factor VII. It also synthesizes clotting factors II, VII, IX and X which all require vitamin K. All are important markers of liver synthetic function. Function can be tested by measuring the prothrombin time, which is dependent on many of the clotting factors and, although insensitive, can be an early indicator of severe acute liver damage. A prolonged prothrombin time can be corrected with vitamin K in some disease states (e.g. vitamin K deficiency results if there is obstructed bile flow, as in cholestasis) but not in severe hepatitis or chronic liver disease. Clotting factors II, IX and X are raised in normal pregnancies.

Miscellaneous functions

The liver is also concerned in the storage of vitamins, particularly A, D and B_{12}, and in the storage of iron:

Apoferritin + Iron $\rightleftharpoons$ Ferritin

Many drugs, chemical substances and body compounds are also metabolized and excreted through the liver with bile, e.g. antibiotics (penicillin, sulphonamides, etc.), steroid hormones (oestrogen, cortisol), alcohol and calcium.

Nervous system

This section outlines the organization and function of the nervous system.

All integrated neural activity is based on the reflex arc, the process whereby the afferent neurone is stimulated, by either a sense organ or another nerve. The stimulus is transmitted at a synapse to the efferent neurone, and conducted either to another neurone or to an effector organ such as muscle cell (Fig. 10.24).

Nervous transmission is an all-or-nothing effect. If there is sufficient depolarization of the nerve membrane, the impulse will be propagated. If the nerve is not sufficiently depolarized, impulse propagation does not occur. Thus the stimulus from the afferent neurone has to be sufficiently strong to stimulate the efferent neurone. The threshold for nervous transmission at the synapse can be up- or downregulated by other neurones impinging on the efferent neurone. Somatic neurones innervate somatic, striped muscle; visceral neurones innervate smooth and cardiac musculature as part of the autonomic nervous system.

Somatic nervous system

Somatic afferent neurones enter the spinal cord via the dorsal roots or cranial nerves, and efferent neurones leave via the ventral roots or the motor cranial nerves.

The simplest reflex is a monosynaptic reflex of which the only example is the stretch reflex. When a muscle is stretched, the spindles within the muscles are stimulated, which causes a discharge in the afferent neurone. The afferent neurone stimulates the efferent motor neurone at a single synapse in the spinal cord; impulses pass down the motor neurone to the muscle, which then contracts.

Motor system

Most reflexes are polysynaptic with several (often hundreds) of synapses between the sensory receptor and the effector cell. Many different afferent neurones may synapse with each efferent neurone. Thus the motor neurone also receives synapses from nerves originating in the cerebral cortex which allow voluntary control of movement. The motor system is conventionally divided into lower motor neurones, spinal and cranial nerves which directly innervate muscles, and upper motor neurones, those of the brain and spinal cord that innervate lower motor neurones. Lesions of lower motor neurones cause a flaccid paralysis with wasting. Lesions of upper motor neurones often cause a spastic paralysis without initial wasting.

The major innervation from the cortex to somatic muscular cells in humans is via the pyramidal system (Figs 10.25–10.27). Nerves which have their cell bodies in the specialized motor area of the cerebral cortex descend via the internal capsule. About 80% cross the midline in the pyramidal decussation to form the lateral corticospinal tract. The remaining 20% descend the anterior corticospinal tract and cross just before their termination at the spinal lower motor neurone. Current evidence indicates that there are several other areas in the brain which can generate voluntary muscular movement apart from the precentral gyrus, the specialized area where movement of each part of the body is spatially located.

The pyramidal tracts are probably responsible for skilled, fine movement. In addition, the lower motor neurone receives innervation from many other sources. The stretch receptors, acting at a local spinal segmental level, have already been mentioned. The action of these stretch receptors is modulated both by local nervous influences (γ efferent system), which in turn are affected by descending fibres from the cerebrum. The lower motor neurone itself is also innervated from the cerebrum via extrapyramidal tracts, responsible for gross movements and posture, and by fibres from the cerebellum, which are concerned with coordination and control.

Sensory system

Sensation can be divided into the modalities of the special sensory organs – vision, hearing, taste and smell – and the more generalized sensations of pain, touch, temperature and joint position sense. The specialized sensory organs are outside the scope of this book. The

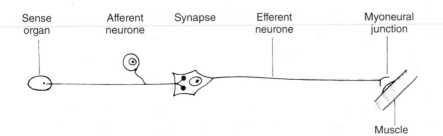

Figure 10.24 • The reflex arc. (Reproduced with permission from Ganong W. Review of medical physiology. Lange Medical, Los Altos, CA.)

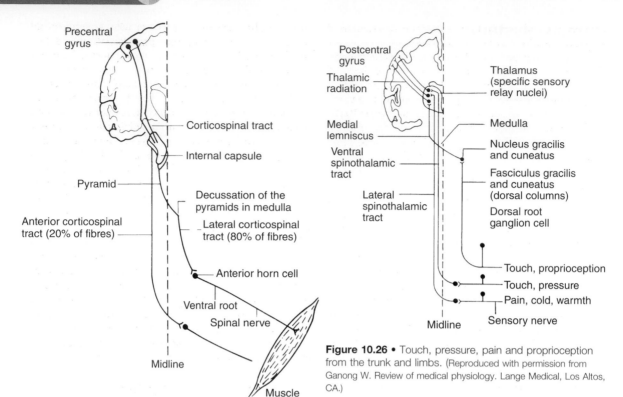

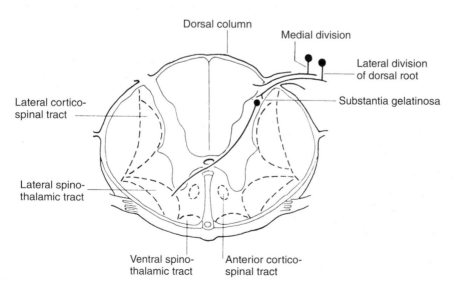

Figure 10.25 • The corticospinal tracts. (Reproduced with permission from Ganong W. Review of medical physiology. Lange Medical, Los Altos, CA.)

Figure 10.26 • Touch, pressure, pain and proprioception from the trunk and limbs. (Reproduced with permission from Ganong W. Review of medical physiology. Lange Medical, Los Altos, CA.)

Figure 10.27 • Major spinal pathways. (Reproduced with permission from Ganong W. Review of medical physiology. Lange Medical, Los Altos, CA.)

organization and cerebral representation of generalized sensation require further consideration.

Primary afferent fibres from specific receptors enter the spinal cord via the dorsal root. They have their cell bodies in the dorsal root ganglion. Those fibres that come from receptors for proprioception and fine touch ascend in the dorsal columns to the medulla (Figs 10.26, 10.27). There they synapse with second-order neurones in the cuneate and gracile nuclei. The second-order neurones cross the midline, at the level of the medulla, and ascend via the medial lemniscus to the thalamus. Neurones project from the thalamus to at least two areas on the cortex. The most precise localization is at somatic sensory area I in the postcentral gyrus. Here each part of the body is specifically represented, and within each area are columns of cells which react to specific sensory modalities (e.g. proprioception and fine touch). A second sensory area, somatic sensory area II, is in the wall of the Sylvian fissure. Here representation of the body is not so complete, nor so specific.

Fibres from pain and temperature receptors and some other touch receptors also enter the spinal cord via the dorsal root, but synapse with nerves in the substantia gelatinosa of the dorsal horn. Fibres from these neurones cross the midline immediately (cf. spinothalamic tracts) and then ascend in the anterolateral system of the spinal cord (lateral columns) (Figs 10.26, 10.27). Touch ascends the ventral spinothalamic tract; pain and temperature ascend the lateral spinothalamic tract. These fibres also project to the thalamus and then synapse with other neurones passing to somatic sensory areas I and II. However, the sensations carried by the anterolateral system are not so exclusively represented in the cerebral cortex as those carried by the spinothalamic tracts. Experimental abla-tion, or observations on patients with spontaneously occurring lesions, show that proprioception and fine touch (spinothalamic tract) are most affected by cortical lesions. Temperature sensation is less affected and pain sensation (lateral columns) is barely affected at all.

The 'gate' theory accounts for the observation that individuals' perception of pain varies enormously both between individuals and within individuals on different occasions. Many external and internal influences, such as hypnosis, acupuncture and analgesic drugs, can affect pain perception, and probably do so by influencing transmission of impulses from pain receptors at many sites within the central nervous system. One site that has been extensively investigated is in the substantia gelatinosa of the spinal cord (Fig. 10.27), where pain afferent neurones synapse with fibres that will ascend in the lateral columns. Transmission here can be inhibited by stimulation of other fibres, mediating touch or proprioception in the adjacent spinothalamic tract. Stimulation of these fibres has been used clinically in the relief of pain. The fibres may be stimulated either in the skin (as in the treatment of trigeminal neuralgia using an electrical stimulator) or by implantation of chronic stimulators in the dorsal columns.

Reticular activating system

Apart from the classical projection of sensory input to the cortex, some sensory fibres activate the reticular activating system. This is a diffuse system of nerve fibres in the ventral portion of the midbrain and medulla which appears to be responsible for consciousness and to require sensory input to maintain consciousness (Fig. 10.28). Thus, blunting of sensory input, either experimentally or when, for example,

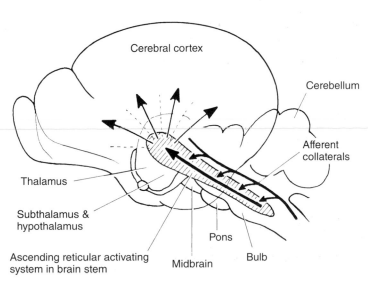

Figure 10.28 • Diagram of ascending reticular activating system. (Reproduced with permission from Starzl TE, Taylor CW, Magoun HW 1951 Collateral afferent excitation of reticular formation of brain stem. Journal of Neurophysiology 14:479–496.)

Cerebral cortex

Cerebellum

Afferent collaterals

Thalamus

Subthalamus & hypothalamus

Pons

Ascending reticular activating system in brain stem

Midbrain

Bulb

prisoners are 'hooded' for interrogation purposes, is associated with disturbed states of consciousness and hallucinations. Patients with tumours that interrupt the reticular activating system are usually unconscious and, if the tumours are small, may be comatose without any other clinical signs. It appears that the reticular activating system integrates all sensory inputs, and that sensory specificity is therefore not important for its function. The reticular activating system contains the respiratory and cardiovascular centres, and can up- or downregulate sensation, motor activity, the electrical activity of the cortex, and many endocrine activities via its hypothalamic connections.

Autonomic nervous system

Like the somatic nervous system, the autonomic nervous system has afferent nerves from receptors, central integrating areas (vasomotor centre and respiratory centre) and efferent neurones which run to effector organs. The receptors may be specific to stimuli, such as pressure (carotid sinus baroreceptor) or PO_2 (carotid body chemoreceptor); there are also non-specific receptors in the viscera which respond to pain. Afferents reach the central nervous system via the facial, glossopharyngeal and vagus cranial nerves, and via the dorsal roots from T7 to L2 and from S2 to S4.

The efferent tract of the autonomic nervous system consists of preganglionic fibres followed by postganglionic fibres. The parasympathetic outflow to the visceral structures of the head is via cranial nerves III, VII and IX, to the thorax and upper abdomen via the vagus nerve, and to the pelvis via the sacral outflow, S2–S4. The preganglionic fibres end in, or very near, the viscus that is innervated. These synapse with short postganglionic fibres that run directly to the effector organ (Fig. 10.29).

By contrast, the sympathetic nervous system is characterized by a chain of ganglia that run outside the spinal cord, but adjacent to it from T1 to L5. The chain is extended towards the head to form three additional cervical ganglia: the superior, middle and inferior or stellate ganglia. The axons of the preganglionic sympathetic nerves leave the spinal cord in the ventral roots of the spinal nerves, and pass via the white rami communicantes to the paravertebral sympathetic ganglion chain. There they synapse with the postganglionic fibres, which run to the viscera. Some postganglionic fibres return to the spinal nerves, via the grey rami communicantes, and then are distributed with the spinal nerves to the autonomic effectors in the appropriate somatic structures innervated by these spinal nerves. Other sympathetic preganglionic fibres do not end in the paravertebral chain, but pass through it to collateral ganglia (coeliac ganglions, superior and inferior mesenteric ganglia) near the viscera that they

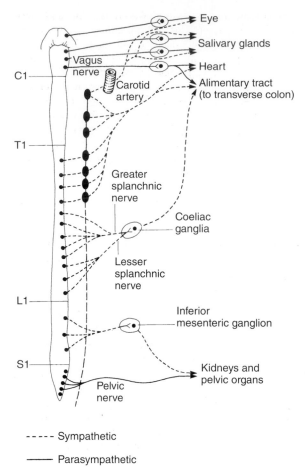

Figure 10.29 • Diagram of the efferent automatic pathways.

innervate. Short postganglionic fibres then run to each viscus.

The uterus is unusual in that the preganglionic sympathetic fibres run all the way to the uterus and anastomose there with postganglionic fibres. The adrenal medulla is also atypical in that it is innervated by preganglionic sympathetic nerves that pass to it through the coeliac ganglion without synapsing. Alternatively, the adrenal medulla may be considered as a specialized postganglionic nerve that secretes adrenaline, as well as noradrenaline, directly into the bloodstream, rather than secreting noradrenaline at the postganglionic nerve ending.

Chemical transmission in the autonomic nervous system and autonomic pharmacology

Parasympathetic nervous system Chemical transmission at ganglia and at the ends of postganglionic fibres stimulating smooth muscle and glands is by acetylcholine. The postganglionic effects of acetylcholine are mimicked by the alkaloid muscarine, and these are therefore known as the muscarine actions of acetylcholine. They are blocked by atropine. Transmission at the ganglia is mimicked by nicotine, the nicotinic action of acetylcholine, and this is not blocked by atropine. It is blocked by very high concentrations of acetylcholine. The acetylcholine is metabolized by cholinesterase. Drugs that interfere with cholinesterase activity, e.g. physostigmine, will potentiate transmission at the autonomic ganglia, and at the postganglionic nerve ending (these drugs will also potentiate somatic neuromuscular transmission).

Sympathetic nervous system Transmission at the ganglia is by the nicotinic action of acetylcholine. Transmission at most postganglionic nerve endings is by noradrenaline (norepinephrine). Some drugs, such as tyramine or ephedrine, increase sympathetic activity by enhancing noradrenaline release at the postganglionic nerve ending.

Those sympathetic postganglionic neurones which innervate sweat glands are cholinergic (acetylcholine as a transmitter), and so are the sympathetic postganglionic fibres which cause vasodilatation in smooth muscle.

Noradrenaline (norepinephrine) is one of a group of substances, the catecholamines. The other principal catecholamine found outside the central nervous system is adrenaline (epinephrine) secreted by the adrenal medulla. Dopamine is on the metabolic pathway of adrenaline and noradrenaline. So far, it has mainly been studied within the central nervous system and hypothalamopituitary axis, where, for example, dopamine inhibits prolactin release. However, it is likely that dopamine also has peripheral actions, e.g. involvement in the control of renal blood flow.

The catecholamine receptors are divided into α- and β-receptors on the basis of the drugs which block transmission at the receptor site. α-Receptors, blocked by phentolamine and phenoxybenzamine, can be separated from β-receptors blocked by propranolol.

In general, α-receptors are excitatory (vasoconstriction, pupillary constriction) and β-receptors are inhibitory (bronchodilatation, decreased uterine activity). An important exception is the heart, where β-receptors are excitatory. Not all β-receptors are the same. Some β adrenergic blocking drugs chiefly affect the heart; these are β_1-adrenergic blocking agents, or cardioselective beta-blocking agents, of which the prototype was practolol. Less toxic agents in current clinical usage are metoprolol and atenolol. Other β-receptors are designated as β_2-receptors. These are found in the bronchi and the uterus, and non-selective β-adrenergic blocking agents (e.g. propranolol) block both β_1- and β_2-receptors. The development of specific α-, β_1- and β_2-receptor blocking agents allowed the differentiation of both naturally occurring and synthetic catecholamines into α, β_1 and β_2 agonists. Thus adrenaline and noradrenaline stimulate both α- and β_1-receptors, but adrenaline also stimulates β_2-receptors. Metaraminol and phenylephrine are specific α agonists. Isoprenaline is a specific β agonist which stimulates both β_1- and β_2-receptors. Salbutamol, orciprenaline, terbutaline and ritodrine, all of which have been used for the treatment of premature labour, stimulate β_2-receptors more than β_1 and so cause relaxation of the uterus. In addition, these drugs cause bronchial dilatation, and most have been used and were developed for the treatment of asthma (the exception is ritodrine).

A list of adrenergic (sympathetic) and cholinergic (mainly parasympathetic) activity is given in Table 10.12. Table 10.13 shows some of the drugs that influence autonomic activity.

Blood

Iron metabolism

Iron is abundant in most soils and waters of the Earth's surface. It is easily and reversibly oxidized or reduced. It has been incorporated into numerous proteins of critical importance for the sustenance of both plant and animal life.

The total body iron content of a normal adult male is approximately 50 mg/kg, that of an adult women about 38 mg/kg. This difference merely reflects the high incidence of reduced iron stores in women; there are no fundamental differences in iron metabolism between the sexes.

The iron is distributed in several physiologically and chemically distinct forms (Table 10.14). Haemoglobin iron comprises about 70% of the total body iron and is the largest iron-containing compartment.

The other haem-containing molecule is myoglobin, a protein present in muscle. It is said to provide a reserve of available oxygen in cases of sudden strenuous exercise.

Storage iron is held available for use as needed in the macrophages of the reticuloendothelial system and is in two forms: ferritin, which is a glycoprotein detectable by chemical analysis, and aggregates of ferritin, which form haemosiderin.

A very small amount of iron is contained in the enzymes – cytochromes, catalases and peroxidases essential for metabolism of all cells in the body.

A minute portion of the total iron (0.19%) is bound to a specific plasma protein – transferrin (Table 10.14).

The total iron content of the body tends to remain fixed within narrow limits; otherwise iron excess (siderosis) or deficiency occurs. Iron is not excreted in the usual sense of the word; it is lost from the body only when cells are lost, especially epithelial cells from the gastrointestinal tract. Urinary iron amounts to

Table 10.12 Responses of organs to cholinergic and adrenergic stimuli

Organ	Response	
	Adrenergic (α/β)	Cholinergic
Pupil	Constriction (α) Dilatation (β)	Constriction
Salivary glands	Scanty viscid secretion (α)	Copious watery secretion
Blood vessels Heart Skin Muscle Pulmonary Kidney	Constrictor (α) Dilator (β_2) Constrictor (α) Constrictor (α) Dilator (β_2) Constrictor (α) Constrictor (α)	Dilator Dilator
Lung Bronchi Bronchial glands	Relaxation (β_2)	Constriction Increased secretion
Heart Rate, contractility, conduction velocity	Increased (β_1)	Decrease
Kidney Renin secretion	Increased (β_2)	
Sweating	Localized, e.g. palms of hands (α)	Generalized
Pregnant uterus	Decreased contraction (β_2) Increased contraction (α)	

<0.05 mg/day in desquamated cells. In women, menstrual flow constitutes an important additional route of iron loss. Average daily loss has been estimated to be about 1.0 mg/day in normal adult men and non-menstruating women. About twice this amount is lost in menstruating women. In normal situations, these losses are balanced by an equivalent amount of iron absorbed from the diet. Therefore, iron balance is unique in that it is achieved by control of absorption rather than control of excretion.

Iron absorption

Since the total body iron content depends so greatly on absorption of iron, the mechanisms by which the rate of absorption is regulated are of critical importance.

Iron is absorbed chiefly in portions of the intestine proximal to the jejunum. Maximum absorption occurs in the duodenum.

Two factors are of prime importance in determining absorptive rate:

1. The amount of storage iron. When it is depleted, iron absorption is increased. When it is excessive, iron absorption is decreased.
2. The rate of erythropoiesis. Iron absorption goes up when red cell production rate is increased and down when production is decreased.

Iron absorption takes place in two distinct steps:

1. Mucosal uptake.
2. Transfer of iron from mucosal cell to plasma.

The uptake of iron by the mucosa is influenced by the overall composition of the diet, which determines how much iron is available for absorption (see below).

A normal mixed diet supplies about 14 mg iron each day, of which only 1–2 mg is absorbed. The availability in food is quite variable. In most foods, inorganic iron is in the ferric form (Fe^{+++}) and has to be converted to the ferrous form (Fe^{++}) before absorption can take place. In foods derived from grain, iron often forms a stable complex with phytates and only small amounts can be converted to a soluble form. The iron in eggs is poorly absorbed because of binding with phosphates present in the yolk. Milk, particularly cow's milk, is poor in iron content. Tea (tannins) inhibits the absorption of iron. Gastric acid and vitamin C promote reduction of ferric iron (Fe^{+++}) to ferrous iron (Fe^{++}) which is more easily absorbed.

Haem iron derived from haemoglobin and myoglobin of animal origin is more effectively absorbed than non-haem iron. Factors interfering with or promoting the absorption of inorganic iron have no effect on the absorption of haem iron. This puts vegetarians at a disadvantage in terms of iron sufficiency.

Iron cycle

The metabolism of iron is dominated by its role in haemoglobin synthesis. In this process iron is utilized repeatedly so that the internal movements of iron may be described as a cycle (Fig. 10.30). Central to this cycle is the plasma compartment in which iron is bound to a transport protein – transferrin. Iron moves from plasma to cells that have the capacity to make haemoglobin. At the end of the red cells' 120-day lifespan, they are ingested by macrophages of the reticuloendothelial system. There, iron is extracted from haemoglobin, delivered to the plasma and bound to transferrin, completing the cycle. A small amount of iron, probably less than 2.0 mg, leaves the plasma each day to enter the hepatic cells and other tissues. Here,

Table 10.13 Some drugs influencing autonomic activity

Site of action	Agents decreasing activity	Agents increasing activity

Sympathetic and parasympathetic ganglia	High concentration of acetylcholine
	Ganglion-blocking agents:
	   Hexamethonium
	   Mecamylamine
	   Pentolinium
	   Trimetaphan
		Acetylcholine
		Carbachol
		Nicotine
		Anticholinesterase drugs, e.g. physostigmine

Endings of parasympathetic neurones	Atropine
	Scopolamine
	Propantheline
		Anticholinesterase drugs:
		   Acetylcholine
		   Carbachol
		   Muscarine
		   Pilocarpine

Sympathetic postganglionic nerve endings	Reserpine
	Guanethidine
		Drugs releasing noradrenaline:
		   Ephedrine
		   Amphetamines
		   Tyrosine

β_1-receptors	Propranolol Atenolol Metoprolol Practolol } Also block β_2-receptors to a lesser extent	Isoprenaline Adrenaline Noradrenaline
β_2-receptors	Propranolol	Adrenaline Isoprenaline Salbutamol Orciprenaline Terbutaline Ritodrine } Also β_1 but mainly β_2
α-receptors	Phenoxybenzamine Phentolamine	Noradrenaline Adrenaline Metaraminol Methoxamine Phenylephrine

Table 10.14 Distribution of iron

Location	Form	Distribution (%)
Haemoglobin iron		70
Tissue iron		30

Storage iron
  Essential iron
	Haemosiderin
	Ferritin
	Myoglobin
	Enzymes
	  Cytochromes
	  Peroxidases
	  Catalases	

Plasma transport iron	Transferrin	0.19

the iron is utilized to make tissue haem proteins such as myoglobin and the cytochromes.

Haemopoiesis and iron metabolism in pregnancy

There is increased erythropoiesis from early pregnancy due to increased erythropoietin production and possibly due to other hormones such as placental lactogen. In spite of this, some degree of anaemia, as judged by normal non-pregnant standards, is manifest by the end of the second trimester. This is due to haemodilution and occurs because the increase in plasma volume (50%) exceeds that of the red cell mass (18–25%). The haemoglobin reaches its lowest level at 32 weeks of gestation, when the haemodilution is maximal

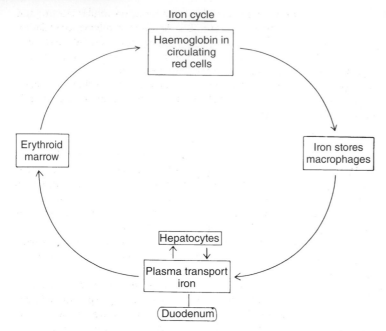

Iron cycle

Figure 10.30 • The iron cycle.

(see p. 186). The haemodilution is exaggerated in twin pregnancies.

In pregnancy, the demand for iron is increased to meet mainly the needs of the expanded red cell mass and, to a lesser extent, the requirements of the developing fetus and placenta. The fetus derives its iron from the maternal serum by active transport across the placenta predominantly in the last 4 weeks of pregnancy. The total requirement of iron is about 700–1400 mg. Overall, the requirement is 4 mg/day, but this rises from 2.8 mg/day in the non-pregnant woman to 6.6 mg/day in the last few weeks of pregnancy. This can be met only by mobilizing iron stores in addition to achieving maximum absorption of dietary iron.

Iron absorption is increased when there is erythroid hyperplasia, i.e. rapid iron turnover and a high concentration of unsaturated transferrin, both of which are part of the physiological response in the healthy pregnant woman. There is evidence that absorption of dietary iron is enhanced in the latter half of pregnancy, but this still does not provide enough iron for the needs of pregnancy and the puerperium for a woman on a normal mixed diet.

The amount of iron absorbed will depend very much on the extent of the iron stores, the content of the diet and whether or not iron supplements are given.

The commonest haematological problem in pregnancy is anaemia resulting from iron deficiency.

Iron deficiency in pregnancy

The changes in blood volume and haemodilution are so variable that the normal range of haemoglobin concentration in healthy pregnancy at 30 weeks of gestation in women who have received parenteral iron is 10.5–14.5 g/dL. However, haemoglobin values of less than 10.5 g/dL in the second and third trimesters are probably abnormal and require further investigation.

Red cell indices

The appearance of red cells on a stained film is a relatively insensitive gauge of iron status in pregnancy. Most hospital laboratories now possess electronic counters, allowing accurate red cell counts to be performed. The size of the red cell (mean cell volume, MCV), its haemoglobin content (mean corpuscular haemoglobin, MCH) and haemoglobin concentration (MCHC) can be calculated from the red cell count (red blood cell count, RBC), haemoglobin concentration and packed cell volume (PCV).

A better guide to the diagnosis of iron deficiency in pregnancy is the examination of these red cell indices. The earliest effect of iron deficiency on the erythrocyte is a reduction in MCV, and in pregnancy, with the dramatic changes in red cell mass and plasma volume, this is the most sensitive indicator of underlying iron deficiency. Hypochromia and a fall in the MCHC only appear with more severe degrees of iron depletion. However MCV is elevated in pregnancy, and in B_{12} or folate deficiency and hypothyroidism.

Some women start pregnancy with already established anaemia due to iron deficiency or with grossly depleted iron stores and they will quickly develop florid anaemia with reduced MCV, MCH and MCHC.

Serum iron and total iron-binding capacity (TIBC)

The serum iron of a healthy, adult, non-pregnant woman lies between 13 and 27 µmol/L. Serum iron levels vary markedly and even fluctuate from hour to hour. The TIBC in the woman in a non-pregnant state lies in the range 45–72 µmol/L. It is raised in association with iron deficiency and is low in chronic inflammatory states. In the non-anaemic individual the TIBC is approximately one-third saturated with iron.

In pregnancy, there is a fall in the serum iron and percentage saturation of the TIBC; the fall in serum iron can be largely prevented by iron supplements. Serum iron, even in combination with the TIBC, is not a reliable indication of iron stores because it fluctuates so widely and is affected by recent ingestion of iron or factors such as infection, which are not directly involved with iron metabolism. With these major reservations, a serum iron of <12 µmol/L and a TIBC saturation of <15% indicates iron deficiency in pregnancy.

Ferritin

Ferritin is a high-molecular-weight glycoprotein, which circulates in the plasma. The normal plasma concentration is 15–300 µg/L. It is stable and not affected by recent ingestion of iron. It appears to reflect the iron stores accurately and quantitatively, particularly in the lower range associated with iron deficiency, which is so important in pregnancy.

Haemostasis

Haemostatic mechanisms have two functions:

1. To confine the circulating blood to the vascular bed.
2. To arrest bleeding from injured vessels.

Both of these aspects of haemostasis probably depend on:

- Normal vasculature
- Platelets – number and function
- Coagulation factors
- Healthy fibrinolysis.

Haemostasis and pregnancy

Normal pregnancy is accompanied by dramatic changes in the coagulation and fibrinolytic systems. There is a marked increase in some of the coagulation factors, particularly fibrinogen. Fibrin is laid down in the uteroplacental vessel walls and fibrinolysis is suppressed. These changes, together with the increased blood volume, help to combat the hazard of haemorrhage at placental separation but play only a secondary role to the unique process of myometrial contraction, which reduces blood flow to the placental site. They also produce a vulnerable state for intravascular clotting and a whole spectrum of disorders involving coagulation which may occur in pregnancy; these fall into two main groups: thromboembolism and bleeding due to disseminated intravascular coagulation.

A short account of haemostasis during pregnancy and how it differs from non-pregnant haemostasis follows.

Vascular integrity

It is not known how vascular integrity is normally maintained but it is clear that the platelets have a key role to play because conditions in which their number is depleted or they function abnormally are characterized by widespread spontaneous capillary haemorrhages. In health, the platelets are constantly sealing microdefects of the vasculature, minifibrin clots being formed; the unwanted fibrin is then removed by a process of fibrinolysis.

Prostacyclin (PGI_2) is an unstable prostaglandin first discovered in 1976. It is the principal prostanoid synthesized by blood vessels and is a powerful vasodilator and potent inhibitor of platelet aggregation. It has been proposed that there is a balance between the production of PGI_2 and thromboxane, a powerful platelet-aggregating agent and vasoconstrictor. Prostacyclin prevents aggregation at much lower concentrations than is needed to prevent adhesion. Therefore, vascular damage leads to platelet adhesion but not necessarily to aggregation and thrombus formation.

When the injury is minor, small platelet thrombi form and are washed away by the circulation as described earlier, but the extent of the injury is an important determinant of the size of the thrombus and whether or not platelet aggregation is stimulated. Prostacyclin synthetase is abundant in the intima and progressively decreases in concentration from the intima to the adventitia. In contrast the pro-aggregating elements increase in concentration from the subendothelium to the adventitia. It follows that severe vessel damage or physical detachment of the endothelium will lead to the development of a large thrombus rather than simple platelet adherence.

Deficiency of prostacyclin production has been suggested in platelet consumption syndromes such as the haemolytic uraemic syndrome.

Prostacyclin production has been shown to be reduced in fetal and placental tissue from pre-eclamptic pregnancies and the current role of prostacyclin in the pathogenesis of this disease is undergoing active investigation.

There have been several conflicting reports concerning the platelet count during pregnancy. There is probably no significant change in uncomplicated, healthy pregnancy even towards term, but a decrease in the platelet count has been observed in pregnancies with fetal growth restriction, whether or not pre-eclampsia was implicated. There is no evidence of changes in platelet function, or differences in platelet lifespan, between healthy non-pregnant and pregnant women, although the lifespan is shortened significantly when pre-eclampsia is present.

Arrest of bleeding after trauma

An essential function of the haemostatic system is a rapid reaction to injury, which remains confined to the area of damage. This requires control mechanisms which will stimulate coagulation after trauma and limit the extent of the response. The substances involved in the formation of the haemostatic plug normally circulate in an inert form until activated at the site of injury or by some factor released into the circulation which will trigger off intravascular coagulation.

Local response

Platelets adhere to collagen on the injured basement membrane. This initiates a series of changes in the platelets themselves, including a change in their shape and release of ADP (adenosine diphosphate) and other substances. ADP release stimulates further aggregation of platelets, the coagulation cascade is triggered off and the action of thrombin leads to the formation of fibrin, which converts the loose platelet plug into a firm, stable wound seal. The role of platelets is of less importance in injury involving large vessels because platelet aggregates are of insufficient size and strength to breach the defect. The coagulation mechanism is of major importance here, together with vascular contraction.

Coagulation system

The end result of blood coagulation is the formation of an insoluble fibrin clot from the soluble precursor fibrinogen in the plasma. This involves a complex interaction of clotting factors and a sequential activation of a series of pro-enzymes, which has been termed the coagulation cascade (Fig. 10.31). When a blood vessel is injured, blood coagulation is initiated by activation of factor XII by collagen (intrinsic mechanism) and activation of factor VII by thromboplastin release (extrinsic mechanism from the damaged tissue). But the intrinsic and extrinsic mechanisms are activated by components of the vessel wall and both are required for normal haemostasis.

Strict divisions between the two pathways do not exist and interactions between activated factors in both pathways have been shown. They share a common pathway following activation of factor X.

The intrinsic pathway, or contact system, proceeds spontaneously and is relatively slow, requiring 5–20 min for visible fibrin formation. All tissues contain a specific lipoprotein, thromboplastin, which markedly increases the rate at which blood clots. It is particularly concentrated in the lung and brain. The placenta is also very rich in tissue factor, which will produce fibrin formation within 12 s, the acceleration of coagulation being brought about by bypassing the reactions involving the contact (intrinsic) system.

Blood coagulation is strictly confined to the site of tissue injury in normal circumstances. Powerful control mechanisms must act to prevent dissemination of coagulation beyond the site of trauma.

The action of thrombin in $vivo$ is controlled by a number of mechanisms, particularly its absorption onto the locally formed fibrin, and the presence of a potent inhibitor, antithrombin, and α_2-globulin, which destroys thrombin activity. Heparin, which potentiates the action of anti-X_a, may be similar to antithrombin. This is the rationale for low-dose heparin therapy as prophylaxis in patients at risk of thromboembolic phenomena postoperatively, and in pregnancy and the puerperium.

Normal pregnancy is accompanied by major changes in the coagulation system with increases in the levels of factors VII, VIII and X, and a particularly marked increase in the level of plasma fibrinogen (Fig. 10.31). The increased fibrinogen concentration is probably the chief cause of the accelerated erythrocyte sedimentation rate observed during pregnancy.

The effect of pregnancy on the coagulation factors can be detected from about the third month of gestation. In late pregnancy, the fibrinogen concentration is at least double that of the non-pregnant state.

Fibrinolysis

Fibrinolytic activity is an essential part of the dynamic interacting haemostatic mechanism and is dependent on plasminogen activator in the blood (Fig. 10.32). Fibrin and fibrinogen are digested by plasmin, a pro-enzyme derived from an inactive plasma precursor, plasminogen.

Increased amounts of activator are found in the plasma after strenuous exercise, emotional stress, surgical operations and other trauma.

Tissue activator can be extracted from most human organs with the exception of the placenta. Tissues especially rich in activator include the uterus, ovaries, prostate, heart, lungs, thyroid, adrenal glands and lymph nodes. Activity in tissues is concentrated mainly around blood vessels, veins showing greater activity than arteries. Venous occlusion of the limbs will stimulate fibrinolytic activity, a fact which should be remembered if tourniquets are applied for any length of time before blood is drawn for measurement of fibrin degradation products (FDPs).

The inhibitors of fibrinolytic activity are of two types: anti-activators (antiplasminogens) and the antiplasmins.

Antiplasminogens include ε-aminocaproic acid (EACA) and tranexamic acid (AMCA). Aprotinin

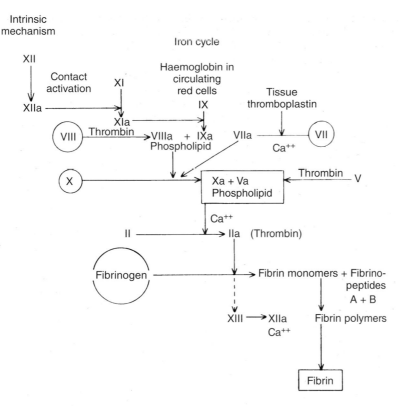

Figure 10.31 • The factors involved in blood coagulation and their interactions. The circled factors show significant increases in pregnancy. (Reproduced with permission from Hytten F, Chamberlain G. Clinical physiology in obstetrics. Blackwell Scientific, Oxford.)

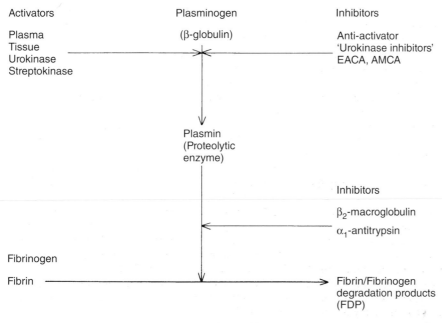

Figure 10.32 • Components of the fibrinolytic system. (Reproduced with permission from F. Hytten F, Chamberlain G. Clinical physiology in obstetrics. Blackwell Scientific, Oxford.)

(Trasylol) is another antiplasminogen commercially prepared from bovine lung.

Platelets, plasma and serum exert a strong inhibitory action on plasmin. Normally, plasma antiplasmin levels exceed levels of plasminogen, and hence the levels of potential plasmin; otherwise we would dissolve away our connecting cement!

When fibrinogen or fibrin is broken down by plasmin, fibrin degradation products are formed which comprise the high-molecular-weight split products X and Y, and smaller fragments A, B, C, D and E (Fig. 10.33). When a fibrin clot is formed, 70% of fragment X is retained in the clot, Y, D and E being retained to a somewhat lesser extent. Therefore, serum under normal circumstances can contain small amounts of fragment X and larger amounts of Y, D and E. All of these components have antigenic determinants in common with fibrinogen and will be recognized by fibrinogen antisera. It is important to be aware of this fact when examining blood for the presence of FDPs. Blood should be taken by clean venepuncture and the tourniquet should not be left on too long (see above). The blood should be allowed to clot in the presence of an antifibrinolytic agent such as EACA to stop the process of fibrinolysis which would otherwise continue *in vitro*.

Plasma fibrinolytic activity is decreased during pregnancy, remains low during labour and delivery, and returns to normal within 1 h of placental delivery.

The rapid return of systemic fibrinolytic activity to normal following delivery of the placenta, and the fact that the placenta has been shown to contain inhibitors which block fibrinolysis, suggest that inhibition of fibrinolysis during pregnancy is mediated through the placenta.

Summary of changes in haemostasis in pregnancy

The changes in the coagulation system in normal pregnancy are consistent with a continuing low-grade process of coagulant activity. Using electron microscopy, fibrin deposition can be demonstrated in the intervillous space of the placenta and in all the walls of the spiral arteries supplying the placenta. As pregnancy advances, the elastic lamina and smooth muscle of these spiral arteries are replaced by a matrix containing fibrin. This allows expansion of the lumen to accommodate an increasing blood flow and reduces the pressure in arterial blood flowing to the placenta. At placental separation, a blood flow of 500–800 mL/min has to be staunched within seconds, or a serious haemorrhage will occur. Myometrial contraction plays a vital role in securing haemostasis by reducing the blood flow to the placental site. Rapid closure of the terminal part of the spiral arteries will be further facilitated by the structural changes within their walls.

The placental site is rapidly covered by a fibrin mesh following delivery. The increased levels of fibrinogen and other coagulation factors will meet the sudden demand for haemostatic components at placental separation.

Thromboembolism

The dramatic changes described above facilitate arrest of bleeding from the placental site at delivery but carry with them an increased risk of thromboembolism. Pregnant women have a four-fold increased risk of thromboembolic disease antenatally, rising to 10-fold in the puerperium. The antenatal increased risk starts in the earlier first trimester and is steady throughout

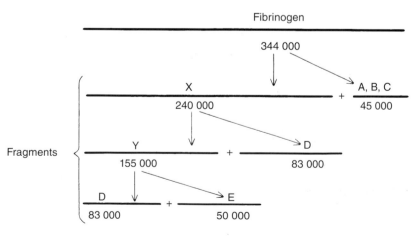

Figure 10.33 • Fibrin degradation products (FDPs) produced by the action of plasma on fibrinogen. The molecular weights are shown. (Reproduced with permission from Hytten F, Chamberlain G. Clinical physiology in obstetrics. Blackwell Scientific, Oxford.)

gestation. The 2000–2002 Confidential Enquiry Audit of maternal deaths showed, as in previous reports, that thromboembolism remains the leading direct cause of maternal mortality in the UK.

Disseminated intravascular coagulation

The changes in the haemostatic system during pregnancy and the local activation of the clotting system during parturition carry with them a risk, not only of thromboembolism, but of disseminated intravascular coagulation (DIC), consumption of clotting factors and platelets leading to severe bleeding – particularly uterine and sometimes generalized. Despite the advances in obstetric care and highly developed blood transfusion services, haemorrhage still constitutes a major factor in maternal mortality and morbidity.

The first problem with DIC is its definition. It is never primary, but always secondary to some general stimulation of coagulation activity by release of pro-coagulant substances into the blood (Fig. 10.34). Hypothetical triggers of this process in pregnancy include the leaking of placental tissue fragments, amniotic fluid, incompatible red cells or bacterial products into the maternal circulation. There is a great spectrum of manifestations of the process of DIC, ranging from a compensated state with no clinical manifestation, but evidence of increased production and breakdown of coagulation factors, to the condition of massive uncontrollable haemorrhage with very low concentrations of plasma fibrinogen, pathological raised levels of FDPs and variable degrees of thrombocytopenia.

Fibrinolysis is stimulated by DIC and FDPs resulting from the process interfering with the formation of firm fibrin clots. A vicious circle is established, which results in further severe bleeding.

Obstetric conditions classically associated with DIC include: placental abruption, amniotic fluid embolism, septic abortion and other intrauterine infection, retained dead fetus, hydatidiform mole, placenta accreta, pre-eclampsia and eclampsia, and prolonged shock from any cause (Fig. 10.34).

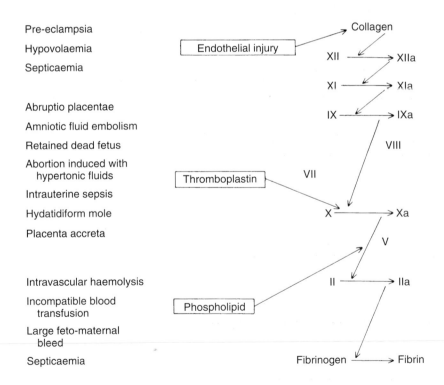

Interactions of the trigger mechanisms occur in many of these obstetric complications

Figure 10.34 • Trigger mechanisms of DIC in pregnancy. (Reproduced with permission from de Swiet M. Medical disorders in pregnancy. Blackwell Scientific, Oxford.)

Rhesus incompatibility

In the late 1930s, it was discovered that red cells from Rhesus monkeys injected into guinea-pigs and rabbits produced an antibody in the animals' sera which reacted strongly with the red cells of 85% of Caucasians. Those individuals whose red cells were agglutinated strongly with the Rhesus (Rh) antibody were called Rh-positive and the remaining 15% were termed Rh-negative.

Soon after the recognition of the Rh factor, it was shown that this antigen had important clinical significance in terms of haemolytic disease of the newborn and transfusion reactions.

The Rh-negative recipients of Rh-positive transfusions could suffer haemolytic transfusion reactions and Rh-positive babies carried by Rh-negative mothers were frequently affected by haemolytic anaemia *in utero* and in the postnatal period.

An immediate recommendation was that Rh-negative female recipients in or below childbearing years should be transfused with Rh-negative blood.

However, there were differences in the specificities of the antibodies produced by the sensitized Rh-negative mothers, and it became clear that the Rh factor was complex and it would be more reasonable to use the term 'Rh blood group system'.

For a basic understanding of the Rh system, only five of the 26 or more recognized antigens need to be considered: C, $\bar{c}$, D, E, $\bar{e}$. The Rh blood group antigens are carried by a series of at least three homologous but distinct red cell membrane associated proteins. Two of these proteins have immunologically distinguishable isoforms designated C, $\bar{c}$ and E, $\bar{e}$. The principal protein, D, has no immunologically detectable isoform d. The RH gene locus (on chromosome 1p34–p36) consists, in RhD-positive individuals, of two similar genes designated C$\bar{c}$ E$\bar{e}$ and D. The first gene, C$\bar{c}$ E$\bar{e}$, encodes both the C/$\bar{c}$ and E/$\bar{e}$ proteins, by alternative splicing of a primary transcript (see Ch. 1). The second gene, D, encodes the major antigen RhD and is absent in RhD-negative individuals. Therefore, the presence or absence of the D gene in the genome determines the genetic basis of the Rh-positive/Rh-negative blood group polymorphism, which explains the absence of a detectable isoform of the D antigen (d) at the red cell surface of Rh negative individuals. Although haematologists will refer to an individual as DD, Dd or dd, the designation 'd' indicates the absence of the 'D' antigen. In the case of C$\bar{c}$ and E$\bar{e}$, both the upper- and lower-case letters indicate the presence of a serologically definable antigen.

The genes encoding the three major sets of antigens are inherited together so that specific sets of antigens are inherited together rather than random inheritance of each of the C/$\bar{c}$, D/d, E/$\bar{e}$ antigens. This suggested to earlier investigators that there would be either one single gene encoding all the C/$\bar{c}$, D/d, E/$\bar{e}$ epitopes, or three genes closely linked on the chromosome so that recombination rarely takes place between them. Whether from Rh-positive or -negative individuals, virtually all normal erythrocytes carry the antithetical antigens C and/or $\bar{c}$ and E and/or $\bar{e}$. The erythrocytes of very rare individuals who lack all these antigens have multiple membrane abnormalities, suggesting that the Rh antigens are of major physiological importance. The RhD-negative phenotype is a trait of Caucasians in whom the incidence is 15%. In Basques, 35% are RhD-negative, while only 1% of North American Indians and 7% of African-Americans are RhD negative. The incidence in Asiatic Chinese and Japanese is almost zero.

It is the D antigens that are the major cause of haemolytic disease of the newborn. In Caucasian populations, 56% of RhD-positive individuals are heterozygous for the D antigen. If an RhD-negative woman has an RhD-positive partner there is therefore an approximately 50% chance that he will be a homozygote, in which case all of their children will be RhD positive (all being heterozygotes), and an approximately 50% chance that he will be a heterozygote, in which case half of their children will be heterozygote RhD positive and half will be RhD negative.

D^u **antigen** A few individuals have antigens on their cells which react weakly and variably with the various forms of anti-D antisera – these are termed group D^u. For transfusion purposes an individual with the blood group D^u should be regarded as Rh(D) negative when receiving blood but as Rh(D) positive when donating blood.

Haemolytic disease of the newborn

Haemolytic disease of the newborn (HDN) is a condition in which the lifespan of the infant's red cells is shortened by the action of specific antibodies derived from the mother. The immune antibodies in the maternal plasma are small molecular immunoglobulins of the IgG subclass and therefore, unlike the large molecule, naturally occurring antibodies of the ABO blood group systems (IgM) are able to cross the placenta.

Although HDN can occur in several situations where the mother lacks an antigen which her baby carries on its red cells, there is no doubt that, prior to the introduction of the specific immunoglobulin for the prevention of Rh(D) haemolytic disease, Rh(D) HDN was by far the most important form of HDN in terms of clinical severity and frequency in Caucasian populations. Other Rh antibodies which can cause HDN are anti-E and anti-c, in which case the mother is usually Rh(D) positive.

Outside the Rh blood group system the most frequently observed immune-induced antibody is anti-Kell. This is more usually transfusion provoked, 95% of the Caucasian population being Kell negative.

Occasionally, this antibody can cause severe HDN where the father is Kell positive (heterozygous or homozygous) and he has transmitted the Kell positive gene to his offspring.

HDN begins in intrauterine life and may result in death *in utero*. In liveborn infants the haemolytic process is maximal at the time of birth and thereafter diminishes as the concentration of maternal antibody in the infant's circulation declines.

During pregnancy, the fetal and maternal circulations are separate. Red cells are not thought to cross the placental barrier in significant numbers in normal circumstances. Oxygen, nutrient and waste exchange takes place by diffusion across the intervillous space. IgG antibodies cross the placenta freely, carrying protection (passive immunity) for the fetus against infective agents to which the mother has had a healthy immune response.

Following delivery and placental separation, rupture of the placental villi and connective tissue allows escape of fetal blood cells into the maternal circulation, prior to constriction of the open maternal vessels. This is when sensitization takes place in the majority of cases unless prevented (see below).

The incompatible Rh(D) fetal cells enter the maternal spleen and the foreign antigen on the fetal red cell triggers off an immune response causing production of antibody.

In a subsequent pregnancy with an Rh(D)-positive fetus, the immune IgG anti-D maternal antibody will cross the placenta and attach to the specific D antigen sites on the fetal red cell. IgG-coated red cells do not have a normal lifespan. They are particularly sensitive to cells of the reticuloendothelial system and are removed from the circulation prematurely. Progressive anaemia *in utero* occurs from about the fourth month of pregnancy and, in the most severe cases, intrauterine death has been recorded from the 20th week of pregnancy, although it is uncommon before the 24th week. Many of the stillborn infants are grossly oedematous and are then described as having hydrops fetalis. Hydropic infants are occasionally born alive and are found to be severely anaemic with cord haemoglobin as low as 3.5 g/dL. There is a great increase in the number of nucleated red cells in the circulating blood, hence the term erythroblastosis fetalis is sometimes used to described the haematological condition.

Jaundice does not occur before delivery because bilirubin produced by the breakdown of cells in the fetal spleen passes via the placenta to the maternal circulation. Albumin transports the fetal bilirubin to the maternal liver where glucuronyl transferase converts it to excretable, direct-reacting bilirubin. The liver of the neonate does not produce glucuronyl transferase and cannot convert bilirubin to an excretable form. Consequently, bilirubin accumulates and if not removed (by exchange transfusion) will collect in the tissues causing jaundice and brain damage. Deeply jaundiced infants often exhibit signs of damage to the central nervous system. These signs usually develop after the age of 36 h.

It has been shown that the brain contains lipid which takes up the unconjugated bilirubin but does not take up conjugated bilirubin. In kernicterus, the yellow-staining material has been shown to be unconjugated bilirubin.

Detection of Rh anti-D antibody
Direct antiglobulin (Coombs') test (baby's red blood cells, one-stage test) When a neonate suffers from HDN the red cells are coated with immune IgG antibody. This is known as incomplete antibody. These cells do not agglutinate but if an anti-IgG antiserum is added to a mixture of sensitized cells the gap is bridged between antibody on individual red cells and visible agglutination occurs. This is known as a positive direct Coombs' test.

Indirect antiglobulin (Coombs') test (maternal serum, two-stage test) The mother produces antibody against the Rh(D)-positive fetal cells. The antibody is free in her serum because her Rh(D)-negative red cells do not carry the appropriate antigen. If her serum is incubated with Rh(D)-positive cells the antibodies will attach to them but, as it is an IgG, agglutination does not occur. However, if anti-IgG antiserum is then added to the sensitized cells (cf. direct Coombs' test), visible agglutination will occur. This is known as the 'indirect Coombs' test' and is used routinely to detect the presence of anti-Rh and other immune antibodies in maternal serum during pregnancy. By serial dilution of maternal serum and reporting the weakest dilution of the serum at which a reaction with the Rh(D)-positive red cell takes place, a crude estimation of the concentration of the antibody can be made. Serial estimations will give an indication of the rate of increase of antibody in a particular pregnancy.

With the advent of automation in blood transfusion laboratories, it has now become routine in large centres to estimate the Rh(D) antibody in international units based on an automated system using the Coombs' test principle.

Amniocentesis
Although measurement of antenatal anti-D concentration has become more exact, correlation between antibody levels and severity of the haemolytic process in the fetus is not sufficient to plan management during pregnancy; however, maternal titres <15 IU/mL are unlikely to cause fetal complications.

By estimation of the bilirubin concentration in the amniotic fluid, the degree of haemolysis of the infant's red cells can be predicted with greater accuracy.

Several methods are in current usage but the most popular is the spectrophotometric measurement of the bilirubin 'bulge' at a wavelength of 450–460 nm (Liley curve). A decision can then be taken on the need for intrauterine transfusion. Donor blood should be compatible with mother and fetus and it should be remembered that the donor RBC will decline by 2% a day.

Amniocentesis is only reliable from 27 weeks of gestation onwards. Fetal Doppler assessment of the middle cerebral artery with hyperdynamic flow seen in anaemic fetuses is an additional, more recently employed assessment tool. However, fetal blood sampling may be necessary to determine the degree to which the fetus is affected.

Reference

Campos O 1996 Doppler echocardiography during pregnancy: physiological and abnormal findings. Echocardiography 13:135–146

Chapter **Eleven**

11

Endocrinology

Mark Johnson

CHAPTER CONTENTS

Introduction

In this chapter the endocrine system will be introduced by describing mechanisms of hormone action and hormone types. Six groups of hormones and/or endocrine systems will then be discussed: (1) hypothalamus, pituitary and pineal glands, (2) reproduction (puberty, menstrual cycle, pregnancy, lactation and menopause), (3) growth, (4) metabolism and the pancreas, (5) thyroid, (6) adrenal.

Mechanisms of hormone action and second messenger systems

Cell surface receptors

Hormones may act in an autocrine (acts on the cells that produced it), paracrine (acting on neighbouring cells) or endocrine manner (acting on cells at a distant site having been transported to that site in the blood or lymphatic system). In the circulation, some hormones such as steroids, insulin-related growth factors and thyroid hormones are bound to carrier proteins. Only the free hormone, that fraction of the total hormone level which is unbound, is active and available to bind to specific receptors to induce its effects. These receptors may be on the cell surface and have associated secondary messenger systems or be in the nucleus and have effects directly on the DNA to alter messenger RNA (mRNA) expression. At each receptor a hormone may be an agonist, a partial agonist or an antagonist.

Neurotransmitters and peptide hormones act predominantly through cell surface receptors. These are divided into four main groups: (1) seven-transmembrane domain (LH, FSH, TSH, β-adrenergic, typically linked to G-protein second messenger system); (2) single transmembrane domain growth factor receptors (insulin, IGFs, linked to tyrosine kinase second messenger system); (3) cytokine receptors (cytokines, GH, prolactin); (4) guanylyl cyclase-linked receptors (natriuretic peptides related to guanyl cyclase second messenger system).

The seven-transmembrane receptors, as their name implies, loop in and out of the cytoplasm (Fig. 11.1). The amino terminus has the hormone binding domain and the carboxy terminus the G-protein transducer. There are multiple types of G-protein which are heterotrimers made up of an α, β and γ subunit (Fig. 11.2). Each type (determined by the α-subunit) may relate to different receptors and be linked to different second messenger systems. For example the β-adrenergic system is linked to α_s G-protein, which in turn is linked to adenylyl cyclase. Thus, β-adrenergic activation is associated with an increase in intracellular

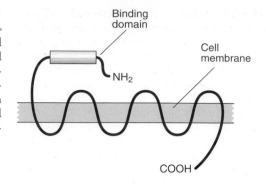

Figure 11.1 • Seven-transmembrane receptor.

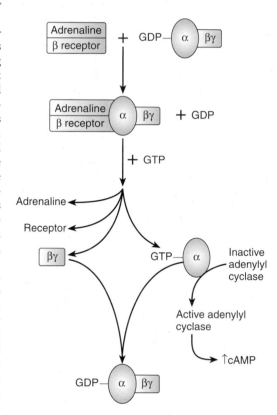

Figure 11.2 • G-protein receptor activation represented by a β-adrenergic receptor.

cAMP (Fig. 11.2). Each G-protein is made up of a GDP–GTP binding domain (the α-subunit), and a β- and γ-subunit. In the absence of stimulation, the G-protein is bound to GDP. With receptor activation the α-subunit binds to the receptor and dissociates from the GDP and the β- and γ-subunit. GTP then binds to the receptor-linked α-subunit initiating its dissociation from the hormone–receptor complex. The activated G-protein then activates its second messenger system (e.g. adenylyl cyclase). The deactivated GDP–α-subunit complex re-associates with the β- and γ-subunit (Fig. 11.2). The G-protein system can be manipulated experimentally by using agents such as cholera toxin, which prolongs the activity of the α-subunit–GTP complex or pertussis toxin, which uncouples the G-protein system and inhibits its activity.

As described earlier, adenylyl cyclase activation generates cAMP which activates protein kinase A (PKA), which then is able to phosphorylate and activate other intracellular proteins such as the cyclic AMP response element binding protein (CREB). This protein mediates many of the transcriptional effects of cAMP. The Gα q is linked to phospholipase Cβ, an initiator of another second messenger system, which when activated cleaves phosphoinositol 4,5-bisphosphonate generating inositol 1,4,5-triphosphate (IP_3) and diacylglycerol (DAG). IP_3 acts via specific receptors to increase intracellular calcium and DAG activates protein kinase C. Activation of phospholipase A releases arachidonic acid, which is a precursor molecule for prostaglandins and leukotrienes.

Growth factor receptors span the cellular membrane once and are linked to tyrosine kinase. Binding to the receptor initiates phosphorylation of the receptor itself and of tyrosines in other molecules. This is thought to trigger a cascade of intracellular responses. The cytokine receptors, like the growth factor receptors, cross the cell membrane once; how they affect intracellular events is not understood.

The guanylyl cyclase-linked receptors can be activated in three ways:

1. They may be activated by nitric oxide (NO) produced by nitric oxide synthase (NOS). NOS exists in either constitutive (endothelial or neuronal, eNOS or nNOS) or inducible (iNOS) forms. In the vasculature, agents such as acetylcholine or bradykinin bind to endothelial cell surface receptors and increase intracellular calcium, which enhances eNOS activity and increases NO production. Increased NO levels diffuse into the smooth muscle cell and activate soluble guanylyl cyclase; this in turn produces cGMP, which stimulates relaxation of the smooth muscle.
2. iNOS is present predominantly in immune cells but is also found in vascular smooth muscle cells. As its name implies it can be induced by various hormones leading to an increase in NO production and so cGMP levels.
3. Guanylyl cyclase is also linked to the peptide receptor directly and so ligand–receptor interaction activates it directly.

Peptide hormones also affect the transcription of the genes through the activation of c-jun and c-fos (via kinases and phosphatases). These are nuclear transcription factors which bind to specific sites on the DNA to alter gene expression. cAMP activates protein kinase A, which, as mentioned above, phosphorylates a number of proteins including CREB, which again alters gene expression.

Nuclear receptors

Several hormones act through nuclear receptors; these include steroid hormones, thyroid hormones, retinoic acid and vitamin D. Some of the receptors exist principally in the cytoplasm (the 'steroid' family includes glucocorticoid, mineralocorticoid, androgen and progesterone receptors) and some primarily in the nucleus (the 'thyroid' family which includes oestrogen, retinoic acid and vitamin D receptors). However, independent of their location, when these hormones bind to their receptors, all act in the nucleus to alter gene expression. The steroid family exists in the cytoplasm as a complex with heat shock protein (HSP). When the ligand binds with the receptor, HSP dissociates revealing a nuclear translocation signal which initiates the transport of the hormone–receptor complex to the nucleus where it binds to the hormone response element to exert its effect (Fig. 11.3). The DNA binding region has two zinc 'fingers'; between the two zinc molecules lies the amino acid sequence which binds to the DNA. The thyroid family exists in the nucleus and, with the exception of the oestrogen receptor, do not associate with HSP. They bind to DNA as dimers; for oestrogen this is a homodimer (i.e. two oestrogen receptor molecules) and for the other members of the family, as heterodimers formed between the receptor molecule and a retinoid X receptor.

Hormone types

Peptide hormones

Most hormones are peptides. A peptide is made up of a chain of a variable number of amino acids. The precise sequence is determined by the DNA coding for it. The process of peptide synthesis is initiated by the transcription of DNA into a specific mRNA. This passes from the nucleus into the cytoplasm, where it binds to ribosomes in the rough endoplasmic reticulum (RER) and is translated into the peptide sequence (illustrated by insulin in Fig. 11.4). Usually this is in the form of a pre-pro-hormone which is then cleaved to form first a pro-hormone and then the hormone itself. Some peptides are secreted immediately while others are stored in secretory granules.

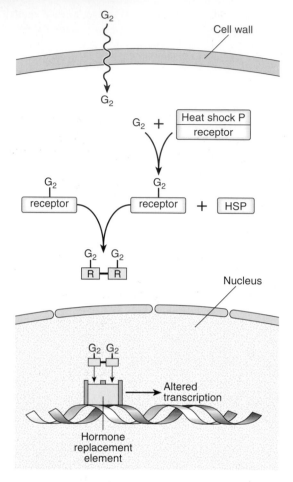

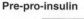

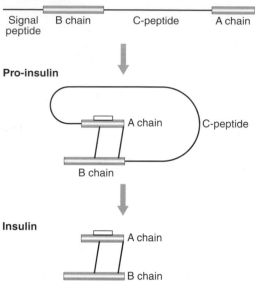

Figure 11.4 • Synthesis of insulin.

Figure 11.3 • Nuclear receptor activation by ligand G_2 which passes through the cell wall, binds to its receptor in the cytoplasm before passing into the nucleus to bind to its response element on DNA.

Steroid hormones

In terms of reproduction, this is the most important group of hormones. They are synthesized from cholesterol and all have the same basic ring structure of 17 carbon atoms with different numbers of carbon atoms added. Glucocorticoids (stress and metabolism), aldosterone (fluid balance) and progesterone (reproduction) have 21 carbon atoms; testosterone and other androgens have 19 carbon atoms while oestrogens have 18 (Fig. 11.5). The synthetic pathways are the same in ovary, testis and adrenal, but the dominant product varies from tissue to tissue (Fig. 11.6). The pathway always starts from cholesterol which is derived either from circulating LDL or from intracellular cholesterol esters.

Ovary

Ovarian steroid production varies during the cycle. Overall, the ovary is the main source of circulating oestrogens, although peripheral conversion of androgens also makes a significant contribution in some situations. During the follicular phase of the cycle, the ovary produces oestrogens predominantly, and both oestrogen and progesterone in the luteal phase.

Adrenal

The adrenal cortex is divided into three zones: (1) the outer zona glomerulosa, (2) the middle zona fasciculata, which consists of cells full of cholesterol and (3) the inner zona reticularis. The first zone is concerned with aldosterone secretion and is under the control of the renin–angiotensin pathway and the last two are controlled by adrenocorticotrophic hormone (ACTH) and are concerned primarily with the secretion of cortisol and, to a lesser extent, adrenal androgens. More details will be given about each in their relevant sections.

Testis

The Leydig cells of the testis produce testosterone in response to luteinizing hormone (LH). This circulates predominantly bound (97%) to sex hormone binding globulin (SHBG) and to a lesser extent to albumin. In some tissues testosterone is active, but in others it has to be converted to dihydrotestosterone (DHT) by the enzyme 5α-reductase. Both testosterone and DHT bind to a cytoplasmic receptor before passing into the cell nucleus to bind to specific areas of DNA to produce their effect.

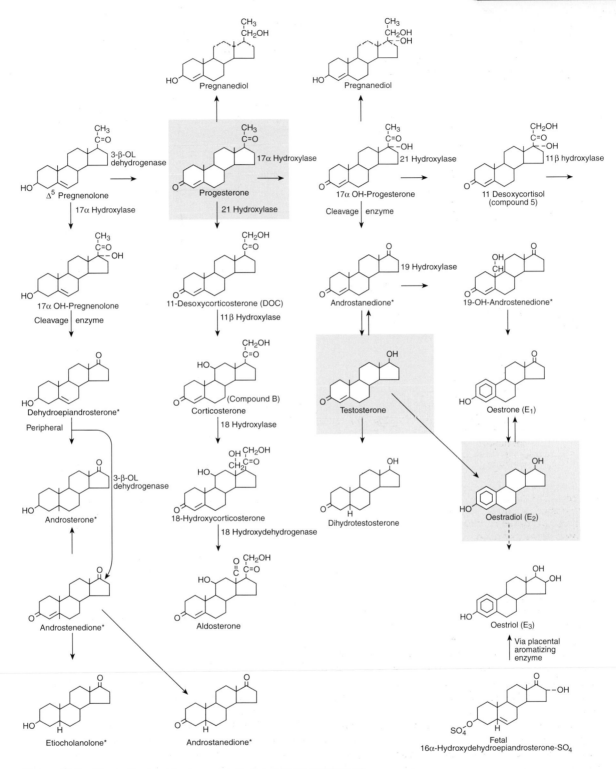

Figure 11.5 • The synthesis of the key reproductive steroids (highlighted).

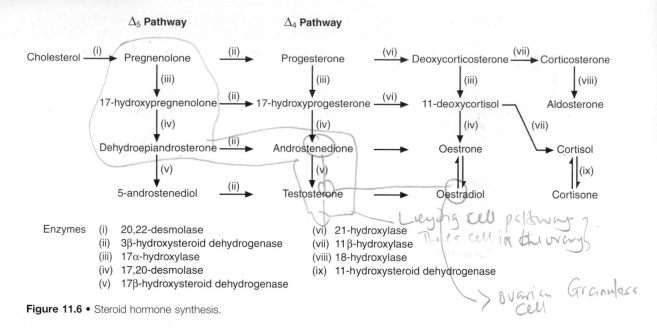

Δ_5 **Pathway** Δ_4 **Pathway**

Enzymes
(i) 20,22-desmolase
(ii) 3β-hydroxysteroid dehydrogenase
(iii) 17α-hydroxylase
(iv) 17,20-desmolase
(v) 17β-hydroxysteroid dehydrogenase

(vi) 21-hydroxylase
(vii) 11β-hydroxylase
(viii) 18-hydroxylase
(ix) 11-hydroxysteroid dehydrogenase

Leydig cell pathway ? The Is cell in the ovarys

→ ovarian Granulose cell

Figure 11.6 • Steroid hormone synthesis.

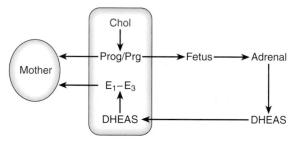

Figure 11.7 • Feto-placental oestrogen production. The fetus lacks sulphatases, 3β-hydroxysteroid dehydrogenase (3βHSD) and aromatase, and therefore produces dehydroepiandrosterone sulphate (DHEAS), which it exports to the placenta, which possesses these enzymes and produces oestrone (E_1), oestradiol (E_2) and oestriol (E_3). Chol, cholesterol; Prog, progesterone; Prg, pregnenolone.

Placenta

During pregnancy, the placenta synthesizes and releases large amounts of progesterone into the maternal circulation. Pregnenolone is also released into the fetal circulation to be converted by the fetal adrenal into androgens, which pass back to the placenta to be aromatized to oestrogens and released into the maternal circulation (Fig. 11.7).

Steroid binding and metabolism

In the circulation, all steroid hormones circulate bound to various proteins (Table 11.1). Steroid hormone metabolism occurs in the liver. For example oestradiol is converted to oestrone, which may re-enter the circulation, be further metabolized to catechol oestrogens or conjugated to form oestrone sulphate, and excreted.

Progesterone is converted to pregnanediol and conjugated to glucuronic acid, and excreted as pregnanediol glucuronide. Androgens are metabolized and excreted predominantly as 17-oxosteroids (which used to be measured to assess androgen synthesis). Cortisol is mainly conjugated to glucuronide and excreted. Its metabolites can be measured in the urine in the form of 17-oxogenic steroids (not to be confused with the androgen metabolites, 17-oxosteroids), but this is rarely measured now, as cortisol can be measured in the urine directly.

Amino acid hormones

Several hormones, thyroid (tyrosine), catecholamines (tyrosine) and melatonin (tryptophan) are derived from amino acids. These hormones are stored in granules.

Their activities are regulated by their release and by the expression of the enzymes necessary for their synthesis.

Prostaglandins and leukotrienes

Collectively known as the eicosanoids, these hormones are derived from arachidonic acid. Synthesis occurs in the cell wall and the hormones pass either into the cell cytoplasm or out of the cell (Fig. 11.8).

Hypothalamus and pituitary

The hypothalamus is at the centre of the different endocrine, autonomic and homeostatic mechanisms

Table 11.1 Steroid binding profiles

Hormone	Plasma conc. (nmol/L)	Free (%)	SHBG (%)	CBG (%)	Albumin (%)
Oestradiol	0.29	1.8	37.3	0.1	60.8
Oestrone	0.23	3.6	16.3	0.1	80.1
Progesterone	0.65	2.4	0.6	17.7	79.3
Testosterone	1.3	1.4	66	2.3	30.4
Androstenedione	5.4	7.5	6.6	1.4	84.5
Cortisol	400	3.8	0.2	89.7	6.3

SHBG, sex hormone binding globulin; CBG, cortisol binding globulin.

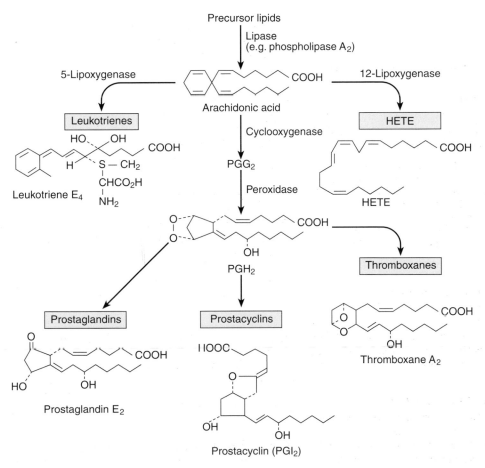

Figure 11.8 • Prostaglandin and leukotriene synthesis from arachidonic acid. (Reproduced with permission from Greenspan FS, Strewler GJ 1997 Basic and clinical endocrinology. 5th edn. Appleton and Lange, London.)

which maintain the body and allows it to reproduce. It directly controls the pituitary, which in turn controls the reproductive axis, lactation, growth, the thyroid and adrenal glands.

Embryology

The thalamus and the hypothalamus develop from the diencephalon, which with the telencephalon (which forms the cerebral hemispheres) forms the proencephalon. Both the thalamus and the hypothalamus develop in the lateral walls of the diencephalon, the cavity that becomes the third ventricle (Fig. 11.9).

The pituitary develops in close association with the hypothalamus and is made up of two parts: (1) the anterior or adenohypophysis and (2) the posterior or neurohypophysis. The anterior pituitary is formed from the ventral ridges of the primitive neural tube, which are pushed forward by the developing Rathke's pouch (Fig. 11.10). By 7 weeks, the sella floor has formed and the pituitary starts to develop under the influence of the hypothalamus. The posterior pituitary is formed by

a downward evagination of the diencephalon called the infundibulum. Thus, the neurohypophysis is in direct contact with the hypothalamus, while the anterior pituitary is connected to the hypothalamus via a rich vascular network called the portal system. The portal system carries all of the hypothalamic hormones which regulate the function of the anterior pituitary (Fig. 11.11). A small part of the anterior pituitary immediately opposed to the neurohypophysis becomes the intermediate lobe (Fig. 11.12).

Anatomy

Boundaries

The thalamus lies superior to the hypothalamus, separated from it by the hypothalamic sulcus. Medially the third ventricle, superiorly the thalamus and inferiorly the pituitary stalk provide anatomical limits for the hypothalamus; anteriorly, posteriorly and laterally the hypothalamus is without distinct boundaries.

The pituitary lies within the sella turcica (the Turkish saddle); anteriorly and inferiorly lies the

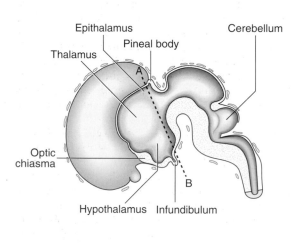

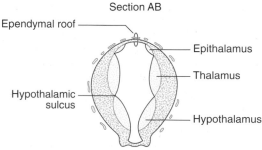

Figure 11.9 • Embryonic development of the hypothalamus. (Reproduced with permission from Moore KL 1993 The developing human – clinically oriented embryology. 5th edn. WB Saunders, Philadelphia.)

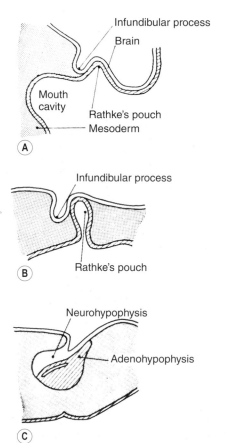

Figure 11.10 • The development of the pituitary.

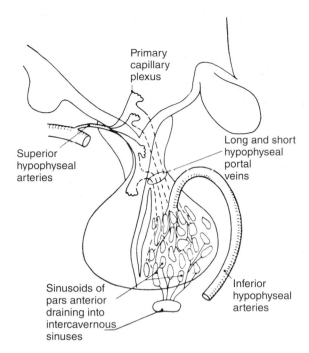

Figure 11.11 • The pituitary portal system and its connections.

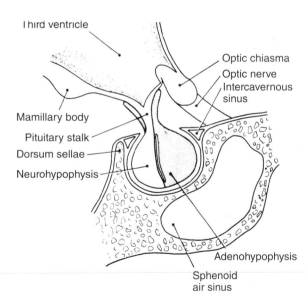

Figure 11.12 • Relations of the pituitary.

sphenoid sinus, laterally the cavernous sinus (containing internal carotid arteries, and sixth cranial nerve), posteriorly the clinoid processes of the sphenoid bone (often eroded on skull X-rays in the presence of a pituitary tumour), and superiorly the pituitary stalk

which merges into the hypothalamus (Fig. 11.12). Anterior to the pituitary stalk lies the optic chiasma, which may be compressed by an expanding pituitary tumour, giving the typical presentation of bi-temporal hemianopia.

Blood supply

The hypothalamus, pituitary stalk and the pituitary are supplied by carotid arteries via the superior and inferior hypophyseal arteries (Fig. 11.11). The superior hypophyseal arteries form a primary plexus in the base of the hypothalamus in a region called the median eminence. The plexus forms into the portal vessels which pass on either side of the pituitary stalk to the anterior pituitary, where they form a secondary plexus. The nerves from the hypothalamic nuclei which regulate anterior pituitary function end close to primary plexus and release their regulatory hormones which are taken up and are carried via the portal vessels to the anterior pituitary. The posterior pituitary is supplied by the inferior hypophyseal artery.

Structure

The hypothalamus is made up of a series of nuclei arranged around the third ventricle. The nuclei consist of the cell bodies of the neurones. In the case of the nuclei which regulate the anterior pituitary, the axons pass to the area of the median eminence (see earlier). The axons of the paraventricular (situated in the lateral wall of the third ventricle) and the supraoptic nuclei (situated above the optic tract) pass down the pituitary stalk to the posterior pituitary. Both synthesize and release oxytocin and vasopressin (Fig. 11.13).

As described earlier, the pituitary develops from two parts. The anterior pituitary is made up of a mixture of cells with different secretory properties. They are divided into three groups on the basis of their staining with haematoxylin and eosin. The chromophobes (which do not stain) are thought to be resting cells, but chromophobe adenomas have been shown to secrete gonadotrophin subunits. The acidophils synthesize prolactin and growth hormone and the basophils, which secrete the gonadotrophins, thyroid-stimulating hormone (TSH) and ACTH. The posterior pituitary is pale and consists of the nerve terminals of the paraventricular and the supraoptic nuclei. The axons are surrounded by glial cells called pituicytes, which regulate the rate of transmission and the cross-talk between neurones.

Hypothalamic products

Table 11.2 summarizes the hormones produced by the hypothalamus which regulate anterior pituitary function. Further details are given in the relevant sections later in this chapter.

Pituitary gland products

Table 11.3A,B summarizes the hormones produced by the anterior and posterior parts of the pituitary gland, respectively. Further details are given in the relevant sections later in this chapter.

Pineal gland

The pineal gland lies in the roof of the third ventricle at the posterior end. Its role in the human is uncertain.

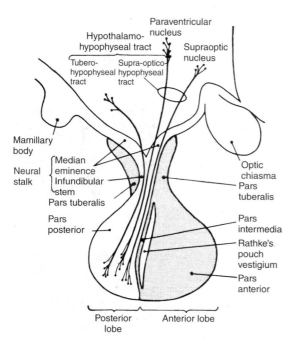

Figure 11.13 • Diagrammatic representation of the hypothalamus and pituitary. The connections of the posterior lobe of the gland with the hypothalamus are indicated. (Figs 11.10–11.13 courtesy of Passmore R, Robson J (eds). Companion to medical studies. Blackwell Scientific, Oxford.)

It produces melatonin, which may have a role in the regulation of the 'body clock' and puberty. Tumours of the pineal gland are associated with the usual symptoms and signs of a space-occupying lesion and a deficiency of hypothalamic hormones or occasionally with precocious puberty. With age, the pineal gland calcifies and may be seen on a skull X-ray.

Reproductive hormones

The reproductive axis is made up of the hypothalamus, pituitary and gonads. The embryology and anatomy of the reproductive tract are discussed elsewhere and in this chapter only the endocrine aspects will be reviewed.

Function

Gonadotrophin-releasing hormone (GnRH) is synthesized in the pre-optic area of the hypothalamus and passes via the median eminence and the portal vessels to the anterior pituitary, where it stimulates the gonadotrophs to synthesize and release LH and follicle stimulating hormone (FSH). It is released in pulses, controlled by the pulse generator in the arcuate nucleus. In the female, the pulse frequency varies with the phase of the cycle, during the follicular phase every 60 min and during the luteal phase every 90 min. The release of GnRH is modulated by opioid and catecholamine inputs. GnRH is synthesized from a 92-amino-acid pro-hormone, which is split into GnRH and a 56-amino-acid GnRH-associated peptide (GAP). The physiological role of GAP is unknown, but it has been shown to inhibit prolactin secretion.

LH and FSH are glycoproteins from the family which includes TSH and human chorionic gonadotrophin (hCG). These hormones consist of a common α-subunit and specific β-subunit. All are glycosylated, which determines their bioactivity and half-life. Both LH and FSH act on the gonads to stimulate gameto-

Table 11.2	Regulators of anterior pituitary function		
Hormone	**Source**	**Amino acids**	**Role**
GnRH	Pre-optic area	10	Stimulates LH and FSH release
CRH	Anterior paraventricular nucleus	41	Stimulates ACTH release
GRH	Arcuate nucleus	44	Stimulates GH release
Somatostatin	Periventricular area	14	Inhibits GH release
TRH	Medial paraventricular nucleus	3	Stimulates TSH release
Dopamine	Arcuate nucleus		Inhibits prolactin release

Table 11.3A   Anterior pituitary hormones

Hormone	Type	Amino acids	Size	Role
LH	Glycoprotein	204	30 000	Stimulates ovarian hormone synthesis and oocyte release
FSH	Glycoprotein	204	30 000	Stimulates follicle maturation
TSH	Glycoprotein	201	28 000	Stimulates thyroid hormone release
ACTH	Protein	39	4500	Stimulates cortisol synthesis in the adrenal
GH⁻	Protein	191	21 500	Stimulates hepatic IGF II synthesis and release
Prolactin	Protein	198	22 000	Stimulates lactation

Table 11.3B   Posterior pituitary hormones

Hormone	Source	Amino acids	Role
Oxytocin	Lateral and superior paraventricular and supraoptic nuclei	9	Stimulates contraction of the myoepithelial cells of the breast causing milk let down, and of the uterine myocytes in labour
Vasopressin	Lateral and superior paraventricular and supraoptic nuclei	9	Retains water by altering the permeability of the collecting ducts in the kidney; cardiovascular regulation; enhances CRH-stimulated ACTH release

genesis and hormone synthesis (see later). The levels of the gonadotrophins vary with age. Before puberty they are low; they rise at puberty, initially at night in both sexes, then continuously in the male and cyclically in the female. With the menopause, the levels of both rise markedly.

During the follicular phase, FSH and LH stimulate oestrogen synthesis by the developing follicle. This initially feeds back to the level of the hypothalamus and possibly to the pituitary to inhibit FSH and LH release. Negative feedback occurs in a short and ultrashort manner too, in that LH and FSH feed back to the hypothalamus to reduce further GnRH; GnRH also feeds back to inhibit its own release.

Positive feedback also occurs at mid-cycle. Oestrogens rise to such a point that their usual negative feedback is reversed and a marked positive effect occurs. GnRH release increases and results in a LH, and to a lesser extent FSH, peak. The former, but not the latter, is responsible for ovulation and initiation of luteinization of the follicle.

Oestrogen and progesterone

Oestrogens have a number of important general effects (Table 11.4), but during the menstrual cycle their most important role is to stimulate endometrial growth. Following ovulation, the corpus luteum continues to

Table 11.4   The properties of oestrogen

Structure	Stimulates endometrial growth, maintenance of vessels and skin, reduces bone resorption, increases bone formation, increases uterine growth
Protein synthesis	Increases hepatic synthesis of binding proteins
Coagulation	Increases circulating levels of factors II, VII, IX, X, antithrombin III and plasminogen; increases platelet adhesiveness
Lipid	Increases HDL and reduces LDL, increases triglycerides, reduces ketone formation, increases fat deposition
Fluid balance	Salt and water retention
Gastrointestinal	Reduces bowel motility, increases cholesterol in bile

synthesize and release oestrogens and progesterone. Their production peaks 7 days after ovulation and thereafter declines unless conception and implantation occur, when the developing embryo releases hCG into the maternal circulation which maintains corpus luteum function. Progesterone also has several effects (Table 11.5), but during the luteal phase it regulates endometrial receptivity.

Androgens

In the female, androgens are synthesized in both the ovary and adrenal glands. Of the circulating testosterone, 25% is formed directly in the ovary. The remainder is derived either directly from the adrenal (25%) or indirectly through the peripheral conversion predominantly of androstenedione (50% from the ovary and 50% from the adrenal) and to a much lesser extent of dihydroepiandrostenedione (DHEA, derived mainly from the adrenal glands). In the female, androgens are probably responsible for the maintenance of pubic and axillary hair and also control libido.

Sex differentiation *in utero*

In the absence of any stimulation, the default phenotype is female. The male phenotype is determined by one key gene called the sex determining region Y (SRY) gene. This is expressed by the support cells of the embryonic testis, which develop into Sertoli cells. It also stimulates the germ cells to become spermatogonia, the steroid secreting cells to become Leydig cells and the connective tissue cells to be peritubular cells. In the absence of SRY, the four cell lineages develop into the granulosa cells, oogonia, thecal cells and stromal cells of the ovary.

The Wolffian and Müllerian systems initially develop in parallel. The secretion of Müllerian inhibitory substance (MIS) by the Sertoli cells causes regression of the Müllerian system. The secretion of MIS is controlled by SRY and epidermal growth factor (EGF). Further sex differentiation occurs with the secretion of

testosterone by the testis. Testosterone promotes development of the Wolffian ducts into vas deferens, seminal vesicles and epididymis. In order for some structures to develop (penis, scrotum and prostate) testosterone has to be converted to dehydrotestosterone by the enzyme 5α-reductase. In the absence of testosterone (and thus of dehydrotestosterone) the embryo will develop into a phenotypic female, at least in terms of the external genitalia.

Puberty

Female

There is variation in the timing and order of the events of puberty. Usually breast growth and the growth spurt occur first, followed by the appearance of pubic, then axillary hair, and then menstruation (Tables 11.6, 11.7). Increase in height prior to puberty is about 5 cm per year. During the growth spurt (lasting 2–3 years), this increases to 8–9 cm per year. Peak growth velocity usually occurs at around 12 years. Breast growth usually begins between 9 and 13 years. The average time to develop from stage II to V (Table 11.6) is 4 years (range 1.5–9 years); for pubic hair the average is 3 years (range 2–5 years). The first menstrual period usually occurs at the age of 13 years (range 11–15 years). In affluent societies, better nutrition and health mean that the age of menarche is decreasing.

Structurally, the reproductive organs change markedly with puberty. The ovaries elongate and become oval in shape due to follicular development and an increase in stroma. Before puberty, the cervix makes up two-thirds of the uterus; with puberty this changes, so that at menarche it makes up half and within 2 years

Table 11.5	The properties of progesterone
Structure	Enhances endometrial receptivity, maintains myometrial quiescence, breast development
Respiration	Increases respiratory drive
Lipid	Reduces HDL and increases LDL
Fluid balance	Promotes sodium exertion
Bowel	Reduces bowel motility
Metabolism	Increases body temperature

Table 11.6	Stages of breast growth
Stage I	The prepubertal stage. No development has yet occurred
Stage II	The breast bud begins to grow beneath the nipple
Stage III	The breast is more rounded and begins to resemble the adult breast in appearance, but is much smaller
Stage IV	Greater development has taken place, and the breast is larger than stage III. In addition, the nipple and areola project forward in front of the contour of the breast as a secondary mound
Stage V	Full adult breast size and form has been achieved

Table 11.7	Stages of pubic hair development
Stage I	Prepubertal stage. No terminal hair is visible
Stage II	Terminal hair appears on the vulva and in the midline of the mons
Stage III	The narrow triangular area of the pubis shows darker hair, which is still sparse in amount
Stage IV	A wider triangular area of the pubis is covered and the density is greater. The lateral angles of the triangle still have to be filled in
Stage V	The adult stage has been achieved

only one-third. This is due to the increase in size of the body of the uterus. The vagina changes from having a thin epithelium, to a thicker stratified multi-layered squamous epithelium, rich in glycogen.

Male

The first sign of puberty in boys is an increase in the size of the testis secondary to an FSH-induced increase in the seminiferous tubules. This is defined as stage II. At stage III, the scrotum reddens and the penis starts to increase in length. At stage IV the process continues with a more marked increase in the size of the penis, testes and scrotum. Stage V is reached when the testes are approximately 5 cm in length, the scrotum is pigmented and thickened and the penis is of adult size and proportions. Pubic hair starts to appear at stage III and is of an adult pattern at stage V. The growth spurt starts 12 months after the increase in testicular volume is noted.

Endocrinology of puberty

The factors controlling the time of onset of puberty are uncertain. It is thought that the hypothalamus in childhood is highly sensitive to sex steroid inhibition of GnRH secretion and that, as puberty approaches, this inhibition reduces resulting in increased secretion of GnRH and consequently of the gonadotrophins. However, in children without gonads, there is still inhibition of gonadotrophin secretion, implying the existence of another mechanism. This may involve leptin (see later), the hormone produced by fat tissue. Once the hypothalamic inhibition is overcome, and/or the inhibition from other factors is released, then, in females, the initial endocrine change is an increase in the nocturnal pulse frequency of GnRH. This stimulates FSH secretion and results in a multicystic appearance in the ovaries (also seen in the recovery phase of anorexia nervosa or exercise-induced amenorrhoea)

and in oestrogen secretion. Later in puberty, the levels of LH also increase. As puberty advances, the peaks in gonadotrophins occur during the day as well as at night, and finally in late puberty the secretion of gonadotrophins loses its diurnal pattern and the levels remain elevated. The next step is the onset of positive feedback of oestrogen on GnRH release, resulting in the LH surge, ovulation and menstruation (see later). Of the initial cycles, 90% are anovulatory. With time, the number falls, so that 4–5 years after menarche, less than 20% of cycles are anovulatory. The increasing levels of oestrogen stimulate the maturation of the female genital tract, breasts, the initial growth spurt followed by fusion of the epiphyses and the redistribution of the body fat. Fusion of the epiphyses limits growth. Therefore, high levels of oestrogen (endogenous or exogenous) in early life are one cause of stunted growth (see later).

Independent of the changes in gonadotrophins and oestrogen, the adrenal gland is increasingly active early in puberty, as shown by the higher circulating levels of dihydroepiandrostenedione sulphate (DHEAS). The factors controlling the onset of adrenal activity (adrenarche) are uncertain.

Leptin

Leptin is the 167-amino-acid product of the ob-gene in white fat cells. It is a helical molecule and a member of the tumour necrosis factor group of cytokines. It was discovered in the ob/ob mouse, where a mutation of the ob-gene results in obesity and hypogonadotrophic infertility. Replacement with leptin results in weight loss and the restoration of fertility, probably by increasing GnRH levels. Leptin expression is increased by insulin, glucocorticoids, noradrenaline and food. Circulating levels are reduced in weight-related amenorrhoea. Leptin is the probable link between body weight and menstruation.

Menstrual cycle

At the time of puberty the ovary contains between 300 000 and 600 000 primordial follicles. These consist of an oocyte (<25 μm) and its associated granulosa cells. Maturation from a primordial follicle is independent of gonadotrophins until the follicle reaches secondary follicle stage, when further maturation is dependent on FSH (Fig. 11.14). The tertiary follicle contains a steroid-rich, fluid-filled antrum and rapidly grows to become a pre-ovulatory, or graafian follicle (2.0–2.5 cm). In each cycle, around 10 secondary follicles are recruited. Eventually one becomes the dominant follicle and the remainder become atretic. Following

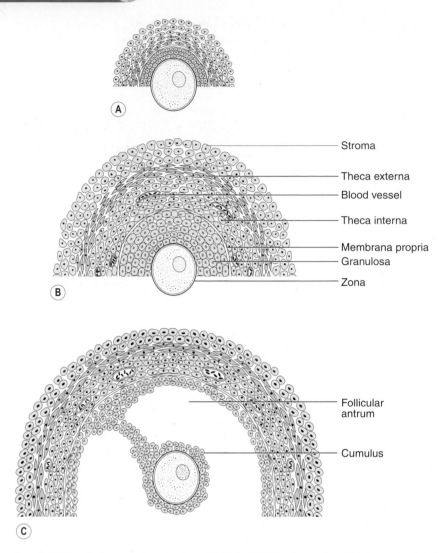

Figure 11.14 • Follicular maturation form (A) 1° to (B) 2° to the mature 3° (C) graafian follicle. (Reproduced with permission from Johnston MH 1988 Essential reproduction. 3rd edn. Blackwell Scientific, Oxford.)

ovulation, the granulosa cells luteinize and vessels from the theca invade as the remnant of the follicle becomes the corpus luteum.

Oestrogen synthesis by the developing follicle is controlled by FSH, which stimulates the production of aromatase by the granulosa cells. Androgens, synthesized by thecal cells in response to LH, pass across the basement membrane to granulosa cells to be converted by aromatase to oestrogens. This, the 'two cell' theory of oestrogen synthesis, developed from observations that granulosa cells do not possess the enzymes to be able to synthesize oestrogen from pregnenolone and progesterone themselves. However, thecal cells can also produce oestrogens and it has been suggested that the thecal cell oestrogen production determines the

circulating level of oestradiol, while the follicular fluid oestrogen is granulosa cell derived. Circulating oestrogen levels rise through the follicular phase of the cycle, peaking between days 12 and 14 (Fig. 11.15). The increasing levels trigger the LH surge, which stimulates ovulation. Progesterone levels increase slightly towards the end of the follicular phase and may also play a role in the LH surge.

After ovulation, the follicle remnant becomes the corpus luteum and produces oestrogen and progesterone. It also produces relaxin, inhibin-A and inhibin-B. The role of relaxin is uncertain, during both the menstrual cycle and pregnancy. Inhibin has been suggested to feed back to the pituitary to inhibit FSH release in both the male and female (see below). If pregnancy

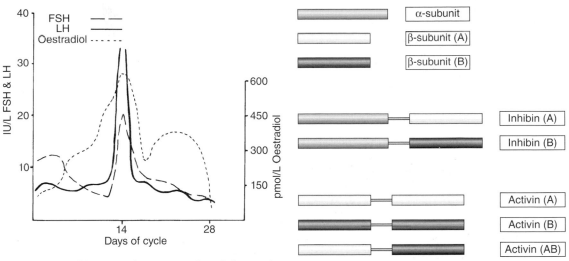

Figure 11.15 • Diagrammatic representation of changes in hormone levels during the menstrual cycle. The LH peak is left open because it is subject to great variation.

Figure 11.16 • The subunits forming activin and inhibin.

occurs, increasing levels of hCG maintain the corpus luteum and its production of oestrogen and progesterone until 8–9 weeks of pregnancy. Thereafter, the placenta becomes the main source of oestrogen and progesterone. The corpus luteum continues to produce relaxin throughout pregnancy.

Inhibin and activin

Inhibin and activin belong to the same family. Inhibin is a heterodimer made up of an α and β subunit. There are two β-subunits – A and B – thus inhibin may exist as either inhibin-A or inhibin-B. Activin is a homodimer of the β-subunit, and thus may exist as activin-A, activin-B or activin-AB (Fig. 11.16). During the menstrual cycle, activin is not detectable or is found at very low levels. Inhibin A and B are present in the circulation and are derived from the ovary. Inhibin is known to inhibit FSH release while activin stimulates it, but as both inhibin and activin are synthesized in the pituitary they may act in a paracrine manner to inhibit or stimulate FSH synthesis and release. During pregnancy, circulating levels of inhibin-A and activin-A are derived from the fetoplacental unit. Circulating levels of inhibin-A peak in early pregnancy and rise again at the end; those of activin increase gradually with gestation. A further marked increase in activin-A levels occurs with the onset of labour and in pregnancies complicated by pre-eclampsia. No changes have been reported in the circulating levels of inhibin-A with the onset of labour, but marked increases have also been reported in pregnancies complicated by pre-eclampsia. The role of either activin or inhibin during pregnancy is unknown.

Pregnancy

The placenta becomes the dominant source of circulating oestrogen and progesterone from 8–9 weeks of gestation. In addition, the placenta produces several peptides (hCG, human placental lactogen [HPL]) and virtually all of the hypothalamic-releasing hormones. hCG is structurally similar to LH but has an additional 30 amino acids. It is detectable in the maternal circulation approximately 10 days after ovulation. The level rises and peaks at 10–12 weeks' gestation (Fig. 11.17). hCG prevents corpus luteum involution. It may also stimulate the maternal thyroid and be responsible for hyperemesis gravidarum. It is produced in excessive amounts by placental tumours and may be used as a marker of therapeutic response.

During pregnancy, progesterone acts to maintain myometrial quiescence. Its importance is confirmed by the efficacy of progesterone antagonists in the induction of abortion in early pregnancy or labour in late pregnancy. In addition, it inhibits other smooth muscles of the body (the GI tract and urinary tract); it stimulates the appetite, fat storage and the respiratory centres (Table 11.5). The role of the three dominant oestrogens, oestrone [E_1], oestradiol [E_2] and oestriol [E_3], during pregnancy is less clear. They may promote uterine blood flow, myometrial growth, stimulate breast growth and at term promote cervical softening and the expression of myometrial oxytocin receptors (Table 11.4).

HPL is a member of the GH–prolactin family. It antagonizes the effect of insulin and so promotes lipolysis, reduces glucose utilization and enhances amino

Human chorionic gonadotrophin levels (IU/L)

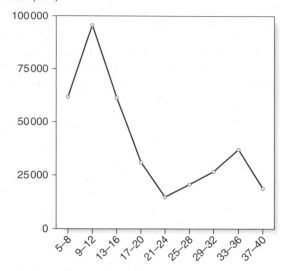

Figure 11.17 • Levels of human chorionic gonadotrophin during pregnancy.

acid transfer across the placenta. These effects may be designed to increase nutrient supply to the fetus. Prolactin levels rise throughout pregnancy probably from both pituitary and decidual sources. It promotes breast development, regulates fat metabolism and may contribute to the maternal immune suppression.

Biochemistry of human labour

During pregnancy, the uterus expands to accommodate the growing fetus and placenta, without increasing contractility, while the cervix remains firm and closed. Throughout pregnancy 'pro-pregnancy' factors operate to inhibit myometrial contractility and allow myometrial hypertrophy until, near to term, 'pro-labour' factors begin to operate to mediate remodelling of the cervix. These factors allow the cervix to efface and dilate, and stimulate the uterus to begin coordinated contractions. Labour is the result of the activation of a 'cassette of contraction-associated proteins' which act to convert the myometrium from a state of quiescence to a state of contractility. These include gap junction proteins, oxytocin and prostaglandin receptors, enzymes for the synthesis of prostaglandins or cytokines, and also components of cell-signalling mechanisms, which affect the way in which the uterus responds to receptor activation. It is likely that the factors which control the activation of the 'cassette of contraction-associated proteins' also activate factors in the fetal membranes that lead to the production of

prostaglandins and cytokines associated with labour, and factors within the cervix which lead to cervical remodelling and ripening.

Pregnancy can be divided into four parturitional phases. The first phase, during the first and second trimesters, is dominated by 'pro-pregnancy factors' and is the period of myometrial growth and quiescence. The second phase, during the early and mid-third trimester, is also a phase of myometrial quiescence, but during which preparation for labour is made by upregulation of myometrial, cervical and fetal membrane proteins which will be needed for labour. The third phase is the phase of labour itself and has the character of an inflammatory reaction. During this third phase of pregnancy, the 'brake' on myometrial contractility caused by 'pro-pregnancy' factors is released and the spontaneous contractility of the uterus is augmented by oxytocic compounds such as prostaglandins and possibly oxytocin itself. The fourth parturitional phase represents the state of the intrauterine tissues after the process of labour.

Pro-pregnancy factors

Progesterone is the principal pro-pregnancy factor. It has a negative regulatory effect upon many of the 'contraction-associated proteins' associated with the formation of myometrial gap junctions (connexins), and the modulation of cervical ripening (interleukin-8). It also decreases uterine sensitivity to oxytocin. In many species, a withdrawal of progesterone immediately precedes the onset of labour either through regression of the corpus luteum (e.g. in rodents) or through changes in placental steroidogenesis (e.g. in sheep). There is no obvious systemic withdrawal of progesterone prior to labour in the human or other primates. However, inhibition of progesterone, using mifepristone (RU486), causes cervical ripening and increases myometrial contractility. It is possible that in the human there is no actual or functional withdrawal of progesterone prior to labour, rather its 'pro-pregnancy' action is simply overwhelmed by 'pro-labour' factors. Alternative hypotheses are that there is a reduction in free, active progesterone, that progesterone withdrawal is a local event seen only within the fetal membranes, or that functional progesterone withdrawal occurs because of a switch from expression of the type 1 to the type 2 progesterone receptor within the uterus near to term. It has also been suggested that functional progesterone withdrawal may occur as a result of competition between progesterone and increased concentrations of cortisol which compete for binding to the same receptor.

In some species, for example the rabbit, nitric oxide synthesis in the endometrium also mediates myometrial quiescence and there is abrupt withdrawal just before labour. This is not seen in primates. Although the human uterus will relax if exposed to high concentrations of nitric oxide, there is no evidence for any physiological role for nitric oxide in human labour.

Placental clock

The timing of human labour is probably controlled by increased placental release of corticotrophin-releasing hormone (CRH), oestrogens, or a combination of both. The concentration of CRH in maternal plasma rises about 90 days prior to the onset of labour while binding protein falls. CRH acts to increase prostaglandin synthesis and may also directly stimulate myometrial contractility. Although maternal oestrogen concentrations do not rise acutely before human labour, as they do in sheep, there is a gradual rise in both oestriol and oestradiol concentrations during the third trimester, reaching a plateau at about 38 weeks. Oestradiol upregulates oxytocin receptors and oxytocin synthesis within the uterus.

The role of oxytocin probably varies from species to species. In the monkey, increased oxytocin release is associated with the switch from pre-labour contractures to labour contractions. In the human, there are no changes in oxytocin concentrations before or during labour, and, although the density of myometrial oxytocin receptors does increase toward term, oxytocin is not thought to signal the onset of human labour.

Labour: an inflammatory reaction

Labour is associated with increased prostaglandin synthesis within the uterus, especially within the fetal membranes. This increase is associated with increased activity of the pro-inflammatory prostaglandin synthetic enzyme cyclooxygenase type 2. Prostaglandins mediate cervical ripening and stimulate uterine contractions. They also act indirectly to increase fundally dominant myometrial contractility, by upregulation of oxytocin receptors and synchronization of contractions. There is also an increase in the production of inflammatory cytokines such as interleukin-1β and of chemokines such as interleukin-8. These are involved in complex feed-forward and feed-back mechanisms, which further increase cytokine and prostaglandin synthesis. At term, near to labour, the collagen of the cervix changes, undergoing collagenolysis. The fibrils become dissociated from their tightly organized bundles and are more widely scattered in an increased amount of ground substance; there is also a loosening of the collagen bundles in the cervical stroma. There is an accumulation of neutrophils which release collagenase into the cervix. Cervical ripening therefore resembles an inflammatory reaction. It is currently thought that neutrophils are attracted into the cervix at term by the combination of increased prostaglandin synthesis and the 'neutrophil attractant peptide' interleukin-8.

A unified hypothesis of the onset of labour in humans

How each of these various factors that are associated with the control of the length of human pregnancy and the onset of labour are linked is currently far from understood. A current hypothesis is that during the first parturitional phase the uterus is under strong progesterone repression. During the second phase, rising oestrogen and CRH concentrations activate proteins such as cell surface receptors and gap junctions, which will be needed for labour itself. CRH also increases the expression of inflammatory cytokines and of type 2 cyclooxygenase.

Labour itself arises because a relatively rapid increase in synthesis of inflammatory mediators and the influx of inflammatory cells leads to cervical ripening and uterine contractions. It is probable that the transition from parturitional phase two to phase three occurs once a certain threshold of CRH, or of cytokines stimulated by CRH, is reached. In addition, the fetus may signal its maturity, either through increased cortisol release, which stimulates placental CRH synthesis, and/or through release of platelet activating factor from the lungs, which also stimulates prostaglandin and cytokine synthesis. Once phase three is entered, there are multiple positive feedback mechanisms which accelerate the processes of labour, which only stops once delivery is complete.

Lactation

During pregnancy, several hormones stimulate breast growth (oestrogen, progesterone, HPL, prolactin, cortisol and insulin). However, the high concentrations of oestrogens inhibit lactation. After delivery, with the fall in oestrogen levels, lactation is initiated by the continuing prolactin stimulation. Prolactin is released from the anterior pituitary under the control of dopamine (inhibitory) and TRH (stimulatory). Prolactin continues to be released in response to suckling and promotes milk formation. The milk let-down reflex involves the release of oxytocin from the posterior pituitary, which stimulates the smooth muscle surrounding the acini to contract and cause milk ejection.

Menopause

The menopause is a retrospective diagnosis made after the absence of periods for 1 year. The average age in the UK is 50 years. It occurs because the ovary has run out of recruitable follicles. *In utero*, the peak number of oocytes is 7 million. By birth, this has fallen to 2 million and by the time of puberty only 3–600 000 remain. The factors which determine the initial number of oocytes and their rate of loss are unknown, but a premature menopause is associated with deletions of the X chromosome, smoking and galactosaemia. In the absence of sex steroids and probably of inhibin, gonado-trophin levels rise and remain elevated for 10 years or more. The ovaries become atrophic, as does the uterus (which reverts to a 1 : 1 ratio of body to cervix) and the vagina. The lack of oestrogen induces a series of vasomotor changes which include hot flushes, night sweats and palpitations. Depression is also more common and all these symptoms may be helped by hormone replacement therapy (HRT). Other structurally important changes occur in the heart, which becomes more susceptible to ischaemic heart disease (probably due to changes in the structure of the vessel wall and reductions in HDL and increases in LDL levels), and in the bones where bone resorption increases and formation reduces, together resulting in osteoporosis.

Growth

Growth *in utero* seems to be determined primarily by the maternal environment rather than any genetic influence. By the first birthday, there is a closer relationship between the current size and the child's final height. Whether a child will fulfil its genetic potential or not will depend on nutrition, health and the expression of the correct growth hormones. Growth is at its most rapid *in utero* and immediately after birth; thereafter a second peak occurs before puberty, but during puberty itself the increased levels of oestrogen and testosterone result in epiphyseal fusion and the cessation of longitudinal growth.

Physiology

Growth hormone (GH) is a 191-amino-acid peptide secreted from the somatotrophs of the anterior pituitary. It has some homology with prolactin and human placental lactogen (HPL) and its synthesis is increased in response to the growth hormone releasing hormone (GHRH) and reduced by somatostatin. Both GHRH and somatostatin are synthesized in the hypothalamus and carried to the anterior pituitary in the portal blood system. GH stimulates the synthesis of the insulin-related growth factors (IGF-I and IGF-II) predominantly in the liver, but also in the chondro-cytes, fat and muscle. It promotes lipolysis in fat and gluconeogenesis in the muscle. Plasma levels of the IGFs are highest in childhood, and fall with age. They act in both a paracrine and endocrine manner to promote bone growth, protein synthesis in muscle and lipolysis in fat cells. GH release is also stimulated by exercise and hypoglycaemia.

Other hormones are important in growth. These include those that: (1) control the availability of materials for growth, such as parathyroid hormone (calcium) and insulin (fats, carbohydrates and amino acids); (2) inhibit GH release such as cortisol; and (3) have effects on cell growth and differentiation themselves such as insulin, thyroid hormones and oestrogen and progesterone.

Dysfunction

Deficiency in GH leads to dwarfism in children and weight loss, lethargy and impaired physical performance in adults. Excess GH leads to gigantism in children and acromegaly in adults. The latter is characterized by excessive growth of soft tissues (tongue, liver, heart) and of bones (hand, feet and jaw); diabetes mellitus and hypertension.

Pancreas

The seat of control of blood glucose levels is the pancreas, working in concert with the liver, which acts as a store. Glucose is the principal energy source of the body and so its level has to be tightly controlled. Excess glucose is stored in the liver and muscle as glycogen and in adipose tissue as fat. At times of fasting, these stores are broken down to provide glucose and fatty acids as sources of energy. Only one hormone, insulin, controls the reduction in blood glucose levels. Several other hormones act to increase blood glucose; these include glucagon, adrenaline, growth hormone and cortisol. Both insulin and glucagon are synthesized and released in the islet cells of the pancreas.

Embryology

The pancreas develops between the layers of ventral mesentery from endodermal buds (ventral and dorsal) which originate from the caudal part of the foregut. The ventral bud forms the uncinate process and some of the head of the pancreas, but the majority of the pancreas is derived from the dorsal bud. The main pancreatic duct is derived from the ventral bud; this usually fuses with the dorsal bud duct, but occasionally the dorsal bud duct persists and opens into the duodenum independently.

Anatomy

The pancreas weighs approximately 80 g and is divided into the head (including the uncinate process), neck, body and tail. It is retroperitoneal, the head lying within the curve of the duodenum and the neck, body and tail extending in front of the vena cava and aorta to the spleen. The stomach lies anterior to the body and tail. The pancreas is made up of glandular acini (which secrete enzymes and bicarbonate) and the islets of Langerhans (1–2% of the pancreas) which synthesize glucagon (α cells), insulin (β cells), somatostatin (δ cells) and pancreatic polypeptide (PP).

Function

Insulin (mol.wt 5734, 51 amino acids) is made up of two chains (A and B). It is synthesized as a pre-pro-hormone and cleaved to pro-insulin and finally to insulin and C-peptide which are released in equal amounts (Fig. 11.4). Its release is stimulated by glucose (oral stimulus is greater than intravenous due to the involvement of the intestinal hormones), basic amino acids, ketones and free fatty acids. Insulin release is further potentiated by glucagon, GH and gut hormones, and inhibited by hypocalcaemia, adrenaline and somatostatin. The release profile of insulin is divided into two phases; the first is a burst lasting <1 min, and the second is more prolonged, persisting as long as does the stimulus to insulin secretion. Insulin promotes the transport of glucose and amino acids across the cell membrane in muscle and adipose tissues. In adipose tissue it inhibits lipolysis, and in the liver it increases glucose uptake and glycogen formation. Insulin is metabolized by the liver and kidney and has a half-life of approximately 10–15 min.

Glucagon (mol.wt 3485, 29 amino acids) is released in response to hypoglycaemia, basic amino acids, gut hormones, exercise and adrenaline. Its release is inhibited by increasing blood glucose, ketones, free fatty acids, insulin and somatostatin. It generally inhibits the uptake of glucose and amino acids, promotes lipolysis and hepatic glycogenolysis, gluconeogenesis and ketone generation.

Pancreatic somatostatin regulates stomach motility and the secretion of gut hormone and pancreatic polypeptide may have a role in the regulation of digestion.

Dysfunction

Insulin deficiency results in hyperglycaemia. The effects of hyperglycaemia are salt and water depletion due to an osmotic diuresis, weight loss, tiredness, vomiting, hypotension, infections, hyperventilation (due to ketoacidosis) and impaired conscious level and coma. Chronic hyperglycaemia results in microangiopathy (affecting the kidney, nerves and retina) and macroangiopathy causing peripheral, coronary and cerebral vascular disease.

Hypoglycaemia (defined as a blood sugar of <2.5 mmol/L) is usually a complication of insulin treatment and rarely the presenting symptom of liver disease, hypoadrenalism or insulinoma. In the early stages of hypoglycaemia, patients are pale, sweaty and tachycardic; they may complain of hunger and palpitations, and later may be confused, in a coma or even convulsing.

Thyroid

Embryology

The thyroid is the first endocrine gland to appear, beginning development at 24 days after fertilization and becoming active in terms of thyroid hormone secretion at about 11 weeks of pregnancy. It is derived from the floor of the primitive pharynx in the form of the 'thyroid diverticulum'. As the embryo grows, the thyroid descends to lie below the hyoid bone in front of the developing tracheal rings. During development the thyroid is connected to the tongue via the thyroglossal duct, a remnant of which may give rise to a thyroglossal cyst. The thyroid diverticulum divides into the left and right lobes and is connected by the isthmus (Fig. 11.18).

Anatomy

The thyroid weighs about 20 g and each lateral lobe is about 4 cm long. Its blood supply is from the superior thyroid artery (external carotid) and the inferior thyroid artery (subclavian artery), and the superior and middle thyroid veins drain into the internal jugular and the inferior into the brachiocephalic vein (Fig. 11.18). The four parathyroid glands lie on its posterior aspect. Microscopically, the thyroid is seen to consist of 1 million or more follicles. Each has a layer of follicular cells surrounding a central colloid. The follicular cells secrete thyroxine (T_4) and tri-iodothyronine (T_3) into the colloid which are then stored, bound to thyroglobulin. Parafollicular cells (C-cells) synthesize and secrete calcitonin.

Thyroid hormone synthesis

The thyroid hormones are iodinated metabolites of tyrosine (T_3 has three iodine molecules and T_4, four). The process of thyroid hormone synthesis (Fig. 11.19) is split into several steps: (1) iodide is actively taken up into the follicular cells by the iodide pump against the concentration gradient (iodide trapping); (2) it is converted to iodine (iodide oxidation); (3) tyrosine is incorporated to form pre-thyroglobulin; (4) which is iodinated to form iodoprethyroglobulin (contains 134 tyrosine residues, of which only 25–30 can be iodinated and 6–8 coupled into hormone residues) (Fig. 11.20); (5) coupling of T_1 and T_2 to form T_3 and of T_2 and T_2 to form T_4, both of which are stored in the colloid in the form of iodothyroglobulin; (6) iodothyroglobulin is

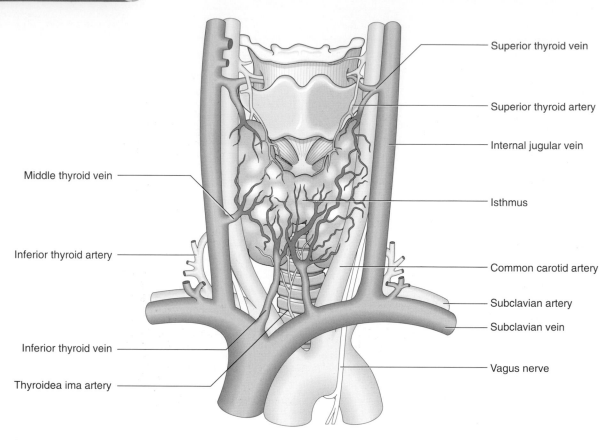

Figure 11.18 • The vascular supply of the thyroid gland.

taken up by the follicular cells and broken down into free T_3 and T_4, which diffuse into the blood. Once in the circulation thyroid hormones are bound (T_4, 99.96% and T_3, 99.4%) either to thyroxine binding globulin (TBG), pre-albumin or albumin (Table 11.8); only the free portion is active. The circulating levels of T_4 are higher than T_3 as the thyroid secretes more T_4 than T_3 and T_4 has a longer half-life. However, T_4 is less active than T_3 and acts more as a storage form; it is also converted peripherally and within cells to T_3. T_4 can be converted to T_3 and to rT_3 (an inactive form). The relative balance in this conversion varies and more T_4 is converted to rT_3 during illness. Also during illness, the feedback effects of thyroid hormones seem to be lost, so that, although the peripheral concentrations are low, the pituitary response seems to be reduced and TSH levels are not elevated, giving rise to the 'sick-euthyroid' picture. T_3 is inactivated by further deiodination or conjugation in the liver. The fetus and neonate also have relatively high levels of rT_3.

The recommended daily intake of iodine is 150 mg; it is found in meat and vegetables. Thyroid uptake of

Table 11.8 Relative binding of T_4 and T_3 to plasma proteins and its effect on their activities

	T_4	T_3
Total in serum (nmol/L)	50	1
Fraction bound (%)		
TBG[a]	85	75
TBPA[b]	14	0
Albumin	0.95	24.5
Fraction free (%)	0.05	0.5
Total free (pmol/L)	25	5
Potency[c] of free hormone	1	8
Activity (total free × potency)	25	40

[a]TBG, thyroxine-binding globulin.
[b]TBPA, thyroxine-binding prealbumin.
[c]Potency, calorigenic effect and prevention of goitre in propylthiouracil-treated animals.

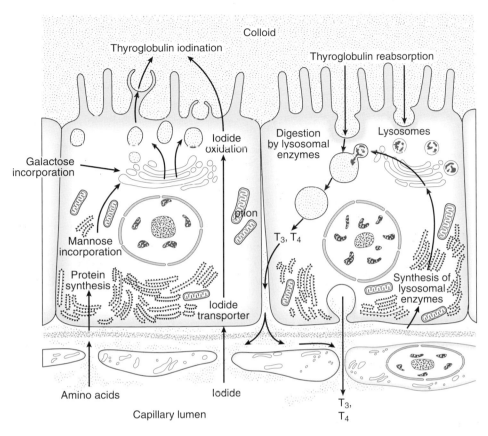

Figure 11.19 • The synthesis, storage and release of thyroid hormones. (Reproduced with permission from Greenpan FS, Strewler GJ 1997 Basic and clinical endocrinology. 5th edn. Appleton and Lange, London.)

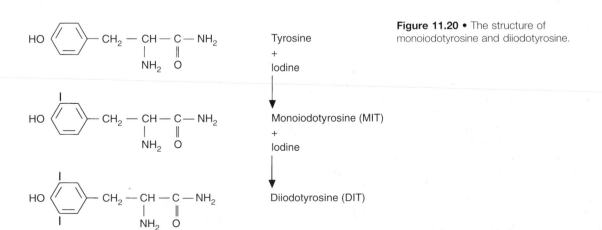

Figure 11.20 • The structure of monoiodotyrosine and diiodotyrosine.

iodine is enhanced by TSH and iodine deficiency, but reduced by an excess of iodine and digoxin. Most iodine is excreted via the kidneys (Fig. 11.21).

Function

Thyroid stimulating hormone (TSH, molecular weight 28 000, 204 amino acids) is released from the anterior pituitary in response to TRH, a tripeptide synthesized in the supraoptic and supraventricular nuclei. TSH has a number of effects on the thyroid: it increases its size, vascularity, iodine uptake, protein synthesis, storage of colloid and the secretion of T_3 and T_4. Thyroid hormones feed back to both the hypothalamus and pituitary.

There are several thyroid receptors which bind to the thyroid hormone response element on DNA. The transcriptional effects of T_3 take hours or days to occur (such as tissue growth, brain maturation, increased heat production and oxygen consumption). Other non-genomic effects are more immediate; these include an increase in glucose and amino acid transport. T_4 and T_3 are essential for normal fetal development. In their absence, brain development and musculoskeletal maturation are markedly impaired resulting in 'cretinism'. Thyroid hormones maintain the normal hypoxic and hypercapnic drives to the respiratory centre and this may account for the occasional need to ventilate patients with severe hypothyroidism. Metabolically, T_4 and T_3 stimulate lipolysis, glycolysis, gluconeogenesis, the absorption of glucose and the metabolism of insulin and cortisol.

In excess, thyroid hormones increase O_2 consumption and heat production by stimulation of Na^+-K^+ ATPase and are positively inotropic and chronotropic on the heart. Part of their cardiovascular effects is mediated through an increase in the expression of β-receptors in the heart and they have similar effects in skeletal muscle and adipose tissue. Thyroid hormones increase gut motility and thus cause diarrhoea. They also increase bone resorption and thyrotoxicosis or excess thyroxine replacement therapy may be associated with osteopenia.

Thyroid function in pregnancy is altered in two ways. The circulating levels of the thyroid binding proteins are increased, resulting in an increase in the total circulating levels of thyroid hormones (but a slight fall in the free component). In addition, pregnancy is associated with stimulation of thyroid hormone production, probably by a direct effect of hCG on the thyroid, so that in some normal pregnancies TSH may be suppressed. This effect is particularly marked in hyperemesis gravidarum, where the TSH is usually suppressed, raising the question of thyrotoxicosis. Also, during pregnancy, maternal thyroid disease can affect the fetus in two ways: (1) the maternal antibodies causing thyrotoxicosis or hypothyroidism may cross the placenta and cause a similar self-limiting problem in the fetus and (2) the therapy used in the treatment of thyrotoxicosis may cross the placenta and cause fetal hypothyroidism.

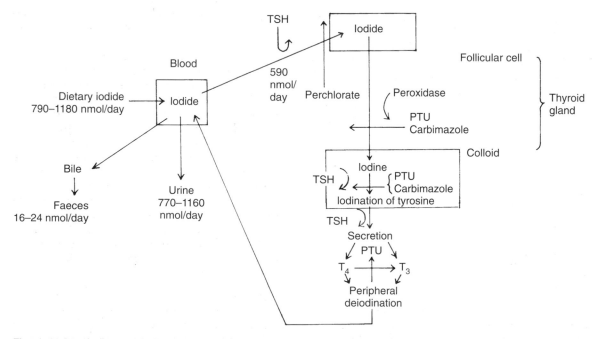

Figure 11.21 • Iodine metabolism.

Table 11.9 The effects of thyroid excess and deficiency

Process	Thyrotoxicosis	Hypothyroidism
Metabolism	High Weight loss	Low Weight gain
Heat production	Increased Heat intolerance	Reduced Cold intolerance
Gut	Increased motility Diarrhoea	Reduced motility Constipation
Heart	Fast heart rate, palpitations	Slow heart rate
General	Sweating, tremor, anxiety	Dry skin, depression, lethargy

Dysfunction

The effects of thyroid hormone deficiency and excess are shown in Table 11.9.

Therapy of thyroid disease

The management of thyrotoxicosis due to Graves' disease is usually with antithyroid drugs, the most common of which are carbimazole and propylthiouracil (PTU). Both act to inhibit the conversion of iodide to iodine, the iodination of tyrosine and the release of both T_4 and T_3; propylthiouracil in addition prevents the deiodination of T_4. Giving iodine also suppresses the thyroid gland via an uncertain mechanism. The dose of antithyroid drugs used during pregnancy should be determined by the maternal free thyroxine and TSH levels. As these drugs readily cross the placenta while a relatively smaller proportion of the maternal thyroid hormones cross the placenta, a block and replace approach is not appropriate. Although both drugs are present in breast milk, the amount of propylthiouracil is relatively less.

In hypothyroid women the replacement dosage of thyroxine should also be titrated to the TSH and for maternal free thyroxine levels using normal ranges for pregnancy.

Adrenal gland

Embryology

The cortex of the adrenal gland develops from mesoderm (the mesothelium of the posterior abdominal wall), the medulla from neural crest cells. The latter is essentially part of the sympathetic nervous system. Differentiation of the cortex begins in late fetal life, but the zona reticularis is not recognizable until 3 years of age. At birth, the adrenal cortex is large due to the presence of the fetal cortex (which produces DHEAS as a substrate for placental oestrogen synthesis). This regresses over the first year of life.

Anatomy

The adrenal glands weigh approximately 4–5 g, are retroperitoneal and lie on top of the kidneys. The yellowish cortex accounts for 90% of the gland weight and the medulla, the remainder. The adrenals are supplied with blood by branches of the aorta, renal and inferior phrenic arteries. Each gland has one vein which drains on the right into the inferior vena cava and on the left into the renal vein.

The cortex is divided into three layers. The outer, zona glomerulosa, produces aldosterone (it lacks 17α-hydroxylase and so cannot produce cortisol or androgens). The middle, zona fasciculata, which is the thickest layer, produces androgens and cortisol. The inner, zona reticularis, also produces androgens and cortisol. Both of the inner zones are controlled by adrenocorticotrophic hormone (ACTH).

Adrenal cortisol synthesis

ACTH controls the synthesis of cortisol (and androgens) by the zona fasciculata and reticularis. ACTH is itself controlled by the hypothalamic hormones CRH and vasopressin. ACTH stimulation of the adrenal results in an immediate increase in the circulating levels of cortisol; it also increases the availability of cholesterol.

ACTH is released in a circadian rhythm, so that cortisol is lowest in the evening and highest in the early hours of the morning. This pattern is lost during illness, stress, Cushing's syndrome and alcoholism. An acute stress, physical or otherwise, results in an increase in ACTH and cortisol levels. Cortisol feeds back at the level of the hypothalamus and the pituitary. At the level of the pituitary, cortisol reduces ACTH release acutely within minutes, and chronically by reducing synthesis of its precursor, pro-opiomelanocortin.

Once released, 95% of cortisol circulates bound to cortisol binding protein (80%) and albumin (15%). Most is metabolized in the liver and a small amount is excreted unchanged in the urine (24-h urine collection and cortisol measurement is used as an initial estimation of cortisol production).

Function

Cortisol, like the other steroid hormones, enters the cell, binds to its receptor and then directly interacts with a response element on DNA to alter gene expression. It is important metabolically and in the management of 'stress'.

Metabolism

Cortisol stimulates gluconeogenesis and lipolysis (increasing glycerol and free fatty acid levels), but inhibits peripheral glucose usage. Overall effect is to maintain glucose levels.

Connective tissue

Fibroblasts are inhibited and collagen lost, resulting in thin skin with easy bruising and poor wound healing. Bone resorption is enhanced and formation inhibited resulting in bone loss, both by a direct effect on bone and indirectly by (1) enhancing the activity of parathyroid hormone and vitamin D, and (2) increasing urinary calcium excretion and reducing calcium absorption in the gut. In the adult, this results in bone loss, and in children this may contribute to the observed reduction in growth.

Haematology and immunology

Cortisol has little effect on haematopoiesis, but it does increase the circulating neutrophil count by increasing their production and half-life, and reducing their movement out of the circulation. Circulating numbers of lymphocytes, eosinophils and monocytes are reduced by increasing their movement out of the circulation. Glucocorticoid steroids are generally immunosuppressive.

Cardiovascular and renal effects

Cardiac output is increased as is peripheral resistance. The combination results in an increase in blood pressure. This effect is augmented by salt and water retention (potassium excretion), which is induced by stimulation of the mineralocorticoid receptors.

Miscellaneous effects

Corticosteroids may cause a change in affect resulting in euphoria; other psychiatric states may also be observed. Gonadal function may be suppressed.

Dysfunction

The typical pictures of Cushing's syndrome (cortisol excess) and Addison's disease (cortisol deficiency) are shown in Table 11.10.

Adrenal androgens

Adrenal androgen synthesis occurs predominantly in the zona reticularis, is controlled by ACTH and starts between 7 and 9 years of age (adrenarche). DHEA and androstenedione, and to a lesser extent testosterone, are synthesized and account for 50% of testosterone in the female and 5% in the male. Excessive secretion results in hirsutism and virilism in the female.

Table 11.10 Features of cortisol excess and deficiency

Process	Cushing's syndrome	Addison's disease
Metabolic	Increased glucose and free fatty acids, central fat deposition	Hypoglycaemia
Connective tissue	Collagen loss causing thin skin, muscle wastage, osteoporosis	
Haematology and immunology	Increased neutrophils Reduced lymphocytes	Reduced neutrophils, increased lymphocytes
Psychiatric	Euphoria and other psychiatric disturbances	Lethargy
Cardiovascular and renal effects	Hypertension, fluid retention and hypokalaemia	Hypotension, hyponatraemia and hyperkalaemia

Adrenal medulla

The adrenal medulla is essentially part of the sympathetic nervous system from which it receives a rich nerve supply. Sympathetic stimulation results in the release of adrenaline and noradrenaline (both synthesized from the amino acid tyrosine) into the blood, where they circulate bound to albumin until metabolized in the liver (by catecholamine-O-methyl transferase and monoamine oxidase into vanillylmandelic acid, VMA). The effects of adrenaline and noradrenaline are mediated through G-protein-linked surface receptors which are classified generally into α and β. Their activation produces the typical 'flight or fight response' (Table 11.11).

In excess, as seen in a phaeochromocytoma, adrenaline causes marked hypertension and anxiety. It may also be associated with sweating, pallor and tremor as expected from its effects listed in Table 11.11. It is possible to measure the circulating levels of catecholamines to make the diagnosis of a phaeochromocytoma, but many units still use 24-h urinary excretion of VMA. If either is elevated, further investigation involves visualization of the adrenals.

Table 11.11 Effects of sympathetic activation

Organ/system	Effect
CVS	Tachycardia, hypertension
Skin	Sweating and vasoconstriction
Muscle	Vasodilatation
Liver	Increased gluconeogenesis
Pancreas	Reduced insulin and increased glucagon release
Adrenal gland	Increased cortisol release
Fat	Increased lipolysis
CNS	Dilated pupils, increased level of alertness

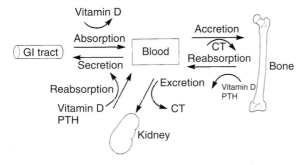

Figure 11.22 • Calcium: secretion into an excretion from the blood to the gastrointestinal tract, bone and kidney. The influences of vitamin D, parathyroid hormone and calcitonin.

Calcium homeostasis

Calcium is essential for many of the body's processes. It is a key intracellular messenger necessary for the maintenance of cell membrane potential in excitable cells (nerve, cardiac), muscle contraction, enzyme action and inhibition, and hormone release; it also is important in bone formation and clotting factor activity. It is not surprising, therefore, that there is a complex mechanism to ensure that its levels are tightly regulated. The key components are parathyroid hormone (PTH), vitamin D and calcitonin, which act on the bone (which contains most of the body's calcium), kidney and gut (Fig. 11.22). The calcium concentration in plasma is 2.5 mmol/L; approximately 45% is protein bound (albumin) and the remainder is either free (47%) and therefore active, or complexed with other compounds.

Parathyroid hormone (PTH)

PTH anatomy and embryology

There are four parathyroid glands which develop from the pharyngeal pouches: the superior glands from the dorsal portion of the third pouch and the inferior glands from the superior portion of the fourth pouch. They are oval shaped, about 0.5 cm in size, 40 g in weight and embedded beneath the capsule in the posterior aspect of the thyroid gland. Their blood supply is derived from the thyroid arteries. They contain two sorts of cell: the chief cells which synthesize, store and secrete PTH, and the oxyphil cells of unknown function.

PTH synthesis

The gene for PTH is located on chromosome 11. It is synthesized as a pre-pro-hormone; the signal peptide is removed to form pro-PTH, which is converted to PTH by the removal of the pro-sequence in the Golgi apparatus prior to storage in the cell cytoplasm. It is an 84-amino-acid peptide with a molecular weight of 9300. Low plasma calcium levels evoke its release, which is suppressed by increased plasma calcium levels.

PTH function

PTH acts via G-protein-linked cell surface receptors in bone and kidney. In the kidney, it acts on the renal tubule to enhance phosphate and bicarbonate excretion (proximal), and calcium and hydrogen ion reabsorption (distal); it also enhances the renal 1α-hydroxylation of vitamin D, increasing vitamin D activity. PTH acts indirectly on the gut through increased vitamin D activity to enhance calcium and phosphate absorption. In the bone, PTH reduces osteoblast collagen synthesis and enhances osteoclast activity, which results in increased osteolysis and release of collagenase and hydrogen ions; the last two enhance bone resorption. The overall effect of PTH is to increase circulating calcium and phosphate.

PTH dysfunction

A deficiency of PTH results in hypocalcaemia and the clinical picture of brisk reflexes – Chvostek's sign, (tapping over the facial nerve causes a facial twitch), numbness and paraesthesia, tetany carpopedal spasm (Trousseau's sign, induced by inflating a blood pressure cuff), and a prolonged QT interval on ECG. An excess causes hypercalcaemia and the clinical picture of 'bones, stones, moans and groans':

1. *Bones* are painful and fragile due to excessive resorption.
2. Renal *stones* are due to increased urinary calcium levels and ectopic calcification secondary to hypercalcaemia in the heart, pancreas, uterus and liver.

3. *Groans* include headache, abdominal pain, anorexia and constipation.

4. *Moans* include weakness and tiredness. Reflexes are sluggish, there is polyuria, dehydration and renal failure, confusion and coma. On ECG, the QT interval is short and cardiac arrhythmias may be seen.

Vitamin D

Vitamin D synthesis

Vitamin D is a sterol hormone (synthesized from cholesterol). It is either synthesized in the skin by photo-isomerization (90%, action of UV light) or absorbed in the diet (10%, fish and eggs). It is activated in the liver and kidney. In the liver, vitamin D is 25-hydroxylated and then stored in body fat. It is transported to the kidney where it is 1-hydroxylated in the proximal tubules. The 1α-hydroxylation is controlled by PTH (see earlier), calcium and phosphate levels, growth hormone, cortisol, oestrogens and prolactin.

Vitamin D function

Vitamin D promotes calcium absorption at various sites (gut, kidney and bone). It does this by binding to a nuclear receptor (VDR) which has a DNA binding domain. Once vitamin D has bound, the complex (vitamin D–VDR) has to bind with retinoic acid receptor to form a heterodimer in order to be able to bind to DNA and to exert its genomic effects. In the gut, vitamin D increases calcium and phosphate absorption in the jejunum and ileum. There are several possible mechanisms: (1) opening of calcium channels, (2) the increased synthesis of two calcium binding proteins (calbindins) which promote the passage of calcium across the cell into the blood and (3) the promotion of mucosal cell division and growth. In the bone, it increases calcium and phosphate release by enhancing osteoclast activity; this effect is indirect as osteoclasts lack VDR. In addition, osteoblast synthesis of osteocalcin is increased. Thus, in the bone, vitamin D has effects which promote formation and resorption and quite what its overall effect is remains uncertain (see later). In the kidney, vitamin D increases tubular calcium and phosphate reabsorption.

Vitamin D dysfunction

A deficiency of vitamin D has varying effects depending on the age of the subject. In children, deficiency results in rickets with bowed legs, chest deformity and hypocalcaemia. In adults, deficiency results in osteomalacia with bone pain, fractures, hypocalcaemia and on X-ray pseudofractures are seen (Looser's zones). The effects of vitamin D deficiency relate to impaired gut absorption of calcium, which results in hypocalcaemia. This increases serum PTH which stimulates bone resorption

and causes the picture of bone demineralization. Vitamin D-resistant rickets rarely occurs and is an X-linked dominant condition, which is the result of an abnormal vitamin D receptor. Vitamin D excess results in hypercalcaemia, the features of which have been described earlier in the section on PTH.

Vitamin D deficiency may arise in a variety of ways: (1) dietary deficiency; (2) malabsorption due either to obstruction of the bile duct or bowel disease as seen in coeliac or Crohn's disease; (3) liver disease that may result in reduced 25-hydroxylation; and (4) renal disease that may result in reduced 1α-hydroxylation.

Calcitonin

Calcitonin is synthesized by the parafollicular C-cells of the thyroid. These are neuroendocrine cells derived from the neural crest, which make up less than 0.1% of the mass of the thyroid.

Calcitonin synthesis

Calcitonin is 32 amino acids in length and its synthesis is regulated by circulating calcium levels, increasing when the levels are higher and reducing when they are lower. The gene encodes two different peptides which are formed by alternative splicing. The first is calcitonin and the second calcitonin gene-related peptide (CGRP). CGRP is a 37-amino-acid peptide with potent vasodilator properties which is thought to be at least in part responsible for the marked vasodilatation of pregnancy.

Calcitonin function

Calcitonin acts via a G-protein-linked receptor which is linked to adenyl cyclase. Its primary site of action is the bone where it reduces osteoclast activity, although it also acts in the renal tubule to reduce phosphate reabsorption and to a lesser extent calcium. The importance of calcitonin in calcium homeostasis is uncertain (see later).

Calcitonin dysfunction

Medullary tumours of the thyroid secrete calcitonin and result in high circulating levels. Despite this, calcium levels are unaltered. Nor are calcium levels altered by a total thyroidectomy, which removes the only source of calcitonin. Thus, in the human it is uncertain whether calcitonin has any role in calcium homeostasis. Nevertheless, therapeutically, calcitonin is useful for the treatment of Paget's disease of bone and as an inhibitor of osteoclast activity.

Osteoporosis

In contrast to osteomalacia, osteoporosis occurs when there is insufficient protein synthesis, i.e. a deficiency of bone trophic hormones, but mineralization is normal.

The most common example is in postmenopausal women, although hypogonadal men have the same problem. Peak bone mass is typically reached at 25–30 years and thereafter declines at an annual rate of 2–5% in women and 0.3–0.5% in men. Bone loss may be prevented or reduced by a number of approaches: (1) hormone replacement therapy, (2) calcium supplements in combination with vitamin D; (3) calcitonin (inhibitors of osteoclast activity such as the bisphosphonate), and (4) weight-bearing exercises.

Chapter Twelve

12

Drugs and drug therapy

Hassan Shehata

Introduction

A drug is broadly defined as any chemical agent that affects living protoplasm. About one-third of women in the UK take drugs at least once during pregnancy, but only 6% take a drug during the first trimester. In the puerperium, the use of drugs increases substantially with no difference in the pattern of prescribing between mothers who breastfeed and those who bottle-feed.

Possible effects of drugs in pregnancy include:

- Teratogenicity (e.g. thalidomide) – readily detected at, or shortly after, birth
- Long-term latency (e.g. diethylstilbestrol (DES) – increased risk of vaginal adenocarcinoma after puberty, or abnormalities in testicular function and semen production)
- Impaired intellectual or social development (e.g. exposure to phenobarbital or sodium valproate).

Language of clinical pharmacy

Prodrugs are pharmacologically inactive derivatives of active drugs. They are designed to maximize the amount of active drug that reaches its site of action through manipulation of the physicochemical, biopharmaceutical or pharmacokinetic properties of the drug. Prodrugs are converted into the active drug within the body through enzymatic or non-enzymatic reactions.

Distribution volume is a hypothetical concept that is defined as the volume that a drug would occupy if the concentration throughout the body were equal to that in plasma. The distribution volume depends on factors like lipid solubility and protein binding.

Clearance is the volume of plasma cleared of the drug in unit time. It determines what dose of drug is necessary to maintain a certain plasma concentration but does not indicate how rapidly the drug disappears when treatment is stopped. Patients with abnormal renal or liver function can have increased clearance times.

A receptor is any cellular molecule to which a drug binds to initiate its effects. Receptors can be proteins (hormones, growth factors and neurotransmitters) or nucleic acids (cancer chemotherapeutic agents). An agonist binds to a physiological receptor and often mimics the regulatory effects of endogenous signalling compounds. An antagonist binds to receptors without regulatory effects and blocks the endogenous agonist. Drugs that stabilize the receptor in its inactive form are called inverse antagonists. Receptors of relevance to clinical practice are summarized in Table 12.1.

Table 12.1 Some receptors involved in the action of commonly used drugs

Receptor	Subtype	Main actions of natural agonist	Drug agonist	Drug antagonist
Adrenoceptor	α_1	Vasoconstriction		Prazosin
	α_2	Hypotension, sedation	Clonidine	
	β_1	↑ Heart rate	Dopamine Dobutamine	Atenolol Metoprolol
	β_2	Bronchodilation; vasodilation Uterine relaxation	Salbutamol, terbutaline Ritodrine	
Cholinergic	Muscarinic	↓ Heart rate ↑ Secretion ↑ Gut motility Bronchoconstriction		Atropine Benztropine Orphenadrine Ipratropium
	Nicotinic	Contraction of striated muscle		Suxamethonium Tubocurarine
Histamine	H_1	Bronchoconstriction Capillary dilation		Chlorpheniramine Terfenadine
	H_2	↑ Gastric acid		Cimetidine Ranitidine
Dopamine		CNS neurotransmitter	Bromocriptine	Chlorpromazine Haloperidol Thioridazine
Opioid		CNS neurotransmitter	Morphine, pethidine, etc.	Naloxone

CNS, central nervous system.

pKa is the pH at which half the drug is in its ionized form.

Henderson–Hasselbalch equation is used to calculate the ratio of ionized to non-ionized drug at each pH.

Absorption is the rate at which a drug leaves its site of administration and the extent to which this occurs.

Bioavailability is the term used to indicate the fractional extent to which a dose of drug reaches its site of action or a biological fluid from which the drug has access to its site of action.

Half-life (t½) is the time taken for the plasma concentration, or the amount of the drug in the body, to be reduced by 50%. The half-life of a drug depends on its rate of clearance and volume of distribution. Highly lipophilic drugs may have an increased clearance but prolonged half-life.

Steady-state concentration is reached when drug elimination is equal to availability with repeated equal doses. It takes repeated dosing for about five half-lives to achieve steady state.

Teratogenesis

This is defined as structural or functional (e.g. renal failure) dysgenesis of the fetal organs. Typical manifestations of teratogenesis include congenital malformations with varying severity, intrauterine growth restriction, carcinogenesis and fetal demise. Lack of understanding of the mechanisms of teratogenicity makes it difficult to predict on pharmacological grounds that a particular drug will produce congenital malformations. The period of highest sensitivity to teratogens is early organogenesis. Later in fetal development, exposure to a teratogen is far less likely to be the cause of a structural defect, but can cause serious functional abnormalities, notably of the neurobehavioural type.

Organogenesis

The major body structures are formed in the first 12 weeks after conception (Fig. 12.1). Interference in this process causes a teratogenic effect. If a drug is given after this time it will not produce a major anatomical defect, but possibly a functional one. The overall incidence of major congenital malformations is around 2–3% of all births, and of minor malformations, 9%. The part played by drugs is probably small. It has been estimated that 25% of congenital malformations are due to genetic or chromosomal abnormalities, 10% due to environmental causes including drugs and 65% are of unknown aetiology. Even known teratogens do not invariably cause anatomical defects and the mechanism of drug-induced teratogenicity remains unclear. The genetic composition of the fetus, the timing of the insult, maternal age, nutritional condition, disease status and the dose of the drug may play a role. The critical time for drug-induced congenital malformations is usually the period of organogenesis. This occurs approximately 20–55 days after conception, i.e. 34–69 days (7–10 weeks) after the first day of the last menstrual period (Fig. 12.1).

Pharmacokinetics

Pharmacokinetics is the mathematical description of the rate and extent of uptake, distribution and elimination of drugs in the body. It mainly concerns time.

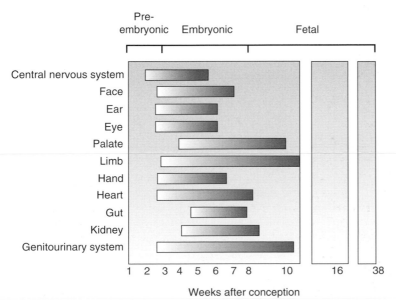

Figure 12.1 • Timing of the development of major body structures in the embryo and fetus. (From Br Med J (Clin Res Ed) 1986;293:1485–8, with permission of BMJ Publishing.)

Pharmacokinetics is important for drugs that are given for more than an isolated dose, and those whose margin of safety is narrow. The pharmacokinetics of a drug depends upon its concentration, structure, degree of ionization, relative lipid solubility and binding to tissue proteins.

Oral absorption is unpredictable and is dependent on various factors such as gastric emptying time, surface area of absorption, blood flow, lipid solubility and physical state of the drug. Venous drainage from the oral mucosa is to the superior vena cava and hence bypasses first-pass metabolism. Rectal administration causes erratic absorption and irritation of the rectal mucosa but 50% of the dose will bypass the liver. Absorption after subcutaneous or intramuscular injection occurs by simple diffusion.

Distribution occurs in two phases: an initial rapid phase to the liver, kidney and brain followed by a slow phase to the muscles, viscera, skin and fat. The distribution of a drug is determined by its lipid solubility and the pH gradient between the intracellular and extracellular fluids.

- Acidic drugs bind to albumin (e.g. salicylates, warfarin, anticonvulsants, NSAIDs)
- Basic drugs bind to α_1-acid glycoprotein (e.g. beta-blockers, opioid analgesics, local anaesthetics)
- Covalent bonding can occur with reactive drugs, e.g. alkylating agents.

Hypoalbuminaemia due to liver disease or nephrotic syndrome results in reduced binding and an increase in the unbound fraction of acidic drugs. An acute-phase response leads to an elevation of α_1-acid glycoprotein levels and therefore to reduced availability of basic drugs. Figure 12.2 summarizes the different compartments in which drugs can be distributed in the materno-fetal unit.

Drugs can undergo different types of transport

Transcapillary movement: this is transfer of the drug with bulk transfer of water due to hydrostatic or osmotic pressure differences and accounts for the majority of unbound drug transfer.

Paracellular transport: this occurs between cell junctions and is the principal mechanism of excretion of drugs by the kidney.

Passive transport: this is diffusion of the drug through the cell membrane along a concentration gradient by virtue of its lipid solubility.

Active transport: this is characterized by a requirement for energy and involves the movement of a drug against an electrochemical gradient.

Facilitated diffusion: this is a carrier-mediated transport process in which there is no input of energy. Enhanced movement is down an electrochemical gradient.

Drugs that are lipid soluble are less likely to be excreted and polar compounds are likely to be excreted more quickly. The kidneys excrete drugs by filtration, tubular secretion and tubular re-absorption. Changes in renal function affect all three functions and are impaired

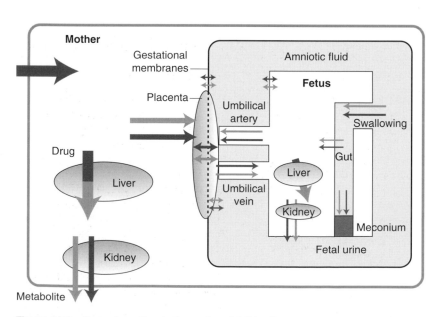

Figure 12.2 • Drug disposition in the maternal–fetal unit.

in the elderly, as adult renal function decreases by 1% per year. Unbound drugs are excreted by filtration. P glycoprotein and multidrug resistance associated protein type 2 secrete ions and conjugated metabolites, respectively, into the tubules. Some of the ways that pregnancy influences pharmacokinetics are summarized in Table 12.2.

Pharmacodynamics

Pharmacodynamics is the study of biochemical and physiological effects of drugs on the body and their mechanism of action. The majority of the drugs pass through cells rather than between them. Broadly speaking, drugs act on four different targets: receptors, enzymes, membrane ion channels and metabolic processes. Drugs commonly act on electrical or chemical signalling pathways and drug action commonly involves a signal transduction pathway, which consists of receptor, cellular target and intermediary molecules.

Factors that influence drug action

Drug metabolism

Drug metabolism will influence the duration and potency of the effect of specific drugs. Drugs are commonly converted to more polar metabolites to facilitate their excretion. This is frequently catalysed by enzymic reactions. While the majority of drug metabolism results in less toxic metabolites, occasionally it can result in the formation of more toxic compounds. A large number of drugs are metabolized by hepatic phase I and II reactions.

Phase I metabolism occurs in the endoplasmic reticulum and involves the formation of more polar metabolites of the original compound. These reactions can involve oxidation (catalysed by cytochrome P450 enzymes), hydrolysis, reduction, cyclization or decyclization. The polar metabolites may be directly excreted, usually in the urine, or may be converted further by phase II reactions.

Phase II reactions occur in the cytoplasm and commonly involve conjugation with sulphates, glucuronides, glutathione or amino acids and result in the formation of metabolites that are usually less toxic and more easily excreted.

The metabolism of a drug can be affected by enzyme induction, protein binding and the liver extraction ratio. Table 12.3 summarizes the common drugs that influence the activity of the liver microsomal enzymes.

Drug interactions

Drugs that are likely to precipitate drug interactions are those that are highly protein bound, alter metabolism of other drugs or alter renal or hepatic metabolism. Drugs that are affected by drug interactions are those that have a steep dose–response curve and those that have a low toxic:therapeutic ratio (e.g. aminoglycosides, anticoagulants, anticonvulsants, antihypertensives, cardiac glycosides, cytotoxic drugs, oral contraceptives).

Table 12.2   The principal factors that influence maternal, fetal and placental pharmacokinetics in normal pregnancy

Maternal pharmacokinetics	Fetal pharmacokinetics	Placental pharmacokinetics
Changes in body fluid volume Changes in CVS parameters Changes in pulmonary function Alterations in gastric activity Changes in serum binding protein concentrations and occupancy Alterations in kidney function	Plasma binding proteins differ from maternal so free fractions of basic drugs are elevated Liver expresses metabolizing enzymes, but capacity less than in mother Drugs transferred across the placenta undergo first pass through the fetal liver The fetal kidney is immature Fetal urine enters amniotic fluid which may be swallowed by the fetus	Blood flow through the placenta (maternal side) increases during gestation (i.e. from 50 mL/min at 10 weeks of pregnancy to 600 mL/min at 38 weeks) Transfer of flow-limited drugs is affected by placental flow Compounds that alter blood flow alter maternal drug disposition and placental transfer Placental metabolism (dealkylation, hydroxylation, demethylation) affects drug transfer across the placenta At term, the surface area of the placenta is at its maximum and nearly all substances can reach the fetus

Table 12.3 Common drugs that influence microsomal enzyme induction and inhibition

Microsomal induction (Cytochrome P450)	Microsomal inhibition
Smoking	Oestrogen
Anticonvulsants	Ciprofloxacin
Progestogen	Fluconazole
Rifampicin	Omeprazole
Theophylline	Quinidine
Ethanol	Erythromycin, sulfonamide
Griseofulvin	Grape fruit juice, metronidazole

Pharmacokinetic interactions can be related to:

- Absorption
  - ○ Drugs that decrease gastric emptying (e.g. morphine, anticholinergics)
  - ○ Chelation of calcium, aluminium, magnesium salts by tetracycline
  - ○ Binding of warfarin and digoxin by cholestyramine
- Protein-binding displacement interactions
  - ○ For example, warfarin and phenytoin are displaced by sulfonamides, salicylates, phenylbutazone and valproate
- Metabolism interactions with induction or inhibition of cytochrome P450 or phase I functionalization reactions (e.g. oral contraceptives decrease anticoagulant effect of warfarin). Table 12.3 summarizes drugs that commonly influence microsomal enzymes
- Excretion interactions
  - ○ Probenecid and penicillin at the renal tubules
  - ○ Quinidine doubles digoxin levels
  - ○ Diuretics causing lithium retention.

Pharmacodynamic interactions could be antagonism at same site (e.g. pethidine/naloxone), synergism at same site (e.g. verapamil/beta-blockers increase arrhythmias) or indirect, e.g. when alterations in coagulation, fluid and electrolyte balance affect drug action.

Impaired liver function

Liver disease can lead to impaired drug metabolism. The severity of the liver damage reflects the extent of the reduced metabolism but clinical liver enzymes are of little value in predicting this. Drugs with high hepatic first-pass metabolism are most severely affected.

Physiological changes that affect drug metabolism in pregnancy

- The distribution volume for all drugs increases
- There is delayed gastric emptying, resulting in slow peak levels of readily absorbed drugs (e.g. paracetamol) and increased bioavailability of slowly absorbed drugs (e.g. digoxin)
- Nausea and vomiting in early pregnancy increases the clearance time affecting the dosage of drugs (e.g. anti-epileptics)
- Increased body fat increases clearance of lipophilic drugs (e.g. thiopental) even though the plasma half-life is prolonged
- Decreased albumin and raised free fatty acids lead to increase in free levels of albumin-bound drugs. Therefore measurement of these drugs may not reflect the actual concentration and saliva monitoring may be needed
- Increased alveolar ventilation and cardiac output seen in normal pregnancy may lead to enhanced alveolar and intramuscular drug absorption
- Renal blood flow increases and GFR increases by 50% leading to enhanced renal clearance of many medications
- α_1-Acid glycoprotein levels do not change, but there is a large transplacental concentration gradient that affects transfer of drugs
- Maternal albumin concentrations progressively decrease during pregnancy and fetal albumin concentrations progressively increase. They achieve equivalence at around week 30 of gestation. Albumin-bound drugs may be transferred to the fetus in a higher concentration. The placenta has cytochrome P450 sulphating and acetylating enzymes that can metabolize drugs.

The placental barrier

Virtually all drugs cross the placenta and achieve equal concentrations on either side over repeated administration. Most drugs have a molecular weight below 1000 daltons (Da), and molecules of this size cross the placenta (<600 Da cross easily). Lipid-soluble drugs are readily transferred across the placenta. Diffusion is the most important mode of transfer of drugs through the placenta. Fetal plasma is more acidic and leads to ion trapping of basic drugs.

Some commonly used drugs

Selective β₂ agonists

Inhalational β_2 agonists are a major breakthrough in treatment of asthma. They relax bronchial smooth muscle but also suppress release of leukotriene and histamine from mast cells, enhancing mucociliary action and inhibiting phospholipase A_2. They are used mainly in the treatment of asthma and chronic obstructive airway disease. Side-effects include tremor, hyperglycaemia, tachycardia and pulmonary oedema with an increased risk in patients with cardiovascular decompensation. Selected drugs like salbutamol, terbutaline and ritodrine can be used for tocolysis.

Vasodilators

α₂-Adrenergic agonists

Clonidine activates α_2-adrenergic receptors in the cardiovascular control centres of the central nervous system and suppresses the outflow of sympathetic nervous system activity from the brain. It is 100% bioavailable with a half-life of 12 h. Side-effects include postural hypotension, dry mouth, sedation and sexual dysfunction. It is considered to be safe in pregnancy, although this is supported by fewer studies than methyldopa.

Methyldopa is a prodrug that is metabolized into alpha-methyl-noradrenaline (norepinephrine) and acts centrally to decrease the adrenergic neuronal outflow from the brain stem. It readily crosses the placenta and achieves fetal concentrations similar to those found in the mother, although it does not affect the fetal vasculature. Methyldopa is used for the treatment of hypertension in pregnancy and 7.5 years of follow-up in children has not shown any adverse effects. Side-effects are transient and include sedation, depression, decreased libido and hyperprolactinaemia. Rarely, hepatotoxicity, granulocytopenia, thrombocytopenia and haemolytic anaemia may occur.

Prazosin is a potent and selective α_1 antagonist with 1000 times more affinity to α_1 than α_2 receptors. It causes blockade of α_1 receptors in arterioles and veins and decreases peripheral vascular resistance leading to a decrease in the venous return to the heart, and hence an absence of reflex tachycardia. Its half-life is 2–3 h and its duration of action is 7–10 h. Profound postural hypotension with the first dose is a well known side-effect and hence it is always started at bedtime. Adverse fetal effects have not been observed as the fetal drug concentration is only 20% of the maternal concentration.

Hydralazine causes direct relaxation of the arteriolar smooth muscle. It causes a selective decrease in vascular resistance in the cerebral, coronary and renal circulations with a less marked effect on skin and muscle, and hence it does not cause postural hypotension. Side-effects include reflex tachycardia and tachyphylaxis. It is used mainly in the acute control of blood pressure; intravenous administration may cause a rapid fall in blood pressure but does not affect placental vessels. Case reports of fatal maternal hypotension, a lupus-like syndrome in mother and offspring, neonatal thrombocytopenia and bleeding have been reported.

β-Adrenoceptor antagonists

Beta-blockers are used in a variety of conditions, including hypertension, angina, secondary prevention of myocardial infarction, cardiac arrhythmias, migraine, thyrotoxicosis, anxiety necrosis and glaucoma. Cardioselective beta-blockers are those that act selectively on β_1 receptors and have effects only on the heart (e.g. atenolol, bisoprolol), while the majority act on both (e.g. labetalol, propranolol, oxprenolol and atenolol).

Labetalol is a competitive antagonist at both α_1 and β adrenergic receptors with partial agonist activity at β_2. α_1 receptor blockade leads to relaxation of arterial smooth muscle and vasodilatation. β_1 blockade contributes by decreasing the reflex sympathetic stimulation of the heart. It is used orally for control of chronic hypertension and intravenously for hypertensive emergencies.

Atenolol is a β_1-selective antagonist with no intrinsic sympathomimetic activity. Its half-life is 5–8 h. It blocks release of renin from the juxtaglomerular apparatus. It has been used for treatment of hypertension and tachyarrhythmias. Its use in the first trimester has not been shown to be teratogenic but adverse perinatal effects have been reported. Intrauterine growth retardation was reported in association with the use of atenolol in some studies, although subsequent randomized trials have not confirmed this. When used in pregnancy atenolol can cause a decreased fetal heart rate and hyperglycaemia occurring shortly after birth.

Calcium channel blockers

Among the calcium channel blockers, the most commonly used is nifedipine. This is a dihydropyridine compound, which inhibits the influx of calcium (voltage-dependent fast channels) in the smooth muscle and causes vascular relaxation. It has no effect on the slow calcium channels, which control the sinoatrial node and hence can cause reflex tachycardia (this does not occur with diltiazem and verapamil). A single dose lasts for 6 h. Although it can be used in the acute control of blood pressure it should not be given sublingually as it can affect the placental vessels with a rapid drop in blood pressure causing fetal distress. It is used to treat hypertension in pregnancy and to inhibit premature labour. The Cochrane review demonstrated that calcium channel blockers have superior effects for delaying delivery and a reduction in the risk of several neonatal morbidities. Side-effects include flushing, headache and tachycardia. Evidence of exposure during the first trimester is limited and animal studies have shown embryotoxicity. Thus, their use should ideally be limited to the second and third trimester.

Ergot alkaloids

Ergot alkaloids are potent α-blockers that cause direct smooth muscle contraction. They are products of the fungus *Claviceps purpurea*. Only products of lysergic acid are of clinical importance. Ergotamine has a 100% first-pass metabolism and hence its derivatives, ergonovine and methyl ergonovine, are commonly used. They are used in the treatment of migraine and for prevention and treatment of postpartum haemorrhage. Side-effects include nausea and vomiting. Also precordial distress and angina-like pain are known to occur after intravenous injection due to coronary spasm. In addition, there have been reports of gangrene of the limbs following repeated doses. Ergot alkaloids are contraindicated in patients with hypertension and cardiac disease.

Bromocriptine is 2-bromo-α-ergocryptine, which is used to control secretion of prolactin due to the dopamine agonist effect of the drug.

General anaesthetics

Mechanism of action

Inhalational anaesthetics can hyperpolarize neurones and hence reduce both pacemaker neurone and postsynaptic neurone action potentials. Inhalational and intravenous anaesthetics affect synaptic function by inhibiting excitatory synapses and enhancing inhibitory synapses. General anaesthetics act by increasing the sensitivity of the gamma-aminobutyric acid (GABA) A receptor to GABA thus enhancing inhibitory neurotransmission and depressing nervous system activity. Glycine receptor-mediated activation of chloride channels is responsible for inhibition of neurotransmission in the spinal cord and brain stem. Ketamine, nitrous oxide and xenon act via N-methyl-D-aspartate (NMDA) receptors and cause long-term modulation of synaptic responses.

Intravenous anaesthetics

Intravenous (i.v.) anaesthetics are unique drugs that induce anaesthesia rapidly as they quickly achieve high concentrations in the central nervous system. Their pharmacological effects are terminated by redistribution to tissues with low blood flow. Commonly used drugs are thiopental and propofol for induction of anaesthesia. Thiopental is an ultrashort-acting agent that has quick entry into the CNS followed by quick redistribution of the drug. After i.v. administration, it causes unconsciousness with amnesia without analgesia or muscle relaxation. It is used mainly as an induction agent and by infusion during short procedures. It is also used to control convulsions in status epilepticus and eclamptic convulsions not responding to magnesium sulphate.

Inhalational anaesthetics

Halothane is commonly used. Due to its high lipid solubility and increased clearance from lungs, induction is slow and speed of recovery is also lengthened. Some 80% is excreted unchanged and 20% is metabolized by cytochrome P450 enzymes to trifluoroacetylate, which can bind to several liver proteins. Hypersensitivity to these proteins leads to halothane-induced hepatotoxicity.

A side-effect of the drug is uterine smooth muscle relaxation and this can be helpful for manipulation of fetus (version) and for manual removal of placenta. It can also lead to an increased risk of postpartum haemorrhage. It is a triggering agent for malignant hyperthermia.

Nitric oxide (NO) is very insoluble in blood and other tissues. Due to its high insolubility, rapid induction and rapid emergence occurs during anaesthesia. On discontinuation of nitrous oxide it can diffuse from blood to alveoli and decrease the concentration of oxygen in alveoli (diffusional hypoxia). Hence 100% oxygen should be administered during recovery from NO. NO is a weak anaesthetic and analgesic at 20%, and is a sedative. A 50% concentration is frequently used to provide analgesia in labour and outpatient dentistry.

A collaborative perinatal project showed no embryonic or fetal effects of NO. Its use during delivery may lead to neonatal depression and fetal accumulation of nitrous oxide, which increases over time; hence, it is safer to keep the induction to delivery time as short as possible.

Neuromuscular blocking agents

These agents are used as an adjunct to anaesthetics to provide muscle relaxation. Based on their mechanism of action they are divided into depolarizing (e.g. succinylcholine) and non-depolarizing (e.g. pancuronium). The actions of neuromuscular blocking agents are reversed by acetylcholine esterase inhibitors (e.g. neostigmine) and muscarinic receptor antagonists (e.g. glycopyrrolate). The only depolarizing agent in use is succinyl choline, which acts by depolarizing the membrane by opening sodium channels. A series of repetitive excitation followed by block transmission and neuromuscular paralysis occurs. Competitive antagonists act by decreasing the frequency of channel opening events that result in an action potential. At increasing doses the drug binds to the channels in a non-competitive manner.

Depolarizing muscle relaxants, e.g. suxamethonium and succinylcholine, can cause histamine release and hyperkalaemia (and therefore should be avoided in patients with heart disease, trauma and burns). Malignant hyperthermia occurs due to calcium release from the sarcoplasmic reticulum of the skeletal muscle. Clinical features include contracture, rigidity and heat production resulting in hyperthermia-accelerated muscle metabolism and acidosis. Malignant hyperthermia is treated with dantrolene which inhibits calcium release.

Local anaesthetics

Local anaesthetics cause a reversible block in the action potential responsible for nerve conduction. They decrease the permeability of the nerve to sodium and block propagation of electrical impulses. Combination with adrenaline (epinephrine) doubles their duration of action. Excessive administration can cause cerebral irritation and convulsions.

Drugs affecting uterine activity

Prostaglandins

Prostaglandins are eicosanoids derived from 20-carbon essential fatty acids of which arachidonic acid is the main precursor. Their role has been established in conception, menstruation and labour. Prostaglandin analogues are widely used for ripening of the cervix (PGE_2), treatment and prevention of postpartum haemorrhage ($PGF_{2\alpha}$ and PGE_1) and as an abortifacient. Their role is being evaluated in emergency contraception (PGE_1).

Oxytocin

Oxytocin is a cyclic nonapeptide, synthesized in the paraventricular nuclei and secreted by the posterior pituitary. After intravenous infusion, oxytocin reaches a steady-state plasma concentration after 20 min, with a half-life of 3 min, and hence hyperstimulation resolves rapidly after stopping the infusion. It increases the frequency and force of uterine contractions. There is less response in the first trimester due to decreased numbers of oxytocin receptors, compared with a more marked response at term, as there is a 30-fold increase in oxytocin receptors. It acts on the breast and helps in milk ejection. Oxytocin acts through G-protein receptor and calcium–calmodulin complex. It is used in induction and augmentation of labour, and treatment and prevention of postpartum haemorrhage. Oxytocin infusion over a prolonged time can cause haemodilution and hyponatraemia due to vasopressin-like effects. High doses may provoke reflex hypotension and tachycardia.

Tocolytics

Tocolytics are drugs that inhibit uterine contractions. They have not been shown to improve perinatal morbidity or mortality and hence their use is restricted until after the administration of steroids or to facilitate *in-utero* transfer.

Beta agonists act through adenylate cyclase to increase cAMP, which inhibits myosin light chain kinase (MLCK) activity by direct phosphorylation and by reducing intracellular free calcium. They also interact with surface receptors on the trophoblast, leading to increased cAMP which increases progesterone production. Tachyphylaxis of the adrenergic receptor occurs throughout the body after prolonged exposure and occurs due to reduced receptor density and adenyl cyclase activity. Side-effects include pulmonary oedema, myocardial ischaemia and cardiac dysrhythmia, hypotension, hyperglycaemia and hypokalaemia. They have been linked to increased risk of neonatal intraventricular haemorrhage, neonatal hypocalcaemia and hypoglycaemia.

Magnesium sulphate acts by competition with calcium either at the motor end plate, reducing excitation, or at the cell membrane, reducing calcium influx into the cell. It is used to prevent eclampsia in women with severe pre-eclampsia. Flushing, nausea, vomiting and headache are common side-effects. It can cause respiratory depression in high doses and this is treated by calcium gluconate intravenously.

Indometacin inhibits cyclooxygenase and reduces synthesis of prostaglandins. Side-effects include gastrointestinal bleeding, alterations in coagulation, thrombocytopenia and asthma in aspirin-sensitive patients. Contraindications include renal or hepatic disease, active peptic ulcer disease, poorly controlled hypertension, asthma and coagulation disorders. In neonates, indometacin may cause constriction of the ductus arteriosus, oligohydramnios and neonatal pulmonary hypertension.

Oxytocin receptor antagonists: atosiban is a peptide analogue which inhibits uterine activity by interacting with oxytocin at its membrane receptor. It is a specific inhibitor of myometrial contractions and does not affect smooth muscles all over the body. It has limited transfer into the fetal circulation and does not have direct effects on the fetus. The disadvantage of atosiban is that administration is complex with different bolus and infusion rates and its use is not cost-effective compared with calcium channel blockers.

Diuretics

Diuretics may cause a reduction in the intravascular volume and decrease placental perfusion. However, reviews of the use of diuretics in pregnancy have not shown any adverse fetal effects, although some diuretics can cause maternal electrolyte imbalances. Table 12.4 summarizes the site and mode of action and the maternal and fetal side-effects of commonly used diuretics.

Opioids

All centrally acting opioids cross the placenta. Pethidine is the most commonly used opioid. It reaches fetal blood within 2 min following intravenous administration and achieves steady-state concentration in the maternal blood within 6 min. Opioids have been used over many decades and are not known to cause any anomalies. Some important facts about specific opioids are outlined below:

- Morphine is not used as it causes more respiratory depression in the fetus and causes histamine release
- Methadone has the longest elimination half-life, i.e. 23 h in the fetus

Table 12.4   Summary of the site and mode of action, maternal and fetal side-effects of diuretics

	Site of action	Mode of action	Maternal side-effects	Fetal side-effects
Carbonic anhydrase inhibitors (acetazolamide)	Proximal tubular cells Inhibition of sodium bicarbonate absorption	Increase urinary pH Metabolic acidosis Bone marrow depression Skin toxicity Calcium phosphate stones	Open-angle glaucoma Acute mountain sickness Familial periodic paralysis	
Loop diuretics (furosemide)	Thick ascending limb of loop of Henle Blockade of the Na-K symporter	Hyponatraemia Volume depletion Ototoxicity – tinnitus Hyperuricaemia Hyperglycaemia	Acute pulmonary oedema Congestive cardiac failure Hypertension Nephritic syndrome	Crosses the placenta and causes a diuretic effect on the fetus; changes in liquor volume not established
Thiazide diuretics	Distal convoluted tubule Inhibition of sodium transport	Hyperuricaemia Sexual dysfunction Fluid and electrolyte imbalance Hyponatraemia Hyperglycaemia	Congestive cardiac failure Cirrhosis Acute glomerulonephritis Reacts with quinidine to prolong QT interval leading to polymorphic ventricular tachycardia (torsade de pointes)	Not associated with malformation Adverse fetal effects are rare Neonatal thrombocytopenia Hyponatraemia and hypotonia have been reported
Potassium-sparing diuretics	Epithelial cells in the late distal tubule and collecting duct Competitive inhibition of binding of aldosterone to its receptor	Hyperkalaemia Metabolic acidosis in cirrhotic patients Gynaecomastia, impotence, decreased libido, hirsutism and menstrual irregularities, breast cancer on chronic administration	Co-administered with loop or thiazide diuretic in treatment of oedema and hypertension Primary hyperaldosteronism Diuretic of choice in patients with liver cirrhosis, hirsutism	Unlikely to cause abnormalities, limited data Consider use only if other treatments fail

- Pethidine is used as a sedative in labour to block the sympathetic response to pain. Respiratory depression in the neonate is common if delivered between 1 and 3 h after intramuscular administration of the drug
- Fentanyl is an opioid used in epidural block and spinal anaesthesia to prolong and decrease the dose of local anaesthetics
- Codeine is widely used as an analgesic and is safe in pregnancy and lactation
- Meptazinol is an agonist–antagonist opioid analgesic believed to be unique in its selectivity for μ_1 (high affinity) receptors and its cholinergic activity. It is partially antagonized by naloxone and is used in the management of postoperative pain. It has recently been licensed for use as a labour analgesic. Meptazinol induces little respiratory depression and has low addictive potential.

Neither intravenous nor inhalational anaesthetics are good analgesics. Opioids are used to decrease the haemodynamic response to painful stimuli and to decrease the anaesthetic requirement. They are given during induction to decrease the pain response to intubation. Opioids act by agonist activity at μ receptors. Meperidine decreases shivering postoperatively due to its κ-receptor agonist activity. Side-effects include hypotension and respiratory depression.

Naloxone is an opioid antagonist with no agonist properties. It is frequently used in neonates to treat respiratory depression secondary to opioids. It can cause severe withdrawal symptoms if given to a baby born to an addicted mother.

Retinoids

Acitretin and isotretinoin are synthetic vitamin A derivatives. They are used for severe resistant or complicated psoriasis and some congenital disorders of keratinization. Vitamin A derivatives reduce sebum secretion and are used for the treatment of nodulocystic and conglobate acne and severe antibiotic-resistant acne. Teratogenic effects are seen in up to 25% of babies born to mothers who took retinoids. Isotretinoin is eliminated from the body within 4 weeks of stopping treatment but acitretin may take up to 2 years.

Cytotoxic drugs

These drugs affect rapidly dividing cells. Methotrexate, chlorambucil and cyclophosphamide are all contraindicated in pregnancy. Cyclophosphamide may be used in life-threatening conditions like progressive proliferative glomerulonephritis because of its immunosuppressant actions.

Azathioprine is used commonly for conditions like SLE, inflammatory bowel disease and in transplant patients. It is a 6-mercaptopurine derivative which interferes with antibody production and halts proliferation of T cells. There is extensive experience of its use in pregnancy and current evidence suggests an increased risk of impaired fetal immunity, but that this is not sustained in the neonate. Fetal growth restriction has been reported, but it is hard to separate the effect of chronic maternal disease on fetal growth from the potential effect of azathioprine. Only a small proportion of azathioprine is transferred into breast milk.

Mycophenolate mofetil is a prodrug that is rapidly hydrolysed to mycophenolic acid (MPA), a selective, uncompetitive and reversible inhibitor of inosine monophosphate dehydrogenase. Since T and B lymphocytes are dependent on this pathway, it causes selective inhibition of antibody formation, cellular adhesion and migration. It is used primarily in prophylaxis of transplant rejection and is used in combination with glucocorticoids and a calcineurin inhibitor but not with azathioprine. Toxicity is mainly gastrointestinal and haematological. Its use is associated with an increased incidence of infections, especially sepsis associated with cytomegalovirus. It is excreted mainly by the kidney as an inactive phenolic glucuronide.

Anticoagulants

Warfarin

Warfarin interferes with cyclic conversion of vitamin K to its active metabolite, which is essential in carboxylation of glutamic acid residues of vitamin K-dependent coagulation factors (II, VII, IX, X). Carboxylation is necessary for binding of these factors to calcium and phospholipids. As protein S levels are also dependent on vitamin K activity, warfarin administration causes a prothrombotic state prior to the onset of an anticoagulant effect. It causes embryopathy in 5–10% of pregnancies where there is first-trimester exposure. The clinical features are similar to those of chondromalacia punctata (stippled epiphysis, nasal and limb hypoplasia). The embryopathy is secondary to vitamin K involvement in the post-translational modification of proteins enabling them to bind calcium. The use of warfarin in the second and third trimester is associated with recurrent micro-haemorrhages in the brain leading to optic atrophy, dorsal midline dysplasia and mental retardation. It is avoided after 36 weeks to prevent maternal and neonatal complications related to delivery.

Heparin

Heparin is the anticoagulant of choice from the fetal perspective as it does not cross the placenta. It is a glycosaminoglycan and acts through interaction with antithrombin III. Antithrombin III inactivates thrombin, factor Xa and factor IXa. Two major side-effects that can occur with heparin treatment are heparin-induced thrombocytopenia and osteoporosis. There are two types of thrombocytopenia that occur in association with heparin treatment. Non-immune heparin-associated thrombocytopenia is associated with a mild reduction in platelet count and occurs 2–5 days after heparin injection. Immune thrombocytopenia occurs due to IgG antiplatelet antibodies, 3–4 weeks after therapy, and increases the risk of thrombus formation.

Anticonvulsants

The pharmacokinetics of all antiepileptics is altered in pregnancy and therapeutic drug monitoring can be of benefit. Phenytoin, primidone, phenobarbital, carbamazepine and sodium valproate all cross the placenta and are teratogenic. Major abnormalities produced by anticonvulsants are neural tube, orofacial and congenital heart defects. Fetal hydantoin syndrome includes prenatal and postnatal growth restriction, motor or mental deficiency, short nose with broad nasal bridge, microcephaly, hypertelorism, strabismus, low-set or abnormally formed ears, limb and positional deformities. Sodium valproate and carbamazepine mainly cause neural tube defects and spina bifida (always lumbar). Phenobarbital appears to be safer than phenytoin. The risk of teratogenicity rises with the use of more than one drug. The newer anticonvulsants are often prescribed along with other drugs, and it is difficult to ascertain teratogenic risk of these drugs in isolation.

Altered pharmacokinetics in pregnancy may lead to changes in drug levels and for most drugs the concentration of the free drug falls. If a woman is fit free, there is usually no need to measure serial drug levels or adjust the dose for most anticonvulsants. An exception is lamotrigine as levels of this drug almost invariably fall in pregnancy. In women who have regular seizures, and who are dependent on critical drug levels, it is worth monitoring drug levels and increasing dosages of anticonvulsants should be guided by serum concentrations. Vitamin K is given in the last 4 weeks of pregnancy to prevent haemorrhagic disease of the newborn. Carbamazepine, phenytoin and valproic acid are safe in breastfeeding. Succinimides, e.g. ethosuximide, are commonly used to treat petit mal epilepsy and are thought to have a low or no teratogenic potential.

Anti-inflammatory drugs

Non-steroidal anti-inflammatory drugs (NSAIDs)

Aspirin and NSAIDs do not produce structural defects. They readily cross the placenta and achieve higher concentrations in the fetus as they are albumin bound. Salicylates and NSAIDs may increase the risk of neonatal haemorrhage via inhibition of platelet function.

NSAIDs may lead to oligohydramnios via effects on fetal kidney. If given in the last trimester, they can cause premature closure of ductus arteriosus and neonatal hypertension. Premature ductus closure and oligohydramnios are reversible. If used, they should be discontinued at 36 weeks. Low-dose aspirin is used in the prophylaxis of early-onset severe pre-eclampsia, migraine attacks and treatment of antiphospholipid syndrome. Aspirin in low doses inhibits thromboxane A_2 resulting in a decrease in vasoconstrictor prostaglandins.

COX-2 inhibitors

Cyclooxygenase (COX) enzymes are responsible for production of the prostaglandin series of bioactive compounds. Specifically COX converts arachidonic acid to prostaglandin H_2. There are three known COX isoforms, designated COX-1, COX-2 and COX-3. COX-1 and 2 are both expressed in tissues and have biological functions. COX-3 is a splice variant of COX-1. COX-1 is found in the gastric mucosa, kidney and platelets. COX-2 is an inducible form, although to some extent it is present constitutively in the central nervous system, juxtaglomerular apparatus of the kidney and placenta during late gestation. Recent development of selective COX-2 inhibitors is of major clinical interest as these have been related to lower incidence of gastrointestinal bleeding. Both COX-1 and 2 inhibitors can cause sodium retention and reduction of the glomerular filtration rate. Fetal COX-2 inhibition can be responsible for neonatal chronic renal failure and therefore maternal usage should be avoided until further studies confirm the safety of this group of drugs.

Colchicine

Colchicine reduces the inflammatory response to the deposition of monosodium urate crystals in joint tissue, in part by inhibiting neutrophil metabolism, mobility and chemotaxis. It also inhibits cell division in metaphase by binding tubulin and thereby interfering with mitosis. It is used to treat gouty arthritis and for prophylaxis of recurrent gout attacks. It also used in familial Mediterranean fever, Behçet's disease and amyloidosis. Colchicine given to either parent within 3 months of the time of conception may result in increased frequency of trisomy 21.

Antimicrobials

Antibiotics

Penicillin crosses the placenta and attains fetal concentrations equal to those found in the maternal circulation. It is considered safe in pregnancy and lactation. It does have the potential to modify the normal bacterial flora of the mother's genital and gastrointestinal tract.

are applied to a large area or on an occlusive dressing, the absorption may be sufficient to cause systemic effects. After absorption, >90% of cortisol is reversibly bound to protein. Two plasma proteins account for almost all of the steroid-binding capacity; corticosteroid-binding globulin (CBG) and albumin. A state of physiological hypercortisolism occurs during pregnancy. The elevated circulating oestrogens induce CBG production, and CBG and total plasma cortisol increase several-fold.

Glucocorticoids are administered in multiple formulations for disorders that share an inflammatory or immunological basis. With the exception of patients receiving replacement therapy for adrenal insufficiency, glucocorticoids are neither specific nor curative, but rather are palliative because of their anti-inflammatory and immunosuppressive actions.

Prednisolone is the biologically active form of prednisone. The placenta can oxidize prednisolone to inactive prednisone or even less active cortisone. Only 10% of the maternal prednisolone dose crosses the placenta. Four large epidemiological studies including steroids that readily cross the placenta (betamethasone and dexamethasone) have looked at the use of corticosteroids in first trimester and found an association with non-syndromic orofacial clefts. However, the overall risk is low. The Michigan Medicaid surveillance study looked at 229 101 patients exposed to prednisolone, prednisone and methylprednisolone during the first trimester; the data did not support an association between these agents and congenital defects. There are isolated reports of cataracts in the newborn if prednisolone was used throughout the pregnancy. During lactation, the infant is exposed to minimal amounts of steroid through the breast milk. At higher doses (>20 mg), it is recommended to wait at least 4 h after a dose before nursing the baby.

Betamethasone administration to women with threatened preterm labour is associated with a decrease in respiratory distress syndrome, periventricular leukomalacia and intraventricular haemorrhage in preterm infants. It can induce hyperglycaemia and may rarely precipitate myasthenic crisis or hypertensive crisis in the mother. Approximately 80% of the maternal betamethasone dose crosses the placenta. Single courses of betamethasone have no effects on the fetus but multiple courses have been associated with lower birth weights and reduced head circumference at birth. Follow-up studies have not shown any differences in cognitive and psychosocial development when compared with controls.

Hydrocortisone and its inactive precursor, cortisone, appear to present a small risk to the human fetus. Approximately 50% of the maternal dose of hydrocortisone crosses the placenta. These corticosteroids produce dose-related teratogenic and toxic effects in genetically susceptible experimental animals consisting of cleft palate, cataracts, spontaneous abortion, IUGR and polycystic kidney disease. However, there are no data to support these effects in the great majority of human pregnancies, although the small increase in incidence of cleft lip with or without cleft palate, is supported by large epidemiological studies.

It is important to remember that in some women the benefits of corticosteroids can far outweigh the fetal risks when used to treat maternal inflammatory and autoimmune disease, and these agents should not be withheld if the mother's condition requires their use.

Antineoplastic drugs

Alkylating agents

Alkylating agents are derived from nitrogen mustard. They become strong electrophiles through formation of carbonium ion intermediates that react with various nucleophilic moieties, such as phosphate, amino, sulfhydryl, hydroxyl, carboxyl and imidazole groups forming covalent linkages and alkylating them.

Cyclophosphamide must be activated metabolically by microsomal enzymes of the cytochrome P450 system. The metabolites phosphoramide mustard and acrolein are thought to be the ultimate active cytotoxic moieties. Cyclophosphamide can be given either orally, intramuscularly or intravenously. It has a half-life of 4–8 h in patients receiving it intravenously. It does not cross the blood–brain barrier and is eliminated primarily by the kidney. It is used to treat lymphoma, myeloma, chronic leukaemia, breast cancer, small cell lung cancer and ovarian cancer, and may be used as an alternative to azathioprine in Wegener's granulomatosis, childhood nephrosis and severe rheumatoid arthritis. Side-effects include bone marrow suppression (affecting white cells more than platelets), alopecia, impaired function of both humoral and cellular immunity. Cystitis is relatively common due to renal excretion of the metabolite acrolein and this disappears after discontinuation of treatment.

Melphalan is an amino acid derivative of mechlorethamine, an alkylating agent. It is used for the treatment of multiple myeloma and cancer of the breast and ovary. It can cause relatively prolonged bone marrow suppression and affects both white cells and platelets but does not cause alopecia.

Ifosfamide is an analogue of cyclophosphamide. Its use is associated with relatively low levels of bone marrow suppression, but more bladder toxicity, and hence it is administered with mesna.

Chlorambucil is an aromatic nitrogen mustard and with an anti-tumour activity similar to melphalan. It is well absorbed orally and is used for palliative treatment of lymphomas, chronic lymphocytic leukaemia and myeloma. Bone marrow toxicity is relatively common.

Dacarbazine: the triazeno group of this alkylating agent causes methylation of DNA and RNA and inhibition of nucleic acid and protein synthesis. It is the most active agent in metastatic melanoma and is combined with doxorubicin for treatment of sarcomas and Hodgkin's disease. Side-effects include bone marrow depression, a flu-like syndrome and alopecia.

Antimetabolites

Methotrexate is an antimetabolite which competes for binding sites on dihydrofolate reductase and inhibits the binding of folic acid. Hence, the essential co-factor tetrahydrofolate for synthesis of thymidylate, purines, methionine and glycine is inhibited. Cells in the S phase of the cell cycle are very sensitive. Resistance can occur due to increase in intracellular dihydrofolate reductase levels or appearance of altered forms of dihydrofolate reductase. It is well absorbed orally and mainly excreted through the kidneys. Methotrexate is used in combination chemotherapy for acute lymphoblastic leukaemia, Burkitt's lymphoma and trophoblastic choriocarcinoma and is used in low doses to cause immune suppression in non-malignant conditions like rheumatoid arthritis and psoriasis. The major dose-limiting toxic side-effect is myelosuppression, and occasionally hepatitis and lung toxicity can occur due to a hypersensitivity reaction. High doses of methotrexate can also cause renal failure.

Purine analogues include thioguanine and mercaptopurine (which is converted to thioguanine). This is incorporated into DNA and prevents cell multiplication by inhibition of purine synthesis. These drugs are used in the treatment of leukaemia. Leukopenia and thrombocytopenia are common adverse effects.

5-Fluorouracil is a pyrimidine analogue that kills cells in the S phase of the cell cycle by competitively inhibiting DNA synthesis. It is metabolized largely in the liver and excreted in urine. Side-effects include myelosuppression, skin rashes, nail discoloration and photosensitivity. 5-Fluorouracil is used in the treatment of breast cancer, gastrointestinal adenocarcinomas, and carcinomas of the ovary, cervix and bladder. Topical treatment has been useful in superficial basal cell carcinoma and treatment of premalignant keratoses of the skin.

Antibiotics

Doxorubicin and daunorubicin are anthracycline antibiotics that have the ability to intercalate between base pairs and hinder DNA synthesis. Cells in the S phase are more sensitive. Drug resistance occurs due to enhanced active efflux of the drug. These drugs are not absorbed orally and cause necrosis if given intramuscularly or subcutaneously. Doxorubicin is used in the treatment of breast, ovary, endometrial, bladder and thyroid cancers. It can cause transient cardiac arrhythmias and depression of myocardial function. Myelosuppression occurs to a lesser extent and the drug may cause radiation recall reactions.

Bleomycin is a glycopeptide that binds to DNA and produces single- and double-strand scission and fragmentation of DNA. It is poorly absorbed orally and excreted mainly from the kidneys. Fatal lung toxicity can occur in 10–20% of cases. Skin toxicity may manifest as hyperpigmentation and erythematous rashes, and low-grade, transient fever is common. It is used in combination with platinum-based drugs to treat advanced testicular carcinomas and ovarian germ cell tumours.

Platinum-based drugs

α-Cisplatin

α-Cisplatin is a platinum coordination complex used in the treatment of epithelial malignancies. α-Cisplatin enters the cell by diffusion and reacts with water to yield a positively charged molecule. Platinum compounds react with DNA to form intrastrand and interstrand cross-links. The cross-linking is most pronounced during the S phase of the cell cycle. α-Cisplatin is used in the treatment of cancers of bladder, head and neck, endometrium and ovary. It is nephrotoxic and ototoxic. Nephrotoxicity can be abrogated by hydration and diuresis. Repeated cycles can cause neuropathy.

Carboplatin has a similar mechanism of action and clinical spectrum to cisplatin. Carboplatin is relatively well tolerated and there is less nausea, neurotoxicity, ototoxicity and nephrotoxicity than with cisplatin. A dose-limiting toxic side-effect is myelosuppression, evident as thrombocytopenia. It is an alternative in patients with responsive tumours who cannot tolerate cisplatin clinically due to impaired renal function, refractory nausea, significant hearing impairment or neuropathy.

Vinca alkaloids

Vincristine and vinblastine are plant alkaloids that bind avidly to tubulin and cause arrest in metaphase of cells. They act in the M phase of the cell cycle. Vinca alkaloids are used in the treatment of methotrexate-resistant choriocarcinoma, myelomas, Hodgkin's and non-Hodgkin's lymphomas, Ewing's sarcoma and neuroblastoma. Vinblastine is more toxic to the bone marrow and vincristine is more neurotoxic.

Taxanes

Paclitaxel is a plant compound which binds to tubulin dimmers and microtubulin filaments and prevents their depolymerization. This causes disruption of mitosis and cytotoxicity. Major side-effects include myelosuppression and peripheral neuropathy. It is used in treatment of breast, ovary, lung and head and neck carcinomas.

Psychotropic drugs

Lithium

Lithium carbonate may rarely be indicated for treatment of the manic phase of bipolar disorder during pregnancy. The precise mechanism of action is unknown, but it is thought to be due to altered ion transport or inhibition of adenyl cyclase, influencing nerve excitation, synaptic transmission and neuronal metabolism in the CNS.

Lithium use is associated with an increased incidence of fetal abnormalities. Since the 1960s, an International Register of Lithium Babies has collected information about lithium-exposed children in the first trimester of pregnancy. It is estimated that 7.8% of lithium-exposed embryos develop abnormalities. Early data showed that the cardiovascular system is most affected, with mitral and tricuspid atresias, coarctation of the aorta and patent ductus arteriosus being reported. The disorder known as Ebstein anomaly (tricuspid valve distortion and displacement) occurs with particular frequency among lithium-exposed infants. There have also been reports suggesting an association between maternal lithium therapy and premature delivery.

Antidepressants

Selective serotonin re-uptake inhibitors (SSRIs)

SSRIs inhibit the re-uptake of serotonin into presynaptic cells, thereby increasing extracellular levels of the neurotransmitter that are available to bind postsynaptic neurones. They have become the agents of first choice in the treatment of depression because of their safe side-effect profile. Several studies have evaluated the safety of SSRIs in pregnancy. The well powered studies have not shown any major teratogenic effect. Some have shown mildly increased risks of right ventricular outflow tract defects in particular, and also of omphalocele, septal defects and craniosynostosis. This is reported more commonly with paroxetine than other SSRIs. There is no evidence that SSRIs cause serious neonatal complications, but likewise there is no clear evidence that they are absolutely safe. The recommendation at present is that they should only be used if the benefit outweighs the potential harmful risks. There is variable transfer of SSRIs into breast milk, but overall transfer is low. Ideally nursing mothers should use SSRIs with a shorter half-life (e.g. sertraline or paroxetine).

Tricyclic antidepressants

Tricyclic antidepressants are thought to act by inhibiting re-uptake of dopamine, serotonin and noradrenaline. There is considerable experience of their use in pregnancy and the older tricyclic antidepressants are not believed to be associated with risks of teratogenicity. They are found in breast milk at levels comparable with those demonstrated in the maternal plasma. Therefore it is recommended that they are used with caution in lactating women and, if they are used, tricyclic antidepressants with a short half-life are recommended.

Oral contraceptives

Combined oral contraceptives are commonly used and contain oestrogen and progestogen.

Mechanism of action of the combined pill

- Progestogen acts on the hypothalamus to inhibit GnRH pulses and on the pituitary to inhibit the oestrogen-induced LH surge
- Oestrogen decreases the pituitary response to GnRH and in the follicular phase inhibits the FSH surge. Oestrogen and progestogen alter the transport of sperm, egg and fertilized ovum due to their effects on the fallopian tube
- Progestogen causes thickening of cervical mucus, thereby decreasing sperm penetration and inhibiting implantation.

Mechanism of action of the progestogen-only pill and depot injections of progestogen

- 60–80% blockade of ovulation due to slowing of the GnRH pulse generator, which prevents the LH surge required for ovulation
- Thickening of cervical mucus and impairment of sperm penetration
- Alteration of the intrauterine environment and impairment of implantation.

Depot medroxyprogesterone injections inhibit ovulation in virtually all patients due to high plasma levels of progesterone.

Metabolic effects of the combined oral contraceptive pill

The metabolic side-effects of the combined pill are dose dependent and are uncommon with the introduction of low-dose preparations. The pill does not increase the risk of infarction/stroke in non-smokers, although it does alter coagulation by decreasing antithrombin III and plasminogen activator, thereby increasing platelet activation and the risk of venous thromboembolism. The magnitude of risk is small and is equated to half the risk in pregnancy. Hypertension is seen more often in patients on high-dose than low-dose preparations. The risk of venous thromboembolism decreases after stopping the pill. The low-dose preparations do not have any effect on HDL or LDL and cause a slight increase in triglycerides. Very long-term use has been shown to increase gall bladder disease and the high-dose pills increase insulin resistance.

The combined oral contraceptive pill and cancer

The combined pill protects against endometrial cancer and ovarian cancer (due to the absence of gonadotropin stimulation of the ovaries). There is a slight increase in hepatic adenoma and hepatocellular carcinoma but no definite association has been proved. The relative risk of developing breast cancer is increased slightly and disappears 10 years after stopping the pill.

Drugs which induce microsomal enzymes (e.g. rifampicin, carbamazepine, phenytoin) decrease the efficacy of the pill. Theoretically, drugs that decrease the enterohepatic circulation (e.g. amoxicillin and other broad-spectrum antibiotics) may cause reduced plasma levels of oestrogens.

Drugs of choice in breastfeeding

The processes that govern the passage of a drug into milk are similar to the placenta. The maternal serum concentration is the main determinant. Maternal milk pH is slightly acidic in comparison to serum pH, so weak bases could become trapped in milk (ion trapping).

Conclusion

The use of drugs during pregnancy requires maintenance of a fine balance. Before prescribing a drug, consideration must be given to any potential harmful effects on the fetus. Equally, no harm must come to the mother or baby because a disease is being inadequately treated. To minimize the fetal risks, the lowest possible effective dose should be used.

In addition to the dangers associated with fetal exposure to teratogenic drugs, there are risks associated with misinformation about the teratogenicity of drugs. This can lead to unnecessary termination of pregnancy or the avoidance of essential treatment. The drug

Table 12.5 Drugs that involve considerable fetal risks when used in pregnancy

Absolute	Relative
Cytotoxic drugs	**Psychotropic drugs**
Busulfan, cyclophosphamide, methotrexate	Antipsychotic drugs – lithium
Vitamin A analogues	**Anticoagulants**
Etretinate, isotretinoin	Warfarin
Thalidomide	**Anticonvulsants**
Cardiovascular drugs	Carbamazepine
Angiotensin-converting enzyme inhibitors	Phenytoin
Angiotensin II inhibitors – losartan	Sodium valproate
Spironolactone	**Endocrinological drugs**
Antifungal drugs	Carbimazole
Griseofulvin	Propylthiouracil
Ketoconazole	Chlorpropamide, sulphonylureas
Triazoles – fluconazole, itraconazole	**Cardiovascular drugs**
Terbinafine	Beta-blockers
Anti-inflammatory drugs	Minoxidil
NSAIDs (third trimester)	**Antibiotics**
COX II inhibitors (limited data)	Tetracycline
Endocrinological drugs	Ciprofloxacin
Radioactive iodine	Aminoglycosides
Sex hormones	Chloramphenicol
Octreotide	Nitrofurantoin
Antihelminthic drugs	Vancomycin
Mebendazole	**Anti-inflammatory drugs**
Others	Colchicine
Misoprostol	**Others**
Mefloquine	Dapsone (third trimester)
Statins	
Bisphosphonates	

manufacturers and medical community should make every effort possible to protect women and their unborn babies from both risks. Implicit in this statement is the need to counsel pregnant women about the safety as well as the dangers of drug use in pregnancy. Table 12.5 lists the drugs that are believed to involve the greatest risk to the fetus when used in pregnancy.

To receive up-to-date, evidence-based information on the safety of drugs during pregnancy, clinicians can consult a teratogen information service. Table 12.6 lists some web addresses and telephone numbers of teratogen services.

Table 12.6   Teratogen information services

United Kingdom

National Teratology Information Service (NTIS)
Newcastle (0191) 232-1525

United States

Organization of Teratology Information Specialists (OTIS)
National toll-free number: (866) 626-OTIS, or (866) 626-6847 during normal business hours, Mountain Standard Time.
web address: http://www.otispregnancy.org/

Canada

Motherisk Program
Toronto: (416) 813-6780
web address: http://www.motherisk.org

Chapter Thirteen

13

Physics

David Talbert

CHAPTER CONTENTS

Diagnostic ultrasound

Very high frequency sound, or ultrasound, is useful in diagnosis because it can be directed and will penetrate the body like X-rays but it does not cause ionization at the energy levels used. Frequencies are in the range of 1–10 MHz, the most common being around 3 MHz, about 200 times the highest frequency the average adult can hear. Sound waves cause particles of the medium through which they are travelling to move a minute distance back and forth along the direction of their path. Such waves are called 'longitudinal' to indicate the direction of displacement of the particles supporting the wave.

The power to produce these waves is generated electrically and the device that transforms it into sound power is called a transducer. A common form of transducer uses a thin slice of piezoelectric ceramic or quartz. These materials alter their thickness according to the voltage (V) applied between their faces. The change in thickness is small, only a few micrometres in the highest-powered machines, producing waves with displacements of about 1 nm which travel through tissues at about 1540 m/s (Fig. 13.1).

Intensity

Intensity describes how much energy is passing through a certain cross-sectional area, usually 1 cm^2. It is usually defined in watts per square centimetre (W/cm^2).

Characteristic impedance and reflections

The characteristic impedance of a material describes how it resists being moved in response to a given sound pressure wave. For soft tissues, it is roughly propor-

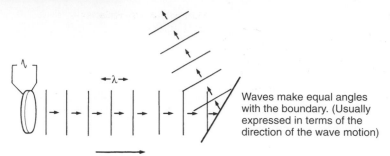

Figure 13.1 • Ultrasound generation and reflection.

Waves make equal angles with the boundary. (Usually expressed in terms of the direction of the wave motion)

Wave crests move at about 1540 m/s in tissue

$$\lambda = \text{distance between crests} = \frac{1540}{\text{Ultrasonic frequency}}$$

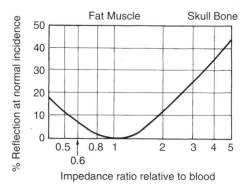

Figure 13.2 • Percentage reflection caused by interfaces of various impedance ratios.

tional to tissue density. When ultrasound encounters a boundary between tissues of different impedances, the mismatch of movements prevents a proportion of the sound energy from being transferred. The rest is reflected and produces the echoes used in diagnostic ultrasound (Fig. 13.2). If the sound meets the boundary at an angle, it will be reflected at the same angle, provided the reflecting surface is large compared with the sound wavelength.

Near the edge of the reflector the local sound pressure pushes particles sideways, rounding off the edge of the reflected wave (Fig. 13.3A) at the centre of the reflector local pressure balance so the reflected wave is flat. If the reflector is reduced in size, as it approaches half a wavelength the flat portion disappears and the reflection spreads in all directions, spherically (Fig. 13.3B). This form of reflection is known as scattering, since the direction of the reflected sound energy bears no relation to the direction of the incident wave.

Absorption

Ultrasound waves lose energy to the tissue by several mechanisms – viscous, relaxation and thermodynamic losses for instance. Viscous losses are increased in non-homogeneous fluids, whose acoustic impedance varies on a microscopic scale. Relaxation mechanisms arise when, at one stage of the sound cycle, associated ions become separated and then require a certain specific minimum time to reassociate. Relaxation mechanisms have characteristic variations with frequency, which may depend on the chemical state of the tissue. Thermodynamic losses occur because, as the tissue is compressed by the sonic pressure, its temperature rises slightly. Nearby, there is another region where the temperature has been reduced by decompression. Any thermal leakage between the two regions is energy lost to the sound wave. In soft tissues at diagnostic frequencies, thermodynamic losses are small compared with viscous and relaxation losses.

Diffraction

The ideal ultrasonic beam for diagnostic purposes would be needle thin to give the finest detail. Unfortunately, this is not possible because of diffraction. A point source transducer would produce spherical waves similar to a point scatterer. Wider transducer faces produce flatter wavefronts but off-axis waves created at one part of the face may cancel or reinforce those from another. This results in sound being emitted at unwanted angles known as side lobes (Fig. 13.4). It is highly desirable to suppress side lobes and make the angle θ at which the first minima occurs (defining the main lobe) as narrow as possible. For a circular transducer this occurs at an angle:

$$\sin^{-1}\theta = 1.22\,\lambda/d$$

where d is its diameter.

Focusing

It is possible to shape the transducer face, fit an acoustic lens, or provide special electronic drive, and thus

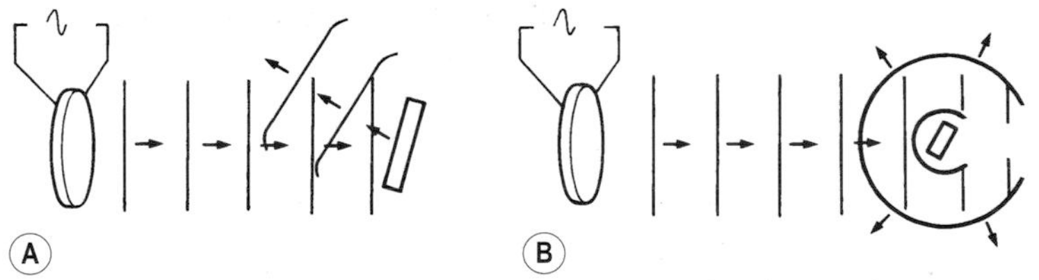
A
B

Figure 13.3 • (A) Reflection. (B) Scattering.

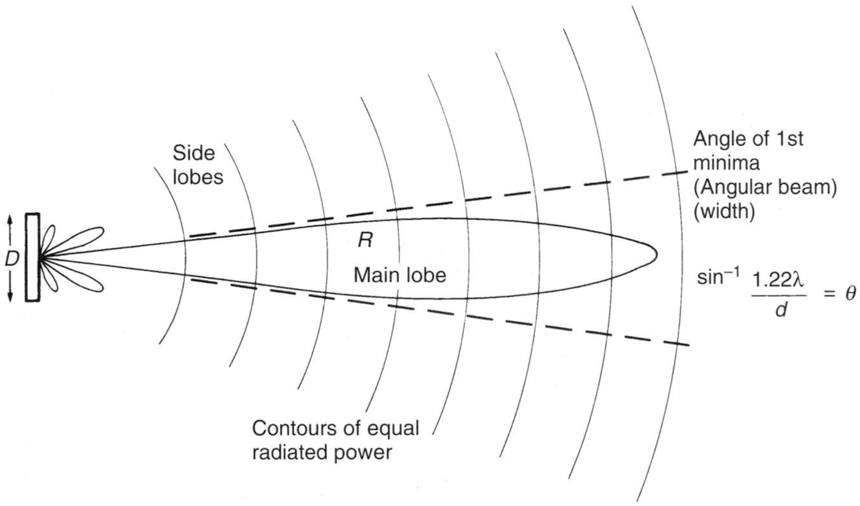
Side lobes
D
R
Main lobe
Angle of 1st minima (Angular beam) (width)
sin⁻¹ 1.22λ/d = θ
Contours of equal radiated power

Figure 13.4 • Polar plot of radiated power vector *R* at angle *d* from a circular transducer of diameter *D*.

generate a concave wave, directed to a point. Diffraction effects still limit the effectiveness of this technique, but nevertheless in the region of this focal point the beam is typically one-half to one-third of that from a flat transducer of the same dimensions, improving lateral resolution and raising the echo strength from the desired target (Fig. 13.4).

Ultrasound reception

Just as applying a voltage between the faces of a slice of piezoelectric material produces a pressure, so pressure on its faces produces a voltage. A slice exposed to the returning ultrasonic echoes produces a corresponding electrical signal. The directional properties of a transducer used as a receiver are usually the same as those used as a transmitter.

Doppler effect

It is well known that, as a police car or fire engine passes, the note of its siren appears to drop. The same effect occurs if sound is reflected off a moving object. If the object is approaching, each sound wave has a shorter distance to travel than the one preceding it. A succession of such waves is received at a higher frequency than the frequency at which it was transmitted. If the reflector moves away from the transducer, the delay will increase and the frequency decrease. Mixing the transmitted signal and the echo can produce a new electrical signal at the difference frequency, representing the velocity of the reflector. Doppler systems therefore detect movement rather than distance, and since the difference frequencies are in the audible range, they may be fed to a loudspeaker directly for simple instruments.

By suitable filtering to select significant sounds, trigger signals for heart rate meters or flow rate indicators can be obtained.

Radioactivity and X-rays

The term 'radioactivity' refers to occurrences in the nuclei of atoms. The nucleus is the positively charged centre around which the negatively charged electrons of the atom circulate in orbits up to 10000 times the nuclear diameter. There is continual exchange of energy between particles constituting the nucleus and, in some atoms, it is possible for sufficient energy to be acquired by a particle to allow it to escape (Fig. 13.5). Protons (carrying one positive charge) or neutrons

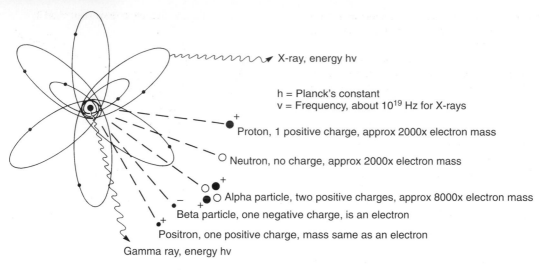

Figure 13.5 • Principal ionizing radiations.

Table 13.1 Principal parameters of some isotopes associated with medicine

Name	Symbol	Half-life	Radiation energy (MeV)[a]	
			Electromagnetic (γ- or X-rays)	Particle (β)
Caesium-137	^{137}Cs	30 years	0.662	0.51[b]
Carbon-14	^{14}C	5760 years		0.155
Cobalt-60	^{60}Co	5.26 years	1.17	0.31[b]
			1.33	0.96
Gold-198	^{198}Au	2.7 days	0.412	
Iodine-125	^{125}I	60 days	0.027	0.61
Iodine-131	^{131}I	8 days	0.36	1.71
Phosphorus-32	^{32}P	14 days		0.167
Sulphur-35	^{35}S	87 days		
Technetium-99m	^{99}Tc^m	6 hours	0.14	0.018
Tritium (hydrogen-3)	^{3}H	12.3 years		

[a] 1 MeV = 1.6×10^{-19} J.
[b] This form of radiation is not utilized for medical purposes.

(uncharged) may leave singly or in a two-plus-two group, which is then known as an α particle. Other particles are electrons (called β particles), electrons with positive charges (called positrons) and miscellaneous others such as neutrinos and mesons, which are not of primary importance in medicine yet. Table 13.1 shows some of the radioactive substances that do have

medical applications and the way in which energy is liberated.

The energy carried away from the nucleus by any particle is limited by wave mechanics to discrete values, and the nucleus may then be left with a surplus energy above its next lowest stable level. The surplus may then be carried away by a burst (quantum) of γ radiation.

Since the energy of a γ quantum is proportional to its frequency, any quantity of energy can be carried by an appropriate frequency.

X-rays are also electromagnetic radiation and differ from γ-rays only in their origin. They are generated by the circulating electrons of the atom instead of its nucleus.

Ionization and excitation

Ionization was the route by which radioactivity was discovered and by which it is usually measured. Excitations may be considered imperfect ionizations, in which sufficient energy is imparted to outer electrons of atoms to put them into orbits of higher energy than usual, but insufficient for them to escape from their parent nucleus.

The biological effects of radiation are due to both phenomena. Both lead to the production of new chemical species inside the cell, some of which lead, in turn, to further chains of damaging chemical reaction. DNA disruption is the most critical mode for cell killing but other fatal or disabling reactions, such as impairment of membrane function leading to osmotic changes, release of lysosome contents, and mitochondrial damage, are also important.

Ionization is usually considered the dominant effect and, as it produces readily detected physical results, it is used as a marker or scalar of radiation activity. The ions referred to are those produced by each particle, not the particles themselves. An ejected proton, for instance, is travelling in a sea of electrons and exerting an attractive force on them as it passes through the orbital shells of various atoms. If the force is large enough and exerted for long enough an electron may be dragged out of orbit round its parent nucleus (Fig. 13.6A). This produces two new ions, positive and negative. It also slows the proton down slightly as it gives up energy to the electron, but only slightly because its mass is some 2000 times that of the electron. The proton will continue ploughing a trail of ion pairs as it goes. As it gradually loses energy, it spends longer in each atom through which it passes and so has greater effect on its electrons, increasing its ionization efficiency. It eventually captures an electron and becomes a neutral hydrogen atom.

Spontaneous radioactive decay favours the emission of a group of two protons and two neutrons as the heavy positive component (α particle). Having twice the charge and four times the mass of a proton, it is even more efficient at ionization. A typical α particle moving through air will leave about 25 000 ion pairs/cm over most of its 7-cm path length rising to 50 000 in the last centimetre. All nuclear particles have definite air path lengths, although it will be tortuous and so effectively reduced in the case of the lighter and so

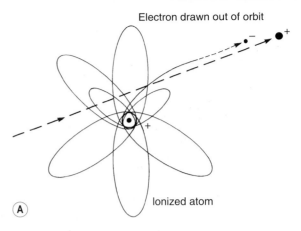

Electron drawn out of orbit

Ionized atom

(A)

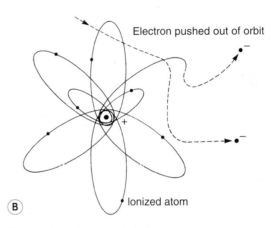

Electron pushed out of orbit

Ionized atom

(B)

Figure 13.6 • Ion pair production.

more easily deflected β and positron particles (Fig. 13.6B).

The electromagnetic X- and γ-rays can also transfer energy to electrons in the material through which they pass, in ways that depend on the frequency of the ray. These mechanisms are pair production, Compton scattering and photoelectric absorption, in order of descending ray frequency and energy. The electrons then escape from their parent atoms and cause the ionization observed, like β particles. The X- or γ-ray continues travelling but its frequency is reduced, corresponding to the loss of energy. Unlike the particles, X-ray velocity is unchanged, the probability of interaction with another electron is largely unaltered, and so it dies away exponentially with distance, rather than having a well-defined range. It is common to use the thickness of a material that will reduce this ionization to half its initial value as a measure of the penetrating power of X- or γ-rays, corresponding to a range in α or β particles. This is known as the half-value layer (HVL).

Quantity of radioactive material

The quantity of a radioactive material can be determined chemically, but one usually needs to know how many atoms will disintegrate per second. This is known as activity and is reported in curies (1 Ci is 3.7×10^{10} transformations/second) or in becquerels (1 Bq is 1 transformation/second).

Any such measurement is only true at the moment it is made since the proportion left capable of transforming is continually decreasing. A second parameter, half-life, defines the rate at which this is happening as the time required for half the initial quantity to have completed its transformation.

To determine these factors it is only necessary to detect when transformations occur. To determine the effect these disintegrations are having requires measurement of the magnitude of the ionization caused by the radiation emitted.

Radiation exposure and dose

Measurement of exposure or beam intensity was initially done by collecting and measuring the charged particles produced in 1 g of air interposed in the beam; 1.61×10^{12} ion pairs was defined as 1 roentgen (R). This was later re-defined in terms of energy (86.9 erg/g).

When measurement was required in biological situations, it was found that the rate of absorption in body tissues varied with the potential used to generate X-rays. A unit to indicate how much energy was actually being absorbed was required and this was the 'rad'. It was defined as the absorbed dose of radiation which imparts 0.01 J/kg of body tissue. When SI units were introduced the 0.01 factor was dropped and the unit 1 J/kg defined as the gray (Gy).

However, the particulate forms of radiation with their various forms of high-density ionizations were being used for their biological effects and it was logical to define a further term to express the relative effectiveness of the way in which the ionization was delivered. A multiplying factor, defined as Q, is used; Q has the value 1 for X-, γ- and β-radiation, but 10 for α particles because of the high density of ions along their tracks. For radiation safety purposes, it is combined with the rad in the product Q rad, which is defined as the 'rem' (radiation equivalent man). With the introduction of SI units the sievert (Sv), defined as Q·Gy, was introduced to replace the rem.

Stable isotopes

Isotope (*iso* same, *topes* place) means occupying the same place in the periodic table, i.e. they are atoms that happen to have the same number of protons in the

Table 13.2	Isotopes and relative abundance		
Isotope	**Relative abundance (%)**	**Isotope**	**Relative abundance (%)**
H-1	99.985	H-2 (D-2)	0.015
C-12	98.892	C-13	1.108
N-14	99.635	N-15	0.365
O-16	99.759	O-18	0.204
S-32	95.0	S-34	4.22
Cl-35	75.79	Cl-37	24.20
K-39	93.22	K-41	6.77

nucleus and hence attract the same number of electrons, giving them the same chemical characteristics. The rest of their nuclei may be thought of as made up of neutrons of similar mass to protons but carrying no charge. Many of these combinations are unstable and break up to form daughter isotopes with different chemical characteristics often producing radioactive effects. Some (Table 13.2), although relatively rare, are perfectly stable, and can be incorporated into compounds as markers without disturbing chemical reactions. Most importantly, they can be detected, distinguished from the more commonly occurring isotopes and do not emit ionizing radiation.

Deuterium is an example. It is relatively cheap and easily incorporated, but is also more easily accidentally 'lost' during processing. C-13 and N-14 are usually bonded more securely but are more expensive to obtain and incorporate. Since these markers are chemically identical to the majority of isotopes, physical methods have to be used to detect their presence by small differences in mass of the molecules into which they are incorporated. The primary tool for this is the mass electromagnetic spectrograph, through which they were first discovered by Aston in 1919 (Fig. 13.7). Just as hairs may be drawn to our clothes by static electricity, so charged atoms can be manipulated by electrostatic fields. If two plates are mounted in parallel and connected to different voltages to set up an electric field across the gap, any positively ionized atom in the space between them will be pulled towards the more negative plate. Making a hole in a negative electrode allows a stream of charged ions to emerge through it. Heavy atoms take longer to reach the negative plate and emerge at a lower velocity in the same way that one's car accelerates more slowly when fully loaded. Aston used an electrical discharge to ionize gases in a bulb ionization chamber, which were attracted to the

Electromagnetic system

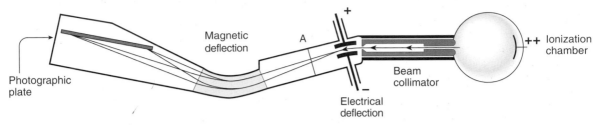

Figure 13.7 • Mass electromagnetic spectrograph.

end of a very fine collimator tube by a high electric field. Some of them then travelled down the tube and emerged at the other end to pass through an electric cross-field between a pair of electrode plates. The sideways force on all the ions was the same, so light atoms were deflected more quickly, but because heavy atoms had reached a lower velocity, they experienced the deflecting force for longer. If the velocity of the atoms were solely due to the initial accelerating voltage, they would all travel along the same path, but superimposed on this velocity is that due to thermal motion. The aperture A selects those ions with a narrow band of initial thermal energy velocities. They then pass into a magnetic field where they experience a force proportional to their velocity through it, deflecting them in the opposite direction. Once again, the deflecting force acts longer on the slower heavy atoms than the faster, lighter ones, but this time the force is not the same because it depends on velocity. The heavy ions are less deflected and end up further down the detecting photographic plate than the light ones. Opposite electrical and magnetic deflections are used because this enables compensation of the divergence caused by thermal velocities in the electrical deflection by a corresponding convergence during magnetic deflection, producing a re-focusing effect. A wider range of thermal velocities can then be used, increasing the ion current and making the machine more sensitive. Modern machines replace the photographic plate with a single highly sensitive electronic detector into which ions of various masses are deflected by incrementing the current through the electromagnet, and plotting the resulting current as a spectrum of isotope abundance in the sample.

For general use, where maximum resolution is not critical, these machines have been largely replaced by the mechanically very much simpler, purely electrostatic quadrupole machine. The beam of mixed isotopes is fired down the gap between four rods and, if no voltages are applied to the rods, will emerge at the far end. To produce selection, two types of electrical deflection are combined: steady (DC) and alternating (RF). The mechanical simplicity hides a mathematically complex design process.

Lasers

The effectiveness of lasers derives from production of a perfectly parallel beam, allowing extremely tight focusing. Concentrating energy into a very small area in a very brief pulse produces very high local temperatures, sufficient to vaporize tissue, surrounded very locally by a cauterizing action which seals the edges and reduces blood loss.

In the following description, the simplified Bohr model of the atom is used, modified where relevant by some of the constraints of wave mechanics. Neodymium-doped yttrium aluminium garnet (Nd-YAG) lasers are rod lasers that are pumped by a flash lamp having a broad spectrum of light. A typical system is shown in Figure 13.8. The flash excites electrons orbiting a nucleus to orbits of higher energy, from where they drop back and may emit a photon of light as they do. In suitable materials, some of these orbits are relatively stable and electrons tend to dwell in them for a relatively long time. The rod has polished squared off ends and is placed between mirrors with surfaces that are exactly parallel, so that any light emitted within the rod is reflected back and forth. Those electrons in unstable orbits soon drop back at random times and take no significant part in the true laser beam. Those in semi-stable orbits accumulate. When they drop back they also emit a photon, although most are not parallel to the axis of the rod and mirrors. When a photon has a wavefront parallel to the mirrors, it is reflected exactly back to the other mirror, which sends it back to the first, etc. Because its wavelength is exactly the same as that represented by the energy difference in all the similar semi-stable electrons, they are stimulated to join in as the wave passes by, adding their energy to the beam in precisely the same direction and phase. The stronger the beam becomes, the more likely any remaining excited electrons are to join in, producing a sudden, very intense, flash of visible or infrared light. This is how lasers get their name: *Light Amplification by Stimulated Emission of Radiation*.

Part of the light is allowed to escape through one of the mirrors, and it is described as 'coherent'. Coherent

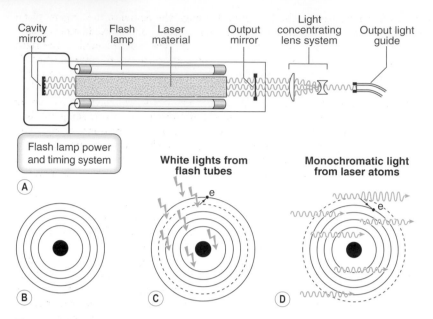

Figure 13.8 • Diagram of laser.

light is monochromatic, highly parallel, sharing the same spatial and temporal phase. Because it is so perfectly parallel it can be focused on to much smaller spots than sunlight. Spots of 0.5 μm can be used to cut into single cells *in vitro*. Although the conversion efficiency from energy in the flash tubes to laser output is very small, typically <1/1000, this fine focusing produces very high local energy deposition, termed irradiance. For instance, a typical CO_2 laser might briefly produce an irradiance of up to 20 kW/cm² over a 0.3-mm diameter spot. The wavelength of the radiation (colour if in the visible range) depends on the material doing the lasering. This has an important bearing on the effect on the tissue. CO_2 lasers produce infrared radiation at a 10.6 μm wavelength, which is strongly absorbed by water in the tissue. Tightly focused intensities of 100 W/cm² produce tissue vaporization depths of 3–4 mm, giving the effect of a laser knife. A laser knife has the further advantage that, at the edge of its beam, blood vessels become coagulated, sealing off the operative field as they cut. Cone excisions from the cervix may be produced by mechanical rotation of the beam. Spreading the beam by partial de-focusing is useful for surface ablation or thermocoagulation.

The physical properties of CO_2 lasers make them unsuitable for operating on thicker tissues, for example to ablate endometriosis. Here the Nd-YAG laser is ideal because its wavelength is in the near infrared range (0.532 μm) at which water is transparent but blood pigments readily absorb. The radiation is conducted to the site via a 0.4-mm diameter fibre light guide. This is a fine glass fibre whose outer surface is coated with a thin layer of another glass of a different refractive index. This ensures that any light not quite parallel to the axis of the fibre is totally reflected back into the fibre as if the fibre were surrounded by a perfect mirror. The fibre is flexible. It can then be passed down endoscopes and positioned using a pilot beam of normal light. When the desired position is attained and the trigger button pressed, a shutter blocks the eyepiece, the flash lamp fires, and the shutter re-opens. It is likely that a whole range of different laser beams will become available, each tailored to a specific surgical application.

Magnetic resonance imaging (MRI)

This method does *not* produce ionization and is called magnetic resonance imaging (MRI) rather than the older 'nuclear magnetic resonance', which had negative associations in patients' minds. No beams of light or sound are produced; instead the nuclei of certain atoms in the patient are induced to report their presence and condition by absorbing or sending out radio waves.

The term 'resonance' is borrowed from the study of sound. A guitar string resonates when it continues making a sound after it has been plucked. It is tuned by altering its tension. Just as the string vibrates at a frequency that depends on its nature and the applied tension, so spinning nuclei produce or absorb radio waves at a frequency that depends on their nature and the steady magnetic field they are in. This frequency is known as the Langmuir frequency. By analogy, this response of nuclei to radio waves, which can be tuned by varying the surrounding magnetic field, is called magnetic resonance.

The converse effect, energy absorption at resonance, can be demonstrated by whistling into a piano while depressing its sustaining pedal. When the whistle ceases, a similar sound is heard coming from the piano. An analogous situation can be set up by supporting a tissue sample in a powerful, steady and very uniform magnetic field to tune the nuclei to the frequency to be absorbed. The whistle is then replaced by a rapidly alternating magnetic field, transverse to the steady main field, referred to as the radiofrequency (RF) field. MR spectroscopy generally measures the energy absorbed from the RF field as its frequency is slowly changed. Since different nuclei have different resonant frequencies for the same main magnetic field, their presence and abundance can be determined from the degree of absorption and the frequencies at which they occur, observed during each frequency sweep. This can be plotted to give a series of spectral lines similar to those in optical spectrometry. More importantly, the small magnetic fields each nucleus generates, and the screening effects the electron clouds surrounding molecules exert, modify the main magnetic field. This causes small variations of resonant frequency to be superimposed on these lines, shifting and splitting them. Thus, not only can the abundance of the various nuclear species be observed, but also changes in their chemical environment. For example tuning into the phosphorus in muscle enables the availability of ATP during repeated contractions to be followed.

While MR spectroscopy normally measures the energy absorbed from the RF field as it happens, imaging (MRI) usually depends on observing the signal still being re-transmitted by the nuclei some time following a short burst or bursts of the RF field. The signal from individual nuclei is too small to be detected; they have to be synchronized by short bursts of the transverse field, referred to as RF pulses. Hydrogen (a single proton) is the usual nucleus selected for imaging applications, as it is by far the most abundant. In imaging, unlike spectroscopy, the main magnetic field is deliberately made non-uniform to vary the tuning of the protons in different parts of the patient. For instance, suppose the field is made high on one side of the patient and low on the other. Then, only one vertical plane in the patient will contain any protons tuned to the same frequency as the RF pulse. If we tune in subsequently with a radio receiver and pick up a signal, we will know that it must have come from that plane.

Suppose that during this period the magnetic field is made high at the head end of the patient and low at the feet end. Although the nuclei in the original plane may all still be transmitting, only those in a new plane, orthogonal to the first, will still be tuned to the right frequency to be picked up by the receiver. If there is some signal it must be coming from where these two planes cross a line through the patient. There are other, more sophisticated ways in which further data can be built into the signal to identify where along the line individual tissue elements are re-transmitting. The intensity of the signal which now represents the quantity of the molecular species is then used to modulate the brightness of a line on a VDU in a position on the screen representing the triple intersection position in the patient. Increasingly complex pulse sequences have been devised, which allow simultaneous reading of the signal from many lines at once and this reduces the time required to scan the patient.

For imaging, some of the spectral detail available in spectroscopy is sacrificed in order to maximize tissue contrast and detail in the image. However, this is partly compensated for by using the dynamic behaviour of the excited protons. Returning to our earlier analogy, if after whistling into the piano the sustaining pedal is released, the vibrational energy of the strings is rapidly removed by the felt dampers, and the sound decays quickly. A corresponding effect results as nuclei give up energy to their surroundings, known as the lattice. This spin–lattice relaxation time (T_1) is generally long in liquids and short in structured tissues. Tissues that have similar concentrations of protons may give similar signal strengths soon after excitation by the RF pulse, but if a delay is allowed before measurement, large differences in the remaining strength may develop.

Within tissues T_1 may be as short as 0.1 s. Fluid-filled cysts have a long T_1, whereas clotted blood and fibrous tissue generally have a short T_1. The longer T_1 of normal blood is generally masked by the fact that it has moved out of the field of view before measurement can be made. Blood vessels usually appear black on the image. The increased T_1 seen in tumours relative to the surrounding tissue is attributed to the increased free water present. Adjustment of measuring delay may increase the contrast between neighbouring tissues of identical proton density but differing internal structure.

Once the RF pulse ceases, some nuclei will resonate slightly faster than average as their local magnetic fields add to the main field, and some slower as the local magnetic field subtracts. Then, although there is no energy loss, the increasing lack of synchronization renders the signal inaccessible to the radio receiver. This is known as spin–spin relaxation, and the time constant describing it is known as T_2. By manipulation of successive RF pulses, those nuclei that were fast can be made slow and vice versa. After a further delay, this results in recovery of synchronization and the signal reappears. By analogy with sound this is described as a spin-echo. It is extensively used to recover the signal after complicated tissue-selective pulse sequence techniques. By altering the repetition rate of the complete cycle, further mixing of multiple RF pulses, and the timing of the final observation relative to them, the method can be made highly selective to the chemical state of observed tissues with differing T_1, T_2 or T_1/T_2 ratios.

Chapter Fourteen

14

Statistics and evidence-based healthcare

Louise Brown

CHAPTER CONTENTS

Introduction

Many doctors often equate statistics with the numbers and equations seen in research papers. But the term 'statistics' does not mean 'numbers'; indeed, a competent statistical analysis of a paper should include non-numerical issues such as the nature of the sampling methods or the validity of a 'gold standard' diagnostic test. Furthermore, papers may be overflowing with numerical data but contain no statistics at all.

Statistics has been defined as the discipline concerned with:

- Data collection and presentation
- Inference from samples or experiments to the population at large
- Modelling and analysis of complex systems
- Broader issues to do with the application and interpretation of the above techniques in politics, management, the law, philosophy and the sciences.

One of the problems in getting to grips with statistics is that, in common with many other branches of medicine, it is becoming an increasingly sophisticated science, where standard textbooks appear to serve only those who are already members of its exclusive club. The analysis of large and complex datasets, and the techniques of mathematical modelling, are generally best left to the experts. But the appraisal of many published articles relevant to the practising obstetrician or gynaecologist can be greatly helped by an understanding of several basic principles, some of which are presented in this chapter.

Some basic statistical principles

Sampling and inference to the population at large

The most fundamental issue of statistics is that one is trying to relate data taken from a relatively small 'sample' to a much larger group where it would be impractical to collect all the available data. In medical statistics, this large and rather nebulous group of subjects is known as 'the population' and it can often be hard to define. This may seem obvious but understanding the concept of sampling is crucial in the interpretation of results from studies. The application of statistics to research is an attempt to ensure that the results from your sample are in general agreement with the results that would have occurred if you had been able to conduct the experiment on all relevant members of the population in question. Figure 14.1 demonstrates this simple relationship and it is intuitive to see that, as the sample size increases, it moves closer to representing the population. In general, as the size of the sample increases, the bias in the study decreases; however, this is not always the case and in some unusual statistical settings the bias will remain, but these are beyond the scope of this chapter.

The most important 'take-home' message for you as an investigator is that, if you repeated your experiment, you would almost certainly get a different result. You may still draw the same conclusions from that result, but the numbers used in the statistical calculations would differ from sample to sample. On average, you would expect the results to be consistent, but when there is disagreement between sample and population the following types of error can occur and these should always be at the front of your mind when interpreting study results.

Type 1 error

This occurs when 'the sample' used in your experiment generates a significant result for your hypothesis but there would not have been a significant result if you had performed the experiment on 'the population'; in other words, it occurred by chance. When we set

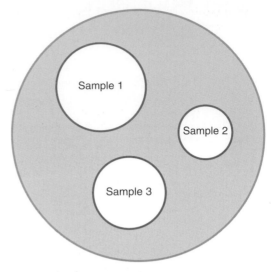

The population – all possible subjects relevant to the study

The samples are ideally selected at random

Figure 14.1 • Representation of sample and population.

a 'significant' p value at 0.05, we are allowing a 5% chance of a type 1 error occurring for our study. To have zero chance of a type 1 error we would need to perform the experiment on 'the population' itself and this is not possible as it infers recruiting an infinite number of subjects. The 5% level is entirely arbitrary and purely a convention that seems 'reasonable' in most research situations. Thus, p values should be interpreted cautiously always bearing in mind the study design and the size of the difference observed between the comparative groups. P values are a continuum that runs from 0 to 1 and thresholds such as 0.05 are only used as a guide.

Another consideration when interpreting the results of a study is whether many comparisons have been made using the same sample. This is known as 'multiple testing' and it is a common flaw seen in a number of studies in the published literature. By setting your p value for significance at 0.05, you are allowing a 5% chance of a type 1 error, i.e. 1 in 20 statistical comparisons will produce a significant result by chance and thus, if a large number of variables in the dataset are tested for significance, there is a considerable risk of getting a type 1 error. Multiple testing often goes hand in hand with an unclear hypothesis and a poorly thought through study design. If you wish to test many outcomes and exposures using the same sample of patients, you need to account for this by setting yourself a more stringent p value for significance, e.g. 0.01. In this case, you would need to make

100 comparisons in order for one of them to be significant by chance.

Type 2 error

This occurs when 'the sample' used in your experiment fails to generate a significant result for your hypothesis but there would have been a significant result if you had performed the experiment on 'the population' , i.e. you have missed a real and possibly important effect. When we require a study to have 90% power, we are allowing a 10% chance that our sample will not detect a significant result that in truth exists in the population. This commonly occurs in small studies where there is insufficient power. Under-powered studies can be frustrating to interpret, particularly when there appears to be quite a large difference between the groups but the p value does not reach the magical threshold for acceptance as a significant result. Some statisticians argue that no under-powered studies should ever be undertaken as they cannot be interpreted and this would probably condense the world's research output to a fraction of its current amount. Most research funders now demand power calculations, but sometimes the assumptions on which power calculations are based are grossly optimistic. However, in many cases a balance can still be achieved between attaining sufficient power and setting a pragmatic target for the sample size.

The null and active hypotheses

It is always important to be able to define the null and active hypotheses for a study and this means having clear definitions for both the outcome and the exposure or treatment. Under the null hypothesis, there is no difference between the groups that are being compared. This will tend to be the 'default' hypothesis unless the study sample accrues sufficient evidence to reject this null hypothesis and show that the active hypothesis is true.

Bias and generalizability

When studies have been sampled in a non-random fashion, differences between the results from the sample and the true population can arise. Similarly, if treatments are allocated to patients non-randomly, estimates for differences between treatment groups can be biased. In other words, bias can arise if the sample is systematically unrepresentative of the population. However, bias and generalizability are not always the same thing. If one runs a well-powered randomized controlled trial, the results comparing randomized groups that are estimated from the sample are unlikely to be biased; however, they will only be generalizable to the sub-group of the population that met the inclu-sion criteria for the study. Thus, when interpreting the results from studies it is important to view them in relation to the study inclusion and exclusion criteria and the sampling methods that were employed when recruiting the subjects. There are many different types of bias and certain study designs are more prone to particular types of bias than others. This will be discussed in more depth in the section about types of study and experimental design (pp 299–300).

Confidence intervals, accuracy and precision

When interpreting a result from a sample, it is useful to express the result with a range of possible values that it might have taken if other samples of the same size had been selected. This range of values is called a confidence interval (CI) and we can set the level of confidence as a percentage; 95% confidence is typically used. For example, if we measure the birth weight of 50 babies and calculate a point estimate for the mean weight of 3360 g and a 95% confidence interval of 3200 to 3520 g, this means that we can be 95% confident that, given this sample size, the true mean birth weight for all babies in the population relevant to this study lies somewhere between 3200 and 3520 g. In general, as the sample size increases, the confidence interval becomes narrower. The term precision is used to describe how wide the confidence interval is around the point estimate, whereas accuracy gives an indication of how close the point estimate from the sample is to the true unmeasurable population value and is therefore more related to bias or generalizability. The calculation of confidence intervals will be discussed in more detail on p. 296.

Independence and matched data

Many statistical tests make assumptions about the independence of the subjects analysed in the study. If data are not independent, e.g. the same mother can be included more than once in a study on childbirth, then account should be taken of this in the analysis. Many commonly used statistical tests assume that all observations are from separate individuals and, by including subjects more than once, you are making your sample less varied than it would be if subjects were only entered once. Similarly, if your study design selected cases and controls by matching them in terms of covariates such as age and ethnic group, then your analysis *must* account for this matching. In general, it is preferable not to match any subjects within a study as it is possible to adjust for potential differences between your groups at the analysis stage. Furthermore, in studies where subjects have been assessed before and after experiencing an exposure, they should be investigated in a 'paired' fashion by analysing the difference between the before and after measurements, as this accounts for the lack of independence between them. This also tends to improve the power of the study as within-patient differences tend to be less variable than absolute variation between patients.

Data types, distribution assumptions and parametric tests

There are many different ways in which we can collate data on a subject of interest but, in general, data can be classified into the following types:

Quantitative or continuous – a continual spectrum of data measurements, e.g. age, blood pressure, height or weight.

Ordinal – subjects are categorized into groups where there is some order to the categories, e.g. mild, moderate or severe symptoms.

Categorical – subjects are categorized into groups but there is not necessarily any particular order to the categories, e.g. eye colour or country of birth.

Binary – this is a sub-group of ordinal and categorical data where there are just two possible categories, e.g. male or female, dead or alive.

Time-dependent data – where subjects have been followed up for different lengths of time, typically in cohort studies and randomized controlled trials when subjects have been recruited over an extended period of time. For example, the classification of a subject as dead or alive may depend upon the length of their follow-up.

When analysing these data types it is often necessary to make assumptions about how the data within our sample are likely to behave in relation to the population from which they came. In order to do this, it is helpful to assume a probability distribution which can be described by a mathematical equation and this can then be used as a template to describe the sample data and make comparisons within it. There are many types of mathematical distribution used in statistics but four of the most common ones are the binomial, Poisson, normal and chi-squared (χ^2) distributions:

> *The binomial distribution* describes the probability distribution for binary data and it relates to the common example of tossing a coin. For large sample sizes, the binomial distribution is very similar to the normal distribution and so the latter is often assumed in the statistical calculations.

> *The Poisson distribution* can be assumed when investigating rates derived from time-to-event data and it represents the idea that a certain event is occurring at a constant rate and thus, as we follow people through time, more events will occur. However, it should be noted that there are also more complex assumptions that are required when analysing time-to-event data, e.g. Cox regression analysis is often used, but these will not be discussed further in this chapter.

> *The normal or Gaussian distribution* is assumed when investigating measurements from continuous data, but it is also used as the basis for many aspects of medical statistics. More detail is provided for this distribution a little further on, as it is so important in understanding the application of statistics. For reasonably large samples of observations (typically >20), another probability distribution known as the *t* distribution is generally used as it a good approximation of the normal distribution and this is the basis for the well known Student's *t*-test.

> *The chi-squared (χ^2) distribution* is derived by squaring the normal distribution and it has particular properties that make it useful for investigating proportions from categorical, ordinal or binary data.

The normal distribution

The normal distribution is one of the most important and widely used probability distributions in medical statistics. It can be described by a rather complex mathematical equation; however, if it is plotted in terms of probability, we can see that it generates the famous 'bell-shaped' curve shown in Figure 14.2. The x-axis is standardized such that the mean corresponds to zero (the most probable value) with units of standard deviation falling above and below this value. It can be seen that 95% of the area under the curve lies between the points that fall 1.96 standard deviations on either side of the mean value and this number is particularly important as we can use it to give us an indicator of the range of values that would incorporate 95% of all possible values. In some cases you may wish to know the range of values that incorporate 90% or even 99% of all values and these ranges correspond to the 1.65 and 2.58 standard deviations on either side of the mean, respectively.

The beauty of the normal distribution is that this symmetrical property around the mean value holds whether we are plotting the actual data points from our sample or whether we are plotting the results of the study if we had repeated it over and over again. In this scenario, we would end up with the 'mean of the mean

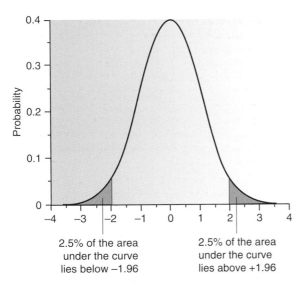

2.5% of the area
under the curve
lies below −1.96

2.5% of the area
under the curve
lies above +1.96

Figure 14.2 • Probability distribution function for the normal distribution. The horizontal axis has been standardized such that zero corresponds to the mean with units of standard deviation above and below the mean.

of the samples' and the range of mean values can be represented by the sampling distribution. The term standard error is essentially the standard deviation of this sampling distribution and it is used throughout statistics to calculate confidence intervals around point estimates. An example of how to calculate a confidence interval for the mean is given on p. 296.

Parametric and non-parametric tests

Parametric statistical tests are ones where assumptions are made about which mathematical distribution best represents the sample and the population from which it was taken. Non-parametric statistical tests are ones where no assumption has been made about the distribution of the data. In general, parametric tests tend to be more powerful and sensitive than non-parametric tests and therefore tend to be preferred as fewer observations are required to provide evidence in favour of the hypothesis if it is true. A typical example of a parametric test is the use of a Student's t-test to compare the mean values of a continuous variable between two groups. One of the test assumptions is that the continuous data measured in the sample can be assumed to follow the normal distribution. If this assumption is not valid, then the non-parametric Mann–Whitney U test can be used which ranks the observations in order of size and compares the proportions that fall above and below the median value for each of the groups in question. Thus, the Mann–Whitney U test is less sensitive to large outlying values

but also less informative as observations above or below the median are all treated in the same way.

Deciding whether to use parametric or non-parametric tests

For binary data, the assumption of a binomial distribution will be valid for small samples of <20, but both the binomial and normal distributions can be assumed for samples of binary data with >20 observations. When comparing proportions across binary, categorical or ordinal data, the chi-squared distribution is often assumed; however, if the numbers in the categories becomes very small then it is often more appropriate to use Yates' correction or Fisher's exact test, both of which are described in any standard statistical textbook.

Probably the most common example of deciding whether to use a parametric or non-parametric test is when you want to know whether the continuous data in your sample can be assumed to follow a normal distribution. In general, for small samples of less than about 15 observations, it is not safe to assume the data are normally distributed and non-parametric methods should generally be employed. However, it should be remembered that these tests are less powerful and the sample size is small, which will make the statistical results hard to interpret. If you have a reasonably large sample size, the first thing to do is to plot your data points on a scattergraph or group the data into bins and plot them on a histogram. Inspection of the graphs or histograms is the simplest way of assessing whether your distribution assumptions are valid. Deviations from the normal distribution can lead to significant skewness or kurtosis. Figure 14.3 demonstrates histograms for data that follow a normal distribution or have a positively or negatively skewed distribution, and Figure 14.4 shows how data can deviate from the classic 'bell-shaped' curve seen in the normal distribution and exhibit kurtosis. Kurtosis is concerned with the shape of the distribution and can have a considerable impact on the statistical analysis that you choose to perform on your data. When kurtosis is extreme, non-parametric tests should be used. It is worth noting that for data that are perfectly normally distributed the mean, median and mode values are all the same, whereas for positively skewed data the mean tends to be larger than the median and vice versa for negatively skewed data. When summarizing skewed data, it is often better to quote the median and interquartile range rather than the mean and standard deviation which are generally used for summarizing normally distributed data. The way to calculate these summary statistics is described in the next section. In some cases, it helps to convert skewed data into another variable that can be assumed to follow the normal distribution (this is called transformation). For example, data that are positively skewed can often be manipulated into a

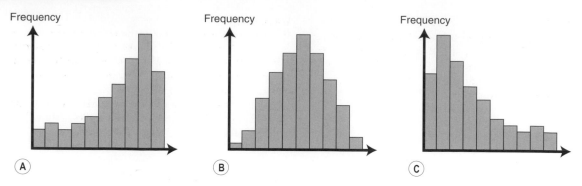

Figure 14.3 • Histograms representing skewness of data. (A) Negatively skewed (median > mean). (B) Normally distributed (median = mean = mode). (C) Positively skewed (median < mean).

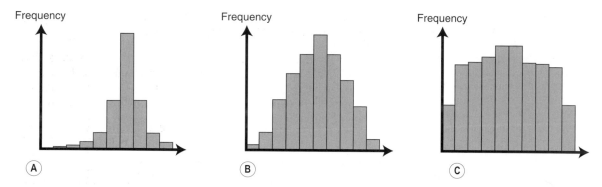

Figure 14.4 • Histograms representing kurtosis of data. Lepto-kurtic (long-tailed). (B) Meso-kurtic (normally distributed). (C) Platy-kurtic (short-tailed).

more normally distributed format by transforming them onto the log scale; the *t*-test can then be used on the log-transformed data. There are more formal ways of testing your assumptions about the normal distribution, such as normal plots and Shapiro–Francia or Shapiro–Wilk tests, but these should be used cautiously and, if there is doubt, you should revert to using non-parametric methods.

Data collection and presentation

There are numerous ways in which data can be summarized and presented and the choice depends on the type of data. The previous section defined the different types of data and the distributions that are often assumed to analyse them. Table 14.1 shows some typical methods for summarizing and presenting different data types. All statistical software packages will perform the analysis for summary statistics, but the following simple example shows how the basic ones can be calculated for a set of data.

Table 14.1 Typical summary statistics and presentation methods for describing data

Data type	Summary statistics	Presentation
Quantitative or continuous	Mean or average, standard deviation, variance, standard error, confidence intervals, mode, median, range, interquartile range	Scatter plots Line plots Box and whisker plots Histograms
Categorical, ordinal or binary	Mode Percentage or risk Odds	Histograms Pie charts Bar charts
Time-dependent event outcomes	Rate Hazard (particular example for Cox modelling)	Life table or Kaplan–Meier curves

Example

A study was conducted to investigate various aspects of systolic blood pressure (SBP), treatment and survival in a sample of 20 people recruited over 1 year and followed for 5 years. The data are given in Table 14.2, arranged in ascending order of SBP.

Mean

This is the sum of all the observations divided by the number of observations.

e.g. Mean systolic blood pressure = (105 + 107 + 107 + ... + 190 + 199)/20 = 144.35 mmHg

Similarly, the mean age = 71.55 years.

Variance

This is an indication of the variability of the observations. Each observation is subtracted from the mean, squared, added up and divided by the number of observations, minus 1.

e.g. Variance of systolic blood pressure = $[(105 -144.35)^2 + (107 -144.35)^2 + ... + (190 -144.35)^2 + (199 -144.35)^2]/(20 -1) = 804.66$ mmHg

Similarly, the variance of age = 136.36 years.

Standard deviation (SD)

This is also an indication of the variability of the observations as it is the square root of the variance.

Table 14.2   Summary of dataset to investigate various aspects of systolic blood pressure, treatment and survival

Age at start of study (years)	Gender	Ethnic group	Systolic blood pressure at start of study (mmHg)	Treated for hypertension	Dead or alive at end of study	Length of time to death or end of study (months)
56	Male	White	105	Yes	Dead	1
74	Male	Afro-Caribbean	107	No	Alive	50
83	Female	White	107	Yes	Dead	55
77	Male	White	109	No	Dead	46
59	Male	White	115	Yes	Alive	50
80	Male	Asian	122	No	Alive	49
67	Male	White	132	No	Dead	6
55	Male	Asian	133	No	Alive	59
80	Male	White	136	Yes	Alive	51
75	Female	White	144	No	Alive	55
64	Female	Afro-Caribbean	148	Yes	Dead	55
64	Female	White	155	No	Dead	32
51	Female	White	155	No	Dead	13
91	Male	White	156	Yes	Alive	49
87	Male	Asian	160	Yes	Alive	53
56	Male	White	167	No	Alive	60
76	Male	Afro-Caribbean	167	Yes	Alive	58
78	Female	White	180	No	Alive	66
77	Male	White	190	No	Alive	65
81	Male	Afro-Caribbean	199	No	Dead	33

e.g. Standard deviation of systolic blood pressure
= $\sqrt{804.66}$ = 28.37 mmHg
Similarly, the standard deviation of age = 11.68 years.

Standard error of the mean (SEM)

The standard error is used to indicate how well the sample mean measurement represents the true population mean value. Standard errors are used to calculate confidence intervals (see next section).

e.g. Standard error of the mean systolic blood pressure = standard deviation divided by the square root of the number of observations = $28.37/\sqrt{20}$ = 6.34 mmHg.

Similarly, the standard error for the mean age is 2.61 years.

Confidence interval for the mean

Earlier in the chapter, the characteristics of the normal distribution were discussed and these properties are central to the construction of confidence intervals. The most common confidence interval is set at 95% as this corresponds to a p value of 0.05. Once the standard error has been calculated, the 95% confidence interval for the mean blood pressure can be constructed using the 1.96 multiplier described on page 292. Thus, the point estimate with the 95% confidence interval for the mean blood pressure is $144.35 \pm (1.96 \times 6.34) = 131.0$ to 157.6 mmHg

Similarly, the 95% confidence interval around the mean age is 66.1 to 77.1 years.

If you wish to be more stringent with your data you can set your p value threshold for statistical significance at 0.01 rather than 0.05 as this corresponds to a 99% confidence interval. In this case, the 1.96 number increases to 2.58. Alternatively, a less stringent threshold would be a p value of 0.1 where the 1.96 value is decreased to 1.65 to generate a 90% confidence interval.

Mode

This is the most common value in the dataset. It is typically used with categorical and ordinal data but can also be used for continuous data. The mode can become a more complicated parameter when the distribution of data has more than one most common value, e.g. bi-modal, but this will not be discussed further here.

e.g. The mode for ethnic group is white, the mode for hypertension treatment is none and the mode for gender is male.

Median

The median is the midpoint of all the observations, indicating that 50% of the observations lie above and 50% lie below the median. Sometimes it is more appropriate to quote the median rather than the mean as it is less sensitive to large outlying values. Similarly, when data are skewed, it is generally better to quote the median rather than the mean.

e.g. The median for blood pressure is midway between the 10th and 11th observation when arranged in rank order, i.e. 146 mmHg

Similarly, the median age is 75.5 years.

Range

This is the total range of values between the largest and the smallest observation. It indicates how widely varied the data are and is often quoted with the median.

e.g. The range for blood pressure is 105–199 mmHg
Similarly, the range for age is 51–91 years.

Interquartile range

This is similar to the median although the lower value indicates that 25% of the observations lie below it and the upper value indicates that 25% of the observations lie above it. Thus, it represents the central 50% range of values and is usually quoted with the median and often used to summarize skewed data.

e.g. The interquartile range for blood pressure is 188.5–163.5 mmHg

Similarly, the interquartile range for age is 61.5–80 years.

Proportion and risk

Table 14.3 shows the results of gender by hypertensive treatment at the start of the study. Providing the status of hypertensive treatment did not alter during the course of follow-up, the percentages can be used to represent the extent of treatment within each gender, i.e. 6/14 males were treated (43%) compared with 2/6 females (33%). Risks and percentages cannot be used

Table 14.3 Results of gender and hypertensive treatment at baseline

	Hypertensive treatment	No hypertensive treatment	Total
Males	6	8	14
Females	2	4	6
Total	8	12	20

for time-dependent data unless subjects have all been followed for the same length of time.

Odds

The odds is calculated as the ratio of the number of subjects classified in one category to the number of subjects classified in another category. Again, using Table 14.3, the odds of hypertensive treatment within each gender are $6/8 = 0.75$ for males and $2/4 = 0.5$ for females. Odds should not be used for time-dependent data unless all subjects have been followed for the same length of time. The reasons for using odds rather than risk are to do with mathematical restrictions which make it more appropriate in certain analysis situations.

Rate

In many situations, subjects are followed for a certain period of time to see if a certain event occurs, e.g. death, surgical intervention, pregnancy, etc. If these events occur at a steady rate over time, the number of events that occurred divided by the amount of time subjects have been followed will generate a rate of events. Person-years are the most common way of calculating the amount of follow-up in a study and this is the sum of the length of time each subject has contributed to the study. For the example given in Table 14.2, there were eight deaths over a total of 906 person-months, which is equivalent to $906/12 = 75.7$ person-years. Thus, the rate of death $= 8/75.5 = 0.106$ deaths per person-year although it is conventional to quote the result per 100 person-years $= 10.6$. This can be interpreted as meaning that, if you follow 100 subjects for 1 year, 10.6 deaths will occur, but this is a very crude summary as it assumes that deaths occur at a constant rate across years, and this may not be the case. Calculation of crude rates in this way makes many assumptions about the frequency of the events over time and alternative methods are often used such as Kaplan–Meier curves for presentation and Cox modelling for generating hazard ratios as a measure of outcome between groups. It is also worth noting in this example that if we had calculated the risk of death as $8/20$ (40%) this would have overestimated the mortality in the study, which is why rates should always be used when subjects have been followed for different lengths of time.

Measures of outcome, exposure and effect

When investigating the relationships between cause and treatment of diseases, it is useful to talk in terms of the exposures (the factors that are thought to relate to the presence or progression of the disease or the treatment that is thought to cure or slow the development of the disease) and the outcome (the variable that describes whether the disease is present or how severe the disease is in terms of some defined symptom or event). At this point, it is worth formally defining the difference between the prevalence and incidence of a disease as these are commonly used as outcome measures in epidemiology.

Prevalence

This refers to the number of individuals with the disease at one point in time as a proportion of the total number of individuals in the population of interest at the same point in time. Thus, the prevalence represents a 'snap-shot' of the proportion of people with the outcome of interest at a given point in time and is therefore dimensionless in terms of time. It therefore relates to the risk of the outcome.

Incidence

This is defined as the number of new cases of a disease that develop in a group of individuals who are at risk during a specified period of time. Thus, as time passes the cumulative incidence of disease will increase and this is dependent on the length of the study and relates to the rate of disease.

Earlier in this chapter, risk, odds and rates were defined and these are commonly used as measures of outcome. Ratios and differences for these outcomes can be used as measures of effect between exposed and unexposed groups. These measures of effect should always be quoted with their confidence intervals and all statistical software packages will calculate these for you, but the methodology describing how to do this is too detailed to provide here. However, interpretation of these types of outcome can be illustrated using the data in Table 14.2 by investigating the relationship between hypertensive treatment, gender and mortality.

Question 1 – Is there any difference in the use of hypertensive therapy between men and women?

This can be investigated by calculating either the risk or the odds ratio.

The risk ratio (RR) for hypertensive treatment between men and women $= 43\%/33\% = 1.30$ [95% confidence interval 0.36 to 4.64].

Thus, the point estimate suggests that men are 30% more likely to be on hypertensive treatment than women but, given the size of our sample, we are 95% confident that the true risk ratio for the population lies somewhere between 0.36 and 4.64. As our 95% confidence interval includes the risk ratio that corresponds to the null hypothesis value of 1.0, we do not have sufficient evidence to reject the null hypothesis and conclude that men are significantly more likely to be on hypertensive treatment than women.

The odds ratio (OR) for hypertensive treatment between men and women = 0.5/0.75 = 0.67 [95% CI 0.09 to 4.93]. Thus, the odds of being on hypertensive treatment is a third less for women than for men, but once again the confidence interval includes the null hypothesis value of 1.0 so there is insufficient evidence to suggest a difference in use of hypertensive therapy.

Question 2 – Is there any difference in mortality between men and women?

This relates to rates rather than risks and a crude rate of death can be obtained.

Rate ratio for mortality between men and women = 7.7/17.4 = 0.44 [95% CI 0.08 to 2.37] where the rates have been calculated as deaths per 100 person-years by dividing the number of deaths within each sex by the total number of years of follow-up in each sex and multiplying by 100. Thus, the rate of death in men is 7.7 per 100 person-years which is 0.44 that of women, but this is also not significant as the confidence interval includes the rate ratio for no difference of 1.0. Note that calculation of risk and odds for mortality would, be incorrect here as subjects have been followed for different lengths of time.

It is also possible to calculate differences in outcomes rather than ratios but these tend to be used more in the realms of public health where absolute numbers tend to be more relevant.

Risk difference (attributable risk) for hypertensive treatment by gender = 43% – 33% = 10% [95% CI –36% to 55%].

Difference in mortality between genders = 7.7 – 17.4 = –9.7 [95% CI –28.3 to 8.9] deaths per 100 person-years. Both of these 95% confidence intervals include the null hypothesis value of zero, and therefore would correspond to *p* values > 0.05.

Confounding and interaction

If one is trying to investigate whether a particular exposure or behaviour is affecting a group of subjects when compared with an unexposed control group, how can one be certain that the difference observed between the groups is attributable to the exposure? If the treated and the control group are different in ways other than the exposure of interest, for example if there are more elderly subjects in the control group, it is very difficult to tease out how much of the difference between the two groups is due to the exposure and how much is due to the younger age of the exposed group. In this case, age is a confounder and it is a classic example as there are very few diseases that do not

show some association with age. In order to be a confounder, the variable must be associated with *both* the outcome and the exposure of interest. Figure 14.5 demonstrates two classic examples where confounding is likely and unlikely to be occurring. Intuitively, it is tempting to think that because smoking and levels of alcohol intake are closely linked, one must always adjust for each of these variables when investigating the effects of the other. However, although this is advisable for studies investigating the effects of smoking and alcohol on heart disease, it is not necessarily required when studying the effects of smoking and alcohol on lung cancer. There is good evidence to suggest both a protective effect of alcohol (low intake) and a damaging effect of alcohol (high intake) on the incidence of heart disease as well as a strong link between smoking and the development of heart disease. It is also known that levels of alcohol intake and smoking are closely related; therefore all three sides of the confounding triangle show significant association. Conversely, in studies investigating the effect of smoking on lung cancer one does not need to adjust for alcohol intake as there is little or no evidence to suggest that increased drinking is associated with an increased risk of lung cancer. Thus, alcohol intake is a confounder in Figure 14.5A but not a confounder in Figure 14.5B.

In the real world, there are probably many variables having a confounding effect on our results and many of them will not be obvious to us, which is why rand-

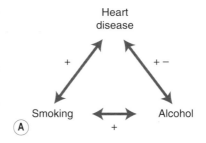

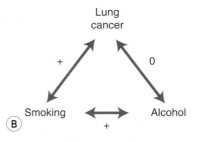

Figure 14.5 • Confounding relationship between alcohol intake and smoking when investigating risk factors for heart disease and lung cancer. (A) Confounding. (B) No confounding.

omized controlled trials are so valuable. By randomly assigning your subjects to either the treatment or the control group, you are minimizing the chance that there are any associations between all the potential confounding variables and the decision to be in the treatment or control group. Thus one side of the triangular relationship that is required for confounding to occur no longer exists. However, there are often times when randomization is not possible as people cannot randomly be assigned to develop a disease and other studies are required to investigate these situations. Thus, in non-randomized comparisons, the tendency for confounding can be high and this often makes interpretation of results very difficult. Adjustment for potential confounders is one way in which the presence of confounding can be assessed. In the heart disease example in Figure 14.5, if you find there is a two-fold increase in the incidence of heart disease between smokers and non-smokers but this risk decreases to 1.5 when adjusted for alcohol intake, it might be interpreted that half of the increase in risk of heart disease is attributable to alcohol and the other half to smoking, providing all other factors are equal. This example raises another issue that often requires investigation and this is called interaction.

Interaction occurs when two risk factors do not combine to produce the expected effect in outcome when they are both present in an individual. For example, if by smoking and not drinking you have a three-fold increase in the risk of developing heart disease, and by drinking but not smoking you have a two-fold increase in the risk of developing heart disease, then one might expect individuals who both drink and smoke to have a six-fold increase in the risk of developing heart disease compared with individuals who neither drink nor smoke. If you tested this hypothesis in an experiment and found that there was a 10-fold increase in the risk of heart disease rather than the expected six-fold, then there might be evidence to suggest that smoking and drinking are interacting in some way that exacerbates the risk of heart disease. Often, investigators are tempted to analyse treatment effects in subgroups, e.g. males and females, but this is not advisable as it is an unpowerful and inefficient use of data, and tests for interaction are recommended. There are formal ways of testing for interaction, but these will not be discussed here; the description is merely included as an alert to the reader that these types of issue should be considered when interpreting results from studies.

Types of study and experimental design

Epidemiology is essentially concerned with the investigation of health and illness across and within populations of people and numerous study design methods have been developed for the analysis of this often complex subject. Figure 14.6 summarizes the most common types of epidemiological study and it can be

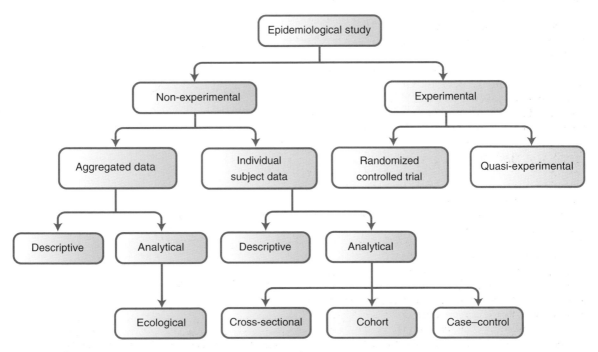

Figure 14.6 • The common types of epidemiological study.

seen that the main division occurs between experimental and non-experimental studies. Non-experimental studies are principally concerned with the causation and progression of disease, while experimental studies are generally concerned with the treatment or prevention of disease. There are also other types of study concerned with diagnosis and testing for disease and each study type is a major subject in its own right. The next section will summarize some of the most common study designs and discuss the pros and cons of each in relation to the research topic in question, and in particular discuss some of the issues relating to bias. There are many different types of bias but some of the most common types are discussed below and the impact that they can have on the different study types is given in Table 14.4. It is also worth stressing that, for all studies, a *consecutive series* should be obtained whenever possible, and if exclusions occur they should be documented with reasons for exclusion so that the generalizability of the results can be considered.

Types of bias

Collectively, most types of bias seen in epidemiological studies can be embraced by the term *measurement bias* as they relate to the incorrect classification of a patient or the inaccurate measurement of some parameter such as blood pressure. Two common types you should consider when designing and interpreting studies are selection bias and responder/observer bias.

Selection bias

When a sample has not been selected at random from the population, selection bias can occur. For example, if you choose to investigate factors associated with blood pressure and you select your subjects from hospital clinics rather than the general public, selection bias may occur in two separate ways. First, blood pressure may be higher for people in hospital clinics than when they are outside of the hospital and, second, patients tend to be in hospital because they are ill and

you do not know whether their condition relates to blood pressure or interacts with any of the factors that you are investigating. Similarly, if you are using hospital records retrospectively to investigate survival following a particular operation you should bear in mind that hospital records for patients who have died are often archived differently from those of patients who are alive, and thus the availability of patients' notes is not random, as it relates to the outcome of interest and considerable bias may creep into your study.

When investigating the impact of treatment on disease, randomized controlled trials are the best way of reducing the effects of selection bias, particularly in trials where subjects and clinicians are blinded to the allocated treatment. The main benefit of randomization is 'concealment', which means that when the decision is made to enter a subject into a trial, nobody knows what the treatment allocation will be. Thus, quasi-randomized trials, where the treatment is decided according to some freely available factor, like month of birth or alternate allocation to treatment or control, are not adequate at reducing levels of selection bias as a clinician may chose not to enter a subject into the trial because he knows what the allocation will be.

Responder or observer bias

Observer bias occurs when the investigator is aware of the disease status, treatment group or outcome of the subject and their ability to interview the subject, collect or analyse the data in an unbiased manner is compromised. Similarly, the subject (responder) may respond differently to questions relating to their levels of exposure if they have been classified as a subject with or without the disease under investigation. A classic example of the latter is also known as *recall bias* and it can be very problematic in cross-sectional and case–control studies. It can often be minimized by keeping the hypotheses of the study undisclosed to the participating subject, although this has become increasingly difficult in recent years as requirements for informed consent tend to mandate the provision of full

Table 14.4 Impact of study design on bias and confounding

Probability of:	Ecological	Cross-sectional	Cohort	Case–control	Randomized trial
Selection bias	N/A	Medium	Low	High	Low
Responder or observer bias	N/A	Medium	Low	High	Low (in blinded trials)
Recall bias	N/A	High	Low	High	Low
Confounding	High	Medium	Low (with adjustment)	Medium	Very low
Loss to follow-up	N/A	N/A	High	Low	Medium

information for the subject. Whenever possible, both the interviewer and subject should be blinded to the treatments and hypotheses of interest.

Types of study

Ecological studies

These tend to be hypothesis-generating studies rather than providing any strong causal evidence. They are concerned with observations made on large groups of the population, e.g. one might postulate that the increase in the incidence of skin cancer over the last 20 years is due to a depletion in the atmospheric ozone layer leading to a more intensive ultraviolet radiation exposure. However, this is entirely speculative and would require a far more detailed study to investigate such a hypothesis. Thus, the tendency for confounding is extremely high in ecological studies as countless other factors may be responsible for the increase in the incidence of skin cancer and, unless data are collected on these as part of a fuller investigation, reliable conclusions cannot be drawn. Nevertheless, these types of study can act as important pointers towards areas of public health that might be worthy of further investigation.

Cross-sectional studies

Cross-sectional studies are often chosen because they tend to be fairly easy to perform and are thus relatively inexpensive. Data are collected from a sample of subjects at a given point in time and comparisons are made between the variables to investigate the extent of the disease of interest or to assess which exposures may be linked with the disease. Thus, these studies represent a 'snap-shot' in time and therefore the prevalence is generally the main outcome measure as no information is obtained on the incidence of the disease over time. Surveys are a typical example of a cross-sectional study and the main problem is that they do not provide good information on the chronology of events as data for both exposure and disease are being measured simultaneously. Thus, it is difficult to assess any temporal relationship between the exposure and the disease as the former should always precede the latter for there to be any evidence of a causal link between the two. Selection bias can also be problematic as people who chose not to complete survey questionnaires can often be the people with the greatest extent of exposure or disease and they end up being excluded from any analysis. Responder bias can also occur as many surveys ask the subjects to give details on various aspects of their life and people are not always very good are estimating these types of data very well, e.g. most smokers tend to underestimate the amount that they smoke. In particular, if you ask people to give details on their retrospective history of smoking when they are aware that the study is investigating the effects of smoking, con-

siderable recall bias may creep into the results and these should be considered when designing the study and inspecting the results.

Cohort studies

Subjects are recruited into a cohort study and followed over time to assess the incidence of a particular disease or the progression of a disease if they have already been diagnosed. A full baseline assessment of data is collected on potential risk factors and other exposures and then follow-up commences to monitor the progress of the subjects. Thus, these studies are far more informative than cross-sectional studies as they provide information on incidence of events and also allow temporal assessments to be made on whether the exposures preceded the outcomes of interest. They are particularly useful for investigating the effects of relatively rare exposures as the classification of being exposed or not occurs at baseline, and they can also be used to investigate a wide range of disease outcomes potentially linked with the exposure of interest. Conversely, cohort studies are not very good at investigating rare diseases as very many people will need to be recruited in order to accrue enough cases for analysis. Thus, cohorts tend to be used when the disease is common and the effects of various exposures are not very well understood, and they are particularly beneficial as data can be collected on many potential confounding variables and these can be used for adjustment in the final analyses at the end of the follow-up period. The main disadvantage is that cohorts are costly in both time and resource and usually require large sample sizes to attain sufficient power for the analyses of interest. There can also be considerable loss to follow-up as it is often hard to keep people involved with the study for many years.

Case–control studies

As discussed in the previous section, cohort studies are not very useful at investigating rare diseases and case–control studies are often performed in this situation. The cohort can be seen as a prospective study following subjects forward through time whereas the case–control study is retrospective in that it recruits cases (subjects with the disease) and then finds a concurrent group of controls (subjects without the disease) and looks back through time to compare their exposures to see if any appear to relate to the development of the disease. Case–control studies tend to be relatively quick and cheap to perform and can be used to investigate a number of different exposures simultaneously. The difficulties often lie in the selection of the control group and this is generally always harder than it may at first appear, hence case–control studies can often experience considerable selection bias problems. They are also particularly prone to recall bias as subjects are being asked about past exposures with the knowledge that they are a case or a control and this may influence their ability to remember the extent of their exposure. This is also the case for the investigator and considerable observer bias can occur. They also differ from cohorts in that they are not good at investigating rare exposures as a large number of subjects need to be recruited to attain enough evidence of the exposure. They cannot be used to make estimates for the incidence of a disease and are not very helpful in trying to investigate the sequence of events leading to the diagnosis of a disease. Confounding can also be problematic in case–control studies and, in some cases, investigators choose to match cases and controls for variables that are thought to be potential confounders, e.g. age and sex. This should be done very cautiously as it is possible to 'over-match' your two groups such that variables of importance are 'matched' out of the analysis and valuable results can be missed. Most importantly, if cases and controls are matched in any way, then it is extremely important that the statistical analysis of the data accounts for this matching as the study has forced the cases and controls to be more similar than they would be in the population and, thus, the precision of the estimates will be incorrect. A simpler method is not to match the cases and controls, but to collect data on potential confounders and adjust for any differences at the analysis stage.

Randomized controlled trials (RCTs)

These are used to investigate the effects of therapies and interventions in a particular treatment situation. Subjects with a particular condition who meet certain trial entry criteria are randomly allocated to either receive the treatment or some form of control (generally no treatment or the current 'gold standard' treatment). The randomization is usually performed by a computer program and should be based separately from the participating centres, usually with a telephone service to request the randomization procedure. Where possible, it is preferable for the subjects and the investigators to be blinded to their randomized allocation and for the control group to be provided with some form of placebo. The groups are then exposed to their allocation and the outcome of interest is measured to see if one group experiences any benefit over the other. There are various types of randomized study, for example cross-over trials, factorial design or cluster randomized trials, and they do not have to be limited to just two comparative groups. The main benefits of randomized trials are the concealment of the treatment allocation and thus minimization of selection bias and also the low chance of confounding (providing the study is of adequate size and power). However, the disadvantages to RCTs are similar to those seen for cohort studies in that they tend to be time consuming and expensive and there can be appreciable loss to follow-up if the infrastructure is not in place to ensure good data collection.

The intention-to-treat principle

Once you have gone to all the effort of conducting a randomized controlled trial, it is very important that your primary analysis keeps the subjects in their randomized group regardless of the treatment that they actually received. By not doing this, you will negate most of the benefits of having randomized your subjects and run the risk of selection bias and confounding occurring. It is very rare that 100% of subjects will comply fully with their randomized allocation and investigators often feel justified in performing a 'per protocol' or 'treatment received' analysis, which excludes subjects who did not receive their intended treatment or who crossed over to the other randomized group. This is generally not advisable and, in the cases where it may be justified, it should be performed with caution and as a secondary analysis to the primary intention-to-treat analysis. The decision to do this additional analysis should also be made in an a priori fashion before any of the data are seen.

Diagnostic testing studies

It is often important to assess how well a particular diagnostic test is detecting people with a particular condition. Table 14.5 shows the standard terms used for describing the usefulness of a diagnostic or screening test, which can be derived from a cross-sectional study of the test against a known 'gold standard' (Figure 14.7). As you can see from Table 14.5, a *sensitive* test has a low false-negative rate (i.e. it successfully identifies most or all of the people with the condition), and a *specific* test has a low false-positive rate (i.e. it successfully excludes most or all of those without the condition). Screening tests, such as the Guthrie test for phenylketonuria in neonates, tend to have a high sensitivity in order not to miss any cases at the first hurdle; a definitive (and more expensive) *diagnostic* test with high *specificity* can be carried out on all those who test positive on the screening test.

The effectiveness of a particular diagnostic test to confirm or exclude a particular diagnosis is known as the *likelihood ratio* of that test; as Table 14.5 shows, it is calculated from the formula *sensitivity/(1 −specificity)*. The likelihood ratio can be thought of as an index of the usefulness of a diagnostic test. The higher the likelihood ratio, the more a positive test result should influence decisions. A likelihood ratio of 1.0 means that the patient is no more or less likely to have the condition than she was before you did the test.

Studies in the USA suggest that any woman of childbearing age attending the emergency department

Table 14.5   Features of a diagnostic test which can be calculated by comparing it with a 'gold standard' in a validation study

Feature of the test	Alternative name	Question that the feature addresses	Formula (see Fig. 14.7)
Sensitivity	True positive rate (**P**ositive in **D**isease)	How good is this test at picking up people who have the condition?	$\dfrac{a}{a+c}$
Specificity	True negative rate (**N**egative in **H**ealth)	How good is this test at correctly excluding people without the condition?	$\dfrac{b}{b+d}$
Positive predictive value	Post-test probability of a positive test	If a person tests positive, what is the probability that (s)he has the condition?	$\dfrac{a}{a+b}$
Negative predictive value	Post-test probability of a negative test	If a person tests negative, what is the probability that (s)he does not have the condition?	$\dfrac{d}{c+d}$
Accuracy	–	What proportion of all tests have given the correct result (i.e. true positives and true negatives as a proportion of all results)?	$\dfrac{a+d}{a+b+c+d}$
Likelihood ratio of a positive test	–	How many times more likely is a positive test to be found in a person with, as opposed to without, the condition?	Sensitivity/(1 − specificity)

Reproduced from Greenhalgh T 1997 How to read a paper: the basics of evidence-based medicine. BMJ, London.

		Result of 'gold standard' test	
		Disease positive a + c	Disease negative b + d
Result of screening test	Test positive a + b	True positive a	False positive b
	c + d Test negative	c False negative	d True negative

Figure 14.7 • 2 × 2 table notation for expressing the results of a validation study for a diagnostic or screening test. (Reproduced from Greenhalgh T 1997 How to read a paper: the basics of evidence based medicine. BMJ, London.)

has a 6% chance of being pregnant, and that those who think they are pregnant have a 40–60% chance of being right. Helpful questions to 'rule in' pregnancy include morning sickness (likelihood ratio: 2.7), breast engorgement (likelihood ratio: 2.7) and uterine size on vaginal examination (likelihood ratio: 3.7). A story of delayed menstrual period is fairly unhelpful (likelihood ratio: 1.56) compared with uterine artery pulsation (likelihood ratio: 11).

These numerical estimates confirm the value of vaginal examination by a competent gynaecologist in the diagnosis of early pregnancy. The world would be a simpler place if all clinical and laboratory tests were safe, readily reproducible by junior staff, and had high likelihood ratios. Unfortunately, clinical signs are often equivocal, definitive investigations impractical or contraindicated, and results of next-best tests incomplete or inconclusive. This is the 'grey area' seen frequently in primary care and the casualty department.

Equations for basic power calculations

For continuous outcomes

$$n \text{ per group} = 2 \times (Z_{alpha/2} + Z_{beta})^2 \times \sigma^2/\delta^2$$

where σ = SD (standard deviation) and δ = d (worthwhile difference).

This intimidating formula consists of four parts. For a continuous variable, δ is the worthwhile difference in mean value (of, e.g., blood pressure). σ is the estimate of variability; specifically it is the standard deviation of the blood pressure.

The other two elements, $Z_{alpha/2}$ and Z_{beta} refer to the type I and type II error rates. The letter Z that precedes alpha and beta in the formula refers to numbers derived from the normal distribution. It is usual practice to require a power of 80% or 90%, and a significance level of 5%. Thus, alpha = 5% and this gives $Z_{alpha/2}$ = 1.96. If beta = 10% (for a power of 90%), then Z_{beta} = 1.28. These values may be taken as constants in the formula.

Suppose the object of appraisal was a study involving a treatment for hypertension which might reasonably be expected to make a difference of 5 mmHg of diastolic blood pressure (DBP) compared with a placebo. This could be taken as the worthwhile difference to be detected (δ). In the population of interest, the standard deviation of DBP might be 10 mmHg – this will be the σ. The aim is to show this difference as statistically significant at the 5% level with 90% power. Thus:

$$n \text{ per group} = 2 \times (1.96 + 1.28)^2 \times 10^2/5^2 = 84.$$

If it was noted that the authors of the study had included only 20 patients per group, we would know that the study was underpowered.

For categorical outcomes

The above formula needs to be modified a little if the outcome of interest is an event. The percentage of subjects who would experience the event in the control group (π_1) must first be estimated, and also the percentage for the group receiving the new treatment (π_2). The δ would now represent the difference in these two percentages, = $\pi_1 - \pi_2$.

However, the notion of a standard deviation is less intuitive for a variable representing an event. In fact, instead of σ^2, it is $[\pi_1 \times (1 - \pi_1)] + [\pi_2 \times (1 - \pi_2)]$.

Thus, the whole formula for a power calculation when the outcome is an event becomes:

$$n \text{ per group} = (Z_{alpha/2} + Z_{beta})^2 \times$$

$$[\pi_1 \times (1 - \pi_1) + \pi_2 \times (1 - \pi_2)]/\delta^2$$

By using the blood pressure example again, if you expected 50% of the treated group to have their DBP reduced by 5 mmHg but only 30% of the control group to experience this drop, the equation indicates that 121 subjects would be required per group (242 in total).

$$n \text{ per group} = (1.96 + 1.28)^2 \times$$
$$[0.5(1-0.5) + 0.3(1-0.3)]/(0.5-0.3)^2 = 121$$

Fortunately, even statisticians rarely have to commit such formulae to memory, but if you are planning a research study yourself you should make a point of consulting this text or a statistician before deciding how many subjects to recruit! It is also recommended to apply inflation factors to your target recruitment to allow for patients 'crossing over' between groups and for loss to follow-up.

Acknowledgement

The sections on diagnostic testing and power calculations were provided previously by Trisha Greenhalgh.

Recommended statistics texts

Altman DG 1990 Practical statistics for medical research. Chapman & Hall, London

Bland M 2000 An introduction to medical statistics, 3rd edn. Oxford University Press, Oxford

Greenhalgh T 2006 How to read a paper: the basics of evidence-based medicine, 3rd edn. Wiley–Blackwell, Chichester

Kirkwood B, Sterne J 2003 Essential medical statistics, 2nd edn. Wiley–Blackwell, Chichester

Chapter Fifteen

15

Clinical research methodology

Andrew Shennan & Annette Briley

Introduction

Research is an organized, systematic and rigorous process of enquiry to develop concepts and theories and describe phenomena. It aims to add to a scientific body of knowledge. A fundamental understanding of how to approach clinical research is now a basic requirement for any specialist. In recent years regulation around research governance has resulted in many mandatory requirements to set up, monitor and execute research in a clinical arena. This chapter will outline the approach required to manage any clinical research, but specific details pertinent to the UK and Europe will be included.

Types of clinical investigation

Evidence that informs knowledge ranges from personal experience of an individual case through to meta-analysis of a number of randomized controlled trials. The quality of research is improved by limiting confounding factors and ensuring the study is large enough to answer the research question. However, best evidence regarding management of a rare disease may be a simple case report. The study design will depend on previous evidence, the rarity of the clinical situation being investigated, and the feasibility and resources available to investigate the question.

Studies that have a control population will help eliminate chance findings unrelated to the research question.

Types of study

A case–control study is a retrospective study (collection of data from past events) investigating the relationship between a risk factor and one or more outcomes. People with a predefined risk factor or outcome are selected (cases) and compared with people who do not have these factors (controls). A case–control study primarily aims to investigate cause and effect. Generally speaking, prospective studies will reduce bias, as the research question is predefined, and then evaluated.

A cohort study is a prospective, observational study looking at a specific effect of a treatment or risk factor, over a period of time.

Systematic research is the process whereby a project is based on an agreed set of rules and processes (protocol) and these are rigorously adhered to. It is against this protocol that the research is evaluated. This will reduce bias, as predefined rules are adhered to, and selecting significant findings of interest from numerous variables that could occur by chance is avoided.

Qualitative research is research undertaken in the field (natural settings) and usually analysed by non-statistical methods.

Quantitative research involves measurements and analysis of observations using statistical methods.

Surveys are based on a representative sample of a population being questioned at one time point.

Randomized controlled trials (RCTs) are viewed as the 'gold standard' for evaluating health services effectiveness and interventions in relation to specific conditions. Participants are randomly allocated to two or

Table 15.1 The differences between audit and research

Research	Audit
Discovers and defines the 'right' thing to do	Determines whether the right thing is being done
Each project 'stands alone'	A cyclical series of reviews
Collects complex and unique data	Collects routine data
Often possible to generalize findings (aims for this to be possible)	Reports individual situation, therefore never possible to generalize findings

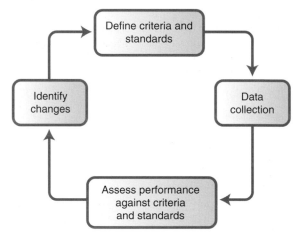

Figure 15.1 • The audit cycle.

more groups, and direct comparisons can be made between the groups. The only difference between the groups should be the investigation intervention. Therefore, any differences found between the groups should be attributable only to the intervention, and a causal relationship is far more likely (rather than association).

What is audit?

Audit is not research. The differences are outlined in Table 15.1. Clinical audit is a quality improvement process that seeks to improve patient care and outcome. This is achieved through systematic review of care against explicit criteria and the implementation of change. Aspects of the structure, processes and outcomes of care are selected and systematically evaluated against explicit criteria (Fig. 15.1). Where indicated, changes are implemented at an individual, team or service level and further monitoring is used to confirm improvement in healthcare delivery (*definition endorsed by the National Institute for Clinical Excellence*, NICE 2002). In short, audit is the process used by health professionals to assess, evaluate and improve care of patients in a systematic way in order to enhance their health and quality of life (www.pdptoolkit.co.uk).

Audit does not require ethical committee review or approval, nor is it under the same regulatory requirements as research. Most hospital trusts will have a robust infrastructure that deals with clinical audit, including registration of projects, which has become an integral part of clinical practice.

The clinical research process

Once a research question is established, a funding source must be identified, an appropriate literature review performed, study design chosen, and the protocol written. There are also a number of mandatory requirements to be undertaken before the project can begin. These will depend partly on the study design and the intervention being investigated. Generally, any research involving human subjects (including analysis of data or samples derived from a human source) requires ethical and, in the UK, research and development (R&D) approval.

Integrated Research Application System (IRAS)

The EU Directive says 'Member States shall take the measures necessary for the establishment and operation of Ethics Committees'. The responsibilities of the ethics committee are to safeguard the rights and well-being of trial subjects, and to ensure proposals meet the requisite standards.

It is stipulated that there must be at least seven members of an ethics committee, including scientific/expert and lay representatives. Research ethics committees (REC) can be either Main or Local (MREC/LREC), depending on their size and the experience of their members. All clinical trials of a medicinal product and multicentre studies need to be ethically reviewed and approved by a Main REC, following which, Local REC approval is granted for Site Specific Information (SSI). Every study should have a chief investigator (CI) and each site must have a local principal investigator (PI), who has overall local responsibility for the trial or study. The ethics committee assesses the suitability of the local PI and support staff in addition to the appropriateness of the local research environment.

An electronic application form (www.myresearch project.org.uk) must be used for applications in the UK. This consists of three parts: part A gives general details of the research project, part B involves information on specialized topics, including the use of existing or newly obtained biological specimens, and part C is SSI (Local Assessor). A separate (duplicate) applica-

tion form can be accessed on the IRAS website for Research & Development (R&D) approval (see below). Once completed, with the requisite signatures, both forms can be processed through the R&D department for the participating Trust or PCT.

Once logged in, the form can be edited any number of times by the individual with the pass code and can be electronically transferred to collaborators for comments and editing.

When complete, the ethics administration should be contacted regarding a unique ethics number, which is assigned to the application (Central Allocation telephone number: 0845 270 4400). The form can then be locked and submitted online and one paper copy, with requisite signatures accompanied by the study protocol, including patient information and informed consent forms, should be delivered to the ethics committee administrator. The administrator will check all the paperwork is present and then send confirmation of receipt of the application. For single-centre studies, parts A and B of the form need to be completed. If the study is undertaken in more than one institution/hospital, SSI will need to be sought in all additional centres. The letter of receipt gives details as to how to ensure this process happens concurrently with MREC consideration.

RECs meet monthly, and the date when the application will be discussed will be notified to the applicant. Each committee will only review a certain number of proposals at each meeting, and an applicant can choose an appropriate committee, according to their commitments and time schedule. A local committee will not therefore always review research from its own institution. A multicentre study (three or more centres) will require a Main REC. Attendance by applicants is not mandatory, but applicants can be invited to attend to clarify any ambiguous or difficult ethical issues. The REC can ask for alteration or clarification of the application on one occasion – at this point the clock stops, and any delay is entirely the responsibility of the applicant. Apart from this delay, a decision will be given within 60 days.

Research and development approval

All projects involving NHS patients, staff or services require approval from the local research and development committee. The form is available online and interconnects with the ethics forms. This needs to be completed at every participating centre, including single-centre sites and academic projects. Most research and development committees expect an early application. Advice is available from RD Direct (www.rddirect.org.uk) or your local Research and Development or Research and Development Support Unit (RDSU).

International Conference on Harmonisation guideline on Good Clinical Practice (ICH GCP)

This document sets out an internationally agreed quality standard for designing, conducting, recording and reporting trials involving human participants. This ensures unified standards of research in the EU, but also covers Japan and the USA. Good clinical practice guidelines from Australia, Canada, the Nordic countries and the World Health Organization (WHO) were also considered in the preparation of these guidelines. The principles of the ICH GCP originate from the Declaration of Helsinki (1964) last updated in 2000. Accordance gives assurance to the public that the rights and wellbeing of the subjects is protected, and that trial data are credible. Information can be found at *www.instituteofclinicalresearch.org*

The European Union (EU) Clinical Trials Directive

The European Union (EU) Clinical Trials Directive (2001/20/EC) is the legislative framework that implements ICH GCP in the EU and also in Iceland, Norway and Liechtenstein, which form the European Economic Area (EEA). The aims of this Directive are three-fold:

1. To protect the rights, safety and wellbeing of trial participants
2. To establish transparent procedures that will harmonize trial conduct in the EU and ensure the credibility of results
3. To simplify and harmonize administrative provisions governing clinical trials.

The EU Directive on Clinical Trials (2001/20/EC) was published in 2001; in the UK, the Directive is implemented by Statutory Instrument 2004 No. 1031 'The Medicines for Human Use (Clinical Trials) Regulations 2004' (MHRA 2004). Full implementation of the regulations became law from 1 May 2004.

Investigational medicinal products

The regulations cover all clinical research on 'investigational medicinal products (IMPs) for human use' (excluding non-interventional trials, see below). The Medical Research Council (MRC 2000) further defines this as: 'Trials designed to ascertain or confirm the safety and/or efficacy of medicinal products involving a clinical intervention conducted to a research protocol'. An investigational medicinal product (IMP) is defined as 'a pharmaceutical form of an active substance or placebo being tested or used as a reference in a clinical trial'. This includes products already with a marketing authorization but which are used or assembled differently from the authorized form, or to gain further information regarding an authorized form. The regulations are required when the trial is designed to support a medical claim, and when the IMP will influence (treat or prevent) a disease process.

Medical devices

A medical device is not recognized as an IMP, i.e. this is when the principal intended action of an intervention in a trial is fulfilled by physical means (device), not pharmacological, immunological or metabolic means (medicinal product). However, medicinal devices may be assisted in their function by a medicinal product (e.g. intrauterine contraceptive [device] with progestogen [medicinal product]), and under these circumsogen will require conformity to these regulations.

Although there is no legislative requirement to follow the exact requirements of ICH GCP when an IMP is not investigated (e.g. in a trial of a surgical procedure), it remains good practice to follow the same basic principles, although reporting requirements to the MHRA may not be mandatory (see below).

A practical implementation of the ICH GCP guidelines can be found in Table 15.2.

Responsibilities of an investigator

The chief investigator (CI) must adhere to the 13 principles of GCP (Table 15.2). In addition, according to ICH CGP the investigator must, by education, training and experience be qualified to fulfil this role, as evidenced through an up-to-date CV or other documentation. They must facilitate monitoring and auditing of the study by the sponsor and inspection by the regulatory authorities. They must maintain a list of the individuals to whom significant trial-related duties have been delegated, demonstrating appropriate qualifications for their relevant tasks.

The investigator must show that recruitment in the agreed time-frame is realistic. They are responsible for ensuring that there is sufficient time to undertake the project, and there is adequate staffing to execute the study. This includes guaranteeing that all staff employed will be adequately trained to undertake the responsibilities expected of them during the course of the study. They also should examine the reason a subject withdraws from a trial prematurely and communicate all significant matters with the ethics committee. They must ensure compliance with the trial protocol. They should be knowledgeable about all aspects of the investigational project, and have responsibility for it. This includes responsibility for randomization procedures and unblinding policies where necessary, as well as for obtaining informed consent from all trial participants.

Table 15.2 Practical implementation of the 13 principles of ICH

1	Clinical trials should be conducted in accordance with the ethical principles that have their origin in the Declaration of Helsinki, and are consistent with GCP and the applicable regulatory requirements.
2	Before a trial is initiated, foreseeable risks and inconveniences should be weighed against the anticipated benefit for the individual trial participant and society. A trial should be initiated and continued only if the anticipated benefits justify the risks.
3	The rights, safety and wellbeing of the trial participant are of utmost importance and should prevail over the interests of science and society.
4	The available non-clinical and clinical information on an investigational product should be adequate to support the proposed clinical trial.
5	Clinical trials should be scientifically sound and described in a clear detailed protocol.
6	A trial should be conducted in compliance with the protocol that has received prior independent ethics committee approval.
7	The medical care given to, and the medical decisions made, on behalf of the participants should always be the responsibility of a qualified physician.
8	Each individual involved in conducting the trial should be qualified by education, training and experience to perform appropriate tasks.
9	Freely given informed consent should be obtained from each subject prior to participation in any clinical trial.
10	All clinical trial information should be recorded, handled and stored to facilitate accurate reporting, interpretation and verification. 'If it's not documented, it did not happen.'
11	The confidentiality of records that could identify subjects should be protected, respecting the privacy and confidentiality rules in accordance with regulatory requirements (Data Protection Act 1998).
12	Investigational products should be manufactured, handled and stored in accordance with Good Manufacturing Practice (GMP), and used as per an approved protocol.
13	Systems with procedures that assure the quality of every aspect of the trial should be implemented.

All trial-related medical decisions are the responsibility of a qualified medical practitioner. Attending clinicians should be aware of a participant's involvement in a trial.

The investigator also has responsibilities regarding records and reports. They have overall responsibility for the accuracy, completeness and timeliness of the data. This includes consistency between data recorded in the case report form (CRF) (study records) and the source documents (medical records). They must be able to explain any discrepancies. Alteration to the CRF should be initialled and should not obscure the original entry. All computer records should be made using programs employing audit trails. Safe storage of the trial records and documentation (including electronically stored data) is necessary during, and after closure of, the trial for the requisite time period (dependent on trial type). This can be up to 25 years for maternity records. The CI is responsible for ongoing mandatory reports during the course and at the end of the trial. This includes progress reports, annually to the MHRA, funding bodies, etc.; safety reporting of SUAES and SUSARs (see below); premature suspension of the trial, e.g. for safety reasons; and final reports to the MHRA, M/LREC, sponsor and funding bodies.

When are studies not covered by the EU directive?

When a medicinal product is used in the manner within the terms of its marketing authorization, or patient allocation is not dictated by protocol but falls within the remit of current practice, the regulations governed by the EU Directive are not required. This also includes when the decision to prescribe the IMP is independent from the decision to include the patient in the trial. This includes mechanistic trials which are not part of clinical research into the efficacy and/or safety of an IMP. Psychotherapy and surgery trials with no IMP comparator, and diet trials with no IMP, are also not covered by these laws. This regulation is also not relevant when a patient undergoes diagnostic or monitoring procedures that are part of normal clinical practice, or when data are analysed using epidemiological methods.

The Medicines and Healthcare products Regulatory Agency

The Medicines and Healthcare products Regulatory Agency (MHRA) is the government agency responsible for ensuring the safety of medicines and medical devices in the UK. It considers no product to be 'risk-free' but applies robust and fact-based judgements to ensure that benefits to patients and the general public justify the risks. The MHRA monitors medicines and devices and ensures, when necessary, that prompt action is taken to protect the public. Within the remit of the MHRA greater access to products and the timely innovation of treatments benefits patients and the public.

The MHRA has produced an algorithm to enable researchers to clarify whether their research question falls within the scope of the EU Clinical Trials Directive. The MHRA will also advise on an individual basis (www.mhra.gov.uk; Tel: 020 7084 2000).

All trials falling into the remit of the EU Directive legally require *Clinical Trials Authorisation* (CTA) from the MHRA (Fig. 15.2). If the trial is international, similar approval will be required from any competent authority in each member state. The MHRA must make a decision within 60 days of application. An Investigator Brochure must be kept for all clinical trials, which is a compilation of all the relevant clinical and non-clinical data available regarding the investigational product in human subjects.

Registration of trials

EudraCT

All trials undertaken within the EU Directive's scope must be registered with EudraCT. It is also wise to register other trials and studies, as editors of journals are increasingly likely to view this as a prerequisite to future publication (see below). This is a European database that issues each trial with a unique identification number, which must be obtained prior to seeking ethical and other regulatory approval before the study can start. There is no fee for this. Registration is the responsibility of the sponsor or CI. Information and registration can be found at www.eurdract.emea.eu.int.

International Standard Randomised Controlled Trial Number (ISRCTN)

In June 2005, the International Committee of Medical Journal Editors (De Angelis et al 2005) issued a state-ment that, after 1 July 2005, all trials must be registered prior to recruiting the first subject as a prerequisite to publication, thus ensuring a comprehensive, publicly available database of clinical trials. Randomized control-led trials and other studies designed to assess the effi-cacy of healthcare interventions should all be registered. The ISRCTN Register is owned by the ISRCTN, a 'not for profit' organization, and the scheme is administered on their behalf by Current Controlled Trials Ltd.

Application for an ISRCTN is the responsibility of the sponsor or CI and is undertaken online at: http://isrctn.org

The form is divided into five sections:

1. Applicant details – the contact details of the person making the application. This should be the person who will deal with any queries regarding the application.
2. Sponsor details – the organization taking primary responsibility for ensuring the study design meets the standards of GCP and that measures are in place to ensure appropriate conduct and reporting.
3. Chief investigator (lead principal investigator) – contact details for the individual with legal and scientific responsibility for the trial (also required for multicentre trials) (Fig. 15.3).
4. Details of the trial – from the protocol.
5. Additional information – general information about where you found out about the ISCTN scheme.

Receipt of the online application will be acknowledged by e-mail, and after the administrators have checked the eligibility of the application, an administrative charge will be made. The 2006 rate is currently GB£156 per entry. This may be reduced or waived for trials in developing countries. There is also a reduced rate for organizations registering more than 100 trials. Once payment is received, the ISRCTN Editorial Office informs the applicant and the CI of the ISCTN assigned to the trial, and the record will appear in the register. This number should then be used on trial documentation.

*meta*Register of Controlled Trials (*m*RCT)

The *m*RCT was initiated in the UK in July 1998 as a result of an initiative involving the UK Medical Research Council, the National Health Service Executive, medical charities, pharmaceutical companies, the UK Cochrane Centre, and journal representatives (i.e. *BMJ* and *Lancet*). This is an international searchable data-base of current ongoing randomized controlled trials in all areas of healthcare. All trial entries are currently in English, although there is an introduction in French,

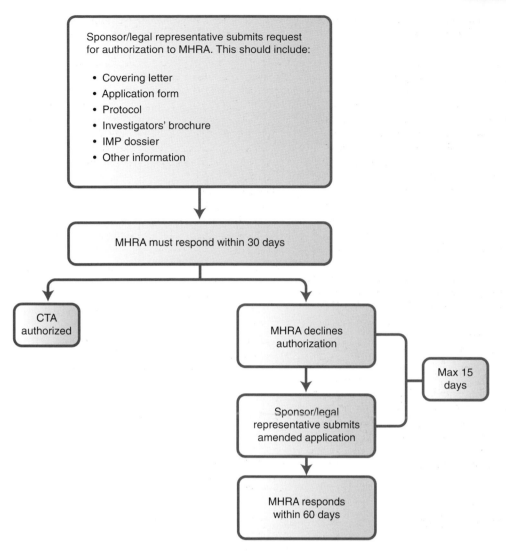

Figure 15.2 • Application process to the Medicines and Healthcare Products Regulatory Agency (MHRA) for Clinical Trials Authorisation (CTA).

German, Spanish and Italian, with other languages to be added at a later date.

The *m*RCT has been formed by combining registers held by trial sponsors from the public, charitable and commercial sectors. It is a free service which aims to:

- Facilitate those wanting to be confident they are aware of all trial evidence available relevant to a particular question (clinicians and scientists)
- Assist research funding bodies who want to make funding decisions in the light of information about ongoing relevant research, thus avoiding duplication and facilitating collaboration
- Inform potential participants regarding ongoing trials they may wish to consider.

Although not compulsory, it would be prudent to register any clinical investigation involving an intervention into all three registers.

Data

While the details of the Data Protection Act (1998) are complex (details can be found at www.dataprotection.gov.uk), within the context of clinical trials all data should be regarded as confidential. Any institution undergoing clinical research must be registered under the Data Protection Act, have an identified custodian of the data, and pay an appropriate annual fee. Special attention should be paid to issues of informed explicit

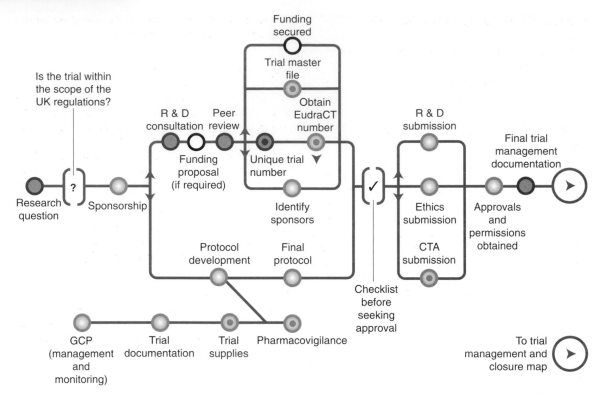

Figure 15.3 • What a researcher needs to set up a multicentre clinical trial (from the Clinical Trials Tool Kit 2006).

consent for participation, data collection and analysis, and anonymization of data. An understanding of the following terms when dealing with data issues is required:

- *Personal information*: refers to all information about individuals (alive or dead), including electronic and written records, opinions, images, recordings and samples
- *Personal data*: comprises information about living people who can be identified from the data, or combinations of the data, which the person in charge of the data has, or may have in the future
- *Anonymized data*: no individual can be identified from these data, although it was generated from personal data
- *Linked anonymized data*: these data are anonymous to the researchers (who hold the information) but contain codes or other information that would enable others to identify people from them. For example, study ID on sample (for researcher) links to hospital number and date of birth (for clinicians)
- *Unlinked anonymized data*: there is no information that could identify an individual to anyone. For example, a multiple choice survey containing no demographic data

- *Coded data*: all information that could identify a participant is concealed in a code, and can be decoded by the researchers
- *Confidential information*: all information obtained on the understanding that it will not be disclosed to others or gathered in circumstances when it is expected that such information will not be disclosed. The law assumes that whenever personal information is imparted to healthcare professionals it is confidential for as long as anyone is identifiable.

Data security

Ensuring data are maintained securely is a legal obligation under the Data Protection Act. Documented procedures to ensure data security must form part of the Standard Operating Procedures (SOP) of each research project. These procedures require regular review; this is especially relevant with IT systems and data transfers.

Procedures should be in place for:

- Overall management and control of data
- Expedient response and reactions to breaches of security
- Back-up policies and recovery procedures

- Minimizing the number of duplicate files in existence
- Limiting access rights, including reacting promptly to staff changes
- Immediate access to chief investigator regarding issues of data security.

Consent, information and sponsors

Informed consent is a process by which a trial subject voluntarily confirms his or her willingness to participate after having been informed of all aspects of the trial that are relevant to the subject's decision to take part. It is the investigator's responsibility to ensure the subject (or his or her legal representative) is informed regarding all pertinent aspects of the trial, in language he or she understands. This includes any new information that comes to light within during the duration of the study.

Patient information sheet

All clinical studies should have a patient information leaflet. This describes the research in lay-person's terms. Many institutions have explicit information to be included in all their patient information leaflets. The DoH publication, Protection & Use of Patient Information (DoH 1996), provides advice and a template for research projects.

All information leaflets should explain:

- The reasons for the research
- Collaborations between universities (and other organizations) and the NHS, and transfer of information between these institutions
- The funding source for the research
- That the research is independently reviewed
- That research staff have the same duty of confidence as the health professionals caring for them
- That there is no obligation to take part in the research and the volunteer is free to withdraw at any time without giving a reason, and that current or future healthcare will not be affected by this decision
- Who to contact for further information about the project
- Who to contact if they have any cause for complaint.

When writing a patient information sheet, it is advisable to keep language simple; the Literacy Trust recommends equivalence to a reading age of 11 years. Avoid jargon and medical terminology, and keep sentences short and concise. By piloting the leaflet on family and friends, many of the pitfalls can be addressed before submission to an ethics committee.

Informed consent form

An Informed Consent Form (ICF) is a form which records that informed consent was given (by the subject) and must include who explained the study and obtained the consent and when. Most institutions insist all trial participants sign a generic consent form, where only the name of the study and very specific lines are altered. General consent to participation and for the researchers to examine medical notes are mandatory. The consent form must be submitted to ethics committee for approval before use, and at each revision. Informed consent guidelines are available on the IRAS website (www.myresearchproject.org.uk).

Sponsorship

Sponsorship is now a legal requirement in all trials that use NHS resources and are under the EU Directive. The responsibilities of the sponsor are listed in Table 15.3.

Trial Steering Committees (TSC) and Data Monitoring and Ethics Committees (DMEC)

All trials should have a committee to oversee the organization and running of the study. The committee includes investigators and other individuals with expertise in the area, usually including appropriate lay representation. A separate data monitoring (and ethics committee) will report to the steering group, but final decisions remain with the TSC. The DMEC will view safety data, including unblinding when necessary at predefined points, although stopping rules should also predefined and be appropriately robust.

Review of the literature

In order to develop the aims and objectives of any research question, the first step is to review the existing literature around the topic. Electronic databases have facilitated comprehensive literature reviews, but hand searching remains valuable, as some articles will not be coded as expected. Grey literature is unpublished non-significant data that tend to remain in internal reports. Therefore it is accessed through 'networking' with experts interested in the area, but is an essential part of developing cutting-edge research.

Table 15.3 The sponsor's responsibilities

Quality assurance and quality control
Contract Research Organization (CRO)
Medical expertise
Trial design
Trial management, data handling and record keeping
Financing
Notification/submission to regulatory authorities
Confirmation of review by institutional review board (IRB)/ independent ethics committee (IEC)
Information on investigational product(s)
Manufacturing packaging, labelling and coding of investigational products
Supplying and handling investigational product(s)
Record access
Safety information
Adverse drug reaction reporting
Monitoring
Audit
Non-compliance
Premature termination or suspension of a trial
Clinical trial study reports
Multicentre trials

Amendments and reports

During the course of the trial it may be necessary to make amendments. This may be the result of protocol change, due to new information becoming available (from other trials or scientific discovery) or because an extension to the trial is required.

Substantial amendments

A notice of substantial amendment needs to be made when a significant alteration to the initial protocol (or any other supporting documentation) is made. This includes aspects that affect the safety or physical or mental integrity of the subjects, impacts on the scientific value of the trial, influences the conduct or management of the trial or affects the quality or safety of any IMP used in the trial. Substantial amendment should be submitted to the REC that gave the favourable opinion. In clinical trials of investigational medicinal products (CTIMPS) use the 'notification of amendment' form from the EudraCT website (see Useful sources).

For all other research, use the 'Notice of substantial amendment' form on the IRAS website: www.myresearchproject.org.uk. This form will need to be completed and signed by the CI. It is then necessary to forward this with altered documentation, with changes tracked, to the ethics committee that originally approved the study. Substantial amendments normally require favourable ethical approval before implementation, the only exceptions being:

* Where urgent safety measures are required
* Where substantial amendments require authorization from the competent authority (MHRA), but are submitted to the main REC for information only.

The MHRA should also be notified of substantial amendments.

Non-substantial amendments

Non-substantial amendments do not have to be notified to the MHRA, but should be recorded centrally, with all the relevant information available for inspection purposes.

In a clinical trial of an investigational medicinal product, it is the legal responsibility of the sponsor to decide whether an amendment is substantial. EU Commission advice regarding this can be found at: www.eudract.emea.eu.int.

Reporting adverse reactions

When reporting any event, adherence to the Data Protection Act is mandatory in all written reports, i.e. retaining the participant's anonymity by using unique code numbers. Within the context of any clinical trial there will be some adverse reactions or events. Many of these will be outlined in the study protocol or investigator brochure, i.e. are known. These are expected adverse events because they are predefined. All other adverse events are usually unexpected, i.e. are not consistent with the information about the medicinal product being investigated or the condition.

When adverse expected events or reactions occur, i.e. those that are outlined in the protocol, they need to be listed and reported in the annual safety report to the MHRA, ethics committee and the sponsor. The exception to this is any adverse event that is identified in the protocol as essential in the safety evaluation of the trial, and these will need to be reported to the sponsor, within the time-frame specified in the protocol.

Serious adverse events and serious unexpected adverse events

Adverse reactions are 'serious' if they result in death; are life-threatening; require hospitalization or prolong existing admission; result in persistent or significant incapacity or disability; or result in a congenital anomaly or birth defect. Both serious adverse events (SAEs) and serious unexpected adverse events (SUAEs) must be reported. The timing will depend on whether they are mentioned in the protocol. If not in the protocol, it must be within 7 days (if they are listed in the protocol they must be included in the Annual Report).

Related and unexpected SAEs must be reported to the REC within 15 days of the CI being aware of it, using the IRAS 'Report of a serious adverse event' form, downloaded from the IRAS website (www.myresearchproject.org.uk). These forms need to be completed in typescript and signed by the CI. In double-blinded trials, SAE reports should be unblinded. The REC administrator acknowledges receipt of these reports within 30 days.

Suspected unexpected serious adverse events/reactions (SUSARs) are defined as an 'adverse reaction' and is 'any untoward and unintended response in a subject to an investigational medicinal product which is related to any dose administered to that subject'. The Medicines for Human Use (Clinical Trials) Regulations 2004 (MHRA 2004).

For those SUSARs that are life-threatening or result in death, the sponsor needs to be informed within 7 days. There will be an agreement between the CI and the sponsor as to who will inform the MHRA. Using forms supplied by the local R&D office, the MHRA must be notified within 7 days following the sponsor being informed, and will require a follow-up report within 8 days. For those SUSARs which are not fatal or life-threatening, the sponsor should be informed as soon as possible, and the MHRA needs to be informed within 15 days of the sponsor knowing.

All adverse events reports and follow-up forms should be sent to the R&D office, and the ethics committee should also be informed. Any reaction should be recorded in the participant's CRF and documented in their medical records.

The end of the trial

The definition of the end of the trial is usually the date the last patient is seen, or reaches the defined endpoint (i.e. date of delivery), this is usually specified in the protocol. The MHRA must be notified within 90 days of the end date, using the 'Declaration of the End of a Clinical Trial' on the EudraCT website: www.eudract.emea.eu.int. If the trial ends early, the MHRA must be notified within 15 days, with a clear explanation of the early termination. In addition to the end of trial declaration to the MHRA, a final report must be sent to the ethics committee (use the 'Declaration of the End of a Clinical Trial' form as used for the MHRA), the R&D Department and the funding body.

Promoting and maintaining a trial

Regular meetings with investigators and management team are an essential part of a successful trial. Regular, realistic targets should be set. Review recruitment, staff issues and outcome data collection regularly, and deal with problems/potential problems as they arise. Keep others informed of progress of the trial, and thank those who help. It is wise to have obvious trial identification, including logos, newsletters and labels to identify participants' notes. Outcome data are as important as recruitment rates – ensure strategies are in place to optimize opportunities to get outcome data.

Common statistical terms used in clinical trials

Power

The power of a study is the probability that it will detect a statistically significant difference. Therefore, if the anticipated effect is large, a small study is required, but if the effect is smaller a larger sample size is required.

Incidence

The number of new cases (of a condition) in a given time-frame.

Intention to treat

This is an analysis that includes all the participants randomized to a group, even if they are subsequently withdrawn and do not receive the allocated intervention.

Likelihood ratio (LR)

This is the likelihood that a test result would be expected in patients with a condition, divided by the likelihood of the same result occurring in patients without that condition.

Sensitivity

This is the number of patients with a condition testing positive for that condition. It describes the effectiveness of a test at picking up a condition.

Specificity

This describes the proportion of people without a condition who test negative – the rate of elimination of a disease by a test.

Positive predictive value

When a person tests positive for a condition the PPV is the chance that they actually have that condition.

Negative predictive value

In the presence of a negative test, this is the chance that the person does not have the condition.

Numbers needed to treat (NNT)

The number of patients who need to be treated, for one to gain benefit.

Numbers needed to harm (NNH)

The number of patients who need to be treated, for one to be harmed by the treatment.

Relative risk reduction (RRR)

The proportion by which the intervention reduced the event rate.

Odds ratio (OR)

Odds are calculated by dividing the number of times an event occurs by the number of times it does not. Odds ratios are calculated by dividing the odds of being exposed to a risk factor with the odds in a control group. Consequently an OR of 1 shows no difference in risk between groups. OR >1 demonstrates benefit, <1 demonstrates harm (Harris & Taylor 2004).

Risk

Risk is the probability of an event happening, and is calculated by dividing the number of events by the number of people at risk.

Risk ratio (can be referred to as relative risk)

Risk ratio is calculated by dividing risk in a treated (or exposed) group by the risk in a control (or unexposed) group (Harris & Taylor 2004).

P values

The probability of any observed difference happening by chance is expressed as a p value. A p value of 0.5 means that the probability of any difference happening by chance is 0.5 in 1, therefore 50:50. The lower the p value, the less likely a difference has occurred by chance; $p = 0.01$ means a difference will only happen by chance 1 in 100 times and therefore is considered significant. Similarly, $p = 0.001$ means a difference will only happen due to chance 1 in 1000 times, and is therefore considered very highly significant.

Type I and type II errors

- Type I errors occur when a correct hypothesis is rejected.
- Type II errors occur when an incorrect hypothesis is accepted.

References

Audit: www.pdptoolkit.co.uk

De Angelis C, Drazon JM, Frizelle FA et al 2005 Is this clinical trial fully registered? – A statement from the international committee of medical journal editors. New England Journal of Medicine 352:2436–2438

Department of Health 1996 Protection & use of patient information. HMSO, London

Department of Health/MRC 2006 Clinical Trials Tool Kit – Planning a new trial. Online. Available: www.ct-toolkit.ac.uk 30 March 2006

Harris M, Taylor G 2004 Medical statistics made easy. Taylor & Francis, London

Medical Research Council 2000 Medical Research Council position statement on research regulation & ethics.

Updated September 2005. Online. Available: www.mrc.ac.uk 30 March 2006

MHRA 2004 Description of the Medicines for Human Use (Clinical Trials) Regulations. HMSO, London

NICE 2002 Principles for best practice in clinical audit (supported by NHS, NICE, CHI, RCN, University of Leicester, Radcliffe Medical Press

Useful sources of information

EudraCT: https://eudract.emea.europa.eu/index.html

Institute of Clinical Research: E-mail: info@instituteofclinicalresearch.org Tel: 01628 899 755

Integrated Research Application System (IRAS): www.myresearchproject.org.uk

Medical Research Council (MRC): www.mrc.ac.uk Tel: +44 (0)20 7636 5422, Fax: +44 (0)20 7436 6179

MHRA: E-mail: info@mhra.gsi.gov.uk Tel: 0207 084 2000

Personal Development Programme, information about audit, reflective practice, evidence-based medicine, clinical governance, significant event analysis and much more, supported by the Eastern Deanery: www.pdptoolkit.co.uk

RD Direct: www.rddirect.org.uk E-mail: info@rddirect.org.uk Tel: 0113 295 1122 (Mon–Fri 8.30am–5pm)

16

Multiple choice questions

CHAPTER CONTENTS

The cell, chromosomes and molecular genetics

Questions

1. In the cell:
   - **A** Lysosomes contain proteolytic enzymes
   - **B** Microtubules are found in the Golgi apparatus
   - **C** Microfilaments attach to desmosomes
   - **D** Centrioles orientate the mitotic spindle
   - **E** Ribosomal RNA is translated into proteins

2. The cell membrane:
   - **A** Is trilaminar
   - **B** Is made up of polypeptide chains
   - **C** Contains the HLA antigens
   - **D** Is attached to the centrosome
   - **E** Synthesizes and stores protein

3. The intercellular matrix:
   - **A** Contains interstitial extracellular fluid
   - **B** Is identical for all cell types
   - **C** May be composed of mucopolysaccharides
   - **D** May contain collagen of four different types
   - **E** Has elastin fibres produced by the glycocalyx

4. In cell damage:
   - **A** Accumulation of normal products is called 'degeneration'
   - **B** Accumulation of abnormal products is infiltration
   - **C** Increased density of the cell chromatin is karyorrhexis

D Pyknosis indicates the digestion of nuclear material
E Cloudy degeneration indicates irreversible cell death

5. In radiation:
   A Cellular effects are potentiated by high oxygen concentrations
   B There may, after a delay, be an increased mitotic rate
   C Multinucleated giant cells may be formed
   D Bones are radiosensitive
   E Damage to blood vessels may cause endothelial proliferation

6. In genetics:
   A The 22 pairs of autosomes are homologous
   B Chromosomes are examined by culturing red blood cells
   C In a metacentric chromosome the centromere is near one end
   D Giemsa staining is required in order to see the chromosomes
   E The long arm of the chromosome is known as 'p'

7. In cell division of somatic cells:
   A During interphase the Y body may be seen
   B During the G1 stage replication takes place
   C Metaphase occurs after anaphase
   D The G1 stage occurs after the S stage
   E During anaphase the chromosomes separate at their centromeres

8. In meiosis:
   A The first division results in diploid cells
   B During zygotene bivalents are formed
   C During pachytene the bivalents contain four strands
   D Terminalization of the chiasmata occurs during diakinesis
   E Crossing over occurs during metaphase

9. Nuclear chromatin:
   A May be seen as a triangular body, the Barr body
   B Is seen at the periphery of the cell
   C Is seen in Turner syndrome
   D Is seen in Klinefelter syndrome
   E May be seen in the buccal smear of a normal male

10. Sex chromosome abnormalities:
    A 47XXX may result from non-disjunction
    B Mosaicism may result from anaphase lag

C May result from a translocation
D Deletion results in the formation of isochromosomes
E 45Y results in mental retardation

11. In Turner syndrome:
    A Congenital lymphoedema may occur
    B Embryos have normal numbers of germ cells
    C There is commonly secondary amenorrhoea
    D Ventricular septal defects are common
    E The metatarsal bones are short

12. In disorders of extra chromosomal material:
    A Patau syndrome is trisomy 13
    B Edward syndrome is trisomy 18
    C 47XXX is compatible with normal life and reproduction
    D 47XYY may be fertile
    E Unbalanced translocations may result in Down syndrome

13. In the chromosome:
    A When genes at one locus are identical they are called 'alleles'
    B Genes occupy homologous loci
    C Each gene consists of two purines and two pyrimidines
    D If genes at a single locus are identical the individual is homozygous
    E DNA polymorphisms are rarely found outside of genes

14. The following genetic disorders are dominant:
    A Achondroplasia
    B Phenylketonuria
    C Multiple polyposis of the colon
    D Tuberose sclerosis
    E Congenital adrenal hyperplasia

15. The following genetic disorders are recessive:
    A Cystic fibrosis
    B Myotonia congenita
    C Duchenne muscular dystrophy
    D Nephrogenic diabetes insipidus
    E Morquio disease

16. The following are examples of X-linked conditions:
    A Osteogenesis imperfecta
    B Glucose-6-phosphate dehydrogenase deficiency
    C Christmas disease (factor IX deficiency)
    D Marfan syndrome
    E Amaurotic family idiocy

17. Sexual differentiation:
    A The H–Y antigen is a plasma membrane protein
    B 46XX may rarely have a male phenotype
    C Müllerian inhibitor appears to have a local action on the side of the testis producing it
    D Androgens prevent development of the paramesonephric duct
    E Wolffian tissues respond only to dihydrotestosterone

18. Sexual differentiation:
    A In the absence of ovaries or testes the embryo has a female phenotype
    B Dihydrotestosterone is converted to testosterone by 5α-reductase
    C In 47XXY an ovotestis develops
    D In 5α-reductase deficiency a female phenotype results
    E The karyotype of true hermaphrodites is commonly 46XX

19. In genetics:
    A The 22 pairs of autosomes are homologous
    B The long arm of the chromosome is the p arm.
    C Mitotic cell division occurs only during gametogenesis
    D The human genome consists of about 300 000 genes
    E Positional cloning does not rely on knowledge of gene function

20. In linkage analysis:
    A Recessive diseases are carried only on the X chromosome
    B At least 12 individuals are needed to link a recessive disease
    C Microsatellite repeats are analysed to follow disease inheritance
    D LOD scores predict the likely location of a disease locus
    E Mendelian diseases are inherited via mitochondrial DNA

21. In molecular biology:
    A PCR can be used to amplify known sequences of DNA
    B Northern blotting is used in the analysis of proteins
    C Restriction endonucleases cut proteins at known sequence sites
    D Ethidium bromide can be used to visualize DNA
    E siRNA can be used to amplify gene expression

22. An individual gene:
    A Is a discrete unit of ribonucleic acid
    B Must be spliced before transcription can occur
    C Is present in two copies in each genome
    D Contains coding information in the introns
    E Usually has an upstream promoter

23. The structure and function of the genome:
    A Chromosomes
    B Alleles
    C Promoter
    D mRNA
    E PCR
    F Splicing
    G Genotype
    H Polyadenylation
    I Wobble
    J Western blotting

23.1 From the above list what would a scientist measure to identify the level of expression of a particular gene?

23.2 From the above list which describes a sequence upstream of a gene that regulates its expression?

23.3 From the above list which is composed of deoxyribose nucleic acid?

Answers

1.	**A**	T	**7.**	**A**	T	**13.**	**A**	F	**19.**	**A**	T
	B	F		**B**	F		**B**	T		**B**	F
	C	T		**C**	F		**C**	F		**C**	F
	D	T		**D**	F		**D**	T		**D**	F
	E	T		**E**	T		**E**	F		**E**	T
2.	**A**	T	**8.**	**A**	F	**14.**	**A**	T	**20.**	**A**	F
	B	F		**B**	T		**B**	F		**B**	F
	C	T		**C**	T		**C**	T		**C**	T
	D	T		**D**	T		**D**	T		**D**	T
	E	F		**E**	F		**E**	F		**E**	F
3.	**A**	T	**9.**	**A**	T	**15.**	**A**	T	**21.**	**A**	T
	B	F		**B**	F		**B**	F		**B**	F
	C	T		**C**	F		**C**	F		**C**	F
	D	T		**D**	T		**D**	F		**D**	T
	E	F		**E**	F		**E**	T		**E**	F
4.	**A**	T	**10.**	**A**	T	**16.**	**A**	F	**22.**	**A**	F
	B	T		**B**	T		**B**	T		**B**	F
	C	F		**C**	T		**C**	T		**C**	T
	D	F		**D**	T		**D**	F		**D**	F
	E	F		**E**	F		**E**	F		**E**	T
5.	**A**	T	**11.**	**A**	T	**17.**	**A**	T			
	B	T		**B**	T		**B**	T			
	C	T		**C**	F		**C**	T			
	D	F		**D**	F		**D**	F			
	E	T		**E**	T		**E**	F			
6.	**A**	T	**12.**	**A**	T	**18.**	**A**	T			
	B	F		**B**	T		**B**	F			
	C	F		**C**	T		**C**	F			
	D	F		**D**	T		**D**	T			
	E	F		**E**	T		**E**	T			

23.1 D mRNA
23.2 C Promoter
23.3 A Chromosomes

Clinical genetics

Questions

1. Chromosomes:
   A Acrocentric chromosomes have a centrally placed telomere
   B For karyotype analysis blood should be taken into a heparinized tube
   C Aneuploidy describes an abnormal number of chromosomes
   D There are usually 46 autosomes
   E Chromosomes have their characteristic H shape during interphase

2. For an autosomal recessive disease:
   A For two carrier parents the risk of having an affected child is 25% or 1 in 4
   B The risk that an unaffected sibling of an affected individual carries a disease causing mutation is 50 : 50 or 1 in 2
   C The risk that an unaffected sibling of an affected individual carries a disease causing mutation is 100%
   D The risk that an unaffected sibling of an affected individual carries a disease causing mutation is 2/3
   E An affected individual has one mutated gene (allele) and one normal gene (allele)

3. For an X-linked recessive condition:
   A All the sons of a carrier female will be affected
   B All the daughters of an affected male will be affected
   C There is a 50% risk that the daughters of carrier females will be a carrier
   D Females never exhibit symptoms of the condition
   E Male-to-male transmission never occurs

4. For chromosomal disorders:
   A Trisomy 21
   B Trisomy 13
   C Trisomy 18
   D XXY
   E XYY
   F 45X0
   G Satellites
   H Telomeres
   I Triploidy
   J Reciprocal translocation
   K Robertsonian translocation

4.1 A couple with recurrent miscarriages have blood taken for karyotyping. The results are a normal karyotype for the woman but the following karyotype for her husband is 46XY,t(5;8)(p14;q25.1). What type of chromosome abnormality is this?

4.2 A baby born at term is noted at birth to have a cleft lip and palate, microcephaly and post-axial polydactyly. What is the likely underlying chromosome abnormality?

4.3 Turner syndrome often causes miscarriage. If the pregnancy survives to term the baby may have short stature, webbing of neck and congenital heart defect. What is the underlying chromosome abnormality?

Answers

1.			2.			3.				
	A	F		A	T		A	F	**4.1 J** Reciprocal translocation
	B	T		B	F		B	F	**4.2 B** Trisomy 13
	C	T		C	F		C	T	**4.3 F** 45 X,0
	D	F		D	T		D	F	
	E	F		E	F		E	T	

Embryology

Questions

1. In spermatogenesis:
   A Four spermatocytes are produced from one spermatid
   B The process occurs continuously from birth
   C A spermatozoon is produced in 30 days
   D Spermatogonia line the basal lamina of the epididymis
   E Every spermatogonium develops into a primary spermatocyte

2. In spermiogenesis:
   A Nuclear material forms the acrosomal cap
   B Mitochondria form a sheath for the neck of the spermatozoon
   C The axial filament derives from the centriole
   D In the endpiece of the tail are found two central and nine peripheral filaments
   E Spermatozoa may remain linked at cytoplasmic bridges

3. In oogenesis:
   A The early development of the primitive germ cells in the ovary during intrauterine life is mitotic
   B Primary oocytes are formed after 37 weeks of gestation
   C Some primary oocytes will remain in prophase for 12–50 years
   D Division of the secondary oocyte occurs at the time of ovulation
   E At puberty there are 1–2 million oocytes present

4. In fertilization:
   A The whole spermatozoon penetrates the ovum
   B The ovum reaches the uterus within 24 h
   C After penetration cortical granules appear around the perimeter of the egg
   D The second meiotic division is completed just before penetration by the spermatozoon
   E The first division of the ovum occurs 6 h after fertilization

5. In early development and implantation:
   A The zygote contains blastomeres
   B The morula is contained within the blastocyst
   C The embryo forms from trophoblast
   D The blastocyst implants about 10 days after fertilization
   E Syncytiotrophoblast arises from the inner cell mass

6. In embryogenesis:
   A The endocervical vesicle becomes the yolk sac
   B The cells adjacent to the amniotic sac form endoderm
   C Ectodermal cells are tall, columnar cells
   D Three layers of cells lie between the amniotic and yolk sacs
   E Mesodermal cells develop principally from ectodermal division

7. In organogenesis:
   A The neural tube develops on the ventral surface of the embryo
   B The vitellointestinal duct may persist as Meckel's diverticulum
   C Paraxial mesoderm divides into splanchnopleure and somatopleure
   D Limb buds develop from splanchnopleure
   E The buccopharyngeal membrane of the stomatodeum breaks down at the 6th week of life

8. In the pharyngeal region:
   A The upper and lower jaws develop from the first arch
   B The styloid process develops from the second pouch

C The inferior parathyroids develop from the third pouch

D The superior parathyroids develop from the third pouch

E The arch of the aorta develops from the fourth arch artery

9. In the pharyngeal region:

A The muscles of the tongue are developed from the first and third arches

B The thyroid gland develops from the distal end of the thyroglossal duct

C A branchial cyst arises following failure of occlusion of the second pharyngeal pouch

D The primitive lungs arise from the fifth pharyngeal pouch

E The fourth and sixth arches contribute to the bones of the larynx

10. In the cardiovascular system:

A The heart develops from angiogenic cells

B The cardinal veins run into the sinus venosus

C The vitelline veins run into the bulbus cordis

D A beating fetal heart tube can be recognized by ultrasound techniques from the 32nd day of intrauterine life

E In the foramen ovale blood passes from left to right

11. In the cardiovascular system:

A The proximal bulbar septum divides the aorta from the pulmonary artery

B Deoxygenated blood passes via the umbilical vein to the left branch of the portal vein

C The ligamentum venosum is the obliterated umbilical vein

D There is a single umbilical artery

E The foramen ovale usually closes 1 month after birth

12. In the alimentary system:

A The foregut ends at the pyloric sphincter

B The spleen is a derivative of the foregut

C The pancreas is a derivative of the midgut

D The stomach forms a sac at the 5th week of intrauterine life

E The hindgut opens into the cloaca

13. The diaphragm:

A Develops from the septum transversum

B Develops from the pleuroperitoneal membrane

C Develops from the costal margin

D Develops from the gastrohepatic ligament

E Has a small contribution from the mesoderm around the aorta

14. In the nervous system:

A The cerebral hemispheres originate from the cerebral vesicles

B The lateral ventricles develop from the side wall of the foremost part of the neural tube

C The neural crest cells give rise to the adrenal medulla

D The commonest form of spina bifida is cervicothoracic

E The notochord is ectodermal

15. In the skeletal system:

A There are three ossification centres in each vertebra

B The nucleus pulposus is derived from a cartilaginous ring

C The vault of the skull is preformed in cartilage

D Limb buds appear at the 7th week of intrauterine life

E Synovial joints arise from endoderm

16. In the development of muscles and skin:

A The muscles of the head and neck develop from the mesenchyme of the pharyngeal arches

B The skin plate arises from proliferation of spindle cells of the dermomyotome

C The involuntary muscles of the bladder arise from the dorsal part of the muscle plate

D Sweat glands arise from the skin plate

E Sebaceous glands are ectodermal structures

17. In the development of the genital organs:

A The pronephros arises in intermediate mesoderm

B The pronephros is found in the thoracic region

C The mesonephros appears in the thoracic and lumbar regions

D The Wolffian duct connects with the tubules of the mesonephros

E The genital ridge appears on the lateral aspect of the mesonephros

18. In the development of the uterus, tubes and vagina:

A The paramesonephric ducts reach the urogenital sinus by week 7

B At 9 weeks both mesonephric and paramesonephric ducts are present

C Muscular walls develop in the uterus in the 6th month

D The vaginal plate is composed of urogenital sinus epithelium and paramesonephric ducts

E The vagina is a solid organ until 30 weeks

19. In the development of the external genitalia:
    A The genital swellings are medial to the genital folds
    B The genital tubercle becomes the clitoris
    C The phallic part of the urogenital sinus reaches cranially to the point where the Müllerian ducts enter the sinus wall
    D The vestibule is derived from both the pelvic and phallic portions of the urogenital sinus
    E Ectopia vesicae results from deficient development of the genital folds

20. In the development of the testis:
    A Primitive germ cells arise from beneath the epithelium of the amniotic sac
    B Gonadal differentiation can be seen at 5 weeks
    C Sex cords develop from coelomic epithelium
    D The interstitial cells of Leydig arise from coelomic epithelium
    E The rete testis arises from the underlying mesoderm

21. In the development of the ovary:
    A Granulosa cells arise from the coelomic epithelium
    B By 20 weeks there are 700 000 germ cells
    C By 20–24 weeks follicle formation can be seen
    D The mesenchyme gives rise to thecal cells
    E The lower part of the gubernaculum becomes the round ligament

22. In the development of the placenta:
    A Syncytiotrophoblast is derived from the cytotrophoblast

B The vessels of the villous stems arise from mesenchyme within the core

C Villous stems are anchored to the basal plate

D The finding of trophoblast into the spiral arteries is abnormal

E The chorion laeve develops into the definitive placenta

23. In the development of the placenta:
    A The placental septa are simply folds of the basal plate
    B The peripheral syncytium degenerates and is replaced by Rohr's layer
    C The number of lobules in a cotyledon varies from 2 to 5
    D Each placental lobule is derived from a single secondary stem villus
    E Terminal villi arise from secondary stem villi

24. In the formation of the membranes:
    A The yolk sac is derived from trophoblast
    B The ectoderm is a continuing source of supply of amniotic cells
    C The vitelline duct is incorporated into the lower end of the body stalk
    D The amniochorionic membrane contains a loose reticular layer
    E The amniochorionic membrane contains a layer of parietal extraembryonic mesenchyme

25. The liquor amnii:
    A Volume is approximately 1 L at 36 weeks
    B In early pregnancy arises by transfer of fluid across the fetal skin
    C The pH is usually >5.6 and <6.5
    D Has bacteriostatic properties
    E Is increased by giving the mother a NSAID

Answers

1.	A	F		8.	A	T		15.	A	T		22.	A	T
	B	F			B	F			B	F			B	T
	C	F			C	T			C	F			C	T
	D	F			D	F			D	F			D	F
	E	F			E	T			E	F			E	F
2.	A	F		9.	A	F		16.	A	T		23.	A	T
	B	F			B	T			B	F			B	F
	C	F			C	T			C	F			C	T
	D	T			D	F			D	F			D	T
	E	T			E	T			E	T			E	F
3.	A	T		10.	A	T		17.	A	T		24.	A	F
	B	F			B	T			B	F			B	T
	C	T			C	F			C	T			C	T
	D	F			D	T			D	T			D	T
	E	F			E	F			E	F			E	T
4.	A	F		11.	A	T		18.	A	F		25.	A	T
	B	F			B	F			B	T			B	T
	C	T			C	F			C	F			C	F
	D	T			D	F			D	T			D	T
	E	F			E	F			E	F			E	F
5.	A	T		12.	A	F		19.	A	F				
	B	F			B	F			B	T				
	C	T			C	F			C	F				
	D	F			D	T			D	T				
	E	F			E	T			E	F				
6.	A	T		13.	A	T		20.	A	F				
	B	F			B	T			B	F				
	C	T			C	T			C	T				
	D	T			D	T			D	F				
	E	T			E	T			E	F				
7.	A	F		14.	A	T		21.	A	T				
	B	T			B	F			B	F				
	C	F			C	T			C	T				
	D	F			D	F			D	T				
	E	F			E	T			E	T				

The fetus

Questions

1. Fetal growth:
   - **A** Crown–rump length is considered to be an accurate ultrasound measurement of fetal growth up until 14 weeks
   - **B** The biparietal diameter is considered to be an accurate ultrasound measurement of fetal growth from 10 weeks
   - **C** The head/abdominal circumference ratio decreases with advancing pregnancy
   - **D** Fetal weight increases with increasing parity
   - **E** In late pregnancy occurs at the same rate as placental growth

2. Fetal circulation:
   - **A** Circulation of blood is present by 21 days
   - **B** The heart originates in splanchnic mesenchyme
   - **C** The fetus responds to hypoxia by increasing the circulation to adrenal glands
   - **D** In response to hypoxia, the fetus can increase the placental circulation by 50%
   - **E** *In utero* only 1% of the cardiac output is directed to the lungs

3. Renal function:
   - **A** Renal agenesis is associated with oligohydramnios
   - **B** The kidney at term is the principal source of amniotic fluid
   - **C** In late pregnancy the amniotic fluid osmolarity rises
   - **D** The concentration of creatinine in amniotic fluid is less than in the fetal plasma
   - **E** The rate of fetal urine production can be measured by ultrasound

4. Nervous system:
   - **A** Nerve cell processes in the cerebrum appear at 8–10 weeks
   - **B** Nerves appear in the fetus between 4 and 5 weeks
   - **C** Limb muscle fibres can contract by 8 weeks
   - **D** Baroreceptor stimulation of the aortic branches of the Xth cranial nerve results in a bradycardia
   - **E** Chemoreceptors in the carotid body respond *in utero* to alterations in pH

5. Alimentary tract:
   - **A** Swallowing commences at 20 weeks
   - **B** Meconium contains vernix
   - **C** Peristalsis is inhibited by hypoxia
   - **D** The stomach bubble on ultrasound is only visible after 20 weeks
   - **E** Digestive enzymes are found by 12 weeks

6. Respiratory system:
   - **A** Breathing movements are present from 20 weeks
   - **B** Alveolar development is complete by 24 weeks
   - **C** Type I pneumocytes produce surfactant
   - **D** Intrathoracic pressures of up to –10 cm H_2O may be required for the baby's first breath
   - **E** As labour approaches, fetal breathing decreases

7. Placental transfer:
   - **A** The placenta is a complete barrier to substances with molecular weights greater than 1500
   - **B** 3–4 L of fluid are exchanged between the mother and fetus per hour
   - **C** The placenta converts phospholipids to simpler forms
   - **D** The concentration of amino acids is less in the fetal blood than in the maternal blood
   - **E** Oxygen delivery occurs by diffusion rate from mother to fetus

8. Oxygen and carbon dioxide transfer:
   - **A** The oxygen dissociation curve for fetal blood is shifted to the right
   - **B** Fetal blood has a larger carrying capacity for oxygen than maternal blood
   - **C** In low oxygen tensions fetal Hb has lesser affinity for oxygen than maternal Hb
   - **D** Carbon dioxide is mostly carried in the blood as carbonic acid or bicarbonate
   - **E** The Haldane effect facilitates release of carbon dioxide from fetal haemoglobin

9. Oxygen:
   - **A** The fetus at 16 weeks of gestation requires 25 mL/min of oxygen
   - **B** Each gram of Hb combines with 1.34 mL of oxygen
   - **C** HbF binds 2, 3-DPG less effectively
   - **D** At P_{50}, the Hb dissociation curve of the fetus is less steep than that of the mother
   - **E** In fetal hypoxia, both metabolic and respiratory acidosis occur

10. Oxygen and carbon dioxide:
    A The fetus requires oxygen at higher tensions than that of the mother
    B A fall in plasma pH decreases the affinity of red blood cells for oxygen
    C Excess fetal lactic acid is metabolized in the placenta
    D Excess carbon dioxide dilates placental vessels
    E The fetus may become polycythaemic in response to low oxygen tensions

11. Placental structure:
    A At term new placental villi continue to be formed
    B There is a positive correlation between placental weight and fetal weight
    C Microvilli are present on the vasculo-syncytial membranes
    D The main factor governing the rate of placental blood flow is the vascular resistance of the spiral arteries
    E At term the total blood flow to the placenta is about 500 mL

12. The following organisms cross the placenta:
    A Variola vaccinia
    B Coxsackie virus
    C Listeria
    D Neisseria meningitidis
    E Toxoplasma

13. The average weight gain at term of:
    A the uterus is 400 g
    B the breasts is 400 g
    C the blood is 1200 g
    D the placenta is 600 g
    E the liquor is 800 g

14. The placenta produces the following substances:
    A oestrone
    B 5α-reductase
    C oxytocinase
    D histaminase
    E progesterone

Answers

1.			5.			9.			13.		
	A	F		A	F		A	F		A	F
	B	F		B	T		B	T		B	T
	C	T		C	F		C	T		C	T
	D	T		D	F		D	F		D	T
	E	F		E	F		E	T		E	T
2.	A	T	6.	A	F	10.	A	F	14.	A	T
	B	T		B	F		B	T		B	T
	C	T		C	F		C	T		C	T
	D	F		D	F		D	T		D	T
	E	F		E	T		E	T		E	T
3.	A	T	7.	A	F	11.	A	T			
	B	T		B	T		B	T			
	C	F		C	T		C	F			
	D	F		D	F		D	F			
	E	T		E	T		E	T			
4.	A	F	8.	A	F	12.	A	T			
	B	T		B	T		B	T			
	C	T		C	F		C	T			
	D	T		D	T		D	F			
	E	T		E	T		E	T			

Anatomy

Questions

1. In the anterior abdominal wall:
   A Rectus abdominis inserts into rib cartilages 7, 8 and 9
   B Pyramidalis is present in 20% of the population
   C The median umbilical ligament is the urachal remnant
   D The ligamentum teres may be connected to ligamentum venosum
   E The lateral umbilical ligaments are the obliterated umbilical arteries

2. The rectus sheath:
   A Anteriorly and suprapubically consists of two layers
   B Below the umbilicus consists of three anterior layers
   C Is supplied by the dorsal rami of the lower sixth or seventh thoracic nerves
   D Encloses an anastomosis between the superficial and deep epigastric vessels
   E When present, contains pyramidalis

3. Abdominal fascia:
   A In the anterior abdominal wall contains the superficial inguinal lymph nodes between its superficial and deep layers
   B Has a superficial layer attached to the linea alba
   C In the iliac region has the lumbar plexus nerves behind it
   D In the lumbar region has two layers
   E As transversalis fascia passes into the inguinal canal

4. In the inguinal ligament:
   A Its pectineal part is called the lacunar ligament
   B The superficial ring lies between the pubic symphysis and the pubic tubercle
   C The deep ring lies medial to the inferior epigastric vessels
   D The round ligament passes along the inguinal canal
   E The lacunar part medially gives rise to the pectineal ligament

5. In the anterolateral group of abdominal muscles:
   A Transversus abdominis arises from the anterior third of the iliac crest

B Transversus abdominis is part of the falx inguinalis

C The conjoint tendon inserts into the crest and pecten pubis

D The internal oblique partially arises from the lumbar fascia

E The internal oblique is attached to the inguinal ligament in its outer two-thirds

6. In the posterior group of abdominal muscles:
  A Psoas major lies behind the anterior layer of lumbar fascia
  B The lateral arcuate ligament is formed by the middle layer of lumbar fascia
  C Psoas major enters the abdomen behind the medial arcuate ligament
  D Psoas major leaves the abdomen medial to iliacus
  E Quadratus lumborum is supplied by the lower six or seven thoracic nerves

7. The diaphragm:
  A Right crus arises from the anterolateral part of the first two lumbar vertebral bodies
  B Is traversed by the inferior vena cava at the level of T12
  C Has an aortic aperture at T10
  D Transmits the sympathetic nerves through the aortic aperture
  E Transmits the superior epigastric vessels between sternal and costal origins

8. The coeliac trunk:
  A Gives rise directly to the right gastric artery
  B Gives rise directly to the left gastric artery
  C Gives rise to the splenic artery
  D Gives rise to the pancreatic artery
  E Gives rise to the common hepatic artery

9. Branches of the superior mesenteric artery include:
  A The common hepatic artery
  B The inferior pancreatic-duodenal artery
  C The superior pancreatic-duodenal artery
  D Middle colic artery
  E Right colic artery

10. The oesophagus:
  A Is supplied by left gastric vessels
  B In the abdomen is covered on anterior and right aspects by peritoneum
  C Is separated from the fundus by the cardiac notch

D Has vagal trunks lying on right and left aspects

E Is contained within the upper part of the lesser omentum

11. The stomach:
  A Is related anteriorly to the liver
  B Antrum is adjacent to the fundus
  C Is supplied by branches of the splenic artery
  D Lies medial to the spleen
  E Is related posteriorly to the left suprarenal gland

12. The duodenum:
  A Forms the floor of the epiploic foramen
  B Is joined halfway down its second part by pancreatic and common bile ducts
  C Is related posteriorly in its second part to the kidney
  D Continues at the level of L2 as the third part
  E Crosses the ureter in its fourth part

13. The portal vein:
  A Lies anterior to the duodenum
  B Lies lateral to the hepatic artery
  C Is related to the cystic duct posterior to the pancreas
  D Drains into the hepatic vein
  E Is formed by superior mesenteric and pancreatic veins

14. Small intestine:
  A Mesentery forms the posterior wall of the lesser sac
  B Mesentery crosses the right ovarian vessels
  C Ileum is more vascular than jejunum
  D Jejunum is related posteriorly to the lower pole of the left kidney
  E Jejunum is thicker than ileum

15. Meckel's diverticulum:
  A Usually arises 5–10 cm from the ileocaecal valve
  B May contain heterotopic gastric mucosa
  C May contain heterotopic pancreatic mucosa
  D May secrete thyroid hormones
  E May be connected to the umbilicus by the vitellointestinal duct

16. The large intestine:
  A The right colic flexure is higher than that on the left
  B Taenia coli arise from the circular muscle coat

C The descending colon runs along the lateral border of the left kidney

D The right colic flexure is related to the second part of the duodenum posteriorly

E The descending colon crosses the left ovarian artery

17. The appendix:
- **A** In every case taenia coli lead to its base
- **B** Is the embryological apex of the caecum
- **C** Arises 2–3 cm below the ileocaecal opening
- **D** Artery runs in front of the terminal ileum to reach the mesoappendix
- **E** Has accessory arteries in 80% of cases

18. The right kidney anterolaterally is related to the:
- **A** Right coronary ligament
- **B** The jejunum
- **C** The suprarenal gland
- **D** The stomach
- **E** The pancreas

19. The left kidney anterolaterally is related to the:
- **A** Left coronary ligament
- **B** Spleen
- **C** Transverse mesocolon
- **D** Stomach
- **E** Pancreas

20. The kidney:
- **A** On the left lies lower than on the right
- **B** Is related to the ilioinguinal nerve posteriorly
- **C** Upper pole is further from the midline than the lower pole
- **D** There may be accessory arteries in up to 30% of cases
- **E** Has a posterior layer of fascia which has attachments to the vertebral bodies

21. On the medial aspect of the kidney:
- **A** The artery runs anterior to the vein
- **B** The ureter passes anterior to the vein
- **C** The artery divides into anterior and posterior branches
- **D** In the sinus there are 12 or 13 minor calyces
- **E** In the sinus each minor calyx includes up to six renal papillae

22. The ureter:
- **A** Is partially retroperitoneal
- **B** Crosses the ovarian vessels
- **C** Passes behind the genitofemoral nerve

D Lies medial to the tips of the transverse processes

E Receives blood supply from the ovarian vessels

23. The pancreas:
- **A** The common bile duct crosses over the anterior surface
- **B** The uncinate process extends behind the superior mesenteric vessels
- **C** The inferior mesenteric vein lies behind the junction of head and neck
- **D** The portal vein lies behind the neck
- **E** The tail is related to the spleen

24. The spleen:
- **A** Is related posteriorly to the left suprarenal gland
- **B** Is supplied by vessels running in the lienorenal ligament
- **C** Has a notch in its anterior border
- **D** Is found between the seventh and ninth ribs
- **E** Must increase in size by 25% before its anterior border passes beyond the left costal margin

25. The liver:
- **A** The caudate lobe lies to the left of the groove for the inferior vena cava
- **B** The quadrate lobe lies to the right of the fissure for ligamentum teres
- **C** The coronary ligament is found on the left
- **D** The ligamentum teres runs from a notch in the inferior border to the left end of the porta hepatis
- **E** The ligamentum venosum runs in a groove between the left and caudate lobes

26. The suprarenal gland:
- **A** On the right is triangular in shape
- **B** On the right lies anterior to the vena cava
- **C** On the left lies on the left crus of the diaphragm
- **D** Has three sources of arterial supply
- **E** Has a zona reticularis in the medulla

27. In renal vessels:
- **A** The inferior phrenic artery is a branch of the renal artery
- **B** The right renal artery passes in front of the vena cava
- **C** The left renal vein lies behind the aorta
- **D** The renal arteries arise immediately below the inferior mesenteric artery

E The right renal artery passes behind the head of the pancreas

28. Peritoneal arrangements:
  A The right and left paracolic gutters communicate with the pelvis
  B Both paracolic gutters continue into subdiaphragmatic spaces
  C The ligamentum teres runs in the falciform ligament
  D The greater omentum forms the anterior wall of the inferior part of the lesser sac
  E The epiploic foramen is related to the gastrophrenic ligament anteriorly

29. The ovarian arteries:
  A Arise just above the renal artery
  B Are crossed by the ureters
  C On the right cross the inferior vena cava
  D On the left cross the left colic artery
  E Reach the ovary through the ovarian ligament

30. The following receive blood supply via the coeliac artery:
  A Pancreas
  B Jejunum
  C Stomach
  D Fourth part of duodenum
  E Gall bladder

31. Branches of the aorta:
  A Coeliac axis gives rise to the hepatic artery
  B Middle mesenteric artery gives rise to the middle colic artery
  C Common iliac artery arises at the left side of L4
  D The inferior mesenteric gives rise to the right colic artery
  E The superior rectal artery arises from the inferior mesenteric

32. The following statements are true:
  A The middle rectal artery arises from the inferior pudendal artery
  B The deep circumflex artery is a branch of the inferior epigastric artery
  C Jejunal straight arteries are longer and less numerous than ileal straight arteries
  D The right common iliac artery crosses the obturator nerve
  E The left common iliac artery is crossed by the superior rectal artery

33. The inferior mesenteric artery:
  A Arises just below the lower border of the horizontal part of the duodenum
  B Crosses the left ureter
  C Gives rise to three sigmoid arteries
  D Enters the pelvis as the superior rectal artery
  E Supplies the transverse colon

34. The external iliac artery is crossed by:
  A The corresponding vein
  B The ovarian vessels
  C The genital branch of the genital femoral nerve
  D The round ligament
  E The ureter

35. The following are branches of the anterior division of the internal iliac artery:
  A The superior lateral sacral
  B The inferior lateral sacral
  C The iliolumbar
  D The obturator
  E The inferior rectal

36. The following are branches of the posterior division of the internal iliac artery:
  A Superior gluteal
  B Middle gluteal
  C Middle rectal
  D Internal pudendal
  E Posterior vesical

37. The uterine artery:
  A Is a branch of the anterior division of the internal iliac artery
  B Runs in front of the ureter
  C Gives a branch to the vagina
  D May anastomose with the obturator artery
  E Divides into arcuate arteries

38. Iliac veins:
  A The left external iliac vein lies lateral to the left external iliac artery
  B The deep circumflex iliac vein drains into the external iliac vein
  C The internal iliac vein is behind and medial to its artery
  D The common iliac vein is formed at the level of L4
  E Rarely the left common iliac vein may receive a renal vein

39. The inferior vena cava:
   A Is related posteriorly to the right middle suprarenal artery
   B Is related posteriorly to the right inferior phrenic artery
   C Is related anteriorly to the right colic vessels
   D Receives the left suprarenal vein
   E Receives the right gonadal vein

40. The hepatic portal system:
   A The hepatic portal vein forms at the level of L1
   B The left branch of the hepatic portal vein receives the cystic vein
   C The superior mesenteric artery runs between the splenic and renal veins
   D The splenic vein receives the short gastric veins
   E The superior mesenteric vein receives the pancreaticoduodenal veins

41. Lymphatics:
   A The cysterna chyli lies in front of L1 and L2
   B The cysterna chyli lies to the right of the azygos vein
   C The ovaries drain to the lateral aortic and preaortic nodes
   D The bladder drains to the lateral and preaortic nodes
   E The urethra drains to the internal iliac nodes

42. Autonomic nerves:
   A Parasympathetic stimulation increases peristalsis
   B There are four lumbar splanchnic nerves
   C The hypogastric plexus is found inferior to the aortic plexus
   D The coeliac plexus distributes autonomic nerve supply along the ovarian artery
   E The preganglionic sympathetic efferent fibres to the cervix derive from T10 and T11

43. In the chest:
   A The thoracic duct drains into the right subclavian vein
   B The hemiazygos drains into the left subclavian
   C The azygos vein drains into the superior vena cava
   D The right subclavian vein runs inferior to the clavicle
   E The thoracic duct arises at the level of the T12 vertebra

44. The following nerves supply the vulva:
   A Genitofemoral
   B Iliohypogastric
   C Perineal branch of S4
   D Pudendal
   E Ilioinguinal

45. The ureter:
   A Is uniform in size except for two slightly constricted portions
   B Enters the pelvis mid-way along the external iliac artery
   C Crosses the ovarian artery
   D Passes about 8–15 mm from the lateral fornix of the vagina
   E Is closed by a true valve, where it enters the bladder

46. Relations of the ovary:
   A The infundibulopelvic ligament is attached to the upper pole of the ovary
   B The ovary lies in front of the ureter
   C The upper pole of the ovary lies beneath the ovary
   D The fimbria of the uterine tube is related to its medial surface
   E The obturator artery and nerve pass across the ovarian fossa

47. In the ovary:
   A The tunica albuginea lies outside the germinal epithelium
   B Some primordial follicles degenerate before birth
   C Oogenesis occurs until the menopause
   D The corona radiata surrounds the liquor folliculi
   E Ovulation occurs 14 days after the start of the last menstrual period

48. In the follicle:
   A The theca externa cells, after ovulation, become the theca-lutein cells
   B The corpus luteum of pregnancy functions until the 6th month of pregnancy
   C The corpus luteum of pregnancy is the corpus albicantes
   D In the follicular phase the theca interna cells synthesize androgens
   E Granulosa cells secrete progesterone in the second half of the cycle

49. The fallopian tube:
    A Isthmus runs a tortuous course within the uterine wall
    B Is 2.5 mm wide in the interstitial portion
    C Has an inner longitudinal muscle coat
    D Has peg cells in the epithelium
    E Has decidual changes in the epithelial tunica propria in pregnancy

50. The uterus:
    A Forward tilt at the cervical isthmus is called anteversion
    B By full-term pregnancy weighs about 900 g
    C Has an outer blend of muscle fibres which encircle the body in spirals
    D Endometrium at mid-cycle is 0.5 mm thick
    E Blood loss at menstruation is usually less than 50 mL

51. The cervix:
    A In infancy a large area is covered with columnar epithelium
    B Has nabothian follicles in the original squamous epithelium
    C Has an increased proportion of fibrous tissue when compared to the body of the uterus
    D Has a fusiform cavity
    E Has ciliated epithelium

52. In the vagina:
    A The left ureter is more closely related to the fornix than the right
    B The lateral walls are in contact with each other
    C The pouch of Douglas extends halfway down the posterior vaginal wall
    D The epithelium is non-keratinized squamous
    E Mucus-secreting glands are present

53. In the vulva:
    A The vestibule lies between the fossa navicularis and the fourchette
    B The skin in the labia minora is keratinized
    C Skene's ducts open into the vestibule
    D The bulbospongiosus muscles run around the vagina
    E Bartholin's gland is 2 cm in diameter

54. The rectum and anal canal:
    A The rectum is below the peritoneal reflection in its lower two-thirds
    B The anal canal is about 7 cm long
    C The junction of the columnar and squamous epithelium in the middle of the anal canal is marked by the white lines of Houston

D The external anal sphincter consists of three parts
E The subcutaneous portion of the external sphincter runs between the anococcygeal ligament and the perineal body

55. The bladder embryology and histology:
    A The urogenital sinus is formed at about the 7th week of embryonic life
    B Caudal portions of the mesonephric ducts are incorporated in the trigone
    C The lining is a mucus-secreting transitional epithelium
    D Is completely surrounded by a loose layer of areolar tissue
    E Has peritoneal attachments superiorly and laterally

56. The urethra:
    A Has an external sphincter at the urethral meatus
    B Is 3–4 cm in length in the adult female
    C Is lined by transitional epithelium in its proximal half
    D Has an inner longitudinal muscle layer
    E Is connected by muscle fibres to the urogenital diaphragm

57. Innervation of bladder and urethra:
    A Cholinergic drugs relax the bladder
    B The pudendal nerve supplies the bladder
    C S3 is the main parasympathetic root for the detrusor muscle
    D Sympathetic nerve supply is via the hypogastric nerves
    E The voluntary urethral sphincter is supplied by the somatic fibres of S2, 3 and 4

58. The uterine supports:
    A The pubocervical ligaments are found lateral to the bladder
    B The round ligament terminally carries some fibres from the internal oblique and transversalis muscles
    C The uterosacral ligaments pass backwards to the 3rd and 4th sacral vertebrae
    D The coccygeus muscle arises from the ischial spine
    E Mackenrodt's ligaments attach to the 'white line' laterally

59. The following statements are true:
    A The canal of Nuck is a patent processus vaginalis

B The endopelvic fascia is continuous with the fascia transversalis lining the abdomen

C The posterior border of the triangular ligament runs across the perineum between the two ischial tuberosities

D Bulbocavernosus forms part of the perineal body

E The deep perineal space is related laterally to the ischiopubic rami

60. Pelvic osteology:
   A The plane of least dimensions is at the level of the ischial spines
   B The arcuate line is part of the iliopectineal line
   C The pubic tubercle lies at the medial end of the pubic crest
   D The obturator crest is the everted superior border of the inferior ramus of the pubis
   E The transversus perinei muscles are attached to the inferior pubic ramus

61. The following statements are true:
   A The pudendal canal lies above the lateral insertion of the levator ani
   B The internal pudendal artery runs behind the pyriformis muscle
   C The internal pudendal artery leaves the pelvis at the lower border of the greater sciatic foramen
   D The pudendal canal lies 2 cm above the ischial tuberosity
   E The pudendal canal runs through the superficial perineal pouch

62. The following statements are true:
   A The inferior rectal artery arises in the pudendal canal
   B The external pudendal artery arises over the sacroiliac joint
   C The superficial perineal pouch communicates anteriorly with the pelvic cavity
   D The obturator internus muscle makes up the lateral wall of the ischiorectal fossa
   E Obturator fascia is found on the inferior aspect of a muscle

63. Pelvic nerve supply:
   A The pudendal nerve lies on the medial side of the pudendal vessels behind the ischial spine
   B The nerve to obturator internus passes through the obturator fossa
   C Levator ani motor supply is from a muscular branch of S2

D The perineal branch of S4 supplies the perineal skin around the anus

E The nerve to obturator internus lies lateral to the internal vessels on the outer aspect of the ischial spine

64. Sacral plexus:
   A The pudendal nerve gives off labial branches into the superficial perineal pouch
   B The pudendal nerve supplies the clitoris
   C The lateral femoral cutaneous nerve gives off a perineal branch
   D The posterior femoral cutaneous nerve arises from S1, 2 and 3
   E The nerve to coccygeus arises from S3

65. The breast:
   A Oestrogen stimulates secretion of colostrum
   B In pregnancy may increase in weight by 2–3-fold
   C Montgomery's glands are sebaceous glands
   D The breast is an apocrine gland
   E The most frequent site of an accessory breast is on the chest wall

66. The femoral triangle:
   A The lateral border is vastus lateralis
   B Pectineus lies in the floor
   C Psoas major laterally rotates the femur
   D The femoral vein lies medial to the artery
   E The femoral vein lies lateral to the nerve

67. The ischiorectal fossa:
   A Has a lateral wall partly formed by the falciform margin of the sacrotuberous ligament
   B Is separated from the perianal space by the perianal fascia
   C Has fat in small loculi separated by complete septa
   D Extends forwards into the urogenital triangle
   E Is separated from the lower surface of the levator and by the lunate fascia

68. Surgical structures of particular importance during surgery:
   A Urachus
   B Superficial circumflex iliac vessels
   C Inferior epigastric vessels
   D Hilton's white line
   E Houston's valves
   F Levator ani muscle
   G Trigone of the bladder
   H Sigmoid mesentery

I   Cardinal ligament
J   Ureter

68.1 When performing a Pfannenstiel incision to enter the abdomen, separating the abdominus recti muscles in the midline by hooking a finger between the muscle and the peritoneum risks injury to this structure.

68.2 When a 4th-degree tear occurs following obstetric trauma a colorectal surgeon should be called if the anal mucosa is torn above the level of this structure.

68.3 When performing an abdominal hysterectomy and securing the uterine pedicle care must be taken to reflect the bladder inferiorly otherwise this structure is threatened.

69. Regarding these ligaments:
   A Broad ligament
   B Round ligament
   C Cardinal ligament
   D Inguinal ligament
   E Arcuate ligament
   F Sacrospinous ligament
   G Sacrotuberous ligament
   H Sacroiliac ligament
   I Median umbilical ligament
   J Medial umbilical ligament

69.1 This ligament forms from the free inferior edge of the external oblique aponeurosis.

69.2 This ligament is a double layer of peritoneum.

69.3 This ligament is the obliterated umbilical artery.

70. The female pelvis:
   A Has an oval inlet
   B The widest diameter of its inlet is in the transverse plane
   C Has a canal which is long and tapered

D Its subpubic angle is normally approximately 60°
E Articulates with two sacral bodies

71. The ureter:
   A Is retroperitoneal throughout its course
   B On the right side lies behind the second part of the duodenum
   C Lies deep to the mesosigmoid on the left side
   D Is crossed by the uterine vessels
   E Enters the pelvis by passing under the bifurcation of the common iliac artery

72. The superior inguinal lymph nodes:
   A Lie along the greater saphenous vein
   B Lie proximal to the inguinal ligament
   C Drain the deep part of the leg
   D Drain the upper part of the uterus
   E Drain the anterior abdominal wall below the umbilicus

73. The fetal skull:
   A The parietal bones meet at the lamboid suture
   B The coronal suture lies between the frontal bones
   C The anterior fontanelle is triangular in shape
   D The sagittal suture runs between the anterior and the posterior fontanelle
   E A face presentation is the largest presenting diameter

74. The inferior epigastric artery:
   A Arises from the external iliac artery
   B Forms the lateral border of the deep inguinal ring
   C Runs superiorly superficial to the rectus abdominis muscle
   D Is extraperitoneal
   E Is vulnerable to damage at laparoscopy

Answers

1.	A	F	11.	A	T	21.	A	F	31.	A	T
	B	F		B	F		B	F		B	T
	C	T		C	T		C	T		C	T
	D	T		D	T		D	T		D	F
	E	T		E	T		E	F		E	T
2.	A	T	12.	A	T	22.	A	F	32.	A	T
	B	F		B	T		B	F		B	F
	C	F		C	T		C	F		C	T
	D	F		D	F		D	F		D	T
	E	T		E	F		E	T		E	F
3.	A	T	13.	A	F	23.	A	F	33.	A	T
	B	F		B	F		B	T		B	F
	C	T		C	F		C	T		C	T
	D	F		D	F		D	F		D	T
	E	T		E	F		E	T		E	F
4.	A	T	14.	A	F	24.	A	T	34.	A	F
	B	T		B	T		B	T		B	T
	C	F		C	F		C	T		C	T
	D	T		D	T		D	F		D	T
	E	F		E	T		E	F		E	T
5.	A	F	15.	A	F	25.	A	T	35.	A	F
	B	T		B	T		B	T		B	F
	C	T		C	T		C	F		C	F
	D	T		D	F		D	T		D	T
	E	T		E	T		E	T		E	F
6.	A	F	16.	A	F	26.	A	T	36.	A	T
	B	F		B	F		B	T		B	F
	C	T		C	T		C	T		C	F
	D	T		D	T		D	T		D	F
	E	F		E	T		E	F		E	F
7.	A	F	17.	A	T	27.	A	F	37.	A	T
	B	F		B	T		B	F		B	T
	C	F		C	T		C	F		C	T
	D	F		D	F		D	F		D	F
	E	T		E	T		E	T		E	T
8.	A	F	18.	A	T	28.	A	T	38.	A	F
	B	T		B	T		B	F		B	T
	C	T		C	T		C	T		C	T
	D	F		D	F		D	T		D	F
	E	T		E	F		E	F		E	T
9.	A	F	19.	A	F	29.	A	F	39.	A	T
	B	T		B	F		B	F		B	T
	C	T		C	T		C	T		C	T
	D	T		D	T		D	F		D	F
	E	T		E	T		E	F		E	T
10.	A	T	20.	A	F	30.	A	T	40.	A	F
	B	F		B	T		B	F		B	F
	C	T		C	F		C	T		C	T
	D	F		D	T		D	F		D	T
	E	T		E	T		E	T		E	T

41.	A	T		50.	A	F		59.	A	T
	B	F			B	T			B	T
	C	T			C	F			C	T
	D	F			D	F			D	F
	E	T			E	F			E	T
42.	A	T		51.	A	T		60.	A	T
	B	T			B	F			B	T
	C	T			C	T			C	F
	D	T			D	T			D	F
	E	F			E	F			E	T
43.	A	F		52.	A	T		61.	A	F
	B	F			B	F			B	F
	C	T			C	F			C	T
	D	T			D	T			D	F
	E	T			E	F			E	F
44.	A	F		53.	A	F		62.	A	T
	B	F			B	F			B	F
	C	F			C	T			C	T
	D	T			D	T			D	T
	E	T			E	F			E	F
45.	A	F		54.	A	F		63.	A	T
	B	F			B	F			B	F
	C	F			C	F			C	F
	D	T			D	T			D	T
	E	F			E	T			E	T
46.	A	T		55.	A	T		64.	A	T
	B	T			B	T			B	T
	C	T			C	F			C	F
	D	T			D	F			D	T
	E	T			E	F			E	F
47.	A	F		56.	A	F		65.	A	F
	B	T			B	T			B	T
	C	F			C	T			C	T
	D	F			D	T			D	T
	E	F			E	T			E	F
48.	A	F		57.	A	F		66.	A	F
	B	F			B	F			B	T
	C	F			C	T			C	F
	D	T			D	T			D	T
	E	T			E	T			E	F
49.	A	F		58.	A	T		67.	A	T
	B	F			B	T			B	T
	C	F			C	F			C	F
	D	T			D	T			D	T
	E	T			E	F			E	T

68.1 F Inferior epigastric vessels
68.2 G Levator ani muscle
68.3 E Ureter
69.1 F Inguinal ligament
69.2 G Broad ligament
69.3 E Medial umbilical ligament

70.	A	T
	B	T
	C	F
	D	F
	E	T
71.	A	T
	B	T
	C	T
	D	F
	E	F
72.	A	T
	B	F
	C	F
	D	T
	E	T
73.	A	T
	B	F
	C	F
	D	T
	E	F
74.	A	T
	B	F
	C	F
	D	T
	E	T

Pathology

Questions

1. In acute inflammation:
   A There is increased capillary permeability
   B There is 'margination' of white blood cells
   C There is rouleaux formation near the centre of the capillaries
   D The exudate may include globulins
   E Bradykinin is released

2. In chronic inflammation:
   A The cells are mostly polymorphonuclear
   B There is associated proliferation of new capillaries
   C Macrophages may form multinuclear giant cells
   D This does not occur as a result of fungal infection
   E There may be a preceding episode of acute inflammation

3. Granulomata may be found in:
   A Hypersensitivity reactions
   B Parasitic infestations
   C Sarcoidosis
   D Primary biliary cirrhosis
   E Crohn's disease

4. Wound healing by regeneration invariably occurs:
   A In the liver
   B In the small intestine
   C In the renal tubular epithelium
   D In the neuronal system
   E In the thyroid

5. Wound healing by organization usually occurs in:
   A The epidermis
   B Infarcts
   C Thrombi
   D Fibrinous inflammatory exudate
   E Chronic inflammation

6. Wound healing is delayed by deficiency:
   A Of vitamin D
   B Of zinc
   C Of calcium
   D Of sulphur-containing amino acids
   E Of glucocorticosteroid hormones

7. Surface epithelium gives rise to:
   A Papillomas
   B Cystadenomas

   C Choriocarcinoma
   D Meningiomas
   E Nephroblastoma

8. Cell injury and death:
   A Cell death is a normal component of embryonic development
   B Necrosis usually affects single cells within a tissue
   C Necrosis is characterized by marked cell swelling and membrane rupture
   D Necrosis is not usually associated with an inflammatory response
   E Apoptosis is mediated by activation of specific intracellular enzyme pathways

9. Tissue response to injury:
   A Acute inflammation results in local vasodilation, increased vascular permeability, and release of mediators
   B The primary inflammatory cell mediator of chronic inflammation is the neutrophil
   C Granuloma formation is a normal component of wound healing
   D Macrophages are not normally present following tissue damage
   E Macrophages are important in granuloma formation

10. Tissue growth and differentiation:
    A Hyperplasia represents an increase in the size of cells in a tissue or organ
    B Atrophy is always pathological
    C Metaplasia represents premalignant abnormality of an epithelium
    D All tumours are not neoplasms
    E Malignant tumours may be primary or secondary

11. Neoplasms:
    A Benign neoplasms do not usually exhibit locally destructive infiltration
    B Malignant neoplasms have the ability to metastasize
    C Carcinomas are malignant mesenchymal neoplasms
    D Staging systems are based on histopathological characteristics
    E Cytological features of malignancy include abnormal nuclear shape and size

12. Gynaecological tumours:
    A Vulval adenocarcinoma represents 90% of malignancies at this site

B Embryonal rhabdomyosarcoma may occur in the vagina

C The cervical transformation zone represents epithelial metaplasia

D Preinvasive abnormalities of cervical epithelium only show minimal local invasion beyond the basement membrane

E Adenocarcinoma may affect the cervix

13. Gynaecological tumours:

   A Endometrial adenocarcinoma may demonstrate a serous morphology

   B Endometrial adenocarcinoma may precede atypical hyperplasia

   C Mesenchymal tumours of the myometrium are common

   D Ovarian carcinoma is the commonest malignant ovarian neoplasm

   E Ovarian germ cell tumours may be benign or malignant

14. Miscarriage:

   A Chromosomal abnormality may be associated with miscarriage

   B Ascending genital tract infection is a common cause of first-trimester miscarriage

   C Defective trophoblast invasion may be associated with first-trimester miscarriage

   D Chorioamnionitis may lead to second-trimester miscarriage

   E Pathological examination of products of conception usually reveals the aetiology of the miscarriage

15. Gestational trophoblastic neoplasia:

   A Hydatidiform moles of all types demonstrate abnormal trophoblast proliferation

   B Partial moles are usually digynic triploidy

   C Complete moles are androgenetic

   D Complete moles do not demonstrate abnormal imprinting

   E Partial mole is a risk factor for development of persistent trophoblastic disease such as choriocarcinoma

16. Congenital anomalies:

   A Malformations are morphological defects of an organ or region of the body as a consequence of extrinsic interference with a developmental process

   B Deformations are abnormalities secondary to mechanical forces

   C May occur during blastogenesis

D An anomaly sequence represents a pattern of multiple abnormalities derived from a single underlying factor

E An association is a non-random occurrence of multiple morphological abnormalities not identified as a sequence or syndrome

17. Placental pathology:

   A Defective trophoblastic invasion of decidual and uterine vessels is associated with pre-eclampsia

   B Defective trophoblastic invasion of decidual and uterine vessels is associated with intrauterine growth restriction

   C Defective trophoblastic invasion of decidual and uterine vessels is the morphological association of abnormal uterine artery Doppler indices

   D In intrauterine growth restriction, the umbilical arteries usually show reduced resistance to flow as a consequence of vasodilation

   E Ascending genital tract infection is associated with chorioamnionitis

18. Regarding placental pathology, match the correct response:

   A Complete hydatidiform mole

   B Choriocarcinoma

   C Chorioamnionitis

   D Partial hydatidiform mole

   E Pre-eclampsia

   F Intrauterine growth restriction

   G Miscarriage

   H Stem vessel thrombosis

   I Massive perivillous fibrin deposition

   J Chronic villitis

18.1 A 40-year-old woman presents with persistent vaginal bleeding 8 weeks post-miscarriage. Histopathological review of the products of conception from the miscarriage reveals a diagnostic abnormality of all the chorionic villi. The serum hCG is raised.

18.2 A 25-year-old woman presents at 21 weeks of gestation with vaginal discharge and pre-term premature rupture of membranes. Delivery ensues and histopathological examination of the placenta reveals numerous polymorphs within the fetal membranes.

18.3 The placenta from a 29-year-old woman is examined following induced delivery for fetal distress at 32 weeks of gestation and maternal proteinuria, and demonstrates multiple placental infarcts and villus features suggesting significant reduction in uteroplacental blood flow.

19. Regarding pathology of neoplasia, match the correct response:

 A Leiomyoma
 B Endometrioid adenocarcinoma
 C Clear cell adenocarcinoma
 D Invasive squamous cell carcinoma
 E Embryonal rhabdomyosarcoma
 F Mature teratoma
 G Cervical intraepithelial neoplasia (CIN)
 H Serous cystadenocarcinoma
 I Atypical complex hyperplasia
 J Leiomyosarcoma

19.1 A 63-year-old obese woman presents with postmenopausal bleeding. Imaging demonstrates an irregular mass at the fundus of the uterus. At hysterectomy, a malignant neoplasm is diagnosed which is invading the myometrium.

19.2 An 80-year-old woman presents with an ulcerating lesion of the labia majora. On examination, there is an inguinal lymphadenopathy in addition to a labial lesion. A biopsy demonstrates a malignant tumour.

19.3 A 29-year-old woman attends for a routine cervical smear test and an abnormal result is noted, but the specimen is unsuitable for further grading. A colposcopy is carried out which demonstrates a macroscopically normal cervix with an area of apparent thickening at the transformation zone. A biopsy is carried out which does not reveal invasive malignancy.

Answers

1.	A	T		7.	A	T		13.	A	T
	B	T			B	F			B	F
	C	T			C	F			C	T
	D	T			D	F			D	T
	E	T			E	F			E	T
2.	A	F		8.	A	T		14.	A	T
	B	T			B	F			B	F
	C	T			C	T			C	T
	D	F			D	F			D	T
	E	T			E	T			E	F
3.	A	T		9.	A	T		15.	A	T
	B	T			B	F			B	F
	C	T			C	F			C	T
	D	T			D	F			D	F
	E	T			E	T			E	T
4.	A	F		10.	A	F		16.	A	F
	B	T			B	F			B	T
	C	F			C	F			C	T
	D	F			D	T			D	T
	E	F			E	T			E	T
5.	A	F		11.	A	T		17.	A	T
	B	T			B	T			B	T
	C	T			C	F			C	T
	D	T			D	F			D	F
	E	T			E	T			E	T
6.	A	F		12.	A	F				
	B	T			B	T				
	C	F			C	T				
	D	T			D	F				
	E	F			E	T				

18.1 A Complete hydatidiform mole
18.2 C Chorioamnionitis
18.3 E Pre-eclampsia
19.1 B Endometrial adenocarcinoma
19.2 D Invasive squamous cell carcinoma
19.3 G Cervical intraepithelial neoplasia (CIN)

Microbiology and virology

Questions

1. Bacteria:
   - **A** Are eukaryotic
   - **B** All have a cytoplasmic membrane
   - **C** All have cell walls
   - **D** All have pili (fimbriae)
   - **E** All have mitochondria

2. *Staphylococcus*:
   - **A** *aureus* forms long chains
   - **B** *aureus* produces coagulase
   - **C** *epidermidis* is coagulase negative
   - **D** Phage group II produces enterotoxins
   - **E** Phage group III produces impetigo and pemphigus neonatorum

3. *Streptococcus* spp.:
   - **A** May be classified on cell wall C-carbohydrate antigens
   - **B** May produce endotoxins
   - **C** May produce haemolysins
   - **D** The majority of dangerous strains are group B, β-haemolytic
   - **E** *S. pneumoniae* may cause peritonitis

4. *Corynebacterium* spp.:
   - **A** Show Chinese lettering on staining
   - **B** Contain many commensal bacteria
   - **C** Infection with C. *diphtheriae* can be shown by the Schick test
   - **D** Are Gram-positive
   - **E** Are sporing

5. *Clostridium* spp.:
   - **A** Produce endotoxins
   - **B** Are Gram-positive
   - **C** Are anaerobes
   - **D** Bear spores
   - **E** Are obligate intracellular bacteria

6. *Clostridium perfringens*:
   - **A** Type A may cause gas gangrene
   - **B** Is a normal commensal in the large bowel of humans
   - **C** Is sensitive to metronidazole
   - **D** May cause food poisoning
   - **E** Is identified by the Nagler reaction

7. *Clostridium tetani*:
   - **A** Produces an exotoxin: tetanospasmin
   - **B** May be found in the gut
   - **C** May infect the fetus via the vagina
   - **D** Neurotoxin interferes with the action of the lower motor neurone
   - **E** Is an obligate anaerobe

8. *Neisseria* spp.:
   - **A** Include a number of normal commensals
   - **B** *N. gonorrhoeae* are free-living bean-shaped diplococci
   - **C** *N. gonorrhoeae* may be isolatable from asymptomatic carriers
   - **D** *N. gonorrhoeae* infection is diagnosed by a high vaginal swab
   - **E** Stain pink on Gram's stain

9. Gram-negative bacteria:
   - **A** *Pseudomonas* is a facultative anaerobe
   - **B** *Klebsiella* is an obligate aerobe
   - **C** *Bacteroides* is an obligate anaerobe
   - **D** Produce lipopolysaccharide endotoxins
   - **E** Drug resistance is due to penicillinase production

10. The normal vaginal flora may include:
    - **A** *Chlamydia trachomatis*
    - **B** *Clostridium perfringens (welchii)*
    - **C** *Bacteroides*
    - **D** *Fusobacterium* spp.
    - **E** Human papilloma virus

11. *Actinomyces* spp.:
    - **A** Are Gram-negative
    - **B** Have acid-fast filaments
    - **C** *A. israelii* is a normal commensal
    - **D** Are sensitive to penicillin
    - **E** May colonize an intrauterine contraceptive device

12. The spirochaetes:
    - **A** *T. pallidum* can be visualized by Giemsa staining
    - **B** *T. pallidum* may be identified by tissue culture
    - **C** *Borrelia* causes undulant fever
    - **D** *Leptospira* causes chancroid
    - **E** Are motile by axial filament

13. Syphilis serology:
    - **A** The Reagin tests depend upon antibody reaction with cardiolipin
    - **B** Cardiolipin is also used in VDRL and WR tests

C The TPHA test makes use of immune fluorescence

D Reagin tests remain positive many years after effective therapy

E FTA-ABS becomes positive earlier in the disease than TPHA

14. False-positive Reagin tests may arise in:
    A Malaria
    B Infectious hepatitis
    C Pregnancy
    D Tuberculosis
    E Rheumatoid arthritis

15. *Chlamydia*:
    A Have cell walls
    B Multiply by binary fission
    C Cause granuloma inguinale
    D Infection results in the formation of cold agglutinins
    E Have ribosomes

16. *Mycoplasma*:
    A May cause pelvic inflammatory disease
    B Are sensitive to penicillin
    C Have cell walls
    D Are obligate intracellular parasites
    E Cause spotted fever

17. Viruses:
    A The capsid is a lipoprotein envelope
    B Herpesvirus is associated with an intranuclear inclusion body
    C Contain a number of capsomeres in the capsid
    D Can be cultivated in appropriate cell cultures
    E Can be identified by polymerase chain reaction

18. The herpesvirus group includes:
    A Papilloma virus
    B Rubella virus
    C Varicella-zoster virus
    D Cytomegalovirus
    E Epstein–Barr virus

19. The following viruses contain DNA:
    A Rubella
    B Measles
    C Mumps
    D Papilloma
    E Parvovirus B19

20. Cytomegalovirus:
    A May cause pneumonitis
    B Is associated with 'owl's eye' inclusion bodies
    C May be transmitted to the fetus transplacentally
    D May be transmitted to the fetus in the birth canal
    E May be transmitted in breast milk

21. *Candida albicans*:
    A Is dimorphic
    B May cause paronychia
    C May be found as a normal commensal in the vagina
    D May cause septicaemia
    E Has Gram-negative pseudohyphae

22. *Trichomonas vaginalis*:
    A Has eight flagella
    B Has two nuclei
    C Forms cysts
    D Has a sexual cycle completed in the cat
    E Has a sucking disc

23. HCV
    A HCV has a characteristic structure by electron microscopy
    B Quantitative HCV PCR is used for monitoring therapy
    C In the UK the risk of transmission from HCV viraemic mothers to infants is <1%
    D Vertical transmission is increased five-fold if the mother is co-infected with HIV
    E Tests for HCV antibody are part of the standard antenatal screen

24. HIV
    A Tests for HIV antibody are offered as part of antenatal screening
    B HIV type 2 is transmitted transplacentally far less frequently than HIV type 1
    C HIV antiretroviral treatment during pregnancy has reduced the rate of HIV transmission
    D Serological techniques are used for monitoring HIV disease in infancy
    E HIV is an RNA retrovirus

25. HBV
    A Presence of anti-HBe indicates an increased risk of transmission
    B Anti HBs levels >100 IU/L designate a good post-vaccine response

C Hepatitis B immunoglobulin is given at birth to babies of HBeAg-positive mothers

D Mother to child transmission of HBV accounts for up to 50% of carriers

E Hepatitis vaccine is given to the infants of HBV carriers at birth, 1 month, 2 months and 12 months

26. *Toxoplasma gondii*

A The normal host of *T. gondii* is the cat

B Antenatal screening tests always include *T. gondii* serology

C Specific IgM indicates recent infection with the organism

D Infection in the early stages of pregnancy may result in disseminated toxoplasma infection

E Cat faeces in litter trays or in the garden are to be avoided throughout pregnancy

27. Varicella-zoster virus (VZV)

A VZV is a herpesvirus

B Immunity can be identified by the detection of specific IgG

C VZV-specific immunoglobulin should be given to susceptible pregnant women in contact with an index case

D Infection gives rise to a persistent infection which can give rise to zoster infection in later life

E Electron microscopy can distinguish between different herpesviruses

28. Viruses which may infect or damage the fetus:

A Cytomegalovirus
B Hepatitis C
C Hepatitis B
D HIV-1
E HIV-2
F Parvovirus B19
G Rubella
H Varicella
I Herpes simplex
J Poliovirus

28.1 A rubella-like rash develops following contact with a child with a 'slap-face' appearance. The fetus is infected in about 33% of cases, and in about 10% of these spontaneous abortion may occur, usually in the second trimester.

28.2 Vaccination and specific immunoglobulin are required for babies born to mothers with infection and e markers, whereas vaccination alone is advised for those born to infected mothers who have antibody to e.

28.3 High carriage rates are detected in injecting drug users but neonatal transmission in the UK is around 6% from mothers who have been shown to be viraemic using quantitative molecular methods.

29. Laboratory methods:

A Direct light microscopy
B Electron microscopy
C Immunofluorescence microscopy
D Bacterial culture
E Detection of specific IgG
F Detection of specific IgM
G Qualitative molecular detection
H Quantitative molecular detection
I Viral culture
J Fungal culture

29.1 A child born to an HIV-infected mother develops pneumonitis. Which routine rapid laboratory method is used to detect *Pneumocystis* in a bronchiolar lavage?

29.2 A mother in contact with chickenpox is unaware of any past history of varicella. Which laboratory method should be used to detect immunity so that VZIG can be given if required?

29.3 Primary maternal cytomegalovirus infection may result in fetal infection. Which laboratory test should be used initially to confirm infection in the mother?

Answers

1.	A	F
	B	T
	C	F
	D	F
	E	F
2.	A	F
	B	T
	C	T
	D	F
	E	F
3.	A	T
	B	F
	C	T
	D	F
	E	T
4.	A	T
	B	T
	C	F
	D	T
	E	F
5.	A	F
	B	T
	C	F
	D	T
	E	F
6.	A	T
	B	T
	C	T
	D	T
	E	T
7.	A	T
	B	T
	C	F
	D	F
	E	T
8.	A	T
	B	F
	C	T
	D	F
	E	T

9.	A	F
	B	F
	C	T
	D	T
	E	T
10.	A	F
	B	T
	C	T
	D	T
	E	F
11.	A	F
	B	F
	C	T
	D	T
	E	T
12.	A	T
	B	F
	C	T
	D	F
	E	T
13.	A	T
	B	T
	C	F
	D	F
	E	T
14.	A	T
	B	T
	C	T
	D	T
	E	T
15.	A	T
	B	T
	C	F
	D	F
	E	T
16.	A	T
	B	F
	C	F
	D	F
	E	F

17.	A	F
	B	T
	C	T
	D	T
	E	T
18.	A	F
	B	F
	C	T
	D	T
	E	T
19.	A	F
	B	F
	C	F
	D	T
	E	T
20.	A	T
	B	T
	C	T
	D	T
	E	T
21.	A	T
	B	T
	C	T
	D	T
	E	F
22.	A	F
	B	F
	C	F
	D	F
	E	F
23.	A	F
	B	T
	C	F
	D	T
	E	F
24.	A	T
	B	T
	C	T
	D	F
	E	T

25.	A	F
	B	T
	C	T
	D	T
	E	T
26.	A	T
	B	F
	C	T
	D	T
	E	T
27.	A	T
	B	T
	C	T
	D	T
	E	F

28.1 F Parvovirus B19
28.2 C Hepatitis B
28.3 B Hepatitis C
29.1 C Immuno-fluorescence microscopy
29.2 E Detection of specific IgG
29.3 F Detection of specific IgM

Immunology

Questions

1. Antibodies:
   - **A** Recognize antigen in the context of MHC class II molecules
   - **B** Are formed of four polypeptide chains
   - **C** Can direct complement components to pathogens
   - **D** Can be transported across the placenta
   - **E** Target NK cells to kill their targets

2. T cells:
   - **A** Are directly activated by pathogens
   - **B** Recognize intact protein antigens on the surface of cells
   - **C** Can secrete reactive oxygen species to kill bacteria
   - **D** Regulate immune responses by secreting cytokines
   - **E** Kill cells that do not express MHC class I molecules

3. The innate immune system:
   - **A** Has a memory of what antigens it has seen before
   - **B** Includes cells that recognize common molecules on pathogen surfaces
   - **C** Interacts and instructs the adaptive immune response
   - **D** Is involved in placentation
   - **E** Secretes antibody molecules

4. Regulation of the immune system:
   - **A** Involves the recognition of danger signals by dendritic cells
   - **B** Can include the degradation of amino acids by cells
   - **C** Involves upregulation of co-stimulatory molecules by dendritic cells
   - **D** Results in immunosuppression in the pregnant woman
   - **E** Alters the nature of the immune response dependent on the situation

5. The fetal allograft normally:
   - **A** Is not rejected because it does not express any foreign antigens
   - **B** Induces a Th1 type response in the maternal immune system
   - **C** Induces apoptosis in infiltrating lymphocytes via CD95L interactions

   - **D** Induces tolerance to itself by deletion of T cells in the thymus
   - **E** Prevents NK cell rejection by expression of HLA-G

6. Maternal antibodies:
   - **A** Can cause autoimmune diseases in the fetus
   - **B** Passively diffuse from the maternal to the fetal circulation
   - **C** Destroy the trophoblast cells via a complement-dependent mechanism
   - **D** Are transferred to the newborn child as IgM antibodies in the milk
   - **E** Provide protection from infection to the newborn child

7. Danger signals:
   - **A** Downregulate immune responses when they are causing damage to the host organism
   - **B** Result in upregulation of co-stimulatory molecules on dendritic cells
   - **C** Can be caused by surgery
   - **D** Are never seen in people who are tolerant to antigen
   - **E** Involve the recognition of pathogen-derived peptides in the context of MHC class I molecules

8. Cells:
   - **A** T lymphocyte
   - **B** B lymphocyte
   - **C** NK cell
   - **D** Neutrophil
   - **E** Dendritic cell
   - **F** Macrophage
   - **G** Endothelial cell
   - **H** Erythrocyte
   - **I** Syncytiotrophoblast
   - **J** Th1 cell

8.1 The expression of indoleamine dioxygenase and HLA-G protects this cell from immune attack.

8.2 This cell recognizes antigen in the form of peptide in the context of molecules of the major histocompatibility complex.

8.3 This cell integrates signals from pathogens and damaged cells in order to initiate immune responses.

9. Molecules of the immune system

   A IgM

   B IgA

   C IgG

   D IL2

   E IL4

   F Tryptophan

   G MHC class I

   H HLA-G

   I FcRn

   J T cell receptor

9.1 The following cytokine is secreted by Th2 cells.

9.2 This molecule transports IgG through cells, and is involved in the transport of IgG from the maternal circulation to the fetus.

9.3 This molecule is produced by B cells early in the immune response.

Answers

1.	A	F		C	T		D	F		D	F
	B	T		D	T		E	T		E	F
	C	T		E	F	6.	A	T			
	D	T	4.	A	T		B	F	8.1	I	Syncytio-trophoblast
	E	T		B	T		C	F	8.2	A	T lymphocyte
2.	A	F		C	T		D	F	8.3	E	Dendritic cell
	B	F		D	F		E	T	9.1	E	IL-4
	C	F		E	T	7.	A	F	9.2	H	I FcRn
	D	T	5.	A	F		B	T	9.3	A	IgM
	E	F		B	F		C	T			
3.	A	F		C	T						
	B	T									

Biochemistry

Question

1. Proteins:
  A The amino acids are always of the D-configuration
  B Most proteins contain between 10 000 and 100 000 amino acid residues
  C Proteins are usually 60% nitrogen
  D In gel filtration large molecules emerge first
  E The way in which protein chains link together is called the quaternary structure

2. Proteins:
  A Haemoglobin changes shape markedly as it functions physiologically
  B There are over 30 different amino acids found in proteins
  C Disulphide bridges occur between glutamine residues
  D The most common type of bond in proteins is the salt bond between acidic and basic amino acids
  E Lipoproteins are not produced by humans

3. Nutrition:
  A During pregnancy an extra 6 g of protein is required daily
  B During lactation an extra 30 g of protein is required daily
  C Protein may be found in potatoes
  D Phenylalanine is an essential amino acid
  E Vegetable protein contains all the essential amino acids

4. Nutrition:
  A Peptidase acts in the stomach
  B Amino acids are absorbed by passive transport
  C Nitrogenous compounds may be excreted in sweat
  D Vitamin K is found in egg yolk
  E Milk increases absorption of iron

5. In carbohydrate metabolism:
  A Insulin is a glycoprotein
  B Human placental lactogen is a steroid hormone
  C Galactose is a pentose monosaccharide
  D Disaccharidases are found in the intestinal lumen
  E Saliva assists absorption of complete carbohydrates

6. In fat metabolism:
  A The action of lipase results in the hydrolysis of fats
  B Chylomicrons contain protein
  C Fatty acids are converted to esters of coenzyme A
  D Animals can convert fatty acids to glucose
  E Fatty acids are synthesized and degraded by different pathways

7. In glycolysis:
  A In anaerobic glycolysis, three molecules of lactate are produced
  B In aerobic glycolysis the end product is acetaldehyde
  C Acetaldehyde undergoes decarboxylation to acetyl-CoA
  D In glycolysis there is a net gain of two ATP molecules
  E Glycogen is the primary source of substrate

8. The following hormones lower the blood sugar:
  A Adrenaline
  B Insulin
  C Glucagon
  D Thyroxine
  E Growth hormone

9. Ketone bodies:
  A Ketone bodies arise from acetyl-CoA
  B Beta-hydroxybutyric acid is a ketone body
  C The liver is the major site of manufacture of acetoacetate
  D Heart muscle metabolizes acetoacetone in preference to glucose
  E The brain cannot utilize acetoacetone to any major degree for its metabolic needs

10. In the tricarboxylic acid (TCA) cycle:
  A Acetyl-CoA condenses with succinate
  B Six pairs of hydrogen atoms are made available
  C Each pair of hydrogen atoms yields three molecules of ATP
  D A six-carbon glucose molecule yields 48 ATPs in total
  E Oxidative phosphorylation results in carbon dioxide and water

11. Enzymes:
  A Increase reaction velocity
  B In a high salt concentration the solubility of enzymes is high
  C In chromatography, acidic enzymes are retained by a positively ionized field

   D Co-enzymes are non-proteins

   E Adenosine triphosphate (ATP) is a co-enzyme

12. Active transport:
   A Takes place in the kidney
   B Takes place in the placenta
   C Takes place in the liver
   D Takes place in the red blood cell
   E Of glucose requires Na^+ to move across the cell membrane in the opposite direction

13. In competitive inhibition of enzyme action:
   A The V_{max} is increased
   B The K_m is decreased
   C There is direct competition between the substrate and inhibitor
   D K_m is a measure of how tightly a substance binds to enzyme
   E Competitive inhibitors typically bear a structural similarity to substrate

14. A paracrine effects results when:
   A A cell releases a hormone which acts on that same cell
   B A cell releases a hormone which has effects on cells of a different type
   C A cell fuses with another cell of the same type
   D A cell fuses with another cell of a different type
   E A nerve cell releases a neurotransmitter

15. Eicosanoid synthesis:
   A Prostaglandins are synthesized in the cell nucleus
   B Eicosanoids are mostly synthesized from arachidonic acid
   C Aspirin inhibits platelet thromboxane synthesis
   D During labour, fetal membranes are the main site of prostaglandin production
   E COX-2 is not inducible

16. Cell signalling:
   A Gap junctions prevent electrical coupling between cells
   B In myometrium gap junction numbers decline at labour
   C Nitric oxide release is increased in response to shear stress
   D Nitric oxide is a vasoconstrictor
   E Nitric oxide is produced in the placenta

17. Calcium signalling:
   A Calcium concentrations are higher inside a cell than outside
   B The endoplasmic reticulum stores calcium
   C Calmodulin mediates many calcium-regulated processes
   D Calcium signalling is not used by nerve cells
   E Calcium signalling is used by smooth muscle cells

18. Hormones:
   A Neurotransmitters are water soluble
   B Water-soluble hormones can cross the plasma membrane
   C Steroid hormones are water soluble
   D Steroid hormones are degraded within seconds in blood
   E Progesterone can cross the plasma membrane

19. Enzymes:
   A Phosphodiesterases destroy cAMP
   B Guanylate cyclase produces cAMP
   C Adrenaline binding to α-adrenergic receptors activates adenylate cyclase
   D Adrenaline binding to β_2-adrenergic receptors activates adenylate cyclase
   E Atrial natriuretic peptide increases cGMP

Answers

1.	**A**	F	**6.**	**A**	T	**11.**	**A**	T	**16.**	**A**	F
	B	F		**B**	T		**B**	F		**B**	T
	C	F		**C**	T		**C**	T		**C**	T
	D	T		**D**	T		**D**	T		**D**	F
	E	T		**E**	T		**E**	T		**E**	T
2.	**A**	T	**7.**	**A**	F	**12.**	**A**	T	**17.**	**A**	F
	B	F		**B**	F		**B**	T		**B**	T
	C	F		**C**	F		**C**	F		**C**	T
	D	F		**D**	T		**D**	T		**D**	F
	E	F		**E**	F		**E**	F		**E**	T
3.	**A**	T	**8.**	**A**	F	**13.**	**A**	F	**18.**	**A**	T
	B	T		**B**	T		**B**	F		**B**	F
	C	T		**C**	F		**C**	T		**C**	F
	D	T		**D**	F		**D**	F		**D**	F
	E	F		**E**	F		**E**	T		**E**	T
4.	**A**	F	**9.**	**A**	T	**14.**	**A**	T	**19.**	**A**	T
	B	F		**B**	T		**B**	F		**B**	F
	C	T		**C**	T		**C**	F		**C**	T
	D	T		**D**	T		**D**	F		**D**	F
	E	F		**E**	T		**E**	F		**E**	T
5.	**A**	F	**10.**	**A**	F	**15.**	**A**	F			
	B	F		**B**	F		**B**	T			
	C	F		**C**	T		**C**	T			
	D	T		**D**	F		**D**	T			
	E	F		**E**	T		**E**	F			

Physiology

Questions

1. Given the atomic weights Na^+ 23, Cl^- 35.5 and Ca^{++} 40, the following statements are true:
   - **A** 1 mole of Na^+ is 46 g
   - **B** 1 mole of NaCl is 58.5 g
   - **C** A normal (molar) solution of NaCl contains 117 g of NaCl
   - **D** The concentration of NaCl in a physiologically 'normal' solution is 6%
   - **E** 1 equivalent of Ca^{++} is 20 g

2. In a normal man weighing 70 kg:
   - **A** 40% of the weight is composed of water
   - **B** 30% of the weight is composed of protein
   - **C** Two-thirds of the body water is intracellular
   - **D** The total blood volume is about 8 L
   - **E** Minerals make up 0.7% of the body weight

3. The distribution of electrolytes:
   - **A** Na^+ and Mg^{++} are the major intracellular cations
   - **B** Phosphate is the major intracellular anion
   - **C** During pregnancy the plasma osmolarity rises
   - **D** In acidosis there is a decrease in the anion gap
   - **E** The concentration of sodium is more in the interstitial fluid than in the plasma

4. Movement of solute and solvent:
   - **A** Osmosis describes the movement of solute across a semi-permeable membrane
   - **B** The pressure that stops osmosis is the osmotic pressure
   - **C** Osmosis describes the process wherein bulk movement of solvent drags some molecules of solute with it
   - **D** In non-ionized diffusion there is preferential transport of molecules of high molecular weight
   - **E** Phagocytosis involves the use of carrier-mediated transport

5. Acid–base:
   - **A** An acid is a proton acceptor
   - **B** The pH is the $-$logarithm$_{10}$ of the hydrogen ion concentration
   - **C** The pH at which 50% of a buffer is changed from acidic to base form is the pK
   - **D** Bicarbonate is the most important buffer in body fluids

   - **E** Plasma protein has at least 6× the buffering capacity of haemoglobin

6. With a pH of 7.4 (and the logarithm$_{10}$ of 4 to be 0.6):
   - **A** The hydrogen concentration is 0.00004 mmol/L
   - **B** The H^+ concentration is 0.00004 mmol/L
   - **C** Body fluids would be slightly acidic
   - **D** Dissociation of O_2 from haemoglobin is increased compared to a pH of 7
   - **E** The pH of urine would be very low

7. Acid–base:
   - **A** Base excess is negative in metabolic acidosis
   - **B** Excessive sedation may give rise to a respiratory alkalosis
   - **C** In pregnancy there is a respiratory alkalosis
   - **D** Prolonged vomiting may cause a metabolic acidosis
   - **E** Metabolic alkalosis frequently accompanies hypokalaemia

8. Cardiac physiology:
   - **A** The dominant tone of control at the sinoatrial node is parasympathetic
   - **B** Blood in the left side of the heart is 99% saturated with oxygen
   - **C** The 'a'-wave in the JVP trace is due to atrial systole
   - **D** A third heart sound may occur at the time of rapid atrial filling
   - **E** The end-diastolic volume is the 'after-load'

9. In pregnancy:
   - **A** The blood volume increases by 1200–1400 mL
   - **B** The cardiac output continues to increase until the end of the third trimester
   - **C** The heart rate is increased by 40%
   - **D** The arteriovenous oxygen gradient decreases
   - **E** The diastolic blood pressure tends to rise slowly throughout

10. Local control of blood flow:
    - **A** Hypoxia causes vasodilatation
    - **B** Carbon dioxide causes vasoconstriction
    - **C** Adenosine is a vasodilator
    - **D** Hydrogen ions cause vasoconstriction
    - **E** Prostaglandin E is a vasoconstrictor

11. Respiratory physiology:
    - **A** The proportion of oxygen in inspired air is 28%

B The proportion of carbon dioxide in inspired air is 3%

C The partial pressure of oxygen in alveolar air is 158 mmHg

D The physiological dead space is increased in pulmonary oedema

E In normal individuals the anatomic dead space nearly equals the physiological dead space

12. Respiratory physiology:
   A The normal tidal volume is 350 mL/breath
   B Under normal circumstances 45% of oxygen delivered to the peripheral tissues is extracted
   C In normal individuals the FEV_1/FVC ratio is at least 75%
   D Deoxygenated haemoglobin is a better buffer than oxygenated haemoglobin
   E The Bezold–Jarisch reflex results in an increased respiratory rate

13. In pregnancy:
   A The total lung volume increases
   B The residual volume decreases
   C Ventilation increases by 40%
   D The total lung capacity decreases
   E Oxygen consumption increases by 50 mL/min by term

14. In pregnancy:
   A The PCO_2 falls
   B There is a decrease in the sensitivity of the respiratory centre to CO_2
   C Respiratory rate increases due to the effect of progesterone
   D Total increase in respiration is 60%
   E Residual volume increases by 200 mL

15. In the neonate:
   A Respiratory distress syndrome (RDS) is due to the absence of type 2 pneumocytes
   B The tidal volume is 10 mL/kg
   C RDS may be prevented by administering dexamethasone to a mother in premature labour before 30 weeks of gestation
   D Intraventricular haemorrhage is most common after 4 days of age
   E Congenital heart disease is the commonest fetal abnormality

16. The haemoglobin dissociation curve:
   A The presence of carboxyhaemoglobin shifts the curve to the right

B Acidosis shifts the curve to the left

C Increased temperature shifts the curve to the right

D The Bohr effect helps haemoglobin to unload oxygen

E 2,3-DPG is produced during glycolysis

17. The levels of 2,3-DPG are:
   A Increased by androgens
   B Decreased by thyroxine
   C Increased by anaemia
   D Decreased in banked blood
   E Decreased by living at altitude

18. Carriage of oxygen and carbon dioxide:
   A The presence of haemoglobin increases the oxygen-carrying capacity of blood 70-fold
   B Cyanosis is only seen when the concentration of deoxygenated haemoglobin is more than 5 g/dL
   C Some carbon dioxide is carried by plasma proteins
   D 2/3 of carbon dioxide is carried by haemoglobin
   E In the chloride shift, chloride ions diffuse out of the red blood cell

19. In the kidney:
   A The capillaries of the glomerulus are a portal system
   B The vasa recta supply the loop of Henle
   C 85% of the tubules are juxtamedullary
   D Juxtamedullary tubules have thickened ascending and descending loops of Henle
   E The loop of Henle is concerned with the reabsorption of chloride ions

20. In the kidney:
   A The normal creatinine clearance is about 1.2 L/min
   B There is an increase in renal blood flow during pregnancy
   C The filtration fraction is the glomerular filtration rate/renal blood flow
   D Glucose is absorbed in the distal tubule
   E Amino acids are absorbed in the proximal tubule

21. Sodium is reabsorbed in the following places:
   A Proximal tubule
   B Loop of Henle
   C Distal tubule
   D Collecting duct
   E Ureter

22. In the kidney:
  A Carbonic anhydrase is found in the brush border of the cells of the loop of Henle
  B Potassium is reabsorbed actively in the proximal tubule
  C In the distal tubule the pH is less than 4
  D Hydrogen ions are actively excreted in the proximal tubule and distal tubule
  E Concentration of urine occurs due to the high osmotic pressure of the medulla

23. Antidiuretic hormone:
  A Increases chloride absorption in the loop of Henle
  B Secretion is stimulated by morphine
  C Secretion is stimulated by alcohol
  D Is a glycoprotein
  E Is secreted from the anterior pituitary gland

24. In the kidney:
  A Urea is actively secreted in the distal tubule
  B At low urine flow, 50–70% of filtered urea is excreted
  C Erythropoietin is a glycoprotein
  D Natriuretic peptide is synthesized in the juxtaglomerular apparatus
  E Natriuretic peptide causes sodium retention

25. In pregnancy:
  A The kidneys increased by 2–3 cm in length
  B The renal blood flow remains constant
  C The renal blood flow is decreased in the erect position
  D The serum creatinine remains at pre-pregnancy levels
  E The creatinine clearance rate falls

26. The bladder and micturition:
  A The normal residual volume of the bladder is 0–100 mL
  B The bladder capacity is 350 mL
  C The maximum urethral pressure in the absence of micturition is 50–100 cm H_2O
  D The maximum urine flow rate is 5 mL/s
  E Detrusor sensation is relayed through the sympathetic nervous system

27. The gastrointestinal tract:
  A During pregnancy the rate of gastric emptying is increased
  B Cholecystokinin is produced by the gall bladder

C Gastrin acts on the parietal cells of the stomach
  D Pepsin is produced by the oxyntic cells of the stomach
  E The pH of the stomach is approximately 3

28. In the intestine:
  A Amylase converts glycogen to glucose
  B Cholecystokinin secretion causes the release of pancreatic enzymes
  C Brunner's glands secrete mucus
  D Goblet cells are present in the large bowel
  E Meissner's plexus is submucous

29. Nutrition:
  A The calorific value of protein and carbohydrate is approximately the same
  B The increase in dietary requirement of pregnancy is 20 kcal/day
  C The average dietary intake of carbohydrate is 400 g/day
  D The pregnancy requirements of protein are 1.5–2 g/kg per day
  E Fat is important for the absorption of vitamin C

30. The following are essential amino acids:
  A Arginine
  B Proline
  C Glycine
  D Valine
  E Histidine

31. Vitamins:
  A Vitamin A is water soluble
  B Vitamin A deficiency predisposes to xerophthalmia
  C Vitamin B_1 is teratogenic
  D Pellagra is due to deficiency of vitamin B_2
  E Vitamin B_6 (pyridoxine) is fat soluble

32. Vitamins:
  A Folic acid is stored in the liver
  B Folic acid levels can only be measured in plasma
  C Vitamin C deficiency results in a microcytic anaemia
  D Vitamin B_6 (pyridoxine) deficiency results in a macrocytic anaemia
  E Vitamin D can be found in egg yolk

33. Vitamin D:
  A Is required for calcium absorption from the gut

B Deficiency causes rickets
C Is water soluble
D 1,25-(OH)$_2$-cholecalciferol concentrations are approximately doubled in pregnancy
E Excess causes hypercalcaemia

34. In pregnancy:
A 1.2 mg of calcium is required/day
B 15 mg of iron is required/day
C The requirements of sodium are increased
D The requirements of iodine are the same
E The requirements of potassium are increased

35. In the liver:
A Galactokinase converts galactose into glucose
B Triglycerides are synthesized from fatty acids and glycerol
C Cephalins are lipoproteins
D Urea is formed from four molecules of ammonia
E 95% of the body's globulin is synthesized

36. In urine the following can be found:
A Unconjugated bilirubin
B Conjugated bilirubin
C Urobilinogen
D Stercobilin
E Bilirubin glucuronide

37. Insulin:
A Is a polypeptide with a molecular weight of more than 5000
B Requires magnesium for its crystallization
C Is stored in quantities of up to 250 units at any one time
D Is produced in α-cells
E Is required for entry of glucose into hepatic cells

38. The hypothalamus:
A Is found below the cavernous sinus
B Has posterior boundaries for the mamillary bodies
C Is medial to the tuber cinereum
D In the supraoptic area contains the dorsomedial nuclei
E Is connected to the posterior pituitary by the pituitary portal system

39. The pituitary gland:
A Oxytocin is produced in the paraventricular nucleus of the hypothalamus
B TRH is a decapeptide

C PIF is dopamine
D The superior hypophyseal artery is a branch of the internal carotid artery
E The inferior hypophyseal artery is a branch of the external carotid artery

40. The pituitary:
A The pars intermedia is derived from the posterior pituitary
B The pituitary gland lies medial to the cavernous sinus
C Prolactin is secreted by the posterior pituitary
D The α unit is the same in all pituitary glycoproteins
E Hypoglycaemia inhibits the release of growth hormone

41. Prolactin secretion is stimulated by:
A Dopamine
B TRF
C Diazepam
D Coitus
E Venepuncture

42. Posterior pituitary:
A Vasopressin is a nonapeptide
B Oxytocin sensitivity of the uterus varies with gestation
C Oxytocinase is found in the uterus
D Oestrogen prevents the action of oxytocin on the breast alveoli
E Oxytocin stimulates production of milk by the alveoli

43. In the menstrual cycle:
A The discus proligerus is found outside the granulosa cells
B Subnuclear vacuole formation occurs in the proliferative phase
C As the cycle proceeds the spiral arteries become less coiled
D Arborization of the cervical mucus can be seen at the time of ovulation
E When progesterone is present a vaginal slide shows large numbers of superficial cells

44. Steroid hormones:
A Before passing into the nucleus a steroid hormone binds to a cytosol receptor
B Androgens are excreted in the urine as 17-oxo steroids
C Ovulation occurs 6 h after the LH peak

D Maximum progesterone levels occur 5 days after the LH peak

E Progesterone is secreted by the testis

45. Gonadotrophins:

A FSH controls the formation of androgen-binding protein in Sertoli cells

B Inhibin stimulates the secretion of GnRH

C The LH surge is in response to the feedback of oestrogen

D Testosterone secretion is controlled by FSH

E Gonadotrophin LH is secreted in 14-min pulses

46. At puberty:

A Generally pubic hair appears after the initiation of breast growth

B At menarche the uterine:cervical ratio is 1:1

C The age of menarche is unrelated to the standard of living

D The earliest changes in puberty are increased adrenal androgens

E The pituitary and hypothalamus become less sensitive to negative feedback

47. After the menopause:

A FSH levels remain high for longer than 2–4 years

B The urinary calcium creatinine ratio slowly falls

C Ovarian follicles do not respond to pituitary stimulation

D LH is increased

E Urinary PO_4^{-3}: creatinine ratio is raised

48. Steroid hormones:

A Are all synthesized from cholesterol

B DHAS is a substrate for oestriol

C ACTH stimulates the secretion of aldosterone

D Corticosteroid metabolites are 17-oxo steroids

E Cortisol secretion shows diurnal variation

49. Adrenaline:

A Has VMA as its principal metabolite

B Stimulates insulin release

C Stimulates glycogen formation

D Increases cyclic AMP levels in the liver

E Is the principal catecholamine affecting the heart

50. Thyroid hormones:

A T_3 is more potent than T_4

B Iodine is better absorbed from the gut as iodine

C Reverse T_3 is more potent than T_3

D Carbimazole prevents conversion of iodide to iodine

E Large doses of iodine suppress thyroid activity

51. Thyroid:

A Iodine-131 may cause fetal hypothyroidism

B In pregnancy plasma levels of iodide rise

C The fetal thyroid glands are inactive until the third trimester

D Carbimazole does not cross the placenta

E Carbimazole is safe for breastfeeding

52. Calcium metabolism in pregnancy:

A Fetal calcium levels are less than maternal

B Parathyroid hormone crosses the placenta by active transport

C Vitamin D_3 crosses the placenta via a binding protein

D The levels of parathyroid hormone increase in pregnancy

E In pregnancy there is an increased turnover of vitamin D

53. Somatic nervous system:

A Efferent fibres pass through the ventral roots of the spinal cord

B 20% of the descending fibres of the motor cortex lie in the lateral corticospinal tract

C Pain and temperature ascend in the lateral spinothalamic tract

D Efferent fibres synapse in the substantia gelatinosa

E Fibres for proprioception ascend in dorsal columns to the medulla

54. The autonomic nervous system:

A Parasympathetic outflow is via cranial nerves IV, VIII and IX

B Sympathetic nerves pass through the grey rami communicantes to the collateral ganglia

C Preganglionic sympathetic fibres run all the way to the uterus

D Atropine blocks transmission at parasympathetic ganglia

E Atropine blocks transmission at sympathetic ganglia

55. The autonomic nervous system:
- **A** Sympathetic neurones to sweat glands are cholinergic
- **B** Sympathetic neurones to vasodilatory smooth muscle are nicotinic
- **C** Phenylephrine is a β-agonist
- **D** β-sympathetic agonists stimulate the uterus
- **E** Labetalol is a β-blocker

56. Iron:
- **A** The fetus derives its iron mainly in the last 4 weeks of pregnancy
- **B** Iron in eggs is well absorbed
- **C** Tea enhances the absorption of iron
- **D** In pregnancy the percentage saturation of the total iron-binding capacity increases
- **E** Ferritin is a high molecular weight lipoprotein

57. Iron:
- **A** Haemoglobin comprises less than 15% of total body iron
- **B** Aggregates of transferrin form haemosiderin
- **C** The total iron body content of the adult female is about 38 mg/kg
- **D** Iron is best absorbed in the ferrous form
- **E** Haem iron is more effectively absorbed than non-haem iron

58. Iron:
- **A** The red blood cell's lifespan is 70 days
- **B** In iron deficiency anaemia, microcytosis appears before hypochromia
- **C** A normal diet contains 40 mg/day
- **D** Is absorbed in the terminal small bowel
- **E** Parenteral iron is more effective than oral iron in correcting severe anaemia

59. Coagulation:
- **A** Prostacyclin prevents platelet adhesion
- **B** Prostacyclin synthetase is found in highest concentrations in the lamina externa of the blood vessels
- **C** Prostacyclin production is increased in pre-eclampsia
- **D** Low platelet count may be associated with intrauterine growth restriction
- **E** Adenosine diphosphate stimulates aggregation of platelets

60. Coagulation:
- **A** Thromboplastin activates the intrinsic system
- **B** The intrinsic pathway is quicker than the extrinsic pathway
- **C** Anti-thrombin III is an α_2-globulin
- **D** In pregnancy factors XI and XII are increased
- **E** Heparin potentiates the action of anti-Xa

61. Fibrinolysis:
- **A** Plasminogen activator is found in raised concentrations in the placenta
- **B** ε-aminocaproic acid stimulates plasminogen activator
- **C** Streptokinase stimulates plasminogen activator
- **D** Plasma fibrinolytic activity returns to normal within 1 h of placental delivery
- **E** The placenta contains inhibitors which block fibrinolysis

62. Disseminated intravascular coagulation may result from:
- **A** Pre-eclampsia
- **B** Factor VIII deficiency
- **C** Idiopathic thrombocytopenic purpura
- **D** Amniotic fluid embolism
- **E** Abruptio placentae

63. Rhesus incompatibility:
- **A** There are three Rhesus antigens
- **B** ABO antibodies are IgG
- **C** In haemolytic disease of the newborn, the haemolytic process is maximal at the time of birth in liveborn infants
- **D** Severe Rhesus sensitization causes recurrent first-trimester abortions
- **E** Causes hydrops fetalis

64. The gastrointestinal tract:
- **A** During pregnancy the rate of gastric emptying is increased
- **B** Cholecystokinin is produced by the gall bladder
- **C** Gastrin acts on the parietal cells of the stomach
- **D** Pepsin is produced by the oxyntic cells of the stomach
- **E** The pH of the stomach is approximately 3

65. In the intestine:
- **A** Amylase converts glycogen to glucose
- **B** Cholecystokinin secretion causes the release of pancreatic enzymes
- **C** Brunner's glands secrete mucus
- **D** Goblet cells are present in the large bowel
- **E** Meissner's plexus is submucous

66. Choose the *single* most appropriate option:

A Administer metoclopramide to speed gastric emptying

B Administer cimetidine

C Administer omeprazole

D Administer metoclopramide to delay gastric emptying

E The operation should be delayed until properly starved

F Administer aspirin

G Immediate caesarean section and transfer baby to the neonatal unit

H Recommend a general anaesthetic

I Reassurance

J Separate mother and baby after delivery

K Transfer to ITU postoperatively

L Treat with antibiotics

66.1 A 26-year-old para 0 has a BMI of 30 kg/m^2 and is having an emergency caesarean section for failure to progress. She last ate 5 h ago. To reduce the risk of aspiration pneumonia what advise should be given?

66.2 A 32-year-old nulliparous woman has taken ranitidine for gastro-oesophageal reflux disease in pregnancy. She is anxious about its safety in pregnancy.

67. Choose the *single* most appropriate option:

A Commence phototherapy to render bilirubin water soluble

B Conjugated and unconjugated bilirubin are present in the urine

C Bilirubin will be unconjugated and insoluble

D Liver failure will ensue

E Administer ranitidine

F Unconjugated bilirubin stains the urine dark

G Steatorrhoea will be absent

H Prophylactic vitamin K should be given to the neonate

I Kernicterus

J Transfer to ITU

K Conjugated bilirubin stains the urine dark

L Treat with antibiotics

67.1 A 30-year-old Afro-Caribbean woman has a sickle cell crisis. She is jaundiced as a result of this.

67.2 A 27-year-old woman is known to have gallstones and presents feeling unwell. She complains of right upper quadrant pain, pale stools and dark urine. An ultrasound reveals a gallstone blocking the common bile duct.

67.3 A neonate born at 40 weeks of gestation presents with jaundice at 36 h of life. There is no sign of infection.

67.4 Hyperbilirubinaemia in a neonate is 350 μmol/L.

Answers

1.	A	F	**11.**	A	F	**21.**	A	T	**31.**	A	F
	B	T		B	F		B	T		B	T
	C	F		C	F		C	T		C	F
	D	F		D	T		D	T		D	F
	E	T		E	T		E	F		E	F
2.	A	F	**12.**	A	F	**22.**	A	F	**32.**	A	T
	B	F		B	F		B	T		B	F
	C	T		C	T		C	F		C	F
	D	F		D	T		D	T		D	F
	E	F		E	F		E	T		E	T
3.	A	F	**13.**	A	T	**23.**	A	F	**33.**	A	T
	B	T		B	T		B	T		B	T
	C	F		C	T		C	F		C	F
	D	F		D	T		D	F		D	T
	E	F		E	T		E	F		E	T
4.	A	F	**14.**	A	T	**24.**	A	F	**34.**	A	F
	B	T		B	F		B	F		B	T
	C	F		C	F		C	T		C	F
	D	F		D	F		D	F		D	F
	E	F		E	F		E	F		E	F
5.	A	F	**15.**	A	F	**25.**	A	F	**35.**	A	T
	B	T		B	T		B	F		B	T
	C	T		C	T		C	T		C	F
	D	F		D	F		D	F		D	F
	E	F		E	T		E	F		E	F
6.	A	F	**16.**	A	F	**26.**	A	F	**36.**	A	F
	B	T		B	F		B	F		B	T
	C	F		C	T		C	T		C	T
	D	F		D	T		D	F		D	F
	E	F		E	T		E	F		E	T
7.	A	T	**17.**	A	T	**27.**	A	F	**37.**	A	T
	B	F		B	F		B	F		B	F
	C	T		C	T		C	T		C	T
	D	F		D	T		D	F		D	F
	E	T		E	F		E	F		E	F
8.	A	T	**18.**	A	T	**28.**	A	F	**38.**	A	F
	B	F		B	T		B	T		B	T
	C	T		C	T		C	T		C	F
	D	F		D	F		D	T		D	F
	E	F		E	F		E	T		E	F
9.	A	T	**19.**	A	T	**29.**	A	T	**39.**	A	T
	B	F		B	T		B	F		B	F
	C	F		C	F		C	T		C	T
	D	T		D	F		D	T		D	T
	E	F		E	T		E	F		E	F
10.	A	T	**20.**	A	F	**30.**	A	T	**40.**	A	F
	B	F		B	T		B	F		B	T
	C	T		C	F		C	F		C	F
	D	F		D	F		D	T		D	T
	E	F		E	T		E	T		E	F

41.	A	F
	B	T
	C	T
	D	T
	E	T
42.	A	T
	B	T
	C	T
	D	F
	E	F
43.	A	F
	B	F
	C	F
	D	T
	E	F
44.	A	T
	B	T
	C	F
	D	F
	E	T
45.	A	T
	B	F
	C	T
	D	F
	E	T
46.	A	T
	B	T
	C	F
	D	T
	E	T
47.	A	T
	B	F
	C	T
	D	T
	E	T
48.	A	T
	B	T
	C	F
	D	F
	E	T

49.	A	T
	B	F
	C	F
	D	T
	E	T
50.	A	T
	B	T
	C	F
	D	T
	E	T
51.	A	T
	B	F
	C	F
	D	F
	E	F
52.	A	F
	B	F
	C	T
	D	T
	E	T
53.	A	T
	B	F
	C	T
	D	F
	E	T
54.	A	F
	B	F
	C	T
	D	F
	E	F
55.	A	T
	B	F
	C	F
	D	F
	E	T
56.	A	T
	B	F
	C	F
	D	F
	E	F

57.	A	F
	B	F
	C	T
	D	T
	E	T
58.	A	F
	B	T
	C	F
	D	F
	E	F
59.	A	T
	B	F
	C	F
	D	T
	E	T
60.	A	T
	B	F
	C	F
	D	F
	E	T
61.	A	F
	B	F
	C	T
	D	T
	E	T
62.	A	T
	B	T
	C	F
	D	T
	E	T
63.	A	F
	B	F
	C	T
	D	F
	E	T
64.	A	F
	B	F
	C	T
	D	F
	E	F

65.	A	F
	B	T
	C	T
	D	T
	E	T

66.1 A Administer metoclopramide to speed gastric emptying
66.2 I Reassurance
67.1 C Bilirubin will be unconjugated and insoluble
67.2 K Conjugated bilirubin stains the urine dark
67.3 A Commence phototherapy to render bilirubin water soluble
67.4 I Kernicterus

Endocrinology

Questions

1. When considering the adrenal gland:
   - **A** The medulla of the adrenal gland develops from neural crest cells
   - **B** In the female it produces 25% of the circulating testosterone
   - **C** The zona glomerulosa is unable to synthesize cortisol
   - **D** Hypoglycaemia may be a feature of Cushing syndrome
   - **E** The adrenal gland is supplied with blood by branches of the aorta, renal and inferior phrenic arteries

2. The following are true of autoimmune thyroid disease:
   - **A** Thyrotoxicosis may present with hyperemesis gravidarum
   - **B** Rarely presents in the first 6 months after pregnancy
   - **C** The fetus is unaffected by maternal thyroid disease
   - **D** A thyroglossal cyst is unrelated to the thyroid gland
   - **E** Heavy periods may be a presentation

3. A patient with a prolactinoma may present with the following problems:
   - **A** Visual field defects
   - **B** Infertility
   - **C** Acromegaly
   - **D** Repeated miscarriage
   - **E** Loss of libido

4. In the control of calcium levels:
   - **A** Parathyroid hormone is secreted by the oxyphil cells of the parathyroid gland
   - **B** A deficiency of parathyroid hormone may be suspected by eliciting Chvostek's sign
   - **C** Looser's zones are seen in calcitonin excess
   - **D** Rickets may be inherited
   - **E** Vitamin D is activated in the kidney only

5. Hirsutism:
   - **A** Is always pathological
   - **B** Is a poor marker of testosterone excess
   - **C** May occur with diazoxide treatment
   - **D** May present in pregnancy
   - **E** Males have more hair follicles than females

6. Swelling of the thyroid:
   - **A** Graves' disease
   - **B** Hashimoto's thyroiditis
   - **C** De Quervain's thyroiditis
   - **D** Thyroid cyst
   - **E** Reidel's thyroiditis
   - **F** Thyroid adenoma
   - **G** Thyroglossal cyst
   - **H** Pregnancy
   - **I** Multinodular goitre
   - **J** Iodine deficiency

6.1 What is the most likely diagnosis in excessive hyperemesis of pregnancy with raised free T_3 and free T_4, suppressed TSH and raised thyroid autoantibodies?

6.2 What is the most likely diagnosis where there was known to have been a pre-pregnancy thyroid swelling, now at 20 weeks she has difficulty swallowing? Ultrasound of the thyroid shows retrosternal extension of a heterogeneous thyroid gland.

6.3 What is the most likely diagnosis for swollen thyroid at 26 weeks pregnant, recent flu-like illness, pain on swallowing, palpitations, sweating more than previously, the neck is tender to touch and diffusely swollen?

7. With regard to calcium homeostasis:
   - **A** Primary hyperparathyroidism
   - **B** Rickets
   - **C** Multiple endocrine neoplasia type 2
   - **D** Sarcoidosis
   - **E** Multiple myeloma
   - **F** Hypoparathyroidism
   - **G** Renal failure
   - **H** Lung cancer
   - **I** Paget's disease of bone
   - **J** Osteoporosis

7.1 An entirely healthy woman has had an uneventful pregnancy culminating in the normal delivery of a healthy baby boy. He starts to have marked tremors in the neonatal period. What is the most likely diagnosis?

7.2 A previously healthy woman presents during pregnancy with a rash on her shins and is found on routine investigation to have a high free calcium level. What is the most likely diagnosis?

7.3 A life-long smoker attends the urogynaecology clinic for stress incontinence and complains of shortness of breath and bone pain and swelling. The heart rate is found to be 120 and a chest X-ray shows diffusely increased basal shadowing. What is the most likely diagnosis?

Answers

1.	A	T
	B	F
	C	T
	D	F
	E	T
2.	A	T
	B	F
	C	F
	D	F
	E	T

3.	A	T
	B	T
	C	T
	D	T
	E	T
4.	A	F
	B	T
	C	F
	D	T
	E	F

5.	A	F
	B	F
	C	T
	D	T
	E	F

6.1 **A** Graves' disease

6.2 **I** Multinodular goitre

6.3 **C** De Quervain's thyroiditis

7.1 **A** primary hyperparathyroidism

7.2 **D** Sarcoidosis

7.3 **I** Paget's disease of bone

Drugs and drug therapy

Questions

1. The following are alkylating agents:
   A Cyclophosphamide
   B Bleomycin
   C Thiotepa
   D Treosulphan
   E Melphalan

2. Cyclophosphamide:
   A Is activated by liver enzymes
   B May cause haematuria
   C Frequently causes profound myelosuppression
   D May cause alopecia
   E Has four alkylating arms

3. These side-effects are recognized complications of the following drugs:
   A Vinblastine – neurotoxicity
   B Vincristine – marrow depression
   C Doxorubicin – cardiomyopathy
   D Methotrexate – diarrhoea
   E 5-Fluorouracil – renal failure

4. The following statements are true:
   A Naloxone is a partial opiate agonist
   B Azathioprine is teratogenic
   C Nalidixic acid may interfere with bilirubin conjugation
   D Oral hypoglycaemic agents are safe in pregnancy
   E Ganglion blockers may be associated with 50% fetal loss

5. These side-effects are recognized complications of the following drugs:
   A Methyldopa – positive Coomb's test in the baby
   B Methyldopa – neonatal ileus
   C Atenolol – fetal overactivity
   D 17-hydroxy-progesterone – virilization of female fetus
   E Lithium – Epstein's malformation

6. The half-life of the drug will be increased by:
   A Increased volume of distribution
   B Increased rate of clearance
   C Increased age, for drugs eliminated mainly by the kidney
   D Pregnancy for drugs metabolized in the liver
   E Shortening the time between doses

7. In pregnancy:
   A The concentration of globulins falls
   B Highly ionized drugs are metabolized more than non-ionized drugs
   C Barbiturates decrease the capacity of the liver to metabolize drugs
   D Antacids enhance drug absorption
   E Anticonvulsants are more slowly eliminated

8. With regard to teratogenicity of drugs in early pregnancy:
   A <5% of anomalies are due to drugs
   B Concurrent use of two antiepileptic drugs increases the chance of anomalies
   C The critical time for teratogenesis is 20–55 days after conception
   D Molecules >1000 Da cross the placenta easily
   E Drug use in early pregnancy potentiates the teratogenic effects of diabetes

9. Pharmacokinetics in pregnancy:
   A Nearly 100% of the drug bypasses the liver after rectal administration
   B Nearly 100% of the drug bypasses the liver after oral sublingual administration
   C Acidic drugs bind to α_1-acid glycoprotein
   D The kidney excretes drugs mainly by paracellular transport
   E Functionalization reactions occur in the cytoplasm and conjugation reactions occur in endoplasmic reticulum

10. The following drugs inhibit microsomal induction:
    A Oestrogen
    B Grapefruit juice
    C Fluconazole
    D Progestogen
    E Griseofulvin

11. Antihypertensives in pregnancy:
    A Thioamides cause intrauterine growth restriction
    B Methyldopa achieves fetal plasma concentrations similar to maternal levels
    C Prazosin causes reflex tachycardia
    D Hydralazine does not affect placental vessels
    E Calcium channel blockers are embryotoxic in animals

12. In relation to adverse drug effects:
    A Halothane-induced hepatotoxicity is a hypersensitivity reaction

B Nitric oxide causes neonatal depression
C Heparin-induced immune thrombocytopenia occurs within a week after administration
D Malignant hyperthermia is due to release of calcium from glycosomes
E Thiazide diuretics cause neonatal thrombocytopenia
F Meptazinol has low addictive potential

13. The drug shown is a drug of choice for the condition mentioned:
    A Potassium sparing diuretic – patients with cirrhosis
    B Sodium valproate – anti-epileptic drug of choice in pregnancy
    C Heparin – anticoagulant of choice in patients with prosthetic heart valves
    D Propylthiouracil – drug to treat hyperthyroidism in pregnancy
    E Loratadine – antihistamine to use when breastfeeding

14. The following statements are true:
    A Azathioprine is transferred into breast milk in high concentrations
    B Mycophenolate mofetil affects T and B cells
    C Warfarin embryopathy is 5–10%
    D Nitrofurantoin is actively secreted into breast milk
    E Metronidazole causes secondary lactose intolerance

15. Oral contraceptives:
    A Progestogen-only pills cause functional cysts
    B Depot medroxyprogesterone blocks ovulation in virtually all patients due to high plasma concentrations of progesterone
    C Progesterone acts on the hypothalamus to inhibit GnRH pulses
    D Newer progestogens cause an increased risk of venous thromboembolism
    E The progestogen-only pill causes acne
    F Amoxicillin decreases efficacy of the oral contraceptive pill by microsomal induction

16. Choose the single most appropriate management strategy:
    A Concerns regarding medication – offer termination of pregnancy
    B Stop medication
    C Reassure, switch to methyldopa
    D Continue on the same medication and allow home
    E Transfer to intensive care unit and consider antihypertensive treatment
    F Admit to antenatal ward, pre-eclampsia bloods, ultrasound to assess fetus, BP monitoring, review antihypertensive treatment
    G Admit to labour ward, commence $MgSO_4$
    H Reassure and allow home
    I Advise to switch to another drug that has the same mode of action but a shorter half-life
    J Immediate caesarean section
    K Carry out visual field assessment
    L Insert central venous pressure line

16.1 A 26-year-old woman (para 1 + 0) at 6 weeks of gestation contacts her GP immediately after finding out that she is pregnant. She has a 3-year history of hypertension and is treated with an ACE inhibitor and a diuretic. She is concerned about the effect of the drugs on the developing fetus.

16.2 Mrs Black is seen in the antenatal clinic at 28 weeks. She has a BP reading of 160/95 mmHg and 2+ protein on urine dipstick. She was started on labetalol by her GP 24 h ago. She otherwise feels well.

16.3 A 35-year-old primigravid woman is 14 weeks' pregnant and has type 2 diabetes. She has a needle phobia that cannot be overcome. Her current treatment is with metformin and chlorpropamide. This combination maintains her blood glucose levels much better than metformin alone. What is the best strategy for sulphonylurea treatment?

Answers

1.	A	T
	B	F
	C	T
	D	T
	E	T
2.	A	T
	B	T
	C	F
	D	T
	E	F
3.	A	F
	B	F
	C	T
	D	T
	E	F
4.	A	F
	B	F
	C	T
	D	F
	E	T
5.	A	T
	B	T
	C	F
	D	F
	E	T

6.	A	T
	B	F
	C	T
	D	F
	E	F
7.	A	F
	B	F
	C	F
	D	F
	E	F
8.	A	T
	B	T
	C	T
	D	F
	E	F
9.	A	F
	B	T
	C	F
	D	T
	E	F
10.	A	T
	B	T
	C	T
	D	F
	E	F

11.	A	F
	B	T
	C	F
	D	T
	E	T
12.	A	T
	B	T
	C	F
	D	F
	E	T
	F	T
13.	A	T
	B	F
	C	F
	D	T
	E	T
14.	A	F
	B	T
	C	T
	D	T
	E	T

15.	A	T
	B	T
	C	T
	D	F
	E	T
	F	F

16.1 C Reassure, switch to methyldopa

16.2 F Admit to antenatal ward, pre-eclampsia bloods, ultrasound to assess fetus, BP monitoring, review antihypertensive treatment

16.3 I Advise to switch to another drug that has the same mode of action but a shorter half-life

Index

thyroid-stimulating hormone, 63, 239, 252
thyrotoxicosis, 253
thyroxine binding globulin, 250
thyroxine releasing hormone, 252
thyroxine (T4), 249, 250, 252
  plasma protein binding, 250
  replacement therapy, 253
tidal volume, 194
  pregnancy-related changes, 195
time-dependent data, 292
tissue injury, 98
tissue plasminogen activator, 191, 224
tissue repair, 98
tissues, 58
tocolytics, 265, 267
total iron-binding capacity, 223
total lung capacity, 194
totipotency, 145
touch sensation, 215, 217
Toxoplasma gondii, 120–121
tranexamic acid, 224
transcription, 4, 149
  regulation, 5, 166
    cyclic AMP-dependent protein kinase (protein kinase A), 169
    protein kinase C, 169
transcription factors, 5, 233
transcriptomics, 10
transfer RNA, 5
transferrin, 219, 220
transient diabetes insipidus of pregnancy, 202, 204
translation, 5
translocations, 17–19
  reciprocal, 17–18
  Robertsonian, 18–19
transport mechanisms, 175–177
  drugs, 262–263
transpyloric plane, 70–71
transverse cervical (cardinal) ligament, 91
transversus (transverse abdominis/transversalis), 72
Treponema pallidum, 110, 116
triacylglycerols *see* triglycerides
trial steering committees, 313
triazole antifungal agents, 272
tricarboxylic acid cycle (citric acid cycle), 152, 153–155, 156
  regulation, 158
Trichomonas vaginalis, 112, 120
Trichophyton, 119

tricuspid valve, 184
tricyclic antidepressants, 275
triglycerides, 155, 157, 161, 162
  liver synthesis, 212, 213
trigone, 93–94
tri-iodothyronine (T3), 249, 250, 252
trimethoprim, 117, 271
triploidy, 14
  partial hydatidiform mole, 103
trisomy, 14, 15, 24
  sex chromosomes, 15
trisomy 13 (Patau syndrome), 15
trisomy 18 (Edward syndrome), 15, 24
trisomy 21 (Down syndrome), 15
  amniotic fluid α-fetoprotein levels, 47
  translocational, 19
trophectoderm, 29
trophoblast, 29, 40
  defective invasion, 55, 104
    miscarriage association, 103
    pre-eclampsia association, 55, 104–105, 141–142
  placental bed invasion, 41, 42, 44
tropical spastic paraparesis, 130
Trousseau's sign, 255
trypsin, 161
tumours, 99, 100–102
  classification, 99
Turner syndrome (45,X), 15, 22
  mosaicism, 16
  X isochromosomes, 17
twinning, 27
type 1 error, 290–291, 316
type 2 error, 291, 316
tyrosine kinase-linked receptors, 5, 170, 233
tyrosine kinases, 170, 171
tyrosine phosphatases, 170

ultrasound, diagnostic, 279–281
  absorption, 280
  characteristic impedance, 279–280
  diffraction, 280
  Doppler effect, 281
  focusing, 280–281
  intensity, 279
  reception, 281
  reflections, 279–280
umbilical artery, 63, 83
umbilical vein, 33, 51, 63
umbilicus, 71

uniparental disomy, 23–24
5′ untranslated region (UTR), 4
upper motor neurones, 215
uracil, 2, 4, 149
urea
  formation, 212
  renal handling, 202
urea cycle, 158–159
Ureaplasma urealyticum, 117
ureter, 80, 94
  pelvic, 88, 91
  relations, 88
ureteric bud, 52
urethra, 94
urinary tract, 79–80, 199–205
urine, 199–200
  concentration, 202
urodynamic data, 205
urogenital sinus, 36, 37, 38, 94
urogenital triangle, 85–86
uterine artery, 84
uteroplacental arteries, formation from spiral arteries, 41, 42, 55, 104, 141, 226
uterosacral ligament, 91
uterovesical pouch, 90
uterus, 90
  blood supply, 84, 90
  development, 36
  drugs affecting activity, 267
  histology, 91–92
  labour, 246, 247
  lower segment, 90, 91
  lymphatic drainage, 90
  nerve supply, 90
  relations, 90
  supports, 90–91
  sympathetic innervation, 218
  upper segment, 90, 91

vacuum autoclaves, 118
vagina, 92
  blood supply, 83, 92
  development, 36, 38
  glycogen metabolism, 27–28
  histology, 92
  lymphatic drainage, 92
  normal bacterial flora, 112
  pH, 28, 112
  relations, 92
vaginal adenocarcinoma, 260
vaginal adenosis, 100
vaginal arteries, 83
vaginal candidosis (thrush), 120